setting of malabsorption, total parenteral nutrition, or zinc supplementation (*Ann Hematol.* 2018;97(9):1527-1534).

Folate or vitamin B12 deficiency are both causes of megaloblastic anemia, a subtype of macrocytic anemia in setting of ineffective DNA synthesis. Severe cases of megaloblastic anemia may also lead to pancytopenia, including neutropenia. Causes of folate and vitamin B12 deficiency include insufficient dietary intake; malabsorption in the setting of surgery, gastrointestinal disease, or medications; increased requirements; among other causes (*Cleve Clin J Med.* 2020;87(3):153-164). Peripheral smear may demonstrate macro-ovalocytes as well as the presence of hypersegmented neutrophils. Bone marrow examination is not typically indicated but classic "megaloblastic changes" are demonstrated. Namely, the bone marrow is markedly hypercellular with erythroid hyperplasia and a reversal of the myeloid:erythroid ratio. Hallmark changes of nuclear-cytoplasmic dyssynchrony (failure of nuclear maturation with open chromatin in the setting of normal mature cytoplasm) are seen in erythroblasts and other erythroid precursors. Other features of dyserythropoiesis may also be seen. Myeloid lineages may demonstrate myeloid hyperplasia with giant band forms and hypersegmentation of neutrophils (*Postgrad Med.* 1978;64(4): 117-122). Because the peripheral cytopenias and cytomorphologic changes of nutritional deficiency-related neutropenia may mimic myelodysplastic syndrome (MDS), evaluation of serum vitamin B12, folate, and copper levels is typically assessed in patients with suspected MDS.

Clinicians should be aware that individuals of certain ancestries (African, Mediterranean, among others) may have lower neutrophil counts without clinical significance. These individuals have normal granulopoiesis and marrow reserves and do not have an increased risk of infection. While this finding was previously referred to as "benign ethnic neutropenia," the terminology has evolved, and it is increasingly being referred to as "Duffy-null antigen count" (*Blood.* 2021;137(1):13). Recent research has shown a strong association between low neutrophil counts in these patients and single-nucleotide polymorphism in the *ACKR1* gene, leading to a loss of expression of Duffy antigens on red blood cells (*PLoS Genet.* 2009;5(1):e1000360). The presence of this finding and the pathophysiology underlying low neutrophil count remain unknown and are active areas of investigation.

Disorders of Neutrophil Function

There are numerous mechanisms that can lead to neutrophil dysfunction given the numerous steps involved in the neutrophil recruitment cascade, including chemotaxis, tethering to the endothelium, rolling, activation, adhesion, crawling, and transendothelial migration with recruitment to the site of inflammation (*Blood.* 2022;139(14):2130-2144). There may be defects in neutrophil function based on abnormal motility or granule function. Furthermore, deficiencies in complement proteins or immunoglobulins may impair neutrophil function, as these components play an important role in opsonization leading to neutrophil-mediated phagocytosis. The major features of disorders of neutrophil function are summarized in Table 4.2-2.

II. LYMPHOCYTES

Disorders of Lymphocyte Number

Abnormalities in lymphocyte number can be detected by a complete blood count and differential, along with a review of the peripheral blood smear. Lymphocytosis is

TABLE 4.2-2 Disorders of Neutrophil Function

Name	Inheritance	Impairment	Gene(s) Affected	Clinical Features	Other Findings
Chédiak-Higashi syndrome	AR	Degranulation	CHS1	Recurrent bacterial infections, oculocutaneous albinism, progressive neurologic abnormalities, bleeding disorder	Large peroxidase-positive cytoplasmic granules in neutrophils
Neutrophil-specific granule deficiency	AR	Granule synthesis	CEBPE and SMARCD2	Pyogenic infections of the skin and other deeper tissues	Granulocytes lack specific granules
Leukocyte adhesion deficiency type 1	AR	Adhesion	ITGB2	Neutrophilia, recurrent bacterial infections delayed separation of the umbilical cord, and periodontitis	Inflammatory infiltrates lacking neutrophils; decreased CD18 expression
Leukocyte adhesion deficiency type 2	AR	Adhesion	SLC35C1	Intellectual disabilities and growth impairment	Inflammatory infiltrates lacking neutrophils; absent CD15a
Leukocyte adhesion deficiency type 3	AR	Adhesion	FERMT3	Severe infections, marked leukocytosis, and a Glanzmann-like bleeding diathesis	Inflammatory infiltrates lacking neutrophils
Chronic granulomatous disease	AR/XL	Respiratory burst	CYBA, CYBB, NCF1, NCF2, NCF4	Recurrent life-threatening bacterial or fungal infections from a young age	Granulomatous lesions in multiple sites

AR, autosomal recessive; XL, X-linked.

typically defined as an absolute lymphocyte count (ALC) greater than 4.0×10^9/L, while lymphocytopenia is defined as an ALC less than 1.0×10^9/L; nevertheless, note that the normal range may vary based on age and laboratory.

Lymphocytosis

Lymphocytosis can be categorized into primary or secondary causes. Primary lymphocytosis refers to conditions in which the increased number of lymphocytes is secondary to an intrinsic defect in the expanded lymphocyte population. These conditions, referred to as lymphoproliferative disorders, are considered monoclonal, as they are characterized by an abnormal clonal expansion of a lymphoid population due to the acquisition of somatic mutations. Clonal proliferation may arise from monoclonal B cells, T cells, natural killer (NK) cells, or less differentiated cells of lymphoid lineage. Immunophenotyping, typically using flow cytometry (FC), is essential for identifying the expression of cell surface markers that can allow for assessment of clonality. Secondary, or reactive, lymphocytosis refers to conditions in which the increased number of lymphocytes is secondary to another disease process, such as infection, toxin exposure, or inflammation.

Primary lymphocytosis

Several T-cell and B-cell neoplasms may present with lymphocytosis. These disorders are discussed in the chapters covering lymphoid malignancies.

Secondary (reactive) lymphocytosis

The most common cause of secondary lymphocytosis is viral infection, specifically infectious mononucleosis (IM). IM is most often caused by the Epstein-Barr virus (EBV), although other viruses may also cause the disease (*Am J Med Sci.* 1978;276(3):325). Infected patients may present with fevers, fatigue, malaise, tender lymphadenopathy, sore throat, and splenomegaly. EBV infects and replicates in B cells, which induces a host immune response involving polyclonal proliferation of $CD8^+$ cytotoxic T cells and $CD16^+/CD56^+$ NK cells (*J Infect Dis.* 2013;207(1):80-88). Lymphocytosis is the most common hematologic manifestation, characterized by polyclonal expansion of atypical lymphocytes in response to EBV-infected B cells (*J Immunol.* 1987;139(11):3802). These atypical "reactive lymphocytes" can be seen on a peripheral blood smear. IM is typically diagnosed clinically, although the heterophile antibody test or serologic testing for antibodies against viral antigens (anti-VCA, anti-EA, anti-EBNA) can be used to confirm the diagnosis (*J Infect Dis.* 1975;132(5):546; *Clin Diagn Lab Immunol.* 2000;7(3):451).

Of note, other viral infections may also lead to lymphocytosis, which can persist for several weeks. Bacterial infection with *Bordetella pertussis* is also known to cause significant lymphocytosis, especially in children (*Pediatrics.* 1997;100(6):E10). Pertussis primarily affects the respiratory tract and causes a disease characterized by paroxysms of severe coughing. Lymphocytosis is mediated by the presence of pertussis toxin, which prevents lymphocytes from trafficking from blood to lymphoid tissues (*Infect Immun.* 1984;46(3):733-739; *Respirology.* 2003;8(2):157-162). Peripheral blood smear examination reveals classic findings of mature lymphocytes with scant cytoplasm, condensed chromatin, and clefted nuclei (*Blood.* 2013;122(25):4012).

Transient lymphocytosis, as a physiologic reaction to severe stress, is commonly seen. It is mediated by the redistribution of lymphocytes and affects all lymphocyte subtypes (*Am J Clin Pathol.* 2002;117(5):819-825). It is typically associated with medical emergencies, including cardiac conditions, status epilepticus, or trauma (*Arch Pathol Lab Med.* 1987;111(8):712).

Drugs are an important cause of lymphocytosis, whether mediated by the drug itself or a systemic reaction. Bruton tyrosine kinase (BTK) inhibitors, such as ibrutinib, are associated with transient lymphocytosis (typically peaking within 24-48 hours) due to the release of previously activated cells from lymph nodes (*Leukemia.* 2014;28(11):2188-2196). Prolonged lymphocytosis is thought to represent the persistence of a quiescent clone and does not have prognostic impact for chronic lymphoid leukemia (*Blood.* 2014;123(12):1810-1817). Interestingly, dasatinib, another BTK inhibitor, also promotes lymphocytosis by an unrelated mechanism, possibly related to splenic contraction (*Blood Adv.* 2022;bloodadvances.2022009279). In patients with chronic myeloid leukemia being treated with dasatinib, clonal expansions of large granular lymphocytes are often seen, but are of unclear significance (*Blood.* 2010;116(5):772-782). Drug hypersensitivity reactions can also lead to lymphocytosis. For example, drug reaction with eosinophilia and systemic symptoms (DRESS) is a well-known yet rare severe adverse drug reaction characterized by an extensive skin rash, visceral organ involvement, and lymphadenopathy (*Br J Dermatol.* 2013;169(5):1071). While the classic hematologic manifestation of DRESS is significant eosinophilia, it may also lead to atypical lymphocytosis due to expansion of both $CD4^+$ and $CD8^+$ T lymphocytes, which stimulate the inflammatory response (*J Dermatol Sci.* 2012;65(3):213).

Lymphopenia

Lymphopenia may be due to either inherited or acquired causes. Inherited causes of lymphopenia are predominantly associated with inherited immunodeficiency disorders resulting in ineffective lymphopoiesis. Examples include severe congenital immunodeficiency disease, common variable immunodeficiency disease, Wiskott-Aldrich syndrome, ataxia-telangiectasia, and other conditions (*Hematology.* 2018;682-690). These conditions classically present in childhood with recurrent infections. FC may be used to identify whether the total number of circulating lymphocytes or a particular subset is decreased, as this may be characteristic of specific disorders.

Acquired lymphopenia is more common and is typically reactive in the setting of infection, systemic diseases, medications, or acute stress. In one study of hospitalized patients with ALC less than 0.6×10^9/L, the most common causes of lymphopenia, in descending order of frequency, were bacterial/fungal sepsis, postoperative state, corticosteroid therapy, malignancy, cytotoxic therapy and/or radiotherapy, trauma or hemorrhage, transplants, viral infections, and human immunodeficiency virus (HIV) infection (*Aust N Z J Med.* 1997;27(2):170-174). There are no defining characteristics on peripheral blood smear examination to differentiate between these causes.

Lymphopenia can contribute to both humoral and cell-mediated immune responses. A Danish population-based study found that lymphocytopenia was associated with an increased risk of hospitalization for infection, as well as an increased risk of infection-related death (*PLoS Med.* 2018;15(11):e1002685).

Infectious causes

While many viral infections lead to lymphocytosis, lymphopenia has also been observed with certain infections. This is classically seen in the setting of HIV infection, related to direct viral attack on $CD4^+$ lymphocytes, chronic immune activation, or apoptosis (*Front Immunol.* 2017;8:580). Lymphopenia is a well-known complication of infections caused by the *Coronaviridae* family, although the underlying mechanism is not entirely clear. This was first demonstrated in patients with severe acute respiratory syndrome caused by the SARS-CoV-1 virus (*J Infect Dis.* 2004;189(4):648-651) and later in patients with Middle East respiratory syndrome caused by the MERS-CoV virus (*J Infect Dis.* 2016;213(6):904-914). Similar lymphopenia later became a hallmark finding of COVID-19 infection caused by the SARS-CoV-2 virus (*Ann Hematol.* 2021;100(2):309-320).

Furthermore, Ebola virus infections are characterized by significant lymphopenia, which has been linked to worse prognosis and survival (*PLoS Pathog.* 2019;15(10):e1008068).

Iatrogenic causes

Lymphopenia is a frequent adverse effect of multimodal cancer therapy. Numerous cytotoxic chemotherapy drugs lead to a predictable decline in lymphocyte count (*J Natl Compr Canc Netw.* 2015;13(10):1225-1231). Radiation therapy frequently depletes lymphocytes as well, as they are considered the most radiosensitive cells of the hematopoietic system (*Crit Rev Oncol Hematol.* 2018;123:42-51). Radiation-related lymphopenia has been associated with suboptimal tumor control and inferior survival (*Radiother Oncol.* 2022;177:81-94). Secondary immunodeficiency induced by monoclonal antibody therapy is a well-known complication. Anti-CD20 monoclonal antibodies, such as rituximab, rapidly deplete B cells in the peripheral blood, and levels remain low or undetectable for 2 to 6 months (*Cancer Treat Rev.* 2005;31(6):456). Monoclonal antibodies to T cells, such as OKT3 (*J Immunol.* 1980;124(6):2708-2713) or alemtuzumab (*JAMA Neurol.* 2017;74(8):961), can also rapidly deplete T cells. As a result, complications can include increased susceptibility to opportunistic infection (*Clin Infect Dis.* 2007;44(2):204).

In addition to numerous effects on the immune system, glucocorticoid administration is also known to cause lymphocytopenia. The mechanism is likely multifactorial, involving the redistribution of circulating lymphocytes to other body compartments (*Immunology.* 1975;28(4):669-680) and induction of apoptosis (*Clin Exp Immunol.* 1996;103(3):482). T cells are more affected by glucocorticoids compared to B cells (*J Lab Clin Med.* 1983;101(3):479). There is also evidence that both short-term (*J Allergy Clin Immunol.* 1978;62(6):340) and long-term (*J Pediatr.* 1996;129(6):898) use of glucocorticoid can lead to hypogammaglobulinemia. Given these effects on lymphoid cells, corticosteroids are often used as a component of treatment regimens for lymphoid malignancies.

Other causes

Idiopathic $CD4^+$ lymphocytopenia (ICL) describes a syndrome in which patients have persistent $CD4^+$ T-cell lymphocytopenia in the absence of infection or other causes of immunodeficiency (*N Engl J Med.* 1993;328(6):380). While heterogeneous immune defects have been identified, the underlying etiology remains unclear (*Blood.* 2008;112(2):287). While some patients may be asymptomatic (*Medicine (Baltimore).* 2014;93(2):61), patients with ICL are at high risk of opportunistic infection, especially with *Cryptococcus* spp. and mycobacteria (*Blood.* 2008;112(2):287).

III. OTHER MORPHOLOGIC WHITE BLOOD CELL ABNORMALITIES

Inflammatory Changes

In inflammatory states, neutrophils may possess characteristic "toxic changes" within the cytoplasm, which refers to coarse dark-colored granules composed of myeloperoxidase and other lysosomal enzymes (*Br J Haematol.* 1983;53(1):15-22). Döhle bodies are also often present, which are small (1-3 μm in diameter) leukocyte inclusions composed of endoplasmic reticulum material, located in the periphery of the cytoplasm (*J Exp Med*. 1969;129(2):267-293; *Br J Haematol*. 1966;12(1):54-60).

The Pelger-Huët Anomaly

The Pelger-Huët anomaly (PHA) is an autosomal dominant condition leading to a defect in terminal neutrophil differentiation due to mutations in the lamin B receptor gene. On a peripheral blood smear, WBCs have dumbbell-shaped bilobed nuclei with two lobes connected by a thin strand of chromatin, giving a "pince-nez" appearance), and structure (coarse clumping of the nuclear chromatin). Pseudo-PHA refers to anomalies resembling PHA that are acquired rather than congenital. These anomalies are most commonly seen in hematologic malignancies (acute myeloid leukemia, chronic myeloid leukemia, MDS), as well as in vitamin B12 and folate deficiencies, viral infections, malaria, and drug reactions.

The May-Hegglin Anomaly

The May-Hegglin anomaly (MHA) is a rare autosomal dominant disorder characterized by abnormal platelet and granulocyte morphology (*JAMA*. 1963;183:737-740). There are fewer than a hundred cases reported in the literature. The pathogenesis is thought to be related to mutations in the gene encoding for nonmuscle myosin heavy chain IIA (*MYH9*). Mutations in this gene are associated with a number of syndromes that represent forms of hereditary macrothrombocytopenia (*Blood*. 2012;119(2):328). MHA is characterized by small, light-blue crescent-shaped inclusions in granulocytes measuring 2 to 5 µm, resembling Döhle bodies (*Br J Haematol*. 1972;22(4):491-496). Thrombocytopenia and associated giant platelets are also present.

The Alder-Reilly Anomaly

The Alder-Reilly anomaly is an inherited abnormality of WBCs, classically associated with mucopolysaccharidoses (*Am J Clin Pathol*. 1982;78(4):544). Patients with this anomaly possess dense azurophilic granules within all leukocytes, resembling toxic granulation in neutrophils (*Am J Dis Child*. 1941;62(3):489-491). In lymphocytes, these granules are surrounded by a clear zone.

Auer Rods

Auer rods are large azurophilic rod-shaped cytoplasmic inclusions that may be found in myeloblasts or other myeloid progenitor cells in cases of myeloid hematologic malignancies, most commonly acute myeloid leukemia (*Blood*. 1950;5(9):847-863).

SUGGESTED READINGS

Frater JL. How I investigate neutropenia. *Int J Lab Hematol*. 2020;42(suppl 1):121-132. doi:10.1111/ijlh.13210

Hamad H, Mangla A. Lymphocytosis. In: *StatPearls* [Internet]. StatPearls Publishing; 2023. Updated July 17, 2023. https://www.ncbi.nlm.nih.gov/books/NBK549819/

Henry B, Cheruiyot I, Vikse J, et al. Lymphopenia and neutrophilia at admission predicts severity and mortality in patients with COVID-19: a meta-analysis. *Acta Biomed*. 2020;91(3):e2020008. doi:10.23750/abm.v91i3.10217

Knight V. The utility of flow cytometry for the diagnosis of primary immunodeficiencies. *Int J Lab Hematol*. 2019;41(suppl 1):63-72. doi:10.1111/ijlh.13010

Ley K, Laudanna C, Cybulsky MI, Nourshargh S. Getting to the site of inflammation: the leukocyte adhesion cascade updated. *Nat Rev Immunol*. 2007;7(9):678-689. doi:10.1038/nri2156

Savoia A, Pecci A. MYH9-related disease. In: Adam MP, Feldman J, Mirzaa GM, et al, eds. *GeneReviews®* [Internet]. University of Washington, Seattle; 1993-2024; 2008 [updated February 18, 2021].

Torrez M, Chabot-Richards D, Babu D, Lockhart E, Foucar K. How I investigate acquired megaloblastic anemia. *Int J Lab Hematol*. 2022;44(2):236-247.

Yu HH, Yang YH, Chiang BL. Chronic granulomatous disease: a comprehensive review. *Clin Rev Allergy Immunol*. 2021;61(2):101-113. doi:10.1007/s12016-020-08800-x

4.3: Platelet Disorders

Joshua Siner, Brooj Abro, and Thomas M. Schneider

Platelets are the terminal unit of megakaryopoiesis, wherein hematopoietic stem cell progenitors differentiate down the common myeloid progenitor line and form large, multinucleated cells that project and bud off approximately 2- to 3-µm platelets lacking DNA (e-Figure 4.3-1). The production of platelets is dependent on thrombopoietin produced by hepatocytes. As platelet counts decrease, the effective thrombopoietin levels increase, stimulating bone marrow megakaryocytes to proliferate and form platelets, which are then released into circulation. Platelets exist in circulation for about 7 days and are critical for primary hemostasis by forming platelet plugs upon exposure to subendothelial collagen and binding to von Willebrand factor (vWF) (Figure 4.3-1). Activation of platelets leads to degranulation of α-granules and dense granules, which release additional hemostatic activators (see Table 4.3-1) and provide a platform for coagulation with increased surface expression of phosphatidylserine (*Semin Thromb Hemost*. 2016;42:185-190). After activation and crosslinking with fibrinogen, the platelet cytoskeleton rearranges to facilitate clot contraction. Additionally, platelets perform nonhemostatic functions, including the proinflammatory response to thrombosis and crosstalk between innate and adaptive immune responses (*Circ Res*. 2022;130:288-308). This chapter predominantly focuses on benign factors contributing to variations in platelet count and morphology. Abnormalities in hemostasis are also discussed but only to a limited extent.

I. LABORATORY ASSESSMENT OF PLATELETS

Methodology

The normal platelet count ranges from 150 to 400×10^9/L and is commonly assessed by automated hematology analyzers, with impedance, optical light scatter, and fluorescence being the most commonly used methods. At low levels, differences and interferences may be seen, and immunologic methods may be used (*Br J Haematol*. 2005;128:520-525). MPV values can vary significantly depending on the instrument used. Therefore, it is necessary to interpret results within the context of laboratory reference ranges (*Cleve Clin J Med*. 2019;86:150).

Faithful assessment of platelet function *in vivo* using *in vitro* techniques is difficult. Platelet aggregation studies (Figure 4.3-2), which test platelet response to a battery of

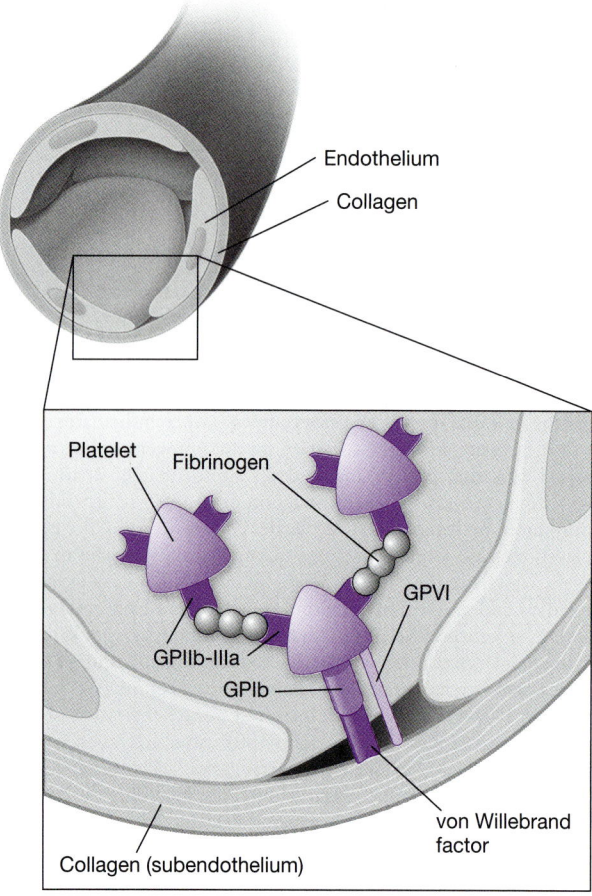

Figure 4.3-1. Platelet adhesion and aggregation. Platelet adhesion to collagen (subendothelial) is mediated by the binding of vWF to GPIb receptors and collagen. In addition, GPVI receptors also facilitate the binding of platelets to collagen. The formation of platelet plug requires platelet cross-linking, which occurs via binding of fibrinogen to GPIIb-IIIa receptors. vWF, von Willebrand factor. (From Armstrong AW, Golan DE. Pharmacology of hemostasis and thrombosis. In: Golan DE, Tashjian AH Jr, Armstrong EJ, Armstrong AW, eds. *Principles of Pharmacology*. 3rd ed. Wolters Kluwer; 2012:372-400.)

platelet-stimulating reagents, are particularly helpful in diagnosing inherited disorders of hemostasis (*Vasc Health Risk Manag*. 2015;11:133-148). Rapid, point-of-care testing (POCT) platelet function analyzers such as PFA-100, PFA-200, and VerifyNow are easier to perform but are nonspecific and not recommended for diagnosing genetic disorders (*Haemophilia*. 2006;12 suppl 3:128-136), but they may be useful for rapidly assessing disrupted platelet function due to antiplatelet medication. Viscoelastic

TABLE 4.3-1 Key Platelet Components Involved in Hemostasis

Components	Function
Glycoprotein (GP) membrane receptors[a]	
GPIIb/IIIa	Bind to fibrinogen
GPIa/IIa and GPVI	Bind to collagen
GPIb/IX/V	Bind to vWF
Other membrane receptors	
ADP receptors ($P2Y_1$, $P2Y_{12}$), thrombin receptors (PAR-1, PAR-4), thromboxane receptors (TPα, TPβ), $α_2$-adrenergic receptor	External receptors coupled to internal G-proteins that are involved in signal transduction and platelet activation following external ligand binding
Granules	
α-Granules	Release platelet factor 4, β-thrombomodulin, fibrinogen, vWF, coagulation factors (V and VIII), P-selectin, fibronectin, and so on
Dense (δ) granules	Release ADP, ATP, serotonin, calcium

ADP, adenosine diphosphate; ATP, adenosine triphosphate; vWF, von Willebrand factor.
[a]GP receptors are involved in platelet adhesion and aggregation by binding to specific ligands as previously mentioned.

assays, notably thromboelastography (TEG) and rotational thromboelastometry (ROTEM), are increasingly utilized for intraoperative evaluation of hemostatic function, including the assessment of platelet-related hemostatic issues (*Transfusion.* 2020;60 suppl 6:S1-S9).

Preanalytical Errors

Pseudothrombocytopenia refers to preanalytical errors that occur when automated cell counters inaccurately measure low platelet levels. When this occurs, they are often mistaken for white blood cells (WBCs) with a resultant higher WBC count. Ethylenediaminetetraacetic acid (EDTA)–dependent platelet antibodies or agglutinins that target glycoprotein IIb/IIIa receptors can cause platelet clumping or WBC satellitism, leading to falsely low platelet counts. Although EDTA is the preferred anticoagulant for hematology tests because it preserves cell shape, it can lead to erroneous results in these rare cases. To address this, blood samples without EDTA, such as those collected in sodium citrate or heparin, should be analyzed (*Clin Chem Lab Med.* 2012;50:1281-1285). Giant platelets, larger than 7 µm, can significantly distort platelet counts due to misinterpretation (*Ann Clin Lab Sci.* 2019;49:554-556). These unusually large platelets can be due to inherited disorders (discussed later) or myeloproliferative disorders. Clotted samples can result in low platelets due to consumption.

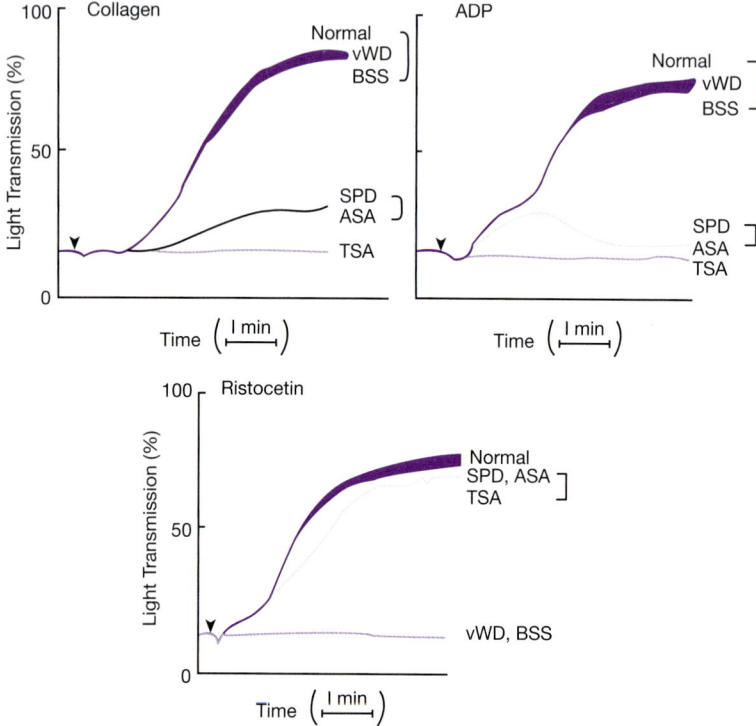

Figure 4.3-2. Schematic representation of normal and abnormal patterns of platelet aggregation and associated disorders. These patterns can be demonstrated using a turbidometric platelet aggregometer and incorporating collagen, adenosine diphosphate (ADP), and ristocetin into stirred platelet-rich plasma samples. A lack of aggregation in reaction to ristocetin is indicative of Bernard-Soulier syndrome (BSS) and von Willebrand disease (vWD). In Glanzmann thrombasthenia (TSA), aggregation is typically absent except when induced by ristocetin. In the context of ADP response, platelet aggregation is characterized by two phases. The initial phase, known as the "first wave," is a direct result of agonist-induced primary aggregation. The subsequent phase, referred to as the "second wave," involves secondary aggregation characterized by the formation of large, irreversible aggregates concurrent with platelet secretion. Notably, the absence of this second wave is a distinguishing feature of storage pool disorders (SPDs) and aspirin (ASA). (From Bennett JS, Rao AK. Inherited disorders of platelet function. In: Marder VJ, Aird WC, Bennett JS, Schulman S, White GC II, eds. *Hemostasis and Thrombosis*. 6th ed. Wolters Kluwer; 2013:805-819.)

Automated instruments can also detect other cellular materials as platelets, leading to spurious elevation of platelet counts. Cytoplasmic fragments, most commonly seen in individuals with acute leukemia or hairy cell leukemia, are small and, therefore, can be misinterpreted as platelets (*Arch Intern Med*. 1981;141:942-944). Schistocytes, seen in thrombotic microangiopathies, and cryoglobulins are other possible contributors to spuriously elevated platelets (*Ann Lab Med*. 2022;42:515-530).

Improvements in instrument flagging mechanisms have played a crucial role in excluding preanalytic errors. When these flags are encountered, strategies such as inspecting samples for clots, conducting slide reviews, requesting redraws using alternative anticoagulants, or switching automated methodologies are all effective for minimizing these preanalytic errors.

Platelet Morphology on Blood Smears

Normal circulating platelets are small, round, and oval in shape. The cytoplasm of platelets is characterized by the presence of azurophilic granules, which can be dispersed across the cytoplasm or centralized in a region known as the granulomere. In contrast, the peripheral region of the platelet cytoplasm, which appears colorless or demonstrates weak basophilic staining and is devoid of granules, is referred to as the hyalomere. In peripheral blood smears, the assessment of platelet size can be effectively performed by comparing the diameter of platelets to that of the red blood cells (7-8 μm). Platelets are typically 2 to 3 μm in size, large platelets are between 3 and 7 μm, and giant platelets are >7 μm (e-Figure 4.3-1B). Abnormal platelet count, size, and color can be associated with various disorders.

II. ACQUIRED DISORDERS OF PLATELET NUMBER

Acquired Thrombocytopenia

Acquired thrombocytopenias are characterized by decreased platelet counts in patients with a documented history of normal platelet counts and the absence of pathologic bleeding. They are generally a result of either (1) poor platelet production, (2) increased platelet consumption, or (3) sequestration into the reticuloendothelial system (Table 4.3-2). Decreased platelet production is typically secondary to liver dysfunction or bone marrow infiltration—such as by hematologic neoplasms, metastatic diseases, or infections.

Heparin-Induced Thrombocytopenia

Heparin-induced thrombocytopenia (HIT) occurs when pathogenic antibodies are directed against a neoantigen that is formed when platelet factor 4 (PF4) is bound to heparins. The diagnosis is primarily clinical following the 4T scoring system (consisting of exposure timing, degree of thrombocytopenia, presence of thrombosis, and potential for other causes of low platelet counts). A 4T score below 3 points is an excellent negative predictive value for ruling out HIT (*Blood*. 2012;120:4160-4167). When results show an intermediate clinical suspicion (4T = 4-5 points), heparin should be replaced by nonheparinoid anticoagulants (ie, argatroban, bivalirudin), and serologic testing is then used to determine if reactive antibodies are present with or without confirmatory testing. A high pretest probability (4T >6) is sufficient for diagnosing HIT. Immunologic HIT antibody testing can be done by enzyme-linked immunosorbent assay (ELISA), immunofiltration, or gel-agglutination assays (*Clin Diagn Lab Immunol*. 2003;10:731-740). The serotonin release assay remains the gold standard (and confirmatory test) in unclear cases. The primary treatment is the removal of heparin and avoidance of future heparinoid exposures.

Vaccine-Induced Thrombocytopenia

Vaccine-induced thrombocytopenia (VITT) is a recently described PF4-based neoantigen-driven disease identified in the vaccination setting of the COVID-19 pandemic. The syndrome's pathologic antibodies are also directed against PF4, however, in a different geographic epitope distribution leading to platelet

TABLE 4.3-2 Causes of Thrombocytopenia

Increased Destruction
Primary ITP
Secondary ITP (drugs, infection, autoimmune)
Transfusion
Thrombotic microangiopathy (TTP, aHUS)
Posttransfusion purpura
Heparin-induced thrombocytopenia
DIC
Infection

Poor Production/Survival
Infection
Medication
Liver disease
B12 deficiency
Neoplastic disorders involving the bone marrow[a]

Inherited Thrombocytopenia
Associated with small or large platelets
Thrombocytopenia-absent radius syndrome (*TAR*)
Radioulnar synostosis with amegakaryocytic thrombocytopenia (*RUSAT1*)
Congenital amegakaryocytic thrombocytopenia (*CAMT*)
Familial platelet disorder with predisposition to AML (*RUNX1*)
ANKRD26, CYCS, ETV6, IKZF5, KDSR, MECOM, STIM1, THPO-related thrombocytopenia

Spurious
EDTA platelet antibodies
Clotted Samples

aHUS, atypical hemolytic uremic syndrome; AML, acute myeloid leukemia; DIC, disseminated intravascular coagulopathy; EDTA, ethylenediaminetetraacetic acid; ITP, immune (idiopathic) thrombocytopenia purpura; TTP, thrombotic thrombocytopenia purpura.
[a]Primary hematologic malignancies, for example, acute leukemias, can present with thrombocytopenia and other cytopenias (discussed in later chapters).

activation (*Nature*. 2021;596:565-569). Cases typically occur 5 to 10 days after administration of an adenovirus-based vaccine. The thrombotic phenotype is characterized by an atypical distribution, including cerebral venous sinus thrombosis, splanchnic vein thrombosis, and arterial thrombosis. Treatment is anticoagulation, preferably with nonheparinoid anticoagulants and high-dose intravenous immunoglobulin (IVIg).

Thrombotic Microangiopathies—Thrombotic Thrombocytopenia Purpura/Hemolytic Uremic Syndrome/Atypical Hemolytic Uremic Syndrome

Thrombotic microangiopathies (TMA) are clinically characterized by the presence of extravascular hemolysis (with elevated lactate dehydrogenase [LDH], indirect bilirubinemia, and undetectable haptoglobin levels) with negative direct antiglobulin testing, and the presence of red cell fragments (schistocytes) on peripheral smear. It is critical to identify TMAs because differentiating the mechanism determines the treatment modality critical to reverse the hemolytic process. One systemic condition that may mimic a TMA with hemolysis present and thrombocytopenia is severe B12 deficiency—one early sign for this scenario is a macrocytosis not driven by a reticulocytosis.

Thrombotic thrombocytopenia purpura

Thrombotic thrombocytopenia purpura (TTP) is a disease characterized by reduced ADAMTS13 activity. ADAMTS13 is crucial for downregulating vWF activity through cleavage of large and ultra-large multimers, which are capable of binding platelets and cause microthrombi under high sheer stress conditions. The high sheer unveils ADAMTS13 cleavage sites in large and ultra-large vWF. ADAMTS13 activity is reduced either through congenital deficiency—known as Upshall-Shulman disease—or acquired via inhibitory autoantibodies (acquired TTP or aTTP). In the evaluation of a new patient with concern for TMA, the PLASMIC score is a diagnostic scoring system that utilizes clinical variables to determine patients with potential TTP who are likely to benefit from plasmapheresis upfront. A delay in the diagnosis and treatment of aTTP can quickly progress and become fatal. The primary modality for treating acquired TTP involves immunosuppression with high-dose steroids +/− rituximab, and plasmapheresis to remove pathologic antibodies. Relapse rates are not uncommon in patients with TTP and are reported at ~30% to 40% in patients presenting with ADAMTS13 activity less than 10% at the highest risk (*Blood*. 2010;115:1500-1511).

Hemolytic uremic syndrome

Hemolytic uremic syndrome (HUS) is a form of microangiopathic hemolytic anemia (MAHA) with thrombocytopenia that is the result of renal endothelial dysfunction, and presents with profound renal injury without loss of ADAMTS13 function. In children, the cause of HUS is predominantly from hemorrhagic diarrheal infections carrying Shiga-toxin, such as the classic *Escherichia coli* strain 0157:H7. In adults, HUS can still be Shiga-toxin–dependent and seen in the setting of foodborne outbreaks, but rare sporadic cases exist. The primary mode of treatment is supportive care during diarrheal illness, renal protection, and dialysis as clinically indicated.

Atypical hemolytic uremic syndrome

Atypical hemolytic uremic syndrome (aHUS), or more appropriately complement-mediated thrombotic microangiopathy, has the same clinical features as HUS. However, instead of being triggered by Shiga-toxin–producing bacteria, aHUS is caused by overactive complement activation leading to MAHA/TMA and acute renal injury. Patients with aHUS typically have an underlying complement deficiency or dysfunction in the alternative pathway, leading to overactivation via congenital mutations or inhibitory anti-complement factor H antibody (*J Autoimmun*. 2022;102979). In both scenarios, the use of terminal complement inhibitors such as eculizumab or ravulizumab has been shown to control overactivation, resulting in renal preservation, reversal of injury, and correction of hemolysis and thrombocytopenia.

Immune Thrombocytopenia Purpura

Accelerated destruction of platelets may occur due to antibody-mediated clearance. In the context of transfusion, this may be due to posttransfusion purpura or acquired platelet alloantibodies, as discussed later. Immune (idiopathic) thrombocytopenia purpura (ITP) is a diagnosis of exclusion in which patients have platelet-directed antibodies, which result in sequestration and destruction within the reticuloendothelial system. Patients typically present with petechial rash, soft tissue bleeding such as epistaxis and gum blisters/bleeding, and splenomegaly. Rarely, patients with ITP may also develop autoimmune hemolytic anemia, known as Evans syndrome. Peripheral blood smear findings show rare platelets that are typically large (4-7 µm) and seldom giant (>7 µm). ITP can be further classified as primary and secondary ITP. Secondary ITP includes autoimmune diseases, infections, and medications. Cross-reactive or molecular mimicry antibodies have been reported in infections such as *Helicobacter pylori*, human immunodeficiency virus (HIV), and hepatitis C virus (HCV) infections. Commonly implicated medications include quinine, quinidine, trimethoprim-sulfamethoxazole, vancomycin, and piperacillin/tazobactam (*J Thromb Haemost.* 2015;13:676-678). Rarely, ITP can be a presenting symptom of a B-cell malignancy. Treatment of primary ITP involves a combination of high-dose steroids and IVIg. In refractory cases there is a role for splenectomy as well thrombopoietin mimetics.

Critical Illness Thrombocytopenia and Disseminated Intravascular Coagulation

Patients admitted to intensive care units (ICU) represent a unique population that develops thrombocytopenia due to heterogeneous and multifactorial mechanisms. Specifically, for patients admitted to a medical ICU, the high presence of severe infections, an inflammatory cytokine milieu, and the use of typical antibiotics may all cause bone marrow suppression, presenting as thrombocytopenia. Additionally, the occurrence of thrombocytopenia upon admission or its development in response to systemic disease serves as an unfavorable prognostic indicator for survival (*Arch Intern Med.* 2008;168:94-102).

Disseminated intravascular coagulation (DIC) is a systemic overactivation of coagulation, endothelial dysfunction, and platelet reactivity in response to infection (severe sepsis, septic shock) and inflammation. DIC is diagnosed clinically and is characterized by thrombocytopenia and coagulopathy (low fibrinogen levels, elevated D-dimer or fibrin split products, and prolonged prothrombin time [PT] and activated partial thromboplastin time [aPTT]). Coagulopathy in DIC typically presents as line-associated bleeding in ICU patients. In patients presenting with fulminant infections, bleeding may be more serious, including intra-abdominal, retroperitoneal, and gastrointestinal bleeding. The ultimate treatment involves reversal of the underlying systemic disease; however, patients should be supported with fresh frozen plasma infusions to supplement consumed fibrinogen and platelet transfusions as needed, with targeting levels based on the presence and location of observed bleeding.

Pregnancy-Associated Thrombocytopenia

Gestational thrombocytopenia is typically encountered in the second trimester of pregnancy. This condition is a benign cause of typically mild to moderate thrombocytopenia (platelet count >80,000/µL) and accounts for 70% to 80% of pregnancy-associated thrombocytopenia (*Blood.* 2013;121:38-47). Gestational thrombocytopenia occurs in response to physiologic changes of pregnancy, including an increased volume of distribution that increases toward term. It is important to note that other causes, such as congenital thrombocytopenias and type 2B von Willebrand disease (vWD), may worsen or become evident during this critical period. Ultimately, in the case of pure gestational thrombocytopenia, supportive care and attention to changes in platelet counts are all that is required through delivery, after which platelet counts should return to their prepregnancy baseline (*Hematology Am Soc Hematol Educ Program.* 2022;2022(1):303).

As pregnancy progresses into the third trimester, the continuum of preeclampsia, eclampsia, and HELLP syndrome (hemolysis, elevated liver enzymes, low platelets) may emerge due to placental endothelial dysfunction. Strictly speaking, delivery of the fetus and all placental tissue will reverse all three conditions. However, more recent data have shown that there is a degree of complement activation that is similar between HELLP and aHUS—which is further complicated by pregnancy being a trigger for aHUS (*Adv Chronic Kidney Dis.* 2020;27:155-164).

Bone Marrow Infiltration/Suppression/Primary Disorders
As the primary location for megakaryocytic production of platelets, bone marrow niche alterations can lead to "crowding out" of necessary precursors or direct suppression of megakaryocytes. Infiltration of bone marrow can be the result of primary bone marrow neoplasms and bone marrow failure syndromes, which are described in later chapters. The presence of thrombocytopenia with a second lineage cytopenia should trigger evaluation with a bone marrow biopsy when there is no obvious systemic cause for the presenting cytopenias. Rarely, such evaluation will demonstrate infiltrative processes including, but not limited to, fungal infections, mycobacterial infections, or noncaseating granulomas. Notably, in the evaluation of fever of unknown origin, bone marrow culture will identify unique culprit organisms (not otherwise diagnosed) in a small percentage of patients, almost exclusively in patients with uncontrolled HIV and cytopenias (*Am J Clin Pathol.* 1998;110:150-153).

Posttransfusion Purpura
Posttransfusion purpura (PTP) is a serious transfusion-associated disorder that manifests as a severe thrombocytopenia ($< 10 \times 10^9$/L) occurring within 2 weeks after a blood transfusion (*J Blood Med.* 2019;10:405-415). PTP is due to the formation of alloantibodies targeting specific platelet antigens, predominantly human platelet antigen-1a (HPA-1a), following the recipient's exposure to these antigens in transfused blood products. In individuals diagnosed with PTP, the generated alloantibodies paradoxically affect the patient's own platelets through a mechanism that is not entirely elucidated. One hypothesis posits that autologous platelets may passively adsorb foreign platelet antigens from transfused blood, thereby becoming targets for the alloantibody-mediated immune response. Alternatively, it has been suggested that both alloantibodies and autoantibodies are concurrently produced, with the latter being more challenging to detect, a phenomenon observed similarly in many patients with immune thrombocytopenic purpura (ITP). PTP is an exceedingly rare event, with an estimated incidence of 1:50,000 transfusions. A mortality rate of 10% to 20% has been documented, predominantly attributed to intracranial hemorrhage. HPA genotyping and platelet antibody workup can be used to make the diagnosis. Management of PTP involves the immediate cessation of further platelet transfusions unless absolutely necessary and the administration of high-dose IVIg. In most cases, the prognosis of PTP is favorable, with platelet counts typically normalizing within a few days following treatment.

Acquired Thrombocytosis

Thrombocytosis can be divided into primary and secondary causes (Table 4.3-3). Secondary causes of thrombocytosis are more common than primary causes (>85%), with infection being the most common cause (*Hematol Oncol Clin North Am.* 2012;26:285-viii). In the case of reactive thrombocytosis, various cytokines, including interleukin 6 (IL-6), thrombopoietin, IL-1, interferon-γ, and tumor necrosis factor-α, are released. Consequently, conditions that lead to an increase in these cytokines can potentially trigger reactive thrombocytosis. In a retrospective analysis conducted at a single institution, primary thrombocytosis exhibited a higher average platelet count of (857×10^9/L), while secondary causes had an average of approximately (650×10^9/L). However, platelet counts exceeding (800×10^9/L) were also observed in this group (*J Clin Med Res.* 2012;4:415-423). Soft tissue, pulmonary, and GI infections were the most common infectious causes, with malignancy and iron deficiency anemia being the most common noninfectious causes. It should be noted that despite its high incidence in the thrombocytosis cohort, specifically in patients with iron deficiency anemia, it may only be seen 10% of the time (*Blood.* 2018;132(suppl 1):4985). Tissue damage also may cause reactive thrombocytosis and may be the result of burns, pancreatitis, myocardial infarction, and surgery. Thrombocytosis is observed in approximately 50% of cases following splenectomy, a condition that typically resolves within a few months. Elevated platelet counts can also result from various inflammatory conditions, including inflammatory bowel disease, vasculitis, rheumatoid arthritis, and celiac disease. Additionally, thrombocytosis may infrequently be induced by certain medications, such as epinephrine, vincristine, gemcitabine, antibiotics, and low-molecular-weight heparin (*Ann Pharmacother.* 2019;53:523-536).

TABLE 4.3-3 Causes of Thrombocytosis

Primary[a]

Myeloproliferative neoplasms
Myelodysplastic syndrome with 5q deletion

Secondary

Infection
Iron deficiency anemia
Malignancy (nonhematologic)
Tissue damage
Inflammatory disorders
Postsplenectomy

Spurious

Cytoplasmic fragments
Cryoglobulinemia

[a]Discussed in detail in later chapters.

III. ACQUIRED NONNEOPLASTIC DISORDERS OF PLATELET SIZE AND MORPHOLOGY

There are a variety of neoplastic and nonneoplastic causes of abnormal platelet volume and morphology (nonneoplastic causes are listed in Table 4.3-4). In the normal physiologic state, megakaryocytes are stimulated by thrombopoietin to produce larger platelets

TABLE 4.3-4 Benign Disorders With Abnormal Platelet Morphology

Large Platelets

Inherited[a]

- *MYH9*-related disorders (*MYH9*)
- May-Hegglin—Dohle-like bodies
- von Willebrand disease type 2B (*VWF*)
- Platelet-type von Willibrand disease (*GP1BA*)
- Bernard-Soulier (*GP1BA, GP1BB, GP9*)
- Gray platelet syndrome (*NBEAL2*)
- Velocardiofacial syndrome (22q11.2 deletion → *GP1BB* deletion)
- *ACTN1, DIAPH1, FLI1, FLNA, GALE, GATA1, GFI1B, GNE, PRKACG, SLFN14, SRC, TPM4, TRPM7, TUBB1*—related thrombocytopenia

Acquired

- Postsplenectomy states and hyposplenism
- Increased destruction: ITP, TMA
- Drug—cholestyramine

Small Platelets

Inherited

- Wiskott-Aldrich syndrome (*WAS*)
- X-linked thrombocytopenia (*WAS*)
- *ARCP1B, FYB, PTPRJ*—related thrombocytopenia

Acquired

- Impaired production: drug toxicity, bone marrow infiltration

Agranular Platelets

- Storage pool disorders (see Table 4.3-5)
- In vitro—venipuncture, implanted devices, cardiopulmonary bypass, EDTA—induced
- In vivo—DIC

DIC, disseminated intravascular coagulopathy; EDTA, ethylenediaminetetraacetic acid; ITP, immune (idiopathic) thrombocytopenia purpura; TMA, thrombotic microangiopathies.
[a]Genes involved in inherited disorders are mentioned in *italics*.

in response to decreased platelet levels. Therefore, disorders with increased platelet consumption have a higher-than-normal MPV, though not as much as seen in inherited platelet disorders (*Br J Haematol*. 2013;162:112-119). Impaired production of platelets due to drug toxicity or bone marrow infiltration may cause low MPV values. Agranular platelets or pale platelets can be seen in states with consistently ongoing platelet activation, leading to "exhausted" granules, such as patients with cardiac devices, on cardiopulmonary bypass, or in DIC. Rarely, these abnormalities may be EDTA-induced and serve as a source of preanalytical error (*Clin Lab Haematol*. 2005;27:336-334).

Acquired von Willebrand Syndrome

Acquired von Willebrand syndrome (aVWS) occurs in the setting of prolonged and extreme thrombocytosis, typically seen in MPN-associated thrombocytosis, or in situations of abnormal high sheer blood flow. In these scenarios, elevated platelet numbers and activity cause increased binding and unraveling of ultra-large vWF molecules, leading to their cleavage by ADAMTS13. This results in a steady consumption of normal vWF, ultimately leading to a bleeding phenotype. This is also seen in Heyde syndrome (aortic stenosis causing aVWS when associated with gastrointestinal arteriovenous malformations), left ventricular assist devices, and extracorporeal membrane oxygenation due to nonphysiologic blood flow. Laboratory examination shows low vWF antigen activity (measured by either ristocetin or GP1b binding) and loss of high-molecule-weight forms on multimer analysis. Treatment strategies focus on cytoreduction for MPN-associated aVWS, with the addition of low-dose aspirin, or correction of underlying stenotic/flow physiology. Additionally, replacement of vWF with either recombinant forms (ie, Vonvendi) or plasma-derived vWF (ie, Humate-P), in combination with factor VIII.

IV. INHERITED DISORDERS OF PLATELET NUMBER, MORPHOLOGY, AND FUNCTION

To date, nearly 50 genes have been identified that are involved in megakaryocytic development and implicated in clinical thrombocytopenia or platelet dysfunction (*Blood*. 2022;139:3264-3277). Inherited causes of thrombocytopenia can be identified by their association with syndromic conditions, such as thrombocytopenia-absent radius (TAR) syndrome. With increased access to genomic sequencing, mutations in known or new genes are often identified, which requires establishing definitive guidelines for interpretation and assessment of future risks (*J Thromb Haemost*. 2021;19:2127-2136). Several syndromes causing thrombocytopenia have been critical in understanding basic platelet development (*MPL* mutations in congenital amegakaryocytic thrombocytopenia causing severe neonatal thrombocytopenia) and cancer predisposition syndromes (*ETV6*, *RUNX1*, and *GATA1* germline mutations causing mild to moderate thrombocytopenia). Based on the functional changes, patients may develop a combination of abnormalities in platelet number, microscopic appearance, and function. Most function disorders that do not affect platelet counts also do not affect platelet size. In storage pool disorders, the generation, formation, or release of signaling vesicles are abnormal (see Table 4.3-5); these disorders result in either hypogranular or agranular platelets. Signaling disorders manifest through altered posttranslational processing, expression, and changes in the ability of platelet receptors to adequately regulate their activation and binding to ligands. While the effect on platelet aggregation is beyond the scope of this chapter, these disorders can

TABLE 4.3-5 Storage Pool Disorders Causing Platelet Defects

Disease	Gene (Inheritance)	Mechanism	Findings
Hermansky-Pudlak syndrome	AP3B1 (AR) AP3D1 (AR) BLOC1S3 (AR) BLOC1S6 (AR) DTNBP1 (AR) HPS1 (AR) HPS3 (AR) HPS4 (AR) HPS5 (AR) HPS6 (AR)	Absence of dense granules due to deficiencies in intracellular trafficking	Normal size and count Bleeding phenotype Hypogranular platelets on smear Reduced number of dense granules identified by electron microscopy Albinism
Chediak-Higashi syndrome	LYST (AR)	Reduced number of dense granules	Normal size and count Bleeding phenotype Oculocutaneous albinism Recurrent pyogenic infections Giant intracellular granules in their neutrophils
Gray platelet syndrome	NBEAL2 (AR)	Absent α-granules	Macrothrombocytopenia Bleeding phenotype Increased plasma B-12
Familial platelet disorder with predisposition to AML	RUNX1 (AD)	Reduced number of platelet dense or α-granules Reduced MYH10 expression in megakaryocytes, persistence in platelets	Thrombocytopenia ~40% lifetime risk for developing a hematologic malignancy

AD, autosomal dominant; AML, acute myeloid leukemia; AR, autosomal recessive.

result in abnormal platelets. For example, Bernard-Soulier syndrome, type 2B vWD, and platelet-type vWD syndrome result in large to giant platelets accompanied by thrombocytopenia.

Features of select platelet receptor and receptor signaling disorders are summarized in Table 4.3-6. Defects in structural or cytoskeletal components include

TABLE 4.3-6 Platelet Receptor and Receptor Signaling Defects

Disease	Gene (Inheritance)	Mechanism	Findings
von Willebrand disease, type 2B	*VWF* (AD)	Increased binding of vWF to platelet receptor GP1b leading to increased vWF-platelet clearance. Reduced aggregation response to ristocetin but increased with low dose	Macrothrombocytopenia. Thrombocytopenia worsened with DDAVP
Bernard-Soulier syndrome	*GP1BA*, *GP1BB* and *GP9* (AR/AD)	Reduced GP1b/V/IX complex expression leading to loss of vWF binding. Reduced aggregation response to ristocetin	Macrothrombocytopenia. Homozygous AR more severe than AD mutations. Neonatal bleeding phenotype
Scott syndrome	*ANO6* (AR)	Reduced calcium-dependent signaling and phosphatidylserine exposure to support coagulation proteases	Normal count and size. Bleeding phenotype
Leukocyte integrin adhesion deficiency, type III	*FERMT3* (AR)	Absent platelet aggregation in response to all stimuli, except ristocetin (Glanzmann thrombasthenia-like)	Normal count and size Bleeding phenotype. Normal integrin IIb/IIIa receptor levels
Glanzmann thrombasthenia	*ITGA2B* (AR)	Absent aggregation to all agonists except ristocetin. Abnormal integrin IIb does not bind IIIa and leads to degradation in the ER	Normal count and size. Severe bleeding diathesis. Lack of GPIIb/IIIa surface expression

AD, autosomal dominant; AR, autosomal recessive; ER, endoplasmic reticulum; vWF, von Willebrand factor.

MYH9-related disorders arising from mutations in the gene encoding nonmuscle myosin heavy chain IIA, which result in thrombocytopenia with platelet macrocytosis and cytoplasmic inclusions in neutrophils (Dohle-like bodes). Wiskott-Aldrich syndrome is caused by variants in the *WAS* gene, resulting in small platelets and low platelet count.

SUGGESTED READINGS

Gulati G, Uppal G, Gong J. Unreliable automated complete blood count results: causes, recognition, and resolution. *Ann Lab Med.* 2022;42(5):515-530.

Pecci A, Balduini CL. Inherited thrombocytopenias: an updated guide for clinicians. *Blood Rev.* 2021;48:100784.

Robier C. Platelet morphology. *J Lab Med.* 2020;44(5):231-239.

Rose SR, Petersen NJ, Gardner TJ, Hamill RJ, Trautner BW. Etiology of thrombocytosis in a general medicine population: analysis of 801 cases with emphasis on infectious causes. *J Clin Med Res.* 2012;4(6):415.

Sulai NH, Tefferi A. Why does my patient have thrombocytosis? *Hematol Oncol Clin North Am.* 2012;26(2):285-301.

Bone marrow

5.1 Bone Marrow Abnormalities in Systemic Conditions

Callie Torres, Brooj Abro, and Anjum Hassan

There are many non-neoplastic conditions that cause bone marrow abnormalities including infections, storage disorders, autoimmune diseases, and other systemic diseases. These disorders can result in changes in marrow cellularity and morphology, granuloma formation, fibrosis, necrosis, atrophy, and hemophagocytosis. It is important to recognize pertinent marrow changes in patients with systemic conditions as it may help to diagnose underlying etiologies and/or further guide treatment.

I. BACTERIAL INFECTIONS

Bacterial infections can lead to nonspecific changes such as left shift and granulocytic hyperplasia. In immunocompromised patients, more pronounced changes may be present. Bacterial infections that may result in granuloma formation include tuberculosis, rickettsiosis, Whipple disease, Q fever, and other tick-borne infections (see Table 5.1-1).

Tuberculosis

There are several mycobacterial species that can cause morphologic changes in the bone marrow, but the most predominant are *Mycobacterium tuberculosis* and *Mycobacterium avium-intracellulare* (MAI). Infection with either species may cause epithelioid granulomas (e-Figure 5.1-1), with occasional central, caseous necrosis. While granulomas are more prevalent in immunocompromised individuals, they may also be present in immunocompetent patients. Granulomas may contain interspersed lymphocytes and be located near bony trabeculae. In severely immunosuppressed patients, distinct granulomas may not be seen, instead loose histiocytic aggregates may form. In MAI infections, histiocytes containing organisms may appear granular or cloudy. A periodic acid-Schiff (PAS) or Ziehl-Neelsen stain can aid in identification of the organisms (e-Figure 5.1-2).

Q Fever

Q fever is caused by infection with the gram-negative bacterium *Coxiella burnetii* and is characteristically associated with the formation of lipogranulomas (also referred to as ring/fibrin ring or donut granulomas) that can be found in the bone marrow and liver (*Lancet*. 2006;367:679-688). Lipogranulomas consist of epithelioid histiocytes

| TABLE 5.1-1 | Etiologies of Granuloma Formation in the Bone Marrow |

Viral
Epstein-Barr virus
Cytomegalovirus
Hepatitis C
HIV
Herpes simplex

Malignancy
Hodgkin lymphoma
MALT lymphoma
Multiple myeloma
Acute lymphoblastic leukemia
Acute myeloid leukemia
Hairy cell leukemia
Chronic myelogenous leukemia
Lung cancer
Colon cancer
Ovarian cancer
Sarcomas

Fungal
Histoplasma
Cryptococcosis
Coccidioides
Aspergillus
Blastomycosis

Bacterial
Brucella
Bartonella
Syphilis
Typhoid
Tularemia
Borrelia
Mycoplasma
Toxoplasmosis
Whipple disease
Tuberculosis

Medication
NSAIDs
Chemotherapy
Procainamide
Sulfonamide
Phenytoin
Methyldopa
Allopurinol
Bacillus Calmette Guérin
Steroids

Parasitic
Leishmaniasis
Malaria

MALT, mucosa-associated lymphoid tissue; NSAID, nonsteroidal anti-inflammatory drug.

and lymphocytes encircling a central lipid vacuole, creating the appearance of a donut ring. Although lipogranulomas are most commonly associated with Q fever, it is important to note that they may also be present in other infections including Epstein-Barr virus (EBV), cytomegalovirus (CMV), and leishmaniasis.

Whipple Disease

Whipple disease is a bacterial infection caused by *Tropheryma whipplei*. It commonly involves the gastrointestinal tract; however, organisms can also be present within the bone marrow, spleen, and lymph nodes (*Br J Haematol*. 2001;112:677). The organism, which is often rod or sickle shaped, can be highlighted by PAS stain and may be present both within and outside of macrophages. Other nonspecific findings include the presence of noncaseating granulomas and increased marrow cellularity.

Tick-Borne Diseases

Tick-borne illnesses such as anaplasmosis, ehrlichiosis, and rickettsioses may manifest changes in the bone marrow such as granuloma formation, dysplastic features, and hemophagocytosis. Anaplasmosis is caused by the intracellular gram-negative organism *Anaplasma phagocytophilum*. It infects myeloid cells and has been shown to cause dyserythropoiesis and dysmegakaryopoiesis, leading to peripheral cytopenias (*J Clin Exp Hematop*. 2017;56:160). Ehrlichiosis, caused by *E. chaffeensis* and *E. ewingii* species, is an intracellular bacterium that primarily infects neutrophils and monocytes. Like anaplasmosis, ehrlichiosis can cause cytopenia and dysplastic changes. Although rare, morula have been identified in bone marrow samples (*Hum Pathol*. 1993;24:391). Rickettsioses such as *Rickettsia rickettsii*, *R. prowazekii*, and *R. typhi* may also cause cytopenias, and granuloma formation in the bone marrow and formation of lipogranulomas have also been reported. Anaplasmosis, ehrlichiosis, and the rickettsioses have all been shown to cause hemophagocytic lymphohistiocytosis (HLH), which will be discussed in a later section of this chapter.

Syphilis

Syphilis, a sexually transmitted infection caused by the bacterium *Treponema pallidum*, may cause nonspecific findings in the bone marrow such as lymphoid aggregates, non-necrotizing granulomas, and hemophagocytosis. It has also been shown to cause HLH (*Eur J Pediatr*. 1999;158:553).

II. PARASITIC AND PROTOZOAL INFECTIONS

Although parasitic infections more commonly manifest in the peripheral blood, there are several organisms that may be present within the bone marrow. Granulomas, changes in cellularity, and necrosis may be the only findings in some infections, while in others identification of the organism itself may be possible.

Leishmaniasis

Leishmaniasis, caused by *Leishmania* species, is an intracellular protozoan parasite. It most commonly infects the skin, but cases of visceral leishmaniasis may affect the bone marrow. Identification of bone marrow involvement by organisms is a vital component in making the diagnosis of visceral spread. Characteristic amastigotes, termed Leishman-Donovan bodies (LDBs), may be present within monocytes/histiocytes. To distinguish LDBs from other inclusions, a nucleus and a smaller rodlike kinetoplast should be visualized. Intracellular amastigotes may be difficult to distinguish from other infections like tuberculosis, cryptococcosis, and brucellosis, thus visualization of the kinetoplast is essential. Special stains such as Grocott methenamine silver (GMS) and PAS will be negative in leishmaniasis. A Giemsa stain may also help to visualize the nucleus and kinetoplast. Other less specific findings may include hypercellular marrow, dyspoiesis, plasmacytosis, granulomas, hemophagocytosis, fibrosis, lymphoid aggregates, and necrosis.

Trypanosomiasis

Trypanosomiasis is caused by *Trypanosoma* species including *T. brucei gambiense*, *T. b. brucei*, *T. b. rhodesiense*, and *T. b. cruzi*. Trypanosomes are a group of parasitic flagellate protozoa that are commonly seen in peripheral blood. However, the presence of trypomastigotes and amastigotes in the bone marrow of immunocompromised patients has been reported.

Toxoplasmosis

Toxoplasmosis is an infection caused by the parasite *Toxoplasma gondii*. In immunocompetent individuals, granulomas may be the only finding present. However, in immunocompromised patients, tachyzoites (also called trophozoites) may be present. Tachyzoites are oblong shaped and contain a single large nucleus. Cysts containing bradyzoites may less commonly be seen. PAS can be performed in which staining will be positive in bradyzoite cysts but negative in tachyzoites.

Malaria

Malaria is a febrile illness caused by *Plasmodium* (including *P. vivax* and *P. falciparum*) parasites. Organisms are usually identified on peripheral blood smears. During infection, bone marrow is commonly hypercellular with macrophage proliferation, hemophagocytosis, and dyserythropoiesis (*J Infect Dis*. 2022;225:1274). During acute attacks, gametocytes, rings, and schizonts may be present. As part of their survival, malaria digests hemoglobin, which releases free heme. Free heme is toxic to cells, and thus it is converted into an insoluble crystal form called hemozoin (also called malaria pigment). Hemozoin can be seen on hematoxylin and eosin (H&E) where it appears as black-brown pigment within red blood cells (RBCs).

Babesiosis

Like malaria, babesiosis is an intraerythrocytic parasite. On peripheral smear, the intraerythrocytic ring is similar to that seen in malaria. However, characteristic tetrads, also called Maltese crosses, may be seen. Babesiosis commonly leads to dyserythropoiesis, thrombocytopenia, subsequent anemia, and has been reported to cause secondary HLH in several case studies (*Ann Clin Microbiol Antimicrob*. 2017;16:6).

Filariasis

Filariasis is caused by infections by nematodes such as *Wuchereria bancrofti*, *Loa loa*, and *Brugia malayi*. Infection causes eosinophilia and circulating microfilariae can be seen in peripheral blood. Although it is uncommon, microfilariae may also be observed in the bone marrow. The length, presence or absence of a sheath, and tail appearance can help classify the type of microfilariae.

III. FUNGAL INFECTIONS

Disseminated fungal infections are more prevalent in immunocompromised patients or in special circumstances such as chemotherapy, total parenteral nutrition, or use of broad-spectrum antibiotics. Prudent examination of peripheral blood and bone marrow, along with the use of special stains such as GMS and PAS, is key to establishing a diagnosis. However, the use of other techniques, such as molecular testing, is required for speciation. In general, fungal infections are associated with the formation of granulomas in the bone marrow.

Coccidioidomycosis and Paracoccidioidomycosis

Coccidioides immitis is a fungal infection endemic to the western United States and Mexico. In disseminated cases the organism may be present in the bone marrow. It has a unique morphology consisting of a large spherule (10-80 μm) containing smaller endospores (2-5 μm). The spherules of endospores are commonly located within granulomas or lymphoid aggregates. Eosinophilia may also be present. A similar dimorphic fungus, *Paracoccidioides brasiliensis*, is endemic in Mexico and South America. Granulomas, lymphoid aggregates, and giant cells may be present in the bone marrow during infection. Both *Coccidioides* and *Paracoccidioides* can be highlighted with a GMS or PAS stain.

Cryptococcosis

In patients with HIV, cryptococcosis is one of the most common fungal infections. It is caused by the fungus *Cryptococcus neoformans*, which is easy to identify due to its characteristic thick capsule. However, one should not use size to help establish the diagnosis of cryptococcosis as it may vary from 3 to 15 μm. Patients with bone marrow involvement by *Cryptococcus* commonly have pancytopenia and granulomas may be present. A Wright stain will highlight fungal elements on aspirate, while PAS, mucicarmine, and GMS will be positive in tissue.

Aspergillosis

Aspergillosis, caused by *Aspergillus fumigatus*, most commonly infects the sinopulmonary tract. However, the bone marrow may be involved in immunocompromised individuals or via anatomic barrier disruption such as after trauma or surgery. Organisms, which are 2.5 to 8.0 μm in size and have characteristic 45° angle branching, may be highlighted with GMS stain. Areas of frank necrosis may be present. In non-necrotic areas, granulomas and increased macrophages may be seen.

Histoplasmosis

Endemic to the Ohio River valley, *Histoplasma capsulatum* is a dimorphic fungus that consists of small budding yeast forms. The helmet-shaped yeasts are usually present within neutrophils and macrophages. They are uniformly small, measuring only 2 to 5 μm. Granulomas and hemophagocytosis may also be present. Fungal elements may be better seen on Giemsa, GMS, and PAS staining.

Blastomycosis

Blastomycosis is caused by the dimorphic fungus *Blastomyces dermatitidis*, which is endemic to the Ohio and Mississippi River valleys. Although it typically infects the skin and respiratory tract, bone marrow involvement can occur, even in immunocompetent individuals. The organisms of size 40 μm have pathognomonic broad-based budding and can be highlighted by a GMS stain.

Mucormycosis

Mucormycosis is a particularly deadly infection caused by angioinvasive fungal species in the order Mucorales. The fungus commonly infects the sinonasal tract and lungs but can disseminate to involve the bone marrow. Morphologically, it has wide ribbon-like filaments that branch at 90° without septae.

III. VIRAL INFECTIONS

HIV/AIDS

HIV/AIDS involvement of the bone marrow is termed HIV myelopathy, and nearly all patients with HIV/AIDS will have changes in their bone marrow. Bone marrow findings may depend on the patient's current viral status, medication use, concurrent infection, etc. A myriad of different manifestations may be seen in HIV myelopathy, although most changes are nonspecific. More common changes include granulomas and/or collections of histiocytes, hypercellular bone marrow, lymphoid aggregates, increased plasma cells, increased fibrosis, and even gelatinous transformation of marrow.

The megakaryocytic cell line is particularly affected by HIV/AIDS as the virus can directly infect the cells. As a result, dyspoietic changes such as small and/or clustered megakaryocytes, large forms, abnormal lobation, and increase in number may be present. Perhaps the most pathognomonic sign of HIV myelopathy is seeing naked megakaryocytes, in which cells are stripped leaving only nuclei remaining. This finding has been reported in over half of patients with HIV myelopathy (*Afr J Med Med Sci*. 2006;35 suppl:85). Other less specific findings can include granulocytes with Pelger-Huet anomalies, myeloid and erythroid cells with vacuolation, and plasma cell inclusions (such as Dutcher or Russell bodies).

One of the reasons bone marrow examination may be necessary in patients with HIV/AIDS is to elucidate a cause of cytopenia, which is a common occurrence. Cytopenia(s) may be due to infection, hematologic neoplasms, medication side effect, or the virus itself (*Hematol Transfus Cell Ther*. 2022;44:542).

Parvovirus B19

Parvovirus B19 is a DNA virus that infects RBC precursors. In patients with underlying disorders associated with a decreased RBC life span (such as hereditary spherocytosis), infection can lead to severe anemia due to RBC aplasia. Bone marrow biopsy during acute infection can show unique and somewhat specific findings of large pronormoblasts with ground glass intranuclear viral inclusions. These are sometimes called lantern cells, due to the shape of the inclusion appearing like a lantern. Immunohistochemistry for the virus can be performed to confirm that the viral inclusions are due to parvovirus and not another viral entity.

Epstein-Barr Virus

EBV is a double-stranded DNA virus that causes infectious mononucleosis. Although it is commonly associated with large, atypical lymphocytes (Downey cells) in peripheral blood, changes may also be present in the bone marrow. During acute infection, lymphocytosis and an increase in myeloid to erythroid ratio may be seen. Granulomas or hemophagocytosis may be present. One possible complication of EBV infection is chronic active EBV infection in which the viral replication is uncontrolled and EBV-infected cells proliferate. During this time, the bone marrow will show infiltrates of infected T or natural killer (NK) cells. Immunohistochemistry or in situ hybridization for EBV will highlight the infected cells.

Cytomegalovirus

CMV is a double-stranded DNA virus that also causes mononucleosis. While infection is commonly mild for immunocompetent individuals, it can affect hematopoiesis in immunocompromised patients. CMV infects monocytes, macrophages, and T cells. In the bone marrow, there may be nonspecific findings such as lymphocytosis, granulomas, and left shifted myelopoiesis. Immunostaining for the virus can help highlight infected cells, although only approximately 30% of cases will have the viral inclusions. A CD15 immunostain can also highlight infected cells.

COVID-19

Although bone marrow findings during acute COVID infection are still being investigated, studies have shown increase in cellularity of the bone marrow, megakaryocytic hyperplasia, myeloid left shift, and hemophagocytosis (*Am J Clin Pathol.* 2021;155:627).

IV. LIPID STORAGE DISORDERS

Lipid storage disorders, which occur due to enzyme defects in lipid metabolism pathway, lead to buildup of different substances that can be seen in the bone marrow. There are a wide variety of storage disorders (Table 5.1-2), but three of the most common are Gaucher, Niemann-Pick, and Fabry disease.

Gaucher

Gaucher disease is an autosomal recessive disorder caused by mutations in beta-glucosylceramidase, which leads to accumulation of glucocerebroside. The pathognomonic Gaucher cells are histiocytes with wrinkled tissue paper cytoplasm that stain positive for PAS and Tartrate-resistant acid phosphatase (TRAP or TRAPase). Additionally, Gaucher disease has been associated with B-cell neoplasms and amyloidosis.

Niemann-Pick

Niemann-Pick disease is an autosomal recessive disorder caused by mutations in *SMPD1*, *NPC1*, or *NPC2*, which leads to a sphingomyelinase deficiency. In the bone marrow, histiocytes filled with many vacuoles, termed foam cells, are often present. Sea-blue histiocytes can also occur, which appear blue due to cytoplasmic

TABLE 5.1-2 Storage Disorders With Marrow Involvement

Gaucher disease
Niemann-Pick disease
Fabry disease
Mucolipidosis
Cystinosis
Tay-Sachs disease
Gangliosidosis
Alpha mannosidosis
Fucosidosis
Faber disease
Acid lipase deficiency
Sialic acid storage disease
Sandhoff disease
Tangier disease

accumulation of PAS-positive sphingomyelin. It is important to note that sea-blue histiocytes are a nonspecific finding and may also be present in other storage disorders.

Fabry Disease

Fabry disease is an X-linked disease caused by mutations in alpha-galactosidase A, which leads to accumulation of ceramide trihexoside (CTH). Fabry disease is another storage disorder that can cause sea-blue histiocytes. The granules can be highlighted with a Sudan Black B or PAS stain.

V. OTHER SYSTEMIC CONDITIONS

Hemophagocytic Lymphohistiocytosis

HLH is a potentially fatal group of disorders caused by a defective and uncontrolled immune response. HLH is divided into two categories, primary and secondary. Primary, also termed familial HLH, is due to genetic mutations, while secondary, also called acquired, is due to a myriad of conditions such as infection, malignancy, and autoimmune diseases (Table 5.1-3).

Primary HLH can be inherited or occur sporadically. Common mutations include *PRF1*, *UNC13D*, *MUNC12-4*, *STX11*, *RAB27*, *STXBP2*. Primary HLH may also be associated with underlying immunodeficiency syndromes, such as Chediak-Higashi or X-linked lymphoproliferative syndrome.

When secondary HLH occurs due to rheumatologic or autoimmune disorders, it is also called macrophage activation syndrome (MAS). HLH/MAS has a strong association with systemic juvenile arthritis (SJIA), but has also been associated with

TABLE 5.1-3 Infectious Etiologies Associated With Hemophagocytic Lymphohistiocytosis (HLH)

Viral	Bacterial
Epstein-Barr virus	Brucella
Cytomegalovirus	Rickettsia
Hepatitis	Leptospira
HIV	Tuberculosis
Parvovirus	Anaplasma
Herpes simplex	Salmonella
Varicella-zoster	Ehrlichia
Measles	Syphilis
Human herpesvirus 8	Typhoid
Influenza virus	Other gram-negative bacteria
Parasitic	**Fungal**
Leishmaniasis	Histoplasma
Malaria	Candida
Babesia	Mucor

other disorders such as systemic lupus erythematosus (SLE). Malignancy-associated HLH most commonly occurs with hematopoietic malignancies such as T/NK-cell lymphoma, B-cell lymphomas, and plasma cell myeloma. It can also occur in conjunction with solid tumors such as thymomas or germ cell tumors. A broad number of infectious agents are associated with secondary HLH.

Clinically, HLH commonly presents with fever, fatigue, myalgia, hepatosplenomegaly, coagulopathy, and lymphadenopathy. Diagnosis requires mutation involving one of the genes associated with HLH or at least five of the eight following criteria (*Pediatr Blood Cancer*. 2007;48:124):

- Fever
- Splenomegaly
- Cytopenia affecting more than two cell lines: hemoglobin less than 90 g/L, platelets less than 100×10^9/L, neutrophils less than 1.0×10^9/L
- Hypertriglyceridemia and/or hypofibrinogenemia: fasting triglycerides 3.0 mmol/L or more (ie, ≥265 mg/dL), fibrinogen 1.5 g/L or less
- Hemophagocytosis in bone marrow or spleen or lymph nodes
- Decreased or absent NK-cell activity (according to local laboratory reference)
- Ferritin 500 µg/L or more
- Soluble CD25 (ie, soluble interleukin [IL]-2 receptor) 2,400 U/m or more

Aspirate smear is commonly hypocellular and may demonstrate hemophagocytosis, ingestion of hematologic cells by macrophages (e-Figure 5.1-3). Macrophages otherwise appear normal in morphology. The most common cells to be phagocytosed are erythrocytes. The bone marrow core may also be hypocellular with fibrosis, plasmacytosis, and hemophagocytosis. If infection-associated HLH is suspected, immunohistochemical or in situ hybridization for studies for EBV or other etiologies can be considered.

Amyloidosis

Amyloid, consisting of abnormally folded proteins, can deposit in the wall of vessels and interstitium of bone marrow. Both primary amyloidosis and amyloid deposition secondary to myeloma may involve the bone marrow. The eosinophilic material can also appear as pink to purple globules on aspirate. Special stains such as PAS, crystal violet, thioflavin T, and Congo red can be performed to confirm the presence of amyloid. Amyloid stained with thioflavin and Congo red will demonstrate birefringence under polarization.

Autoimmune Diseases and Collagen Vascular Disorders

In general, collagen vascular disorders present with several nonspecific findings in the bone marrow including lymphoid aggregates, granulomas, sea-blue histiocytes, and megaloblastic erythroid changes. Bony abnormalities such as osteosclerosis or osteopenia may also be present. Bone marrow cellularity is highly variable.

SLE is associated with cytopenias including anemia, thrombocytopenia, and leukopenia. Marrow findings include increased marrow fibrosis, lymphoplasmacytic infiltration, and hemophagocytosis. The erythroid lineage may show dysplastic changes including nuclear budding, multinucleation, and abnormal nuclear contours. Small immature megakaryocytes may also be seen (*Am J Hematol*. 2006;81:590).

Rheumatoid arthritis can cause large granular lymphocytosis (LGL) and is also associated with LGL leukemia. Immune thrombocytopenia (idiopathic thrombocytopenic purpura [ITP]), which leads to the destruction of platelets via antibodies, causes an increased number of small megakaryocytes. Additionally, rosette-like formations consisting of megakaryocytes surrounded by lymphocytes can rarely occur with ITP.

Autoimmune myelofibrosis commonly results in an acellular aspirate. The bone marrow core will generally appear normal apart from fibrosis. In the early stages, fibrosis may not be identifiable in H&E. Use of a reticulin stain can help to highlight early fibrosis while trichrome will highlight advanced stage fibrosis.

SUGGESTED READINGS

Diebold J, Molina T, Camilleri-Broët S, Le Tourneau A, Audouin J. Bone marrow manifestations of infections and systemic diseases observed in bone marrow trephine biopsy review. *Histopathology*. 2000;37(3):199-211.

O'Malley DP, Smith L, Fedoriw Y. Benign causes of bone marrow abnormalities including infections, storage diseases, systemic disorders, and stromal changes. In: Hsi ED, ed. *Foundations in Diagnostic Pathology, Hematopathology*. 3rd ed. Elsevier; 2018.

5.2 Bone Marrow Failure Syndromes

Ying-Chen Claire Hou and Julie Ann Neidich

Bone marrow failure (BMF) is caused by ineffective hematopoiesis of the bone marrow and is attributed to either acquired or inherited causes. BMF commonly manifests as pancytopenia in the peripheral blood. Differentiating inherited bone marrow failure syndromes (IBMFS) from acquired aplastic anemia (AA) is important for accurate diagnosis, disease-specific management, surveillance, and risk evaluation of relatives. IBMFS include Fanconi anemia (FA), dyskeratosis congenita (DC), Diamond-Blackfan anemia (DBA), and Shwachman-Diamond syndrome (SDS), which are frequently observed in children, constituting roughly 25% to 30% of constitutional/inherited bone marrow aplasia cases.

I. ACQUIRED CAUSES OF BONE MARROW FAILURE

Aplastic Anemia

Acquired AA is characterized by peripheral blood pancytopenia and hypocellular bone marrow. Anemia and thrombocytopenia are the most frequent manifestations, and neutropenia is less common. Hepatosplenomegaly and lymphadenopathy are typically not observed. Most patients are diagnosed between 10 and 25 years of age with presentations of bleeding tendency, fatigue, and infection. The incidence of AA is estimated at 1 to 2 cases per million population per year in the United States. The incidence rate is two or three times higher in Asia (*Haematologica*. 2008;93:518-523). Most acquired AA occurs without any identifiable causes. Autoimmune disorders or environmental factors, including infections, drugs, chemicals, or nutrition deficiency, have been linked to acquired AA as etiologies. Immunosuppressive therapy and hematopoietic stem cell transplantation (HSCT) are treatment options for patients with AA (*Pediatr Clin North Am.* 2013;60:1311-1336).

II. INHERITED BONE MARROW FAILURE SYNDROMES

Fanconi Anemia

- **Clinical Features**
  FA is the most common IBMFS. The hallmark of FA pathogenesis is defective homologous recombination of double-stranded DNA repair pathways in response to alkylating agents or cytotoxic drugs. FA is characterized by physical abnormalities, progressive BMF, and an increased risk of cancer. Physical abnormalities, including short stature, abnormal skin pigmentation (hypo- and hyperpigmentation or café-au-lait spots), and skeletal malformations of the upper and/or lower limbs, are commonly observed in patients with FA. Microcephaly, microphthalmia, genitourinary tract anomalies, endocrine disorders, and hypogonadism are also observed. Approximately 60% of patients with FA were reported to have at least one physical abnormality (*Blood Rev.* 2010;24:101-122).

  The prevalence of FA is estimated from 1 in 100,000 to 250,000 births and has been observed in all races. Populations, including Ashkenazi Jews, Afrikaners, northern Europeans, sub-Saharan Blacks, and Spanish Gypsies, with founder variants have increased carrier frequencies. The ratio of males to females is 1:1.2 (Fanconi anemia. In: *GeneReviews*. 2002 [Updated 2021]). The age of onset of BMF for patients with FA is highly variable, and the median age at diagnosis was 6.5 years (*Blood Rev.* 2010;24:101-122). BMF has been reported in 80% of patients with FA, and the cumulative incidence was 90% by age 40. Head and neck, skin, and genitourinary tract cancers are common in patients with FA (*Blood.* 101;4:1249-1256).

- **Histologic Features**
  The bone marrow of FA patients usually shows hypocellularity for age depending on the stage of the disease, and dyserythropoiesis in more than 90% of patients (*Blood.* 1994;84:1650-1655). In the early stages, bone marrow might be normocellular. With disease progression, bone marrow becomes hypocellular, indistinguishable from AA. FA-related myelodysplastic syndromes (MDS) are associated with an increase in blasts and the presence of dysgranulopoiesis (*Am J Clin Pathol.* 2010;133:92-100).

- **Diagnosis and Genetic Testing**
  The chromosomal breakage test is the diagnostic testing method for FA. Clinical diagnosis of FA is established when lymphocytes treated with diepoxybutane (DEB) and mitomycin C (MMC) show increased chromosomal breakage and radial forms on cytogenetic testing (Fanconi anemia. In: *GeneReviews*. 2002 [Updated 2021]). FA is inherited in an autosomal recessive pattern and rarely inherited in an X-linked recessive pattern. FA is caused by pathogenic variants in one of 23 FA-associated genes that encode proteins involved in DNA damage response (Table 5.2-1) (*Exp Hematol.* 2022;105:18-21). Patients with FA with *FANCA* pathogenic variants are the most commonly observed (60%). Patients with FA with *FANCC* and *FANCG* variants are the next most common, consisting of 15% and 10%, respectively (Fanconi anemia. In: *GeneReviews*. 2002 [Updated 2021]). Therefore, sequencing analysis of *FANCA*, which detects missense, nonsense, splice site variants, and small intragenic deletions/insertions, can be performed first. Gene-specific deletion and duplication analysis can be performed to detect exon and whole-gene deletions

1.3 Spleen

Callie Torres, Brooj Abro, and Anjum Hassan

The spleen is a convex organ that sits under ribs 9, 10, and 11. It has two primary functions—that of a lymphoid organ and the filtration of blood. Although it is an uncommon organ to come across in pathology, there are several important diseases, disorders, and neoplasms that may manifest in the spleen. Schematic illustration of splenic architecture is shown in Figure 1.3-1.

I. GROSS ANATOMY

Within the body, the convex portion of the spleen rests against the diaphragm while the concave portion of the organ sits on the posterior wall of the stomach and the tail of the pancreas. The posterior portion of the spleen is also in contact with the kidney. The hilum of the spleen contains the gastrosplenic ligament, splenic artery, splenic vein, as well as other nerves and vessels. In healthy adults, the spleen weighs 50 to 250 g.

II. MICROSCOPIC ANATOMY

Histologically, the spleen is made up of red pulp and white pulp surrounded by a dense connective tissue capsule. However, there is no division of cortex and medulla, unlike many other organs. The spleen parenchyma is divided into red pulp and white pulp separated by an ill-defined interface, the marginal zone (e-Figures 1.3-1A and B).

- **White Pulp**
  The white pulp contains periarterial lymphatic sheaths (PALS) that contain lymphoid nodules. These lymphoid nodules have similar components to that of a lymph node, including primary follicles, germinal centers (particularly in children), mantle zones, marginal zones, and perifollicular zones. These nodules may also be referred to as Malpighian corpuscles (not to be confused with the kidney, where the same term is used interchangeably with renal corpuscles).
- **Red Pulp**
  The red pulp is a complex network of venous sinuses and splenic cords (termed cords of Billroth). The cords house most of the splenic macrophages while the sinuses contain endothelial cells termed littoral cells. Distinguishing cords and sinuses histologically may not be easy. However, if viewed on high power, sinusoids may be seen in transverse axes and are lined by endothelial cells that sit parallel to the long axis of the vessel. The ring or reticular fibers and basal laminae of sinusoids can be better highlighted using a periodic acid-Schiff (PAS) stain.

III. FUNCTION

Filtration of the cellular components of the blood is an important function of the spleen. To accomplish this process, blood first enters the splenic artery. It then travels into the capillaries, which end in the red pulp, an interstitium-like space that fills up with blood like a sponge. Red blood cells pass through sinusoids filled with macrophages

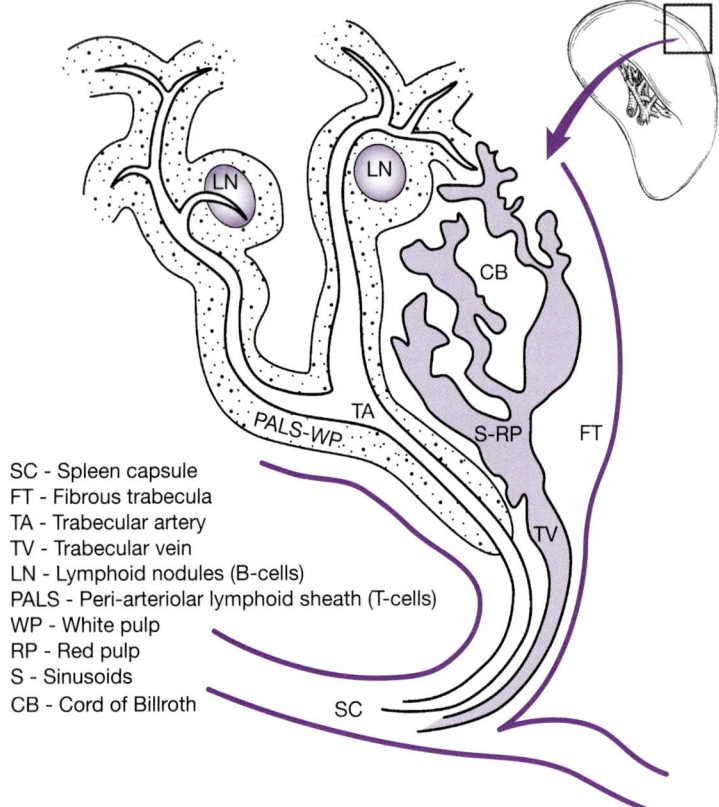

Figure 1.3-1. Diagram of the spleen showing important anatomic landmarks and B- and T-cell distribution.

From Pfeifer JD, Humphrey PA, Ritter JH and Dehner LP, Eds. *The Washington Manual of Surgical Pathology*, 3rd Edition. Lippincott Williams and Wilkins. Philadelphia 2020.
From Pfeifer JD, Dehner LP, Humphrey PA. *The Washington Manual of Surgical Pathology*. 3rd ed. Wolters Kluwer Health; 2019.

before exiting the spleen through the splenic vein. While in the red pulp, macrophages clean up cells by removing fragments, particles, microorganisms, and antibody-coated cells. They also play a role in iron recycling.

The spleen is also involved in antigen presentation. This takes place in the PALS, a network of lymphoid tissue surrounding the splenic arterioles. Antigens are presented within the white pulp by antigen-presenting cells. This initiates the activation of T and B cells leading to the production of opsonizing antibodies, which allows the recruitment of macrophages, neutrophils, and dendritic cells.

Of note, as the red pulp is in direct continuity with the bloodstream, neoplasms associated with the peripheral blood or bone marrow may extend into the red pulp. In addition, fetal hematopoiesis occurs in the spleen. Although this process usually ceases after birth, extramedullary hematopoiesis may be present in a variety of scenarios.

IV. GROSS EXAMINATION AND TISSUE PROCESSING

- **Biopsy**
  Splenic biopsies are performed rarely due to the risk of hemorrhage. Needle core biopsies are occasionally performed in scenarios where a full splenectomy procedure may be associated with morbidity. Histologic examination combined with flow cytometry improves the diagnostic yield (*Am J Hematol.* 2001;67:93).
- **Splenectomy**
  First, the spleen should be measured in three dimensions and weighed. The external surface should then be examined. This entails looking for capsular defects such as lacerations, plaques, or other lesions. The splenic capsule is normally very thin and pale to white-gray in color. In cases of splenic congestion, the capsule may appear tightly stretched over the surface of the organ. Next, the hilum should be examined including the splenic artery and vein(s). Clips or sutures on the vessels within the hilum should be noted. The presence of nodules near the hilum should be recorded and may be representative of lymph nodes or an accessory spleen.

  Following external examination of the organ, the spleen should be sliced through at 1-cm intervals. Sections of the parenchyma should be thoroughly examined for masses or lesions. Normal splenic parenchyma is red-purple with small tan-white speckles. However, the white speckles of the white pulp may not always be seen grossly. Slices of splenic parenchyma may also show white- or gray-appearing blood vessels.

  Processing a spleen specimen correctly can be challenging due to the organ's thick capsule and soft interior. For this reason, it is recommended to slice and fix the spleen before taking sections. It is additionally recommended to have the organ immediately transferred to pathology following surgery due to a high rate of autolysis. If a spleen is received morcellated (in fragments), due to a laparoscopic procedure, it should still be weighed and measured in aggregate, properly fixed, with sections of normal- and abnormal-appearing spleen submitted for histologic examination.

2. Approach to the Bone Marrow and Lymph Node Biopsy

Brooj Abro and Anjum Hassan

This chapter highlights the fundamentals of evaluating bone marrow (BM) and lymph node (LN) biopsy samples. While it is important to have adequate knowledge of common hematologic disorders, it is also essential to know the critical components and steps involved in the evaluation of a BM and LN sample that would help formulate a differential diagnosis and guide further workup to reach an accurate diagnosis.

I. TISSUE SAMPLING, PROCESSING, AND GROSS EXAMINATION

Bone Marrow

The BM biopsy procedure commonly involves obtaining an aspirate, core biopsy, and clot. The most common location to perform a BM biopsy is the external iliac crest. The aspirate is generally performed before the biopsy. The aspirate sample is used to prepare smears for morphologic assessment and is also sent for ancillary studies including flow cytometry (FC), cytogenetics, fluorescence in situ hybridization (FISH), and molecular studies. Two or more of the aspirate smears are stained using the Wright-Giemsa technique. One of the smears can be used for an iron stain using the Prussian blue technique, and few unstained smears are saved for additional studies (eg, cytochemistry) if needed. Core biopsy samples require decalcification and formalin fixation before tissue sections can be prepared for hematoxylin and eosin (H&E) staining and other ancillary studies including immunohistochemistry (IHC) and special stains such as reticulin and trichrome. EDTA solution is used to decalcify BM cores. Formalin-fixed paraffin-embedded (FFPE) sections of a clot that contains marrow particles are better suited for molecular studies when needed as it is not decalcified.

Lymph Node

Fresh LN and lymphoid tissue samples should be evaluated for gross abnormalities and a portion of tissue saved for ancillary studies, particularly FC, before formalin fixation. LNs are commonly bisected to evaluate for any gross abnormalities. A touch preparation (TP) is generally performed to assess sample adequacy and presence of lymphoid tissue. TPs can be wet- or air-dried. Wet TPs are fixed in 95% alcohol or formalin, for Papanicolaou or H&E staining. Air-dried TPs are stained with Wright-Giemsa.

A representative sample should be kept in RPMI solution for FC. Care should be taken to avoid submitting associated fat and fibrotic tissue in order to get the best yield from FC analysis.

Sections of LN are fixed in formalin and embedded in paraffin. FFPE tissue can be used for H&E staining, IHC, special stains, and molecular studies. Procuring tissue for histology usually takes priority over other studies.

II. APPROACH TO THE BONE MARROW BIOPSY

While morphologic evaluation is the cornerstone in the practice of pathology, BM examination is complex, and several other components are essential in the appropriate assessment and workup of BM samples (see summary in Table 2.1).

Clinical History

BM biopsy is an invasive procedure and is often done to investigate BM pathology in a patient with abnormal blood counts, ideally after a thorough workup has been performed to investigate other causes. BM biopsy is also performed for the staging of various malignancies and other conditions such as working up a patient suspected to have hemophagocytic lymphohistiocytosis (HLH). Often, without clinical history, evaluation of a BM sample can be difficult and certain findings may be missed. For example, in a patient suspected to have HLH, it is important to look closely for hemophagocytosis and mention it in the report. Hemophagocytosis is otherwise a nonspecific finding and not reported without the appropriate clinical context. When reviewing the patient's clinical chart, pertinent information should be gathered, which can help answer the following key questions: Why was a BM biopsy performed? What

TABLE 2.1 Essential Components in the Evaluation and Workup of a BM Biopsy

Components	Role
Clinical history	Gather pertinent info from the patient's chart: • Why was a BM biopsy performed? • What other pertinent workup was performed? • What clinical questions do I need to address in my report?
CBC	CBC values are critical to the diagnosis of certain conditions.
Morphologic examination	Morphologic examination includes evaluation of PB smear, BM aspirate smear or touch prep, and core biopsy or clot section to generate a comprehensive BM report.
Flow cytometry and immunohistochemistry	Identify abnormal hematologic cell populations and assess immunophenotype.
Cytogenetics, FISH, and NGS studies	Reviewing the results of these tests is often very useful in a patient with prior BM evaluation. In cases with first-time BM biopsy, this information is not available at the time of morphologic assessment; however, in some cases, the final diagnosis and/or disease classification requires the results of these tests, which should be mentioned in the report.

BM, bone marrow; CBC, complete blood count; FISH, fluorescence in situ hybridization; NGS, next-generation sequencing; PB, peripheral blood.

are the clinical questions that should be addressed in my BM report? Pertinent positive and negative findings should be noted in the report.

Complete Blood Count

A complete blood count (CBC) with differential counts is often performed at the time of BM biopsy. The CBC report provides valuable information including red blood cell (RBC) indices (mean corpuscular volume [MCV], red cell distribution width [RDW], etc), hemoglobin and hematocrit levels, and white blood cell (WBC) and platelet counts. This information is very useful and can help formulate a differential diagnosis even before looking at the BM slides.

Microscopic Examination

Peripheral Blood Smear

A peripheral blood (PB) smear is usually received with a BM biopsy sample. Screening the PB smear can provide clues to certain diagnoses, for example, presence of blasts in acute leukemia, dysplastic neutrophils in myelodysplastic syndrome (MDS), lymphocytosis with small mature lymphocytes in chronic lymphocytic leukemia (CLL), etc. Many clinical laboratories use the Sysmex CellaVision, which is an automated cell counting system and also provides images of blood cells that can be viewed remotely. In certain cases, a preliminary diagnosis can be rendered on the PB smear (eg, presence of blasts in suspected acute leukemia) while awaiting BM biopsy results.

Bone Marrow Aspirate Smear

The BM aspirate smear is utilized for the assessment of cytomorphologic features of hematopoietic lineages and performing a manual differential count. A total of 200 to 500 cells are usually counted by a laboratory technologist or pathologist. The aspirate can also give an impression of the marrow cellularity; however, this aspect is more accurately evaluated in the core biopsy.

When evaluating an aspirate smear, the adequacy of the sample should be noted and mentioned in the report. An adequate aspirate contains marrow particles known as spicules (e-Figure 2.1A). An aspirate without spicules is hemodilute and may not be representative of the marrow cellularity (e-Figure 2.1B).

The aspirate is most useful for evaluating the hematopoietic lineages (e-Figure 2.2). Metastatic tumors may be subtle or difficult to assess on the aspirate and better visualized in the core biopsy.

Steps for evaluating a BM aspirate smear are summarized in Table 2.2.

Touch Preparation

A TP provides similar information as the BM aspirate and can be very useful in cases when the aspirate is inadequate. The cytomorphologic features are not always as clear on the TP as in the aspirate smear and cells may artifactually appear more immature. Care should be taken to avoid misclassifying cell types. A good quality TP can also be used to perform a manual differential count.

Bone Marrow Core Biopsy

The BM core biopsy (e-Figures 2.3A and B) is important for the assessment of marrow cellularity, overall architecture, abnormal hematopoietic (e-Figure 2.4) and non-hematopoietic infiltrates, marrow fibrosis, etc. The assessment of dysplasia is limited on the core biopsy and certain cytomorphologic features are difficult to assess,

TABLE 2.2	Steps of Evaluating an Aspirate Smear
At low power (40-200×)	• **Assess adequacy:** Does the smear contain spicules or is it hemodilute?
	• **Evaluate for multilineage hematopoiesis:** Are all lineages present and show maturation? At medium power (10-20×), a normal marrow aspirate shows a heterogeneous population of hematopoietic cells at various stages of maturation.
	• Scan the entire slide and look for any abnormal cell aggregates.
At high power (400-1,000×)	• **Evaluate cytomorphology of individual cells:** presence of blasts, dysplasia, abnormal lymphoid cells, plasma cells, etc
	• **Perform manual cell differential count** (200-500 cells).

particularly for myeloid and erythroid lineages; however, megakaryocytic dysplasia can be readily assessed on the core (clustering, abnormal size, and nuclear lobation).

Clot Section

The clot section is prepared in addition to the core biopsy in many labs. An adequate clot section shows abundant marrow particles (e-Figure 2.5), and in certain situations, this can be very useful, for example, when the core biopsy is inadequate or when a molecular test needs to be performed on FFPE tissue (clot is not decalcified and hence is preferred for molecular testing).

Iron Stain

The iron stain is most commonly performed on an aspirate smear using the Prussian blue stain. Some labs also perform it on the clot sections and core biopsy. The iron stain can be used to assess iron stores; however, the results are not always reliable. The most important use of the iron stain is to evaluate for ringed sideroblasts, which can help in the diagnosis of MDS.

Immunophenotypic Studies

Immunophenotypic studies include FC and IHC. FC is performed on the BM sample using a portion of the aspirate, and IHC studies can be performed on the core and/or the clot section. Ideally, all BM biopsies should have the appropriate FC studies performed. FC is very useful in assessing abnormal myeloid and lymphoid cell populations (see Chapter 32 for details). However, FC analysis should be interpreted with caution in cases when the aspirate smear is hemodilute (not representative of the marrow cellularity). In such cases, IHC studies should be considered on either the core or the clot section as needed.

Cytogenetics, Fluorescence In Situ Hybridization, and Molecular Studies

Cytogenetics, FISH, and molecular studies including polymerase chain reaction (PCR) and next-generation sequencing (NGS) are critical to the final classification of many hematologic diseases, particularly myeloid neoplasms (see Chapters 33 and 34 for details). In some cases, the appropriate studies may not have been ordered at the time of BM collection. When reviewing a BM case, it is important to note which molecular studies are essential and if not already ordered by the clinical team, efforts should be made to ensure that these studies are performed on the remaining BM sample while it is still viable. For example, in a case of new acute myeloid leukemia (AML) diagnosis, it is of utmost importance to send sample for certain molecular studies including an AML FISH panel, *FLT3* mutation analysis, and myeloid mutation NGS panel. The results of these studies can be used for therapeutic purposes, disease prognostication, and future follow-up for residual disease or disease recurrence.

III. APPROACH TO THE LYMPH NODE BIOPSY

Clinical History

Reviewing the clinical history including physical examination and imaging findings can be very helpful when evaluating a LN biopsy or lymphoid tissue sample. While reviewing a patient's chart, a few important things to note include the following:

- Demographics: certain diseases are more common in specific age groups and races. For example, adult T-cell leukemia/lymphoma is more common in Asians; Burkitt lymphoma is more common in children.
- Reason for biopsy (concern for lymphoma, metastatic carcinoma, infection, etc)
- Other sites of potential disease: does the patient have lymphocytosis (review CBC), lymphadenopathy, hepatosplenomegaly, or other organ involvement (review radiology reports, particularly positron emission tomography [PET] scan if available)?
- Does the patient have a previous diagnosis of a hematologic malignancy? If a diagnosis is known, a limited workup may be enough to confirm disease recurrence.

Microscopic Evaluation

An algorithmic approach can be applied to the morphologic assessment of a LN specimen (see Table 2.3).

Immunophenotypic Studies

Both FC and IHC studies are essential for the workup of LN biopsies (see Chapters 31 and 32 for details). FC helps identify abnormal B- or T-cell populations and is particularly useful in assessing B-cell clonality in non-Hodgkin B-cell lymphomas. IHC studies provide the opportunity to assess abnormal lymphoid populations in an architectural context that is essential for the final/definitive classification of most lymphoid neoplasms.

Genetic Studies

Certain genetic studies are essential or helpful in the final classification of lymphoid malignancies and can be performed using either fresh or FFPE tissue. For example, when a diagnosis of diffuse large B-cell lymphoma (DLBCL) is suspected, FISH analysis of *MYC* and *BCL2* rearrangement is essential to rule out high-grade B-cell lymphoma with *MYC* and *BCL2* rearrangements. In a case of suspected follicular lymphoma with nonclassic phenotype, *IGH/BCL2* FISH can be helpful to confirm the diagnosis.

TABLE 2.3   Algorithm for the Workup of Lymphomas

Examination of H&E sections under low power:
  i. In the tissue section, what is the low-power architecture?

Examination of H&E sections under high power:
  ii. **Cell type:** Are the cells lymphoid?
  iii. **Cell size:** Are the majority of cells small (same as a normal lymphocyte)? Or large (~3 times as big as a lymphocyte, or even bigger)?
  iv. **Nuclear shape:** Do the cells have round nuclei with a smooth contour (noncleaved)? Or a round shape with a bumpy or notched contour (irregular)? Or a variable shape with deeply folded or grooved nuclei (cleaved)?
  v. **Characteristics of the infiltrate:** Is the infiltrate composed of similar cells or different sizes and shapes (monomorphic vs pleomorphic)? Are they blastoid, anaplastic, etc?
  vi. **Histologic grade:** Is necrosis present? Is there a "starry sky" appearance? Are mitoses easy to find?

Identify lineage and maturation:
- Lineage and maturation can be identified using FC and IHC studies.

Final disease classification:
- In many cases, lymphoid neoplasms can be classified using FC and IHC techniques; however, additional techniques such as FISH are warranted in some cases (eg, final diagnosis of DLBCL, NOS requires FISH tests to rule out high-grade B-cell lymphoma).

DLBCL, diffuse large B-cell lymphoma; NOS, not otherwise specified; FC, flow cytometry; FISH, fluorescence in situ hybridization; H&E, hematoxylin and eosin; IHC, immunohistochemistry.
Adapted from Pfeifer JD, Dehner LP, Humphrey PA. *The Washington Manual of Surgical Pathology.* 3rd ed. Wolters Kluwer Health; 2019.

Approach to Fine Needle Aspiration of Hematologic Malignancies
Cody Weimholt

I. INTRODUCTION TO FINE NEEDLE ASPIRATION

Fine needle aspiration (FNA) is a widely used, simple, reliable, and accurate means of tissue acquisition that has notable advantages over core needle biopsy (CNB) and surgical biopsy as it is generally considered safer, faster, and more cost-effective. FNA can be utilized to access lesions anywhere in the body. Palpation or ultrasound (US) guidance is generally used in superficial sites and the head and neck region. CT-guided percutaneous FNA is used to sample lesions deep within the mediastinum, abdomen, pelvis, and retroperitoneum. The flexibility of thin needles facilitates transbronchial and endoscopic FNA, which can access pulmonary, hilar, and mediastinal lesions, and lesions within and adjacent to the alimentary tract, respectively. FNA is often preferred over CNB in certain high-risk patient populations or when lesions are deeply seated or adjacent to vital structures. It poses a lower risk of pneumothorax and needle tract seeding. For superficial lesions, FNA can be performed in outpatient and bedside settings with or without the use of US guidance. It can obviate the need for expensive surgical intervention following a diagnosis of a benign entity or an advanced-stage malignancy. A cytology smear can be processed and interpreted in a matter of minutes. A key advantage is the ability to couple FNA with rapid on-site evaluation (ROSE) by cytopathologists that enables the determination of whether or not the lesion has been sampled, if the sampled tumor is viable, if larger biopsies are necessary, and if ancillary studies are needed (eg, culture, flow cytometry, cytogenetics). If collecting for flow cytometric immunophenotyping (FCI), FNA has been shown to significantly outperform CNB in obtaining material (*Cytometry B Clin Cytom.* 2015;88:64-68). With ROSE one can produce a preliminary diagnosis that enables the direction of further diagnostic and therapeutic clinical planning within the first visit. The processing modalities for FNA consist of direct smears, liquid-based monolayer preparations, and formalin-fixed paraffin-embedded (FFPE) cell blocks. These preparations all share the advantage of retaining cellular material for the potential application of special, immunocytochemical (ICC), or immunohistochemical (IHC) stains, as well as for molecular genetic assays such as fluorescence in situ hybridization (FISH), polymerase chain reaction (PCR), and next-generation sequencing (NGS) (*Arch Pathol Lab Med.* 2018;142:291-298). Smears and liquid-based preparations notably yield higher quality genetic material than FFPE tissues.

FNA is not without disadvantages. It produces smaller tissue volumes that are more readily exhausted, tends to produce fewer and smaller true tissue fragments by which to assess tissue architecture and the spatial relationship of tumor to adjacent structures, and generally yields a lower sensitivity compared to CNB and surgical biopsy (see Table 3.1).

TABLE 3.1	**Advantages and Disadvantages of Fine Needle Aspiration Biopsy**
Advantages	**Disadvantages**
Easier to access deep-seated lesions	Lower sensitivity
Ability to perform ROSE for sample adequacy	Lack of tissue architecture
Cost-effective	Challenging to subclassify certain lymphoproliferative disorders

ROSE, rapid on-site evaluation.

II. THE ROLE OF FINE NEEDLE ASPIRATION IN HEMATOLOGIC MALIGNANCIES

The evaluation of lymphoproliferative disorders in the discipline of cytopathology is an especially challenging area, even in academic settings where cytology cases are interpreted by subspecialty-focused, fellowship-trained cytopathologists. This difficulty is given additional weight in community-based settings where it is not uncommon for cytology cases to be interpreted by general pathologists lacking specific fellowship training in cytopathology.

Hematologic malignancies seen by FNA are encountered most frequently in nodal tissues, but they can also be seen in extranodal sites for which a lymphoproliferative process may not be a clinical suspicion. In lymph node FNA, four common scenarios or indications are typical: (1) evaluation of lymphadenopathy (LAD) of unknown etiology or suspected hematologic malignancy; (2) detection of metastasis for primary staging of nonhematologic malignancy; (3) detection of recurrent hematologic or nonhematologic malignancy, and (4) identifying a lesion as non-nodal when submitted as "lymph node." The accuracy of FNA in the evaluation of nodal metastasis by nonhematologic malignancy is well established, but it is notably less sensitive in regard to identifying lymphomatous processes (*Lancet Respir Med.* 2015;3:282-289; *Clin Endosc.* 2021;54:722-729). Given the lower sensitivity (despite a high positive predictive value) when compared to CNB or surgical biopsy, there is much controversy regarding the appropriate use of FNA in the primary diagnosis of hematologic malignancy. An additional factor is the limited ability to subclassify and grade a well-defined subset of hematologic malignancies that generally require evaluation of the tissue context and architecture. Other troublesome areas, challenging also with CNB, include hematologic malignancies with aberrant immunophenotypes, aspirates of lymph nodes with only partial involvement by lymphoma, composite lymphomas, and lymphomas with focal transformation. While surgical biopsy remains the gold standard for the diagnosis of primary and recurrent lymphoma, this is not always feasible to obtain. Similarly, interventionalists may prefer the use of FNA over CNB when the risk of complications is deemed sufficiently high. When utilizing FNA it is recommended that it be performed in conjunction with ROSE as this approach has been shown to improve adequacy rates (*Am J Clin Pathol.* 2013;139:300-308).

Cytomorphologic analysis alone is not recommended for primary lymphoma diagnosis, but diagnostic metrics are significantly improved when cytomorphology is used in conjunction with FCI and/or IHC. FCI in particular is essential to establish monoclonality. Cell blocks, also, are essential not only for the application of IHC to enable subclassification but also to visualize tissue architecture if a sufficient volume of true tissue fragments is captured. A recent literature review of 16 studies evaluating performance of FNA plus FCI in diagnosing non-Hodgkin lymphoma (NHL) showed sensitivity ranged from 75% to 99%, specificity ranged from 87% to 100%, and classification accuracy ranged from 48% to 95% (*Acta Cytologica*. 2016;60:302-314). These metrics are generally considered lower for Hodgkin lymphoma (HL). These findings indicate FNA can be well-suited for diagnosing and subclassifying hematologic malignancies. On the other hand, the heterogeneity of the results highlights the difficulties inherent to lymphoma diagnosis and the high degree of expertise required. Communication and consultation with hematopathology and clinical colleagues is a prerequisite to avoid erroneous diagnoses.

Awareness of the clinical context is likewise a prerequisite. The patient's age, time course and evolution of the lesion(s), presence or absence of systemic symptoms, prior history of malignancy or infection, location and extent of involvement, serologic findings, and radiographic findings all must be taken into consideration.

Perhaps part of the problem in regard to the controversy over FNA utility may be the lack of a standardized reporting system with well-defined diagnostic categories and clinical guidelines, which have long been established in other areas of cytopathology (eg, Bethesda Systems for cervical and thyroid cytopathology, Paris System for urinary cytopathology). Efforts are currently underway to address this issue by way of the recently proposed Sydney System for reporting lymph node FNA cytopathology (*Acta Cytologica*. 2020;64:306-322). If widely accepted it would be instrumental for improving diagnostic reproducibility and enhancing clinician understanding and utilization of FNA for patients with suspected hematologic malignancy. As it stands, concurrent or subsequent CNB or surgical biopsy is recommended to confirm a primary diagnosis of lymphoma rendered by FNA (*Arch Pathol Lab Med*. 2021;145:269-290). For the evaluation of lymphoma recurrence, FNA plus FCI and/or IHC may be sufficient for yielding actionable diagnoses without the need for CNB (*Am Soc Cytopathol*. 2017;6:114-119).

III. THE APPROACH TO FINE NEEDLE ASPIRATION IN HEMATOLOGIC MALIGNANCIES

Cytomorphologic analysis of lymphoid tissues utilizes both Romanowsky and Papanicolaou stains. A cell block is usually prepared by concentrating the cells via a centrifuge and processing the cell pellet in paraffin. The utility of each component is listed in Table 3.2.

TABLE 3.2 Key Components of Cytomorphologic Evaluation of Lymphoid Tissues

Component	Utility
Romanowsky-stained smear	Assess cytoplasmic details
Papanicolaou-stained smear	Assess nuclear details
Cell block	Assess cytomorphology using H&E stain and evaluate immunophenotype using IHC studies

H&E, hematoxylin and eosin; IHC, immunohistochemistry.

Smears from normal lymph nodes are characterized by singly distributed lymphoid cells with scant cytoplasm. The background frequently shows lymphoglandular bodies (cytoplasmic fragments of disrupted lymphocytes), lymphoid tangles (small fragments of lymph tissue with prominent crush artifact), and dendritic-lymphocytic aggregates (clusters of macrophages and lymphocytes held together by dendritic cells) that represent germinal center fragments. The cells present in a normal lymph node consist of varying proportions of small lymphocytes, centrocytes, centroblasts, immunoblasts, plasma cells, plasmacytoid cells, tingible body macrophages (TBMs), dendritic cells, mast cells, neutrophils, and eosinophils. Small lymphocytes are on average 8 μm in diameter, show course chromatin, round nuclear contours, inconspicuous nucleoli, and very scant cytoplasm. Centrocytes are similar but show cleaved nuclear contours and vary in size from small to intermediate (1-2 times the diameter of a small lymphocyte). Centroblasts are large in size (3 times the diameter of a small lymphocyte), show fine chromatin, round nuclear contours, and contain several small nucleoli. Immunoblasts are similar to centroblasts but show a single, prominent nucleolus and increased cytoplasm imparting a plasmacytoid appearance. TBMs and dendritic cells have large oval nuclei and voluminous pale cytoplasm, with the dendritic cells showing fibrillary cytoplasmic processes and TBMs showing engulfed cellular debris.

Assessment of lymphoma by cytomorphology is typically centered on the identification of cytologic atypia coupled with a pattern-based approach organized around predominant nuclear size. In general, lymphomas can be divided into small cell and large cell categories. From these patterns a differential diagnosis can be generated and the appropriate ancillary techniques can be applied. Some lymphomas can show a mixture of small and large cells or may display one pattern or the other based on grade or variant morphology. Therefore, the pattern-based approach should not be rigidly applied. Correlation with ancillary studies is essential.

Reactive Lymphoid Hyperplasia

This finding is nonspecific as an etiology is unknown in most cases. It is the most common cause of LAD and thus the most commonly seen on FNA. The aspirate is characterized by a polymorphous population of lymphocytes that are predominantly small and mature in appearance, with a smaller proportion of intermediate and large lymphocytes interspersed in the background. TBMs and dendritic-lymphocytic aggregates are conspicuous (e-Figure 3.1). Certain NHLs can mimic this pattern so knowledge of the clinical context is extremely important; application of FCI is crucial for equivocal cases to exclude monoclonality (as a note of caution, some reactive hyperplasias can show a small monoclonal B-cell proliferation by FCI). HL typically shows a dense background of reactive hyperplasia in which Reed-Sternberg cells can be easily overlooked and FCI is often noncontributory; high-power assessment is key to avoid a false-negative diagnosis.

Lymphadenitis. Etiologies of lymphadenitis are diverse and can be infectious (eg, fungal, mycobacterial, viral) or noninfectious (eg, sarcoidosis, various autoimmune disorders, drugs). Neutrophilic and necrotic debris often indicates mycobacterial or fungal infection for which acid-fast bacilli (AFB) and Grocott methenamine silver (GMS) histochemical stains should be obtained; granulomas may or may not be seen in these settings and their absence should not preclude the ordering of these special stains. Smears showing dense and tightly cohesive granulomas, small and loose clusters of epithelioid histiocytes, and scattered multinucleated giant cells in a non-necrotic background of small lymphocytes are indicative of sarcoidosis (e-Figure 3.2).

Follicular lymphoma is the most common NHL in the United States. The aspirate is composed predominantly of small cleaved centrocytes intermixed with large cleaved and noncleaved centroblasts (e-Figure 3.3). Grading, ranging from 1 to 3, is determined by histology via the proportion of centroblasts in neoplastic follicles. There is no standardized method of grading by cytologic means; however, it may be possible to favor low (grades 1 and 2) versus high grade (grade 3) based on the proportion of large cells in the aspirate (*J Am Soc Cytopathol.* 2017;6:80-88). The distinction between high-grade follicular lymphoma and diffuse large B-cell lymphoma (DLBCL) also hinges upon histologic evaluation and is in theory not possible via cytology, although follicular center fragments can occasionally be captured in cell blocks and can suggest the presence of follicular architecture. However, this distinction may not be clinically relevant. Ancillary studies typically show expression of CD10 and BCL6 with a lack of CD5 expression. Most cases demonstrate a *BCL2* gene rearrangement.

Marginal zone lymphoma may be nodal or extranodal and typically occurs in older women, often in the setting of autoimmune disease. The aspirate shows a polymorphous population of predominantly small cells with characteristically round nuclei and moderate amounts of pale cytoplasm imparting a monocytoid or plasmacytoid appearance (e-Figure 3.4). Admixed plasma cells are often seen. Lymphoepithelial lesions are a key diagnostic clue in the extranodal type, and while this may be difficult to identify by cytologic means, it has been described (*Cytopathology.* 2011;22:346-349). Cytomorphologic distinction from reactive hyperplasia can be problematic. FCI is needed to identify a light chain restriction. CD10, CD5, BCL6, and cyclin D1 are consistently negative.

Lymphoplasmacytic lymphoma is a rare and indolent B-cell lymphoma. Most patients have evidence of paraproteinemia. The aspirate consists of a mixed population of small lymphoid cells, plasmacytoid cells, and plasma cells (e-Figure 3.5). Ancillary studies show intracytoplasmic and surface monoclonal immunoglobulin M (IgM), and are generally negative for CD5, CD10, and CD23. Difficulties arise in the distinction from marginal zone lymphoma and lymphoplasmacytic lymphoma. Molecular testing for *MYD88* mutation can be helpful.

Small lymphocytic lymphoma is an indolent B-cell lymphoma typically occurring in middle-aged to older adults. The aspirate contains a monotonous population of small lymphoid cells with round nuclear contours, characteristic checkerboard-like clumpy chromatin, and indistinct nucleoli. Scattered large prolymphocytes/paraimmunoblasts with vesicular chromatin, prominent central nucleoli, and pale cytoplasm are present (e-Figure 3.6). A light chain restriction with dim expression is typical, as is positivity for CD5, CD200, and CD23. CD10 and cyclin D1 are characteristically negative.

Mantle cell lymphoma is an aggressive B-cell lymphoma that occurs in older adults with a male predominance and typically presents with widespread disease. The aspirate is composed of a monotonous population of small- to intermediate-sized lymphoid cells with variable nuclear membrane irregularity, dispersed chromatin, and inconspicuous nucleoli (e-Figure 3.7). The blastoid variant, which portends a worse prognosis, is notable for its resemblance to blasts. Cytologic confirmation is based upon demonstrating a B-cell clone with moderate to strong light chain restriction and positivity for cyclin D1 and CD5, and negativity for CD10 and CD23. A *CCND1* gene rearrangement can be detected in most cases by FISH. SOX11 positivity by IHC can be helpful in cases with aberrant immunophenotypes.

Burkitt lymphoma is a highly aggressive B-cell lymphoma with endemic, sporadic, and immune deficiency–associated variants. The aspirate contains a monotonous population of intermediate-sized lymphoid cells with round nuclei, finely dispersed chromatin, and multiple distinct nucleoli. The cytoplasm is scant, deep blue, and contains small lipid-filled vacuoles (e-Figure 3.8). TBMs and mitoses are prominent and are indicative of brisk cell turnover. The characteristic immunophenotype shows positivity for CD10 and BCL6, and negativity for CD5, terminal deoxynucleotidyl transferase (TdT), and BCL2. Rearrangements involving *MYC* are consistently found, which aids in its classification by FNA (*Cancer Cytopathol.* 2005;25: 310-318).

Diffuse large B-cell lymphoma (DLBCL) can arise de novo or upon transformation from an indolent B-cell lymphoma. It is the second most common NHL and while it generally affects older adults there is a wide age range that includes children. The aspirate shows a monotonous population of large atypical lymphoid cells with variably prominent nucleoli (e-Figure 3.9). FCI occasionally results as false negative due to cell fragility; however, surface immunoglobulin can be demonstrated in the majority of cases. Genetic subtyping aids in predicting response to therapy, the germinal center B-cell type and the activated B-cell type, which can be identified by IHC with the application of CD10, BCL6, and MUM1 (*Cancer Cytopathol.* 2016;124:135-143). There are many different types of large B-cell lymphomas (LBCLs) and DLBCL not otherwise specified (NOS) is the most common. The T-cell/histiocyte-rich LBCL (THRLBCL) poses a challenge in cytopathologic evaluation due to the rarity of neoplastic cells within the aspirate, but reports exist demonstrating the ability of FNA in its identification (*Acta Cytol.* 2002;46:893-898).

High-grade B-cell lymphoma (HGBCL) is a distinct entity with morphologic and immunophenotypic similarities to DLBCL and a worse prognosis. The diagnosis requires FISH studies. HGBCL is characterized by the presence of a *MYC* and *BCL2* rearrangement. HGBCL with *MYC* and *BCL6* rearrangement is removed from the recent WHO-HAEM5, while it is retained as a provisional entity in the International Consensus Classification (ICC).

Precursor T- and B-cell lymphoblastic leukemia/lymphoma is a neoplasm of immature lymphoid cells that occurs in a wide age range, preferentially involving children and young adults. The aspirate shows medium- to large-sized atypical lymphoid cells with high nuclear to cytoplasmic ratio, fine chromatin, and conspicuous nucleoli (see e-Figure 3.5). Convoluted nuclear contours are occasionally seen and the cytoplasm is generally less prominent than that seen in Burkitt lymphoma. TdT is an extremely useful diagnostic stain to distinguish it from blastic mantle cell lymphoma and Burkitt lymphoma. Diagnosis by FNA has extremely high accuracy with the use of ancillary studies (*Acta Cytol.* 2016;60:344-353).

Anaplastic large cell lymphoma (ALCL) is a malignancy of mature T cells that occurs in all ages, predominantly in children, with an unpredictable clinical course. Aspirates typically show both singly dispersed and poorly cohesive groups of malignant cells with large and pleomorphic nuclei, prominent nucleoli, and moderate amounts of cytoplasm. Horseshoe- and doughnut-shaped nuclei, as well as binucleated and multinucleated Reed-Sternberg-like tumor cells may also be seen. The immunoprofile is characterized by positivity for CD30 (strong and diffuse), ALK, CD45, and CD3. *ALK* rearrangements are found in most, with ALK-negative cases often showing rearrangements in *DUSP22* and *TP63* (*Biomark Med*. 2015;9:719-722). Mistaking this entity for HL, carcinoma, or other nonhematologic malignancies is a diagnostic pitfall due to cellular cohesion and pleomorphism. Although difficult, ALCL can be accurately diagnosed by FNA if the entity is considered and appropriate ancillary studies are performed (*J Cytol*. 2018;35:37-40).

Other T-cell lymphomas comprise a diverse group of mature T-cell malignancies that include peripheral T-cell lymphoma NOS, angioimmunoblastic T-cell lymphoma, mycosis fungoides, adult T-cell lymphoma, and other extranodal T-cell lymphomas. The aspirates of these entities are generally polymorphic and contain scattered small to large atypical lymphocytes. The background typically shows a reactive pattern with mixture of various other cell types including plasma cells, neutrophils, eosinophils, and macrophages. A wide panel of T-cell-specific markers is required for distinction. Confirmation of clonality is often necessary using PCR or NGS analysis to identify rearrangements of the T-cell receptor genes.

Classic Hodgkin lymphoma (CHL) is a malignancy of B-cell origin with a bimodal age distribution. The aspirate contains rare to scattered Reed-Sternberg cells. The classic binucleated Reed-Sternberg cells have markedly enlarged nuclei, macronucleoli, and a moderate amount of basophilic cytoplasm (e-Figure 3.10). The mononuclear forms (Hodgkin cells) have markedly enlarged, irregular, and multilobated nuclei with macronucleoli. The characteristic reactive lymphoid background includes mainly mature lymphocytes, scattered eosinophils, neutrophils, plasma cells, and occasional epithelioid histiocytes (e-Figure 3.11). Diagnosis can be challenging due to obscured Reed-Sternberg cells and FCI is typically not helpful. IHC for CD30, CD15, and PAX5 is a necessity as it yields a positive predictive value over 90% in some studies (*Cytopathology*. 1994;5:226; *Acta Cytol*. 2001;45:300). Low sensitivity is a limiting factor, typically due to extensive sclerosis yielding scantly cellular aspirates.

Nodular lymphocyte-predominant Hodgkin lymphoma (NLPHL) aka nodular lymphocyte-predominant B-cell lymphoma. Given new understanding of its biologic and clinical differences from CHL and association with THRLBCL, this entity has been renamed "nodular lymphocyte-predominant B-cell lymphoma" by the ICC (*Blood*. 2022;140(11):1229-1253). Historically, it accounts for approximately 5% of HL and typically occurs in young adult males. The characteristic neoplastic cells are markedly enlarged, with one highly convoluted nucleus referred to as popcorn cells. The neoplastic cells are outnumbered by numerous reactive small lymphocytes that tend to be a mixture of T cells and B cells, with B-cell predominance. The immunophenotype consists of positivity for CD20, CD45, OCT2, and BOB1, and negativity for CD30 and CD15. FCI is of limited utility in detecting the neoplastic cells but increased portions of double-positive (CD4 and CD8 positive) reactive

T cells is a clue to the diagnosis. Reported diagnoses by FNA show a high rate of false-negative results (*Cancer Cytopathol.* 2012;120:254-260). Accurate identification may rely on awareness of the clinical context coupled with high-power review of the FNA material.

Miscellaneous Hematologic Malignancies

- **Myeloid sarcoma** is an extramedullary collection of myeloblasts, presenting as a mass lesion. Tumor may be a harbinger of leukemia or evidence of relapsed acute myeloid leukemia (AML). Aspirates show blasts and other precursor myeloid cells, but predominantly blasts. CD43 is a useful screening tool. CD13, CD31, CD117, CD14, CD11c, and myeloperoxidase are variably expressed.
- **Plasma cell neoplasms** uncommonly involve lymph nodes and are typically a sign of advanced extramedullary spread of a known multiple myeloma. Monoclonal gammopathy is seen in the vast majority of cases. Aspirates show numerous well-differentiated plasma cells; however, immature, plasmablastic, or anaplastic variants may be challenging to identify. Kappa and lambda in situ hybridization and immunophenotypic expression of CD38, CD79A, and CD138, with negative expression of CD20, is characteristic.
- **Histiocytic and dendritic cell neoplasms** represent a diverse group of typically slow-growing malignancies derived from either myeloid or mesenchymal cell lineages. Aspirates display histiocytoid to spindled cytomorphology and often display a densely admixed lymphoid or granulocytic infiltrate. These lesions are differentiated by a panel of IHC stains, which includes S-100, CD1a, CD21, CD35, and langerin. Diagnostic accuracy by FNA has been demonstrated in various case reports; however, these entities are often misdiagnosed due to their rarity.

SECTION II

Non-neoplastic

4 Peripheral blood

4.1: Red Blood Cell Disorders

Oladipo B. Cole and John L. Frater

I. NORMAL RED BLOOD CELL RHEOLOGY

Red blood cell (RBC) rheology refers to the characteristic flow properties of healthy RBCs within the bloodstream. RBCs are highly specialized cells that play a crucial role in oxygen transport throughout the body. Their unique biconcave disc shape and deformability enable them to navigate through capillaries and microcirculation. In normal rheology, RBCs exhibit optimal flexibility and resilience, allowing them to pass through small vessels and maintain smooth blood flow. This flexibility is attributed to the structural integrity of the RBC membrane and its cytoskeletal components, which include spectrin, actin, and other proteins regulating the shape and deformability of the cell. The overall viscosity of the blood is influenced by the flow properties of individual RBCs, their aggregation tendencies, and the presence of plasma proteins. In a healthy state, normal RBC rheology ensures efficient oxygen delivery to tissues and organs, contributing to overall physiologic functioning.

II. NUTRITIONAL ANEMIAS

Folate

Folic acid deficiency can arise from multiple causes, including inadequate dietary intake and destruction during cooking. Since folate is absorbed in the jejunum through active and passive transport mechanisms across the intestinal wall, diseases such as celiac disease, tropical sprue, short bowel syndrome, amyloidosis, gastric bypass, or mesenteric vascular insufficiency can hinder folate absorption, leading to deficiency. Elevated pH levels, as seen in achlorhydria, can also impair folate absorption. Medications such as methotrexate, phenytoin, sulfasalazine, and trimethoprim can antagonize folate utilization, inhibit its absorption, or hinder its conversion to its active form, resulting in folate deficiency. Congenital deficiencies of enzymes required in folate metabolism can also lead to folate deficiency. Folic acid deficiency may occur after vitamin B12 deficiency due to an impairment of methionine synthase, resulting in the trapping of folate as methyltetrahydrofolate. This leads to the accumulation of methylene tetrahydrofolic acid (THFA) in serum, known as the folate trap phenomenon, and increased urinary excretion of folate. Alcoholism is a significant cause of folate deficiency. Pregnancy, hemolytic anemia, and dialysis can also result in folate deficiency.

Patients being evaluated for folic acid deficiency should also be assessed for vitamin B12 deficiency, as both conditions can lead to macrocytic anemia, characterized by an increased mean corpuscular volume (MCV) exceeding 100 fL. This finding is consistent with a diagnosis of macrocytic anemia. Additionally, a peripheral smear would reveal macrocytic RBCs, megaloblasts, and hypersegmented neutrophils.

Initial laboratory tests should include a complete blood count (CBC) and a peripheral smear (PS). Laboratory tests in folic acid deficiency would reveal anemia, manifested as a decrease in hemoglobin and hematocrit levels. The initial test for diagnosing folate deficiency is the presence of low serum or plasma folate levels (<3 ng/mL). Although increased homocysteine levels often precede low plasma folate levels, they are less specific indicators. Another useful indicator for identifying folate deficiency is red cell folate, which remains relatively unaffected by sudden changes in folate intake since it reflects folate status over the life span of RBCs. Testing serum vitamin B12 and folate levels can help differentiate between the two deficiencies.

Differential diagnosis: Vitamin B12 deficiency, alcoholic liver disease, hypothyroidism, and aplastic anemia

Key points and diagnostic caveats: Folic acid supplementation, typically 1 to 5 mg/d orally, is usually sufficient to correct anemia. Parenteral preparations (5 mg/mL) of folate should be used in patients with malabsorption. Treatment of tropical sprue typically involves folate supplementation along with antibiotics and additional doses of vitamin B12 as indicated.

Vitamin B12

Symptoms generally develop in severely anemic patients. The main symptoms include weakness, heart palpitations, fatigue, lightheadedness, and shortness of breath, caused by a low hematocrit. Jaundice may occur due to intramedullary and extravascular hemolysis. Leukopenia or thrombocytopenia are generally present but do not typically cause significant clinical concerns. Neurologic symptoms and autonomic gastrointestinal disturbances are also often associated with vitamin B12 deficiency. Neurologic symptoms include symmetric paresthesia, numbness, and impaired vibratory and positional sense, leading to gait disturbances. Approximately 10% of patients with vitamin B12-deficiency show hyperpigmentation, and some patients with pernicious anemia may have associated autoimmune vitiligo. Cerebral manifestations such as mental confusion, paranoia, dementia, and psychosis can also occur in B12 deficiency. Other rarely encountered symptoms of vitamin B12 deficiency include generalized malabsorption caused by intestinal megaloblastosis, infertility, glossitis, and cerebral venous thrombosis. Severe B12 deficiency can lead to a greater risk of thrombosis due to hyperhomocysteinemia.

Megaloblastic anemia is suspected based on clinical features. A blood smear examination reveals anisocytosis, poikilocytosis, hypersegmented neutrophils, and schistocytes. The CBC and examination of the peripheral blood smear show anemia along with increased MCV and mean corpuscular hemoglobin. Additional tests may show low haptoglobin and elevated bilirubin and lactate dehydrogenase levels due to hemolysis. In cases of functional vitamin B12 deficiency, plasma or serum levels of vitamin B12 are elevated, along with folate, red cell folate, homocysteine, methylmalonic acid, and intrinsic factor antibodies.

Differential diagnosis: Acute leukemia, myelodysplastic syndrome (MDS), and folate deficiency

Copper

Copper is an essential nutrient for humans and plays a vital role in cellular transport and hemoglobin synthesis. Most adults obtain adequate copper levels through food consumption. The recommended daily intake ranges from 2 to 3 mg. Multiple factors, including hereditary or acquired deficiencies, contribute to clinically observed copper deficiency. The epidemiology of copper deficiency depends on its underlying causes, and the incidence of comprehensive disease is quite low.

Copper is required for nervous system development and function. Clinical features can mimic subacute combined degeneration, spastic paresthesia, optic neuropathy, and central nervous system demyelination.

Anemia can present as microcytic, normocytic, or macrocytic, with neutropenia being relatively rare. Bone marrow findings may resemble myelodysplasia, and for this reason, testing for serum copper is indicated in patients with a clinical suspicion of a myelodysplastic syndrome. Cytoplasmic vacuolization can be observed in erythroid and myeloid precursors.

Serum copper, serum ceruloplasmin, 24-hour urine copper, and zinc levels should be checked if copper toxicity is suspected. Cytogenetic studies can help rule out a myelodysplastic syndrome, and testing for anti-tissue transglutaminase antibodies and anti-endomysial antibodies can help identify celiac disease.

Differential diagnosis: Myelodysplastic syndrome (MDS) and zinc toxicity

Iron

Iron deficiency anemia (IDA) is the most common micronutrient deficiency and the most common cause of anemia worldwide. It is most frequently seen in women of reproductive age, pregnant women, and premature infants. In developing countries, nearly 50% of all anemia cases are due to IDA. The primary causes of iron deficiency anemia are inadequate dietary intake, blood loss, and infection.

Symptoms suggestive of anemia include fatigue, headache, paresthesia, and a burning sensation, often preceded by depletion of iron stores. There is a poor correlation between the severity of symptoms and blood levels, suggesting that some symptoms may be caused by a deficiency of iron-containing enzymes. Pica may be an early clinical indicator.

Bone marrow examination is not generally indicated, but may be performed in ambiguous cases or to exclude malignancy. Examinations reveal mild to moderate hypercellularity with a predominance of erythrocytes. Storage iron in the bone marrow aspirate, demonstrated by Prussian blue stain, by definition is absent. In most cases, examination shows anisocytosis, elevated red cell distribution width (RDW), decreased MCV, microcytic and hypochromic RBCs, and the presence of target cells.

Tests to aid in identifying IDA include CBC, total iron-binding capacity (TIBC), MCV, mean corpuscular hemoglobin concentration (MCHC), RDW, ferritin, hepcidin, iron levels, iron saturation, erythrocyte protoporphyrin, and bone marrow iron stain. Serum iron and ferritin levels are low, and serum transferrin or total iron-binding capacity is elevated. The concentration of erythrocyte protoporphyrin is increased. Serum ferritin is invariably low in IDA but can be elevated in anemia of chronic disease, sideroblastic anemia, and thalassemia. A serum ferritin level below 12 µg/L is virtually diagnostic of iron deficiency.

Differential diagnosis: Anemia of chronic disease, sideroblastic anemia, thalassemia, lead poisoning

III. RED BLOOD CELL ENZYME DEFICIENCY

Glucose-6-Phosphate Dehydrogenase

Glucose-6-phosphate dehydrogenase (G6PD) deficiency, the first identified red cell enzymopathy, is a polymorphic genetic trait with a worldwide distribution. It affects over 500 million people, but the prevalence varies greatly, ranging from absent in Amerindian populations to over 20% in parts of Africa and Asia.

G6PD is an oxidoreductase enzyme that catalyzes the conversion of glucose-6-phosphate to 6-phosphoglucono-lactone while reducing nicotinamide adenine dinucleotide phosphate (NADP) to its reduced form (NADPH). NADPH serves as a reducing agent in defense against oxidative stress. G6PD activity naturally decreases as red cells age, since mature red cells lack protein synthesis. Reticulocytes have higher G6PD activity, while older red cells retain only about one-tenth of the original activity.

The most common trigger for hemolysis in individuals with G6PD-deficiency is the consumption of fava beans. Additionally, various drugs such as dapsone, primaquine, chloroquine, quinidine, quinine, sulfonamide drugs, and fluoroquinolones can induce hemolysis. Severe bacterial infections including pneumonia, brucellosis, rickettsiosis, and maxillary abscesses caused by *Streptococcus* or *Staphylococcus*, as well as infections like *Clostridium difficile*, hepatitis (A, B, and E), cytomegalovirus, and dengue fever, can trigger acute hemolytic anemia (AHA) in individuals with G6PD deficiency. AHA triggered by an infection can be severe, and its resolution upon controlling the infection helps confirm the role of infection as the trigger.

Clinical features of G6PD deficiency include pallor, jaundice, abdominal pain, and sometimes fever. Supravital staining with methyl violet can reveal the presence of Heinz bodies. Other common findings include neutrophil leukocytosis, decreased platelet count, elevated unconjugated bilirubin and lactate dehydrogenase levels, and low or undetectable haptoglobin levels. Examination of the peripheral blood smear may show microspherocytes, eccentrocytes or "bite" cells, and "blister cells" where hemoglobin accumulates to one side.

Pyruvate Kinase Deficiency

Pyruvate kinase deficiency (PKD) is the most common glycolytic enzyme defect causing red cell hemolysis and is associated with hereditary nonspherocytic anemia. PKD is an autosomal recessive disorder caused by mutations in the *PK-LR* (pyruvate kinase-liver and red cell) gene. Individuals may be homozygous or compound heterozygous for different PK-LR mutations. The population prevalence of PK deficiency among Caucasians is approximately 50 cases per 1 million. PK is one of the key enzymes involved in adenosine triphosphate (ATP) generation in RBCs. Impaired ATP production is the central pathophysiologic abnormality in PK deficiency. PK converts phosphoenolpyruvate to pyruvate, accounting for 50% of RBC ATP production. PK also modulates nicotinamide adenine dinucleotide (NADH) production for methemoglobin reduction and leads to the accumulation of 2,3-diphosphoglycerate (2,3-DPG), resulting in a rightward shift in the hemoglobin-oxygen dissociation curve. Reticulocytosis is often observed and may be more pronounced after splenectomy. Spheroacanthocytes are characteristic but not specific to PKD. In vitro studies suggest that PK deficiency provides protection against *Plasmodium falciparum* infection and replication in human RBCs, potentially due to reduced ATP levels. PK deficiency has also been shown to be protective in a mouse model of *Plasmodium* infection.

Clinical signs and symptoms of PKD include chronic hemolytic anemia, splenomegaly, jaundice, gallstones, increased reticulocytes, indirect hyperbilirubinemia, mild hyperferritinemia, hemochromatosis, pulmonary hypertension, endocrinopathy, extramedullary hematopoiesis, bone fractures, skin ulcers, poor growth, easy fatigability, and jaundice. PK enzymatic activity is usually determined through spectrophotometric assays using RBC lysates. PKD should be confirmed through PK-LR genotyping, as reticulocytosis or transfusion can sometimes lead to falsely normal PK levels in affected patients.

IV. CELL MEMBRANE DISORDERS

Red cell membrane disorders are inherited conditions caused by mutations in various membrane or cytoskeletal proteins. These mutations result in decreased red cell deformability, reduced life span, and premature removal of erythrocytes from circulation. Examples of red cell membrane disorders include hereditary spherocytosis, hereditary elliptocytosis, hereditary ovalocytosis, and hereditary stomatocytosis. To diagnose these disorders, a fundamental step is examining a blood film, which provides important information about RBC morphologic changes. The suggested initial screening for red cell membrane defects includes osmotic fragility tests and an eosin-5-maleimide (EMA)-binding panel.

Hereditary Spherocytosis

Hereditary spherocytosis is the most common congenital hemolytic anemia in Caucasians, with an estimated prevalence ranging from 1:2,000 to 1:5,000. Approximately 75% of cases follow an autosomal dominant pattern of inheritance, while the remainder consists of recessive forms and de novo mutations. The molecular defect is highly heterogeneous, involving genes encoding spectrin, ankyrin, band 3, and protein 4.2.

Clinical features of hereditary spherocytosis include hemolytic anemia, which can vary from compensated to severe, sometimes necessitating exchange transfusion at birth and/or repeated blood transfusions. Other features may include variable jaundice, splenomegaly, and cholelithiasis.

Defective protein detection can be accomplished through sodium dodecyl sulfate-polyacrylamide gel electrophoresis (SDS-PAGE), the NaCl osmotic fragility test on fresh and incubated blood, the standard glycerol lysis test, the acidified glycerol lysis test (AGLT), and the pink test. Sensitivities may vary.

Hereditary Elliptocytosis

Hereditary elliptocytosis is an autosomal dominant disorder characterized by the presence of elliptically shaped red cells on a peripheral blood smear. It is most prevalent in malaria-endemic regions of West Africa, in which approximately 2% of the population is affected. The condition is caused by so-called weakened horizontal linkages in the membrane skeleton, resulting from a defective spectrin dimer-dimer interaction or a defective spectrin-actin-protein 4.1R junctional complex.

Most individuals with hereditary elliptocytosis are asymptomatic, but approximately 10% exhibit moderate to severe anemia, with rare cases including hydrops fetalis and the severe variant known as hereditary pyropoikilocytosis. The latter is characterized by significant membrane fragmentation and reduced membrane surface area.

Splenectomy can reduce the severity of anemia by increasing the circulatory life span of fragmented red cells. However, very few patients with hereditary elliptocytosis require surgery.

Hereditary Stomatocytosis

Hereditary stomatocytosis is an autosomal dominant disorder characterized by decreased intracellular potassium content, loss of intracellular water, increased cytoplasmic viscosity, and an increased mean cell hemoglobin concentration. Molecular analysis has identified two mutations associated with overhydrated hereditary stomatocytosis in *RHAG*, resulting in the Ile61Arg and Ser65Phe variants. These mutations are dominantly inherited and lead to widening of the membrane pore and passage of cations. The genetic basis of dehydrated hereditary stomatocytosis remains unknown, but linkage analysis suggests segregation with chromosome 16q23-q24.

Stomatocytes with increased sphericity are sequestered by the spleen. However, while splenectomy is highly beneficial in managing patients with hereditary spherocytosis and hereditary elliptocytosis, it is contraindicated in overhydrated hereditary stomatocytosis due to an increased risk of venous thromboembolic complications.

Ovalocytosis

Ovalocytosis is an autosomal dominant disease characterized by the presence of oval-shaped RBCs with one or two transverse ridges or a longitudinal slit on a blood smear. It is particularly common in Southeast Asia, with a prevalence ranging from 5% to 25%.

The condition results from decreased membrane deformability, as assessed by ektacytometry. A genomic deletion of 27 base pairs, encoding amino acids 400 to 408 of the erythrocyte anion exchange protein AE1 (band 3), has been identified in the disease. However, the mechanism leading to a marked increase in membrane rigidity has yet to be established.

V. IMMUNE HEMOLYTIC ANEMIAS

Autoimmune hemolytic anemia (AIHA) is characterized by the destruction of RBCs due to an immune regulatory autoantibody mechanism that abnormally recognizes self RBC surface antigen. AIHA is a common term for several diseases that differ from one another with respect to cause, pathogenesis, and clinical presentation, and the individual disorders should be addressed according to these differences. Table 4.1-1 summarizes the various types of immune hemolytic anemias.

TABLE 4.1-1 Immune Hemolytic Anemias

Type	Clinical Features	Antibody	Immunoglobulin Class	Complement Activation	Type of Hemolysis	Typical Laboratory Findings	Associations
Warm antibody agglutinin	5-10:10^6 Frequently in old individuals	Warm-reactive, panreactive	IgG (polyclonal)	Frequently none; classical (++), terminal (+)	Extravascular (spleen predominantly)	DAT (IgG +) Rare cases IgA, IgM C3d−	50% Secondary process 50% Idiopathic
Cold antibody agglutinin	0.5-2:10^6 Frequently in old individuals. Found in lymphoproliferative bone marrow disorder	IgM	IgM binds C1q on the red cell membrane, activating the classical complement pathway but disassociating from the red cells centrally	Classical (+++), terminal (+), hemolysis is extravascular (in acute intravascular exacerbations)	AIHA and a DAT positive for C3d with/without IgG, with a consistent clinical picture and a high-titer cold reactive antibody (titer ≥ 1:64 at 4 °C). Assessment of the antibodies' thermal amplitude can be useful and is usually ≥30 °C when red cells are suspended in 30% bovine albumin. Serum electrophoresis will usually detect a monoclonal paraprotein, typically IgMκ, but serum must be kept at 37 to 38 °C from the time of sampling until serum is removed from the clot.	Bind red cells in the cooler peripheral circulation, causing agglutination that leads to acrocyanosis or Raynaud disease	Occurs in association with secondary disorders, such as infection, SLE, or aggressive lymphoma

| PCH | IgG | Biphasic IgG antibody that binds to red cells at low temperature and causes complement-mediated lysis as the temperature is increased. | Classical (+++), terminal (+++) | Severe hemolysis; intravascular, typically following an infection | Positive Donath-Landsteiner test. Testing should be considered in patients with AIHA and a DAT positive for C3d with/without IgG (the DAT is sometimes negative) hemoglobinuria, cold-associated symptoms, atypical serological features, or patients younger than 18 years old | Seen in tertiary syphilis, hematologic cancers in adults, and postviral in children |

(continued)

TABLE 4.1-1 Immune Hemolytic Anemias (*continued*)

Type	Clinical Features	Antibody	Immunoglobulin Class	Complement Activation	Type of Hemolysis	Typical Laboratory Findings	Associations
Mixed AIHA		Warm IgG, cold IgM				DAT is usually positive for IgG and C3d. Combination of a warm IgG antibody and a cold IgM antibody	A cold antibody with a thermal amplitude ≥30 °C, and an appropriate clinical picture. Cold-associated symptoms rarely appear, and the cold antibody may have a low antibody titer (eg, <1:64) but with a thermal amplitude up to 30-37 °C.

AIHA, autoimmune hemolytic anemia; DAT, direct antibody test; PCH, paroxysmal cold hemoglobinuria; SLE, systemic lupus erythematosus.

VI. DISORDERS OF HEMOGLOBIN

Hemoglobin disorders encompass a group of genetic diseases affecting hemoglobin. They are categorized into two main groups: thalassemia syndromes ("amount" disorders) and structural hemoglobin variants (abnormal hemoglobins). The primary types of thalassemia are α- and β-thalassemia, while major structural hemoglobin variants include HbS, HbE, and HbC. Each group has various subtypes and combined forms. Clinical manifestations of hemoglobinopathies vary widely, ranging from mild hypochromic anemia to moderate hematologic disorders, and to severe, lifelong transfusion-dependent anemia with multiorgan involvement. Hemoglobinopathies are highly prevalent worldwide, affecting approximately 7% of the global population.

α-Thalassemia

α-Thalassemia presents in two clinically significant forms: hemoglobin Bart hydrops fetalis (Hb Bart) syndrome, caused by the deletion or inactivation of all four α-globin genes ($--/--$), and hemoglobin H (HbH) disease, most commonly resulting from the deletion or inactivation of three α-globin genes ($--/-α$). Deletion or inactivation of two α-globin genes, either in *cis* ($--/αα$, or $-α0$ carrier) or in *trans* ($-α/-α$), leads to an α-thalassemia trait/carrier. α-Thalassemia silent carrier is characterized by the deletion or inactivation of one α-globin gene ($-α/αα$ or α+ carrier).

1. **Hb Bart syndrome** is the most severe form, characterized by prenatal onset of generalized edema, pleural and pericardial effusions, and congestive heart failure due to severe anemia. Extramedullary erythropoiesis, hepatosplenomegaly, and an enlarged placenta are common. Neonatal mortality is typical.

   The diagnosis of Hb Bart syndrome is confirmed through characteristic hematologic and hemoglobin (Hb) findings, as well as molecular genetic testing that identifies pathogenic variants in both *HBA1* and *HBA2* genes, resulting in the deletion or inactivation of all four α-globin genes.

   Treatment for Hb Bart syndrome includes intrauterine blood transfusions, improved transfusion strategies, and, rarely, curative hematopoietic stem cell transplantation.

2. **HbH disease** presents with a broad phenotypic spectrum, with clinical features typically appearing in early childhood. However, in some cases, the disease may remain undiagnosed until adulthood or be asymptomatic. Most individuals experience splenomegaly (and less commonly hepatomegaly), mild jaundice, and thalassemia-like bone changes. Gallstones and acute hemolytic episodes may occur in response to infections or exposure to oxidant drugs.

   HbH disease is diagnosed based on hematologic and Hb findings, as well as molecular genetic testing that identifies pathogenic variants in *HBA1* and *HBA2* resulting in the deletion or inactivation of three α-globin alleles.

   In HbH disease, most individuals remain clinically well and do not require treatment. However, occasional RBC transfusions may be necessary during hemolytic or aplastic crises. Severe anemia affecting cardiac function, severe bone changes, and extramedullary erythropoiesis may require RBC transfusions, although this is rare. Nondeletional HbH disease may have more severe manifestations and be transfusion-dependent.

β-Thalassemia

β-Thalassemia results from reduced or absent production of the β-globin subunit, leading to excess production of α-globin. The severity of β-thalassemia can vary from near-complete absence of β-globin synthesis to partial impairment, resulting in different clinical presentations. More than 200 point mutations have been reported, but the deletion of both genes is rare. β-Thalassemia can be classified into three categories. The presence or absence of β-globin production determines the severity of β-thalassemia (by convention, a "β0" mutation indicates the complete absence of β-globin production and causes the more severe form, while a "β+" mutation indicates some retained function).

1. **β-Thalassemia trait.** Also known as β-thalassemia minor, this disease is characterized by one defective gene resulting in individuals being normal or mildly anemic (β0/β or β+/β). These patients have increased Hb A2 levels, and elevated Hb F may also be present. They are not transfusion-dependent.
2. **β-Thalassemia intermedia.** Individuals have two defective genes, but some β-globin production is still observed (β0/β or β+/β+). Individuals with β-thalassemia intermedia have a less severe clinical course than those with β-thalassemia major. Nonetheless, they may experience significant health problems that require intermittent transfusion.
3. **#-Thalassemia major (Cooley anemia).** Individuals have two defective genes, resulting in almost no β-globin function (β0/β0 or β+/β0). This severe form necessitates lifelong transfusions and may result in a shortened life span. Symptoms typically manifest after 6 months of age due to the persistence of fetal hemoglobin. Patients have elevated Hb A2 and Hb F levels, although Hb F may be normal in some cases. In β-thalassemia major, excess α-globin chains precipitate, causing hemolytic anemia. These patients require lifelong transfusions and chelation therapy to manage iron overload.

Clinical characteristics of β-thalassemia include reduced synthesis of the β-hemoglobin chain, resulting in microcytic hypochromic anemia, abnormal peripheral blood smear with nucleated RBCs, and decreased amounts of hemoglobin A (HbA) on hemoglobin analysis. Thalassemia major usually becomes apparent within the first 2 years of life, presenting with severe anemia and hepatosplenomegaly. Without treatment, affected children experience failure to thrive and have a shortened life expectancy. Regular transfusions and chelation therapy help achieve normal growth and development and improve overall prognosis. Thalassemia intermedia presents later and features milder anemia that does not require regular transfusions; however, individuals are at risk of iron overload due to increased intestinal iron absorption resulting from ineffective erythropoiesis.

The diagnosis of β-thalassemia is based on RBC indices revealing microcytic hypochromic anemia, presence of nucleated RBCs on peripheral blood smear, decreased HbA levels, and increased hemoglobin F (HbF) after 12 months of age, elevated hemoglobin A2, and the clinical severity of anemia. Molecular genetic testing can identify biallelic pathogenic variants in the *HBB* gene, which encodes the β-hemoglobin subunit, and may be useful for diagnosis in at-risk individuals under 12 months of age with a positive or suggestive newborn screening result, unexplained microcytic hypochromic anemia, anisopoikilocytosis, and nucleated RBCs on peripheral blood smear. Molecular diagnosis is generally not indicated for the diagnosis of β-thalassemia trait, since presumptive diagnosis can be made on the basis of CBC and hemoglobin electrophoresis.

Sickle Cell Disease (HbSS and HbSC Disease)

Around 70,000 to 100,000 Americans have sickle cell disease (SCD), the most common form of an inherited blood disorder. SCD is a generalized term for a group of autosomal recessive inherited RBC disorders characterized by a point mutation in the β-globin gene, predominantly the presence of hemoglobin S. This defect is present in affected individuals at birth. Common examples of SCD include sickle cell anemia (homozygous Hgb SS), sickle β-thalassemia syndromes (Hgb S-β+ or S-β0), and Hgb

SC disease. Many additional compound sickle cell syndromes have been described in which hemoglobin S is inherited in combination with a range of other globin gene mutations. In sickle cell disease, the hemoglobin is abnormal, causing the RBCs to be rigid and shaped like a "C" or sickle, the shape from which the disease takes its name.

The majority of the complications of sickle cell disease are due to vaso-occlusion, with the sickled cells blocking blood flow to specific organs leading to ischemic events. Other complications are associated with chronic hemolytic anemia. Clinical manifestation include acute and chronic conditions and are typically based on the degree of anemia, genotype, and use of disease-modifying therapies. Some major complications include stroke, acute chest syndrome, organ damage, other disabilities, and in some cases premature death. Chronic conditions are characterized by persistent end-organ damage and include silent cerebral infarcts, pulmonary hypertension, cardiomyopathy, avascular necrosis of bones, renal disease, and retinopathy. It is noteworthy that complications to therapy can cause significant morbidity in relation to chronic transfusion, iron chelation therapy, effects of opioid medications, and toxic effects of hydroxyurea.

SCD is identified through laboratory testing alone. There are no findings on physical examination that suggest the presence or absence of SCD. Neonatal screening resulting in timely definitive diagnosis and appropriate comprehensive care has been shown to reduce the morbidity and mortality of SCD in early childhood. In the United States, all states provide universal screening for newborns. In addition, the American College of Obstetrics and Gynecology recommends hemoglobin testing of all pregnant Black women. When a screening test indicates SCD, a definitive diagnosis is established through further blood testing. The peripheral smear is normal in sickle cell trait (Hgb AS), but sickle cells are seen in each of the major SCD syndromes (Table 4.1-2). Solubility testing is abnormal in all syndromes having at least one sickle cell gene and thus detects all carriers of the *Hgb S* gene as well as those with the SS phenotype. Hgb electrophoresis can provide the clinician with the exact phenotype of SCD. When unclear, RBC genotyping may be utilized to clarify ambiguous hemoglobin states.

TABLE 4.1-2 Hematologic Findings in Sickle Cell Disease and Common Variants

Morphology	Hemoglobin Electrophoresis (%)				Hematologic Parameters		
	S	F	A2	A	Hb (g/dL)	MCV	Smear Findings
SS	>90	<10	<3.5	0	6-8	>80	Sickle cell, target cells
SC	50	<5	a[a]	0	10-15	75-95	Sickle cell, target cells, RBC crystals, poikilocytosis
AS	40-45	<5	>3.5	55-60	12-15	>80	Normal
S-B0	>80	<20	>3.5	0	6-10	<80	Sickle cells, target cells
S-B+	>60	<20	>3.5	10-30	9-12	<80	Target cells, no sickle cells

Hb, hemoglobin; MCV, mean corpuscular volume, RBC, red blood cell.
[a]50% Hb C.

SUGGESTED READINGS

ACOG Committee on Obstetrics. ACOG Practice Bulletin No. 78: hemoglobinopathies in pregnancy. *Obstet Gynecol*. 2007;109(1):229-237. doi:10.1097/00006250-200701000-00055

Bender DA. Megaloblastic anaemia in vitamin B12 deficiency. *Br J Nutr*. 2003;89(4):439-441. doi:10.1079/BJN2002828

Camaschella C. Iron deficiency (published correction appears in *Blood*. 2023;141(6):682). *Blood*. 2019;133(1):30-39. doi:10.1182/blood-2018-05-815944

Cappellini MD, Musallam KM, Taher AT. Iron deficiency anaemia revisited. *J Intern Med*. 2020;287(2):153-170. doi:10.1111/joim.13004

Close A, Malec LM. Copper deficiency. *Blood*. 2017;130(suppl 1):4742. doi:10.1182/blood.V130.Suppl_1.4742.4742

Green R, Datta Mitra A. Megaloblastic anemias: nutritional and other causes. *Med Clin North Am*. 2017;101(2):297-317. doi:10.1016/j.mcna.2016.09.013

4.2: White Blood Cell Disorders

Imran A. Nizamuddin and John L. Frater

This chapter will focus on nonneoplastic disorders of white blood cells (WBCs) in the peripheral blood, primarily those affecting neutrophils and lymphocytes. These disorders include both inherited and acquired conditions contributing to leukopenia, leukocytosis, or qualitative WBC defects.

I. NEUTROPHILS

The neutrophil is the most abundant type of WBC, making up 40% to 70% of all WBCs in humans. A normal neutrophil typically has a multilobulated nuclear shape with three to five segments, with the separate lobes connected by chromatin. The cytoplasm contains numerous granules with contents containing antimicrobial properties.

Neutrophil disorders can be separated from each other based on abnormalities in neutrophil number or function. These abnormalities commonly present with recurrent and severe bacterial and fungal infections, often involving the skin, respiratory tract, and deep tissue sites.

Disorders of Neutrophil Number

Neutrophilia, or an increased neutrophil count, is typically defined as an absolute neutrophil count (ANC) greater than 7.5×10^9/L, while neutropenia, or a decreased neutrophil count, is typically defined as ANC less than 1.5×10^9/L. While neutrophilia typically arises as a consequence of underlying inflammatory disease without any significant consequences, neutropenia can have more severe consequences due to an increased risk of infection. This risk is more profound with severe neutropenia (ANC $< 0.5 \times 10^9$/L).

Neutrophilia

Neutrophilia typically arises as a consequence of inflammation, infection (typically bacterial), tissue necrosis (eg, burns, shock, or trauma), neoplasm, autoimmune disease, drugs/toxins (eg, epinephrine, glucocorticoids, or lithium), asplenia, endocrinopathies, or other underlying conditions. Common findings of neutrophilia include a "left shift" (an increase in the proportion of less differentiated neutrophils and band forms) and toxic granulation. The increased number of neutrophils in the peripheral blood may originate from multiple sources, including increased cell production, accelerated release from bone marrow reserves, demargination of neutrophils from the marginal pool, or decreased spread into the tissue pool (*Trends Immunol.* 2010;31(8):318-324). An exaggerated neutrophilia with an ANC greater than 50×10^9/L is often referred to as a "leukemoid reaction," given that the degree of elevation mimics that of clonal neoplastic disorders such as leukemia (*Int J Lab Hematol.* 2020;42(2):134-139).

In certain cases, patients may have chronic idiopathic neutrophilia (CIN), which refers to an elevation in neutrophil count persisting for months or years without a clear underlying cause or symptoms (*Blood Rev.* 2021;46:100739). Care must be taken to identify any potential causes of neutrophilia that would exclude true CIN. For instance, studies have documented associations of obesity (*Eur J Haematol.* 2006;76(6):516) and smoking (*Eur Heart J.* 2003;24(14):1365) with neutrophilia.

While neutrophilia is typically acquired, rarely patients may have congenital abnormalities leading to this finding.

Neutropenia

Neutropenia may be secondary to disorders of production, distribution, or turnover. Some conditions, such as systemic lupus erythematosus, may induce neutropenia by multiple mechanisms. Congenital neutropenia is typically secondary to bone marrow failure syndromes and will be discussed in a later chapter. Acquired neutropenia can be due to a variety of causes, including infection (typically viral), nutritional deficiencies, autoimmune disorders, medications, and malignancy.

Immune-mediated neutropenia

The major clinicopathologic findings of immune-mediated neutropenias are summarized in Table 4.2-1. In all cases of immune-mediated neutropenias, the detection of antibodies in the serum is not used for diagnosis or management (*Immunohematology.* 2010;26(1):11). Although laboratory tests are available for the detection of antineutrophil antibodies (eg, agglutination, immunofluorescence assays, direct and indirect antiglobulin assays), they lack sensitivity and specificity (*J Pediatr Hematol Oncol.* 2020;42(2):107).

Drug-induced neutropenia

The major clinicopathologic findings of drug-induced neutropenia are summarized in Table 4.2-1. Both immune-mediated and nonimmune-mediated mechanisms (such as direct damage to myeloid precursors) have been described (*Am J Hematol.* 2009;84(7):428-434). The culprit agent should be withdrawn.

Other causes of neutropenia

In contrast to most causes of acquired neutropenia, nutritional deficiency–related neutropenia may demonstrate abnormal morphology in the bone marrow. For example, copper deficiency is characterized by the presence of ring sideroblasts and cytoplasmic vacuoles in myeloid and erythroid precursors in the bone marrow. Bone marrow aspirate can mimic myelodysplastic syndrome (*Am J Clin Pathol.* 1992;97(5):665-668). Copper deficiency can lead to both anemia and neutropenia, as well as neurologic deficits (including neuropathy, ataxia, and muscle weakness). It may develop in the

TABLE 4.2-1 Major Causes of Neutropenia

Name	Frequency	At-Risk Populations	Mechanism	Other Features	Morphologic Findings
Immune-mediated (primary)	Common	Most common cause of neutropenia in infants/children	Antineutrophil antibodies; HNA-1 (HNA-1a or HNA-1b) or HNA-4	Spontaneous remission in ~90% of cases; BM bx not usually indicated	Normocellular/hypercellular BM with decreased mature PMNs
Immune-mediated (secondary)	Common	Autoimmune disorders (RA, SLE); adults	Antineutrophil antibodies	Target antigen unknown in most cases; often accompanied by other cytopenias; BM bx not usually indicated	Normocellular/hypercellular BM with decreased mature PMNs
Alloimmune	Rare (<0.1% of births)	Newborns	Transplacental passage of maternal IgG antibodies binding to paternally inherited infant neutrophil-specific antigens	Sepsis; patients may be asymptomatic	Normocellular BM with normal PMN maturation
Drug-induced	Common	Adults	(a) Dose-related (chemotherapy, radiation therapy); (b) idiosyncratic (1-2 wk after exposure)	Most common drugs: antithyroid drugs, sulfasalazine, and trimethoprim-sulfamethoxazole	BM bx not usually performed
Nutritional	Common	All ages	Nutrient deficiencies (Cu, B12, folate)	Insufficient dietary intake; malabsorption in the setting of surgery, gastrointestinal disease, or medications; increased requirements	BM bx not usually performed
Duffy-null	Rare	African and Mediterranean ethnic populations	Unknown	Normal granulocyte preserves	BM bx not usually performed

BM, bone marrow; bx, biopsy; Cu, copper; PMNs, polymorphonuclear neutrophils; RA, rheumatoid arthritis; SLE, systemic lupus erythematosus; wk, weeks.

setting of malabsorption, total parenteral nutrition, or zinc supplementation (*Ann Hematol.* 2018;97(9):1527-1534).

Folate or vitamin B12 deficiency are both causes of megaloblastic anemia, a subtype of macrocytic anemia in setting of ineffective DNA synthesis. Severe cases of megaloblastic anemia may also lead to pancytopenia, including neutropenia. Causes of folate and vitamin B12 deficiency include insufficient dietary intake; malabsorption in the setting of surgery, gastrointestinal disease, or medications; increased requirements; among other causes (*Cleve Clin J Med.* 2020;87(3):153-164). Peripheral smear may demonstrate macro-ovalocytes as well as the presence of hypersegmented neutrophils. Bone marrow examination is not typically indicated but classic "megaloblastic changes" are demonstrated. Namely, the bone marrow is markedly hypercellular with erythroid hyperplasia and a reversal of the myeloid:erythroid ratio. Hallmark changes of nuclear-cytoplasmic dyssynchrony (failure of nuclear maturation with open chromatin in the setting of normal mature cytoplasm) are seen in erythroblasts and other erythroid precursors. Other features of dyserythropoiesis may also be seen. Myeloid lineages may demonstrate myeloid hyperplasia with giant band forms and hypersegmentation of neutrophils (*Postgrad Med.* 1978;64(4):117-122). Because the peripheral cytopenias and cytomorphologic changes of nutritional deficiency-related neutropenia may mimic myelodysplastic syndrome (MDS), evaluation of serum vitamin B12, folate, and copper levels is typically assessed in patients with suspected MDS.

Clinicians should be aware that individuals of certain ancestries (African, Mediterranean, among others) may have lower neutrophil counts without clinical significance. These individuals have normal granulopoiesis and marrow reserves and do not have an increased risk of infection. While this finding was previously referred to as "benign ethnic neutropenia," the terminology has evolved, and it is increasingly being referred to as "Duffy-null antigen count" (*Blood.* 2021;137(1):13). Recent research has shown a strong association between low neutrophil counts in these patients and single-nucleotide polymorphism in the *ACKR1* gene, leading to a loss of expression of Duffy antigens on red blood cells (*PLoS Genet.* 2009;5(1):e1000360). The presence of this finding and the pathophysiology underlying low neutrophil count remain unknown and are active areas of investigation.

Disorders of Neutrophil Function

There are numerous mechanisms that can lead to neutrophil dysfunction given the numerous steps involved in the neutrophil recruitment cascade, including chemotaxis, tethering to the endothelium, rolling, activation, adhesion, crawling, and transendothelial migration with recruitment to the site of inflammation (*Blood.* 2022;139(14):2130-2144). There may be defects in neutrophil function based on abnormal motility or granule function. Furthermore, deficiencies in complement proteins or immunoglobulins may impair neutrophil function, as these components play an important role in opsonization leading to neutrophil-mediated phagocytosis. The major features of disorders of neutrophil function are summarized in Table 4.2-2.

II. LYMPHOCYTES

Disorders of Lymphocyte Number

Abnormalities in lymphocyte number can be detected by a complete blood count and differential, along with a review of the peripheral blood smear. Lymphocytosis is

TABLE 4.2-2 Disorders of Neutrophil Function

Name	Inheritance	Impairment	Gene(s) Affected	Clinical Features	Other Findings
Chédiak-Higashi syndrome	AR	Degranulation	CHS1	Recurrent bacterial infections, oculocutaneous albinism, progressive neurologic abnormalities, bleeding disorder	Large peroxidase-positive cytoplasmic granules in neutrophils
Neutrophil-specific granule deficiency	AR	Granule synthesis	CEBPE and SMARCD2	Pyogenic infections of the skin and other deeper tissues	Granulocytes lack specific granules
Leukocyte adhesion deficiency type 1	AR	Adhesion	ITGB2	Neutrophilia, recurrent bacterial infections delayed separation of the umbilical cord, and periodontitis	Inflammatory infiltrates lacking neutrophils; decreased CD18 expression
Leukocyte adhesion deficiency type 2	AR	Adhesion	SLC35C1	Intellectual disabilities and growth impairment	Inflammatory infiltrates lacking neutrophils; absent CD15a
Leukocyte adhesion deficiency type 3	AR	Adhesion	FERMT3	Severe infections, marked leukocytosis, and a Glanzmann-like bleeding diathesis	Inflammatory infiltrates lacking neutrophils
Chronic granulomatous disease	AR/XL	Respiratory burst	CYBA, CYBB, NCF1, NCF2, NCF4	Recurrent life-threatening bacterial or fungal infections from a young age	Granulomatous lesions in multiple sites

AR, autosomal recessive; XL, X-linked.

typically defined as an absolute lymphocyte count (ALC) greater than 4.0×10^9/L, while lymphocytopenia is defined as an ALC less than 1.0×10^9/L; nevertheless, note that the normal range may vary based on age and laboratory.

Lymphocytosis

Lymphocytosis can be categorized into primary or secondary causes. Primary lymphocytosis refers to conditions in which the increased number of lymphocytes is secondary to an intrinsic defect in the expanded lymphocyte population. These conditions, referred to as lymphoproliferative disorders, are considered monoclonal, as they are characterized by an abnormal clonal expansion of a lymphoid population due to the acquisition of somatic mutations. Clonal proliferation may arise from monoclonal B cells, T cells, natural killer (NK) cells, or less differentiated cells of lymphoid lineage. Immunophenotyping, typically using flow cytometry (FC), is essential for identifying the expression of cell surface markers that can allow for assessment of clonality. Secondary, or reactive, lymphocytosis refers to conditions in which the increased number of lymphocytes is secondary to another disease process, such as infection, toxin exposure, or inflammation.

Primary lymphocytosis

Several T-cell and B-cell neoplasms may present with lymphocytosis. These disorders are discussed in the chapters covering lymphoid malignancies.

Secondary (reactive) lymphocytosis

The most common cause of secondary lymphocytosis is viral infection, specifically infectious mononucleosis (IM). IM is most often caused by the Epstein-Barr virus (EBV), although other viruses may also cause the disease (*Am J Med Sci*. 1978;276(3):325). Infected patients may present with fevers, fatigue, malaise, tender lymphadenopathy, sore throat, and splenomegaly. EBV infects and replicates in B cells, which induces a host immune response involving polyclonal proliferation of $CD8^+$ cytotoxic T cells and $CD16^+$/$CD56^+$ NK cells (*J Infect Dis*. 2013;207(1):80-88). Lymphocytosis is the most common hematologic manifestation, characterized by polyclonal expansion of atypical lymphocytes in response to EBV-infected B cells (*J Immunol*. 1987;139(11):3802). These atypical "reactive lymphocytes" can be seen on a peripheral blood smear. IM is typically diagnosed clinically, although the heterophile antibody test or serologic testing for antibodies against viral antigens (anti-VCA, anti-EA, anti-EBNA) can be used to confirm the diagnosis (*J Infect Dis*. 1975;132(5):546; *Clin Diagn Lab Immunol*. 2000;7(3):451).

Of note, other viral infections may also lead to lymphocytosis, which can persist for several weeks. Bacterial infection with *Bordetella pertussis* is also known to cause significant lymphocytosis, especially in children (*Pediatrics*. 1997;100(6):E10). Pertussis primarily affects the respiratory tract and causes a disease characterized by paroxysms of severe coughing. Lymphocytosis is mediated by the presence of pertussis toxin, which prevents lymphocytes from trafficking from blood to lymphoid tissues (*Infect Immun*. 1984;46(3):733-739; *Respirology*. 2003;8(2):157-162). Peripheral blood smear examination reveals classic findings of mature lymphocytes with scant cytoplasm, condensed chromatin, and clefted nuclei (*Blood*. 2013;122(25):4012).

Transient lymphocytosis, as a physiologic reaction to severe stress, is commonly seen. It is mediated by the redistribution of lymphocytes and affects all lymphocyte subtypes (*Am J Clin Pathol*. 2002;117(5):819-825). It is typically associated with medical emergencies, including cardiac conditions, status epilepticus, or trauma (*Arch Pathol Lab Med*. 1987;111(8):712).

Drugs are an important cause of lymphocytosis, whether mediated by the drug itself or a systemic reaction. Bruton tyrosine kinase (BTK) inhibitors, such as ibrutinib, are associated with transient lymphocytosis (typically peaking within 24-48 hours) due to the release of previously activated cells from lymph nodes (*Leukemia.* 2014;28(11):2188-2196). Prolonged lymphocytosis is thought to represent the persistence of a quiescent clone and does not have prognostic impact for chronic lymphoid leukemia (*Blood.* 2014;123(12):1810-1817). Interestingly, dasatinib, another BTK inhibitor, also promotes lymphocytosis by an unrelated mechanism, possibly related to splenic contraction (*Blood Adv.* 2022;bloodadvances.2022009279). In patients with chronic myeloid leukemia being treated with dasatinib, clonal expansions of large granular lymphocytes are often seen, but are of unclear significance (*Blood.* 2010;116(5):772-782). Drug hypersensitivity reactions can also lead to lymphocytosis. For example, drug reaction with eosinophilia and systemic symptoms (DRESS) is a well-known yet rare severe adverse drug reaction characterized by an extensive skin rash, visceral organ involvement, and lymphadenopathy (*Br J Dermatol.* 2013;169(5):1071). While the classic hematologic manifestation of DRESS is significant eosinophilia, it may also lead to atypical lymphocytosis due to expansion of both $CD4^+$ and $CD8^+$ T lymphocytes, which stimulate the inflammatory response (*J Dermatol Sci.* 2012;65(3):213).

Lymphopenia

Lymphopenia may be due to either inherited or acquired causes. Inherited causes of lymphopenia are predominantly associated with inherited immunodeficiency disorders resulting in ineffective lymphopoiesis. Examples include severe congenital immunodeficiency disease, common variable immunodeficiency disease, Wiskott-Aldrich syndrome, ataxia-telangiectasia, and other conditions (*Hematology.* 2018;682-690). These conditions classically present in childhood with recurrent infections. FC may be used to identify whether the total number of circulating lymphocytes or a particular subset is decreased, as this may be characteristic of specific disorders.

Acquired lymphopenia is more common and is typically reactive in the setting of infection, systemic diseases, medications, or acute stress. In one study of hospitalized patients with ALC less than 0.6×10^9/L, the most common causes of lymphopenia, in descending order of frequency, were bacterial/fungal sepsis, postoperative state, corticosteroid therapy, malignancy, cytotoxic therapy and/or radiotherapy, trauma or hemorrhage, transplants, viral infections, and human immunodeficiency virus (HIV) infection (*Aust N Z J Med.* 1997;27(2):170-174). There are no defining characteristics on peripheral blood smear examination to differentiate between these causes.

Lymphopenia can contribute to both humoral and cell-mediated immune responses. A Danish population-based study found that lymphocytopenia was associated with an increased risk of hospitalization for infection, as well as an increased risk of infection-related death (*PLoS Med.* 2018;15(11):e1002685).

Infectious causes

While many viral infections lead to lymphocytosis, lymphopenia has also been observed with certain infections. This is classically seen in the setting of HIV infection, related to direct viral attack on $CD4^+$ lymphocytes, chronic immune activation, or apoptosis (*Front Immunol.* 2017;8:580). Lymphopenia is a well-known complication of infections caused by the *Coronaviridae* family, although the underlying mechanism is not entirely clear. This was first demonstrated in patients with severe acute respiratory syndrome caused by the SARS-CoV-1 virus (*J Infect Dis.* 2004;189(4):648-651) and later in patients with Middle East respiratory syndrome caused by the MERS-CoV virus (*J Infect Dis.* 2016;213(6):904-914). Similar lymphopenia later became a hallmark finding of COVID-19 infection caused by the SARS-CoV-2 virus (*Ann Hematol.* 2021;100(2):309-320).

Furthermore, Ebola virus infections are characterized by significant lymphopenia, which has been linked to worse prognosis and survival (*PLoS Pathog.* 2019;15(10):e1008068).

Iatrogenic causes

Lymphopenia is a frequent adverse effect of multimodal cancer therapy. Numerous cytotoxic chemotherapy drugs lead to a predictable decline in lymphocyte count (*J Natl Compr Canc Netw.* 2015;13(10):1225-1231). Radiation therapy frequently depletes lymphocytes as well, as they are considered the most radiosensitive cells of the hematopoietic system (*Crit Rev Oncol Hematol.* 2018;123:42-51). Radiation-related lymphopenia has been associated with suboptimal tumor control and inferior survival (*Radiother Oncol.* 2022;177:81-94). Secondary immunodeficiency induced by monoclonal antibody therapy is a well-known complication. Anti-CD20 monoclonal antibodies, such as rituximab, rapidly deplete B cells in the peripheral blood, and levels remain low or undetectable for 2 to 6 months (*Cancer Treat Rev.* 2005;31(6):456). Monoclonal antibodies to T cells, such as OKT3 (*J Immunol.* 1980;124(6):2708-2713) or alemtuzumab (*JAMA Neurol.* 2017;74(8):961), can also rapidly deplete T cells. As a result, complications can include increased susceptibility to opportunistic infection (*Clin Infect Dis.* 2007;44(2):204).

In addition to numerous effects on the immune system, glucocorticoid administration is also known to cause lymphocytopenia. The mechanism is likely multifactorial, involving the redistribution of circulating lymphocytes to other body compartments (*Immunology.* 1975;28(4):669-680) and induction of apoptosis (*Clin Exp Immunol.* 1996;103(3):482). T cells are more affected by glucocorticoids compared to B cells (*J Lab Clin Med.* 1983;101(3):479). There is also evidence that both short-term (*J Allergy Clin Immunol.* 1978;62(6):340) and long-term (*J Pediatr.* 1996;129(6):898) use of glucocorticoid can lead to hypogammaglobulinemia. Given these effects on lymphoid cells, corticosteroids are often used as a component of treatment regimens for lymphoid malignancies.

Other causes

Idiopathic $CD4^+$ lymphocytopenia (ICL) describes a syndrome in which patients have persistent $CD4^+$ T-cell lymphocytopenia in the absence of infection or other causes of immunodeficiency (*N Engl J Med.* 1993;328(6):380). While heterogeneous immune defects have been identified, the underlying etiology remains unclear (*Blood.* 2008;112(2):287). While some patients may be asymptomatic (*Medicine (Baltimore).* 2014;93(2):61), patients with ICL are at high risk of opportunistic infection, especially with *Cryptococcus* spp. and mycobacteria (*Blood.* 2008;112(2):287).

III. OTHER MORPHOLOGIC WHITE BLOOD CELL ABNORMALITIES

Inflammatory Changes

In inflammatory states, neutrophils may possess characteristic "toxic changes" within the cytoplasm, which refers to coarse dark-colored granules composed of myeloperoxidase and other lysosomal enzymes (*Br J Haematol.* 1983;53(1):15-22). Döhle bodies are also often present, which are small (1-3 μm in diameter) leukocyte inclusions composed of endoplasmic reticulum material, located in the periphery of the cytoplasm (*J Exp Med*. 1969;129(2):267-293; *Br J Haematol*. 1966;12(1):54-60).

The Pelger-Huët Anomaly

The Pelger-Huët anomaly (PHA) is an autosomal dominant condition leading to a defect in terminal neutrophil differentiation due to mutations in the lamin B receptor gene. On a peripheral blood smear, WBCs have dumbbell-shaped bilobed nuclei with two lobes connected by a thin strand of chromatin, giving a "pince-nez" appearance), and structure (coarse clumping of the nuclear chromatin). Pseudo-PHA refers to anomalies resembling PHA that are acquired rather than congenital. These anomalies are most commonly seen in hematologic malignancies (acute myeloid leukemia, chronic myeloid leukemia, MDS), as well as in vitamin B12 and folate deficiencies, viral infections, malaria, and drug reactions.

The May-Hegglin Anomaly

The May-Hegglin anomaly (MHA) is a rare autosomal dominant disorder characterized by abnormal platelet and granulocyte morphology (*JAMA*. 1963;183:737-740). There are fewer than a hundred cases reported in the literature. The pathogenesis is thought to be related to mutations in the gene encoding for nonmuscle myosin heavy chain IIA (*MYH9*). Mutations in this gene are associated with a number of syndromes that represent forms of hereditary macrothrombocytopenia (*Blood*. 2012;119(2):328). MHA is characterized by small, light-blue crescent-shaped inclusions in granulocytes measuring 2 to 5 µm, resembling Döhle bodies (*Br J Haematol*. 1972;22(4):491-496). Thrombocytopenia and associated giant platelets are also present.

The Alder-Reilly Anomaly

The Alder-Reilly anomaly is an inherited abnormality of WBCs, classically associated with mucopolysaccharidoses (*Am J Clin Pathol*. 1982;78(4):544). Patients with this anomaly possess dense azurophilic granules within all leukocytes, resembling toxic granulation in neutrophils (*Am J Dis Child*. 1941;62(3):489-491). In lymphocytes, these granules are surrounded by a clear zone.

Auer Rods

Auer rods are large azurophilic rod-shaped cytoplasmic inclusions that may be found in myeloblasts or other myeloid progenitor cells in cases of myeloid hematologic malignancies, most commonly acute myeloid leukemia (*Blood*. 1950;5(9):847-863).

SUGGESTED READINGS

Frater JL. How I investigate neutropenia. *Int J Lab Hematol*. 2020;42(suppl 1):121-132. doi:10.1111/ijlh.13210

Hamad H, Mangla A. Lymphocytosis. In: *StatPearls* [Internet]. StatPearls Publishing; 2023. Updated July 17, 2023. https://www.ncbi.nlm.nih.gov/books/NBK549819/

Henry B, Cheruiyot I, Vikse J, et al. Lymphopenia and neutrophilia at admission predicts severity and mortality in patients with COVID-19: a meta-analysis. *Acta Biomed*. 2020;91(3):e2020008. doi:10.23750/abm.v91i3.10217

Knight V. The utility of flow cytometry for the diagnosis of primary immunodeficiencies. *Int J Lab Hematol*. 2019;41(suppl 1):63-72. doi:10.1111/ijlh.13010

Ley K, Laudanna C, Cybulsky MI, Nourshargh S. Getting to the site of inflammation: the leukocyte adhesion cascade updated. *Nat Rev Immunol*. 2007;7(9):678-689. doi:10.1038/nri2156

Savoia A, Pecci A. MYH9-related disease. In: Adam MP, Feldman J, Mirzaa GM, et al, eds. *GeneReviews®* [Internet]. University of Washington, Seattle; 1993-2024; 2008 [updated February 18, 2021].

Torrez M, Chabot-Richards D, Babu D, Lockhart E, Foucar K. How I investigate acquired megaloblastic anemia. *Int J Lab Hematol.* 2022;44(2):236-247.

Yu HH, Yang YH, Chiang BL. Chronic granulomatous disease: a comprehensive review. *Clin Rev Allergy Immunol.* 2021;61(2):101-113. doi:10.1007/s12016-020-08800-x

4.3: Platelet Disorders

Joshua Siner, Brooj Abro, and Thomas M. Schneider

Platelets are the terminal unit of megakaryopoiesis, wherein hematopoietic stem cell progenitors differentiate down the common myeloid progenitor line and form large, multinucleated cells that project and bud off approximately 2- to 3-µm platelets lacking DNA (e-Figure 4.3-1). The production of platelets is dependent on thrombopoietin produced by hepatocytes. As platelet counts decrease, the effective thrombopoietin levels increase, stimulating bone marrow megakaryocytes to proliferate and form platelets, which are then released into circulation. Platelets exist in circulation for about 7 days and are critical for primary hemostasis by forming platelet plugs upon exposure to subendothelial collagen and binding to von Willebrand factor (vWF) (Figure 4.3-1). Activation of platelets leads to degranulation of α-granules and dense granules, which release additional hemostatic activators (see Table 4.3-1) and provide a platform for coagulation with increased surface expression of phosphatidylserine (*Semin Thromb Hemost.* 2016;42:185-190). After activation and crosslinking with fibrinogen, the platelet cytoskeleton rearranges to facilitate clot contraction. Additionally, platelets perform nonhemostatic functions, including the proinflammatory response to thrombosis and crosstalk between innate and adaptive immune responses (*Circ Res.* 2022;130:288-308). This chapter predominantly focuses on benign factors contributing to variations in platelet count and morphology. Abnormalities in hemostasis are also discussed but only to a limited extent.

I. LABORATORY ASSESSMENT OF PLATELETS

Methodology

The normal platelet count ranges from 150 to 400 × 10^9/L and is commonly assessed by automated hematology analyzers, with impedance, optical light scatter, and fluorescence being the most commonly used methods. At low levels, differences and interferences may be seen, and immunologic methods may be used (*Br J Haematol.* 2005;128:520-525). MPV values can vary significantly depending on the instrument used. Therefore, it is necessary to interpret results within the context of laboratory reference ranges (*Cleve Clin J Med.* 2019;86:150).

Faithful assessment of platelet function *in vivo* using *in vitro* techniques is difficult. Platelet aggregation studies (Figure 4.3-2), which test platelet response to a battery of

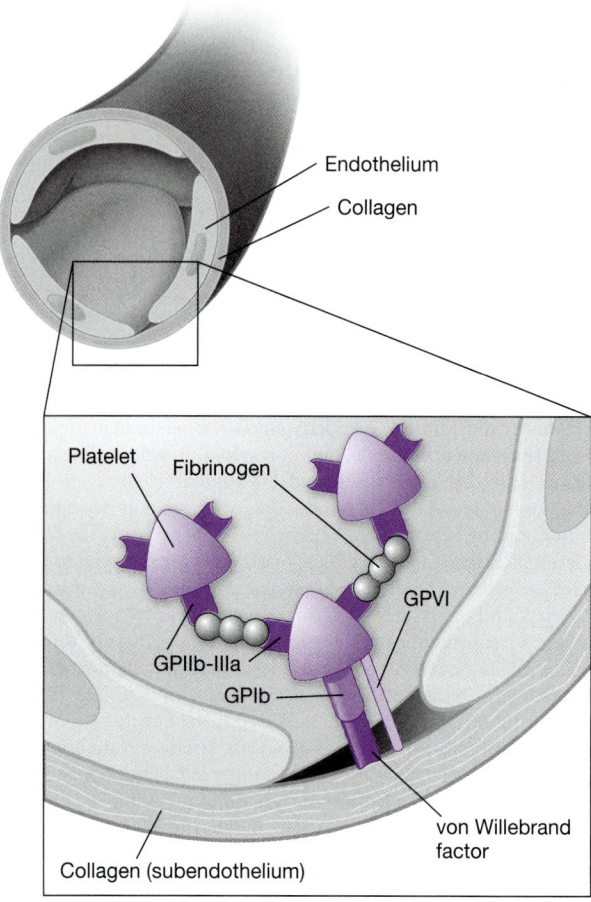

Figure 4.3-1. Platelet adhesion and aggregation. Platelet adhesion to collagen (subendothelial) is mediated by the binding of vWF to GPIb receptors and collagen. In addition, GPVI receptors also facilitate the binding of platelets to collagen. The formation of platelet plug requires platelet cross-linking, which occurs via binding of fibrinogen to GPIIb-IIIa receptors. vWF, von Willebrand factor. (From Armstrong AW, Golan DE. Pharmacology of hemostasis and thrombosis. In: Golan DE, Tashjian AH Jr, Armstrong EJ, Armstrong AW, eds. *Principles of Pharmacology*. 3rd ed. Wolters Kluwer; 2012:372-400.)

platelet-stimulating reagents, are particularly helpful in diagnosing inherited disorders of hemostasis (*Vasc Health Risk Manag*. 2015;11:133-148). Rapid, point-of-care testing (POCT) platelet function analyzers such as PFA-100, PFA-200, and VerifyNow are easier to perform but are nonspecific and not recommended for diagnosing genetic disorders (*Haemophilia*. 2006;12 suppl 3:128-136), but they may be useful for rapidly assessing disrupted platelet function due to antiplatelet medication. Viscoelastic

TABLE 4.3-1 Key Platelet Components Involved in Hemostasis

Components	Function
Glycoprotein (GP) membrane receptors[a]	
GPIIb/IIIa	Bind to fibrinogen
GPIa/IIa and GPVI	Bind to collagen
GPIb/IX/V	Bind to vWF
Other membrane receptors	
ADP receptors (P2Y$_1$, P2Y$_{12}$), thrombin receptors (PAR-1, PAR-4), thromboxane receptors (TPα, TPβ), α$_2$-adrenergic receptor	External receptors coupled to internal G-proteins that are involved in signal transduction and platelet activation following external ligand binding
Granules	
α-Granules	Release platelet factor 4, β-thrombomodulin, fibrinogen, vWF, coagulation factors (V and VIII), P-selectin, fibronectin, and so on
Dense (δ) granules	Release ADP, ATP, serotonin, calcium

ADP, adenosine diphosphate; ATP, adenosine triphosphate; vWF, von Willebrand factor.
[a]GP receptors are involved in platelet adhesion and aggregation by binding to specific ligands as previously mentioned.

assays, notably thromboelastography (TEG) and rotational thromboelastometry (ROTEM), are increasingly utilized for intraoperative evaluation of hemostatic function, including the assessment of platelet-related hemostatic issues (*Transfusion.* 2020;60 suppl 6:S1-S9).

Preanalytical Errors

Pseudothrombocytopenia refers to preanalytical errors that occur when automated cell counters inaccurately measure low platelet levels. When this occurs, they are often mistaken for white blood cells (WBCs) with a resultant higher WBC count. Ethylenediaminetetraacetic acid (EDTA)–dependent platelet antibodies or agglutinins that target glycoprotein IIb/IIIa receptors can cause platelet clumping or WBC satellitism, leading to falsely low platelet counts. Although EDTA is the preferred anticoagulant for hematology tests because it preserves cell shape, it can lead to erroneous results in these rare cases. To address this, blood samples without EDTA, such as those collected in sodium citrate or heparin, should be analyzed (*Clin Chem Lab Med.* 2012;50:1281-1285). Giant platelets, larger than 7 μm, can significantly distort platelet counts due to misinterpretation (*Ann Clin Lab Sci.* 2019;49:554-556). These unusually large platelets can be due to inherited disorders (discussed later) or myeloproliferative disorders. Clotted samples can result in low platelets due to consumption.

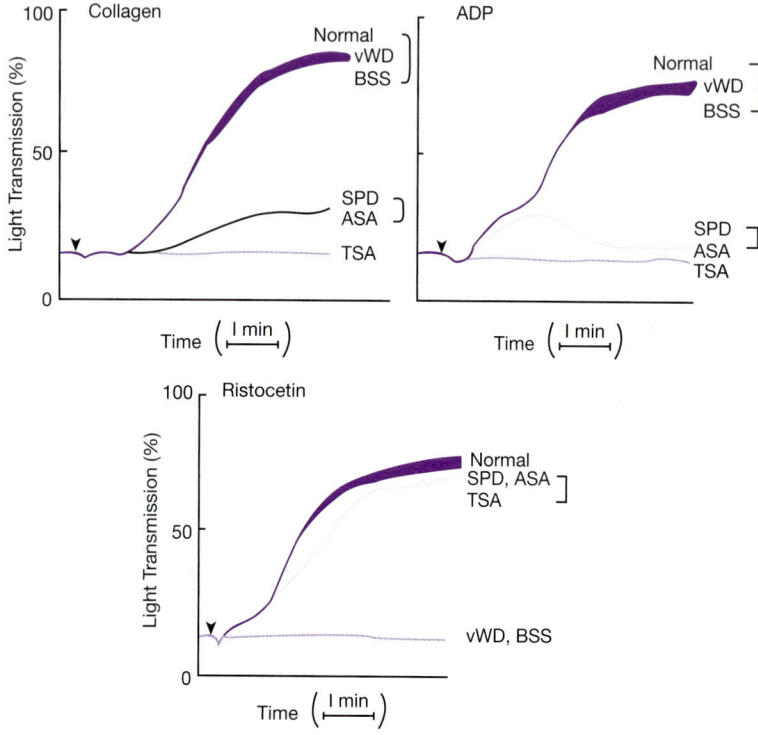

Figure 4.3-2. Schematic representation of normal and abnormal patterns of platelet aggregation and associated disorders. These patterns can be demonstrated using a turbidometric platelet aggregometer and incorporating collagen, adenosine diphosphate (ADP), and ristocetin into stirred platelet-rich plasma samples. A lack of aggregation in reaction to ristocetin is indicative of Bernard-Soulier syndrome (BSS) and von Willebrand disease (vWD). In Glanzmann thrombasthenia (TSA), aggregation is typically absent except when induced by ristocetin. In the context of ADP response, platelet aggregation is characterized by two phases. The initial phase, known as the "first wave," is a direct result of agonist-induced primary aggregation. The subsequent phase, referred to as the "second wave," involves secondary aggregation characterized by the formation of large, irreversible aggregates concurrent with platelet secretion. Notably, the absence of this second wave is a distinguishing feature of storage pool disorders (SPDs) and aspirin (ASA). (From Bennett JS, Rao AK. Inherited disorders of platelet function. In: Marder VJ, Aird WC, Bennett JS, Schulman S, White GC II, eds. *Hemostasis and Thrombosis*. 6th ed. Wolters Kluwer; 2013:805-819.)

Automated instruments can also detect other cellular materials as platelets, leading to spurious elevation of platelet counts. Cytoplasmic fragments, most commonly seen in individuals with acute leukemia or hairy cell leukemia, are small and, therefore, can be misinterpreted as platelets (*Arch Intern Med*. 1981;141:942-944). Schistocytes, seen in thrombotic microangiopathies, and cryoglobulins are other possible contributors to spuriously elevated platelets (*Ann Lab Med*. 2022;42:515-530).

Improvements in instrument flagging mechanisms have played a crucial role in excluding preanalytic errors. When these flags are encountered, strategies such as inspecting samples for clots, conducting slide reviews, requesting redraws using alternative anticoagulants, or switching automated methodologies are all effective for minimizing these preanalytic errors.

Platelet Morphology on Blood Smears

Normal circulating platelets are small, round, and oval in shape. The cytoplasm of platelets is characterized by the presence of azurophilic granules, which can be dispersed across the cytoplasm or centralized in a region known as the granulomere. In contrast, the peripheral region of the platelet cytoplasm, which appears colorless or demonstrates weak basophilic staining and is devoid of granules, is referred to as the hyalomere. In peripheral blood smears, the assessment of platelet size can be effectively performed by comparing the diameter of platelets to that of the red blood cells (7-8 μm). Platelets are typically 2 to 3 μm in size, large platelets are between 3 and 7 μm, and giant platelets are >7 μm (e-Figure 4.3-1B). Abnormal platelet count, size, and color can be associated with various disorders.

II. ACQUIRED DISORDERS OF PLATELET NUMBER

Acquired Thrombocytopenia

Acquired thrombocytopenias are characterized by decreased platelet counts in patients with a documented history of normal platelet counts and the absence of pathologic bleeding. They are generally a result of either (1) poor platelet production, (2) increased platelet consumption, or (3) sequestration into the reticuloendothelial system (Table 4.3-2). Decreased platelet production is typically secondary to liver dysfunction or bone marrow infiltration—such as by hematologic neoplasms, metastatic diseases, or infections.

Heparin-Induced Thrombocytopenia

Heparin-induced thrombocytopenia (HIT) occurs when pathogenic antibodies are directed against a neoantigen that is formed when platelet factor 4 (PF4) is bound to heparins. The diagnosis is primarily clinical following the 4T scoring system (consisting of exposure timing, degree of thrombocytopenia, presence of thrombosis, and potential for other causes of low platelet counts). A 4T score below 3 points is an excellent negative predictive value for ruling out HIT (*Blood.* 2012;120:4160-4167). When results show an intermediate clinical suspicion (4T = 4-5 points), heparin should be replaced by nonheparinoid anticoagulants (ie, argatroban, bivalirudin), and serologic testing is then used to determine if reactive antibodies are present with or without confirmatory testing. A high pretest probability (4T >6) is sufficient for diagnosing HIT. Immunologic HIT antibody testing can be done by enzyme-linked immunosorbent assay (ELISA), immunofiltration, or gel-agglutination assays (*Clin Diagn Lab Immunol.* 2003;10:731-740). The serotonin release assay remains the gold standard (and confirmatory test) in unclear cases. The primary treatment is the removal of heparin and avoidance of future heparinoid exposures.

Vaccine-Induced Thrombocytopenia

Vaccine-induced thrombocytopenia (VITT) is a recently described PF4-based neoantigen-driven disease identified in the vaccination setting of the COVID-19 pandemic. The syndrome's pathologic antibodies are also directed against PF4, however, in a different geographic epitope distribution leading to platelet

TABLE 4.3-2 Causes of Thrombocytopenia

Increased Destruction
Primary ITP
Secondary ITP (drugs, infection, autoimmune)
Transfusion
Thrombotic microangiopathy (TTP, aHUS)
Posttransfusion purpura
Heparin-induced thrombocytopenia
DIC
Infection

Poor Production/Survival
Infection
Medication
Liver disease
B12 deficiency
Neoplastic disorders involving the bone marrow[a]

Inherited Thrombocytopenia
Associated with small or large platelets
Thrombocytopenia-absent radius syndrome (*TAR*)
Radioulnar synostosis with amegakaryocytic thrombocytopenia (*RUSAT1*)
Congenital amegakaryocytic thrombocytopenia (*CAMT*)
Familial platelet disorder with predisposition to AML (*RUNX1*)
ANKRD26, CYCS, ETV6, IKZF5, KDSR, MECOM, STIM1, THPO-related thrombocytopenia

Spurious
EDTA platelet antibodies
Clotted Samples

aHUS, atypical hemolytic uremic syndrome; AML, acute myeloid leukemia; DIC, disseminated intravascular coagulopathy; EDTA, ethylenediaminetetraacetic acid; ITP, immune (idiopathic) thrombocytopenia purpura; TTP, thrombotic thrombocytopenia purpura.
[a]Primary hematologic malignancies, for example, acute leukemias, can present with thrombocytopenia and other cytopenias (discussed in later chapters).

activation (*Nature*. 2021;596:565-569). Cases typically occur 5 to 10 days after administration of an adenovirus-based vaccine. The thrombotic phenotype is characterized by an atypical distribution, including cerebral venous sinus thrombosis, splanchnic vein thrombosis, and arterial thrombosis. Treatment is anticoagulation, preferably with nonheparinoid anticoagulants and high-dose intravenous immunoglobulin (IVIg).

Thrombotic Microangiopathies—Thrombotic Thrombocytopenia Purpura/ Hemolytic Uremic Syndrome/Atypical Hemolytic Uremic Syndrome

Thrombotic microangiopathies (TMA) are clinically characterized by the presence of extravascular hemolysis (with elevated lactate dehydrogenase [LDH], indirect bilirubinemia, and undetectable haptoglobin levels) with negative direct antiglobulin testing, and the presence of red cell fragments (schistocytes) on peripheral smear. It is critical to identify TMAs because differentiating the mechanism determines the treatment modality critical to reverse the hemolytic process. One systemic condition that may mimic a TMA with hemolysis present and thrombocytopenia is severe B12 deficiency—one early sign for this scenario is a macrocytosis not driven by a reticulocytosis.

Thrombotic thrombocytopenia purpura

Thrombotic thrombocytopenia purpura (TTP) is a disease characterized by reduced ADAMTS13 activity. ADAMTS13 is crucial for downregulating vWF activity through cleavage of large and ultra-large multimers, which are capable of binding platelets and cause microthrombi under high sheer stress conditions. The high sheer unveils ADAMTS13 cleavage sites in large and ultra-large vWF. ADAMTS13 activity is reduced either through congenital deficiency—known as Upshall-Shulman disease—or acquired via inhibitory autoantibodies (acquired TTP or aTTP). In the evaluation of a new patient with concern for TMA, the PLASMIC score is a diagnostic scoring system that utilizes clinical variables to determine patients with potential TTP who are likely to benefit from plasmapheresis upfront. A delay in the diagnosis and treatment of aTTP can quickly progress and become fatal. The primary modality for treating acquired TTP involves immunosuppression with high-dose steroids +/− rituximab, and plasmapheresis to remove pathologic antibodies. Relapse rates are not uncommon in patients with TTP and are reported at ~30% to 40% in patients presenting with ADAMTS13 activity less than 10% at the highest risk (*Blood*. 2010;115:1500-1511).

Hemolytic uremic syndrome

Hemolytic uremic syndrome (HUS) is a form of microangiopathic hemolytic anemia (MAHA) with thrombocytopenia that is the result of renal endothelial dysfunction, and presents with profound renal injury without loss of ADAMTS13 function. In children, the cause of HUS is predominantly from hemorrhagic diarrheal infections carrying Shiga-toxin, such as the classic *Escherichia coli* strain 0157:H7. In adults, HUS can still be Shiga-toxin–dependent and seen in the setting of foodborne outbreaks, but rare sporadic cases exist. The primary mode of treatment is supportive care during diarrheal illness, renal protection, and dialysis as clinically indicated.

Atypical hemolytic uremic syndrome

Atypical hemolytic uremic syndrome (aHUS), or more appropriately complement-mediated thrombotic microangiopathy, has the same clinical features as HUS. However, instead of being triggered by Shiga-toxin–producing bacteria, aHUS is caused by overactive complement activation leading to MAHA/TMA and acute renal injury. Patients with aHUS typically have an underlying complement deficiency or dysfunction in the alternative pathway, leading to overactivation via congenital mutations or inhibitory anti-complement factor H antibody (*J Autoimmun*. 2022;102979). In both scenarios, the use of terminal complement inhibitors such as eculizumab or ravulizumab has been shown to control overactivation, resulting in renal preservation, reversal of injury, and correction of hemolysis and thrombocytopenia.

Immune Thrombocytopenia Purpura

Accelerated destruction of platelets may occur due to antibody-mediated clearance. In the context of transfusion, this may be due to posttransfusion purpura or acquired platelet alloantibodies, as discussed later. Immune (idiopathic) thrombocytopenia purpura (ITP) is a diagnosis of exclusion in which patients have platelet-directed antibodies, which result in sequestration and destruction within the reticuloendothelial system. Patients typically present with petechial rash, soft tissue bleeding such as epistaxis and gum blisters/bleeding, and splenomegaly. Rarely, patients with ITP may also develop autoimmune hemolytic anemia, known as Evans syndrome. Peripheral blood smear findings show rare platelets that are typically large (4-7 µm) and seldom giant (>7 µm). ITP can be further classified as primary and secondary ITP. Secondary ITP includes autoimmune diseases, infections, and medications. Cross-reactive or molecular mimicry antibodies have been reported in infections such as *Helicobacter pylori*, human immunodeficiency virus (HIV), and hepatitis C virus (HCV) infections. Commonly implicated medications include quinine, quinidine, trimethoprim-sulfamethoxazole, vancomycin, and piperacillin/tazobactam (*J Thromb Haemost*. 2015;13:676-678). Rarely, ITP can be a presenting symptom of a B-cell malignancy. Treatment of primary ITP involves a combination of high-dose steroids and IVIg. In refractory cases there is a role for splenectomy as well thrombopoietin mimetics.

Critical Illness Thrombocytopenia and Disseminated Intravascular Coagulation

Patients admitted to intensive care units (ICU) represent a unique population that develops thrombocytopenia due to heterogeneous and multifactorial mechanisms. Specifically, for patients admitted to a medical ICU, the high presence of severe infections, an inflammatory cytokine milieu, and the use of typical antibiotics may all cause bone marrow suppression, presenting as thrombocytopenia. Additionally, the occurrence of thrombocytopenia upon admission or its development in response to systemic disease serves as an unfavorable prognostic indicator for survival (*Arch Intern Med*. 2008;168:94-102).

Disseminated intravascular coagulation (DIC) is a systemic overactivation of coagulation, endothelial dysfunction, and platelet reactivity in response to infection (severe sepsis, septic shock) and inflammation. DIC is diagnosed clinically and is characterized by thrombocytopenia and coagulopathy (low fibrinogen levels, elevated D-dimer or fibrin split products, and prolonged prothrombin time [PT] and activated partial thromboplastin time [aPTT]). Coagulopathy in DIC typically presents as line-associated bleeding in ICU patients. In patients presenting with fulminant infections, bleeding may be more serious, including intra-abdominal, retroperitoneal, and gastrointestinal bleeding. The ultimate treatment involves reversal of the underlying systemic disease; however, patients should be supported with fresh frozen plasma infusions to supplement consumed fibrinogen and platelet transfusions as needed, with targeting levels based on the presence and location of observed bleeding.

Pregnancy-Associated Thrombocytopenia

Gestational thrombocytopenia is typically encountered in the second trimester of pregnancy. This condition is a benign cause of typically mild to moderate thrombocytopenia (platelet count >80,000/µL) and accounts for 70% to 80% of pregnancy-associated thrombocytopenia (*Blood*. 2013;121:38-47). Gestational thrombocytopenia occurs in response to physiologic changes of pregnancy, including an increased volume of distribution that increases toward term. It is important to note that other causes, such as congenital thrombocytopenias and type 2B von Willebrand disease (vWD), may worsen or become evident during this critical period. Ultimately, in the case of pure gestational thrombocytopenia, supportive care and attention to changes in platelet counts are all that is required through delivery, after which platelet counts should return to their prepregnancy baseline (*Hematology Am Soc Hematol Educ Program.* 2022;2022(1):303).

As pregnancy progresses into the third trimester, the continuum of preeclampsia, eclampsia, and HELLP syndrome (hemolysis, elevated liver enzymes, low platelets) may emerge due to placental endothelial dysfunction. Strictly speaking, delivery of the fetus and all placental tissue will reverse all three conditions. However, more recent data have shown that there is a degree of complement activation that is similar between HELLP and aHUS—which is further complicated by pregnancy being a trigger for aHUS (*Adv Chronic Kidney Dis.* 2020;27:155-164).

Bone Marrow Infiltration/Suppression/Primary Disorders
As the primary location for megakaryocytic production of platelets, bone marrow niche alterations can lead to "crowding out" of necessary precursors or direct suppression of megakaryocytes. Infiltration of bone marrow can be the result of primary bone marrow neoplasms and bone marrow failure syndromes, which are described in later chapters. The presence of thrombocytopenia with a second lineage cytopenia should trigger evaluation with a bone marrow biopsy when there is no obvious systemic cause for the presenting cytopenias. Rarely, such evaluation will demonstrate infiltrative processes including, but not limited to, fungal infections, mycobacterial infections, or noncaseating granulomas. Notably, in the evaluation of fever of unknown origin, bone marrow culture will identify unique culprit organisms (not otherwise diagnosed) in a small percentage of patients, almost exclusively in patients with uncontrolled HIV and cytopenias (*Am J Clin Pathol.* 1998;110:150-153).

Posttransfusion Purpura
Posttransfusion purpura (PTP) is a serious transfusion-associated disorder that manifests as a severe thrombocytopenia ($< 10 \times 10^9$/L) occurring within 2 weeks after a blood transfusion (*J Blood Med.* 2019;10:405-415). PTP is due to the formation of alloantibodies targeting specific platelet antigens, predominantly human platelet antigen-1a (HPA-1a), following the recipient's exposure to these antigens in transfused blood products. In individuals diagnosed with PTP, the generated alloantibodies paradoxically affect the patient's own platelets through a mechanism that is not entirely elucidated. One hypothesis posits that autologous platelets may passively adsorb foreign platelet antigens from transfused blood, thereby becoming targets for the alloantibody-mediated immune response. Alternatively, it has been suggested that both alloantibodies and autoantibodies are concurrently produced, with the latter being more challenging to detect, a phenomenon observed similarly in many patients with immune thrombocytopenic purpura (ITP). PTP is an exceedingly rare event, with an estimated incidence of 1:50,000 transfusions. A mortality rate of 10% to 20% has been documented, predominantly attributed to intracranial hemorrhage. HPA genotyping and platelet antibody workup can be used to make the diagnosis. Management of PTP involves the immediate cessation of further platelet transfusions unless absolutely necessary and the administration of high-dose IVIg. In most cases, the prognosis of PTP is favorable, with platelet counts typically normalizing within a few days following treatment.

Acquired Thrombocytosis

Thrombocytosis can be divided into primary and secondary causes (Table 4.3-3). Secondary causes of thrombocytosis are more common than primary causes (>85%), with infection being the most common cause (*Hematol Oncol Clin North Am.* 2012;26:285-viii). In the case of reactive thrombocytosis, various cytokines, including interleukin 6 (IL-6), thrombopoietin, IL-1, interferon-γ, and tumor necrosis factor-α, are released. Consequently, conditions that lead to an increase in these cytokines can potentially trigger reactive thrombocytosis. In a retrospective analysis conducted at a single institution, primary thrombocytosis exhibited a higher average platelet count of (857×10^9/L), while secondary causes had an average of approximately (650×10^9/L). However, platelet counts exceeding (800×10^9/L) were also observed in this group (*J Clin Med Res.* 2012;4:415-423). Soft tissue, pulmonary, and GI infections were the most common infectious causes, with malignancy and iron deficiency anemia being the most common noninfectious causes. It should be noted that despite its high incidence in the thrombocytosis cohort, specifically in patients with iron deficiency anemia, it may only be seen 10% of the time (*Blood.* 2018;132(suppl 1):4985). Tissue damage also may cause reactive thrombocytosis and may be the result of burns, pancreatitis, myocardial infarction, and surgery. Thrombocytosis is observed in approximately 50% of cases following splenectomy, a condition that typically resolves within a few months. Elevated platelet counts can also result from various inflammatory conditions, including inflammatory bowel disease, vasculitis, rheumatoid arthritis, and celiac disease. Additionally, thrombocytosis may infrequently be induced by certain medications, such as epinephrine, vincristine, gemcitabine, antibiotics, and low-molecular-weight heparin (*Ann Pharmacother.* 2019;53:523-536).

TABLE 4.3-3 Causes of Thrombocytosis

Primary[a]
Myeloproliferative neoplasms
Myelodysplastic syndrome with 5q deletion

Secondary
Infection
Iron deficiency anemia
Malignancy (nonhematologic)
Tissue damage
Inflammatory disorders
Postsplenectomy

Spurious
Cytoplasmic fragments
Cryoglobulinemia

[a]Discussed in detail in later chapters.

III. ACQUIRED NONNEOPLASTIC DISORDERS OF PLATELET SIZE AND MORPHOLOGY

There are a variety of neoplastic and nonneoplastic causes of abnormal platelet volume and morphology (nonneoplastic causes are listed in Table 4.3-4). In the normal physiologic state, megakaryocytes are stimulated by thrombopoietin to produce larger platelets

TABLE 4.3-4 Benign Disorders With Abnormal Platelet Morphology

Large Platelets
Inherited[a]
- *MYH9*-related disorders (*MYH9*)
- May-Hegglin—Dohle-like bodies
- von Willebrand disease type 2B (*VWF*)
- Platelet-type von Willibrand disease (*GP1BA*)
- Bernard-Soulier (*GP1BA, GP1BB, GP9*)
- Gray platelet syndrome (*NBEAL2*)
- Velocardiofacial syndrome (22q11.2 deletion → *GP1BB* deletion)
- *ACTN1, DIAPH1, FLI1, FLNA, GALE, GATA1, GFI1B, GNE, PRKACG, SLFN14, SRC, TPM4, TRPM7, TUBB1*—related thrombocytopenia

Acquired
- Postsplenectomy states and hyposplenism
- Increased destruction: ITP, TMA
- Drug—cholestyramine

Small Platelets
Inherited
- Wiskott-Aldrich syndrome (*WAS*)
- X-linked thrombocytopenia (*WAS*)
- *ARCP1B, FYB, PTPRJ*—related thrombocytopenia

Acquired
- Impaired production: drug toxicity, bone marrow infiltration

Agranular Platelets
- Storage pool disorders (see Table 4.3-5)
- In vitro—venipuncture, implanted devices, cardiopulmonary bypass, EDTA—induced
- In vivo—DIC

DIC, disseminated intravascular coagulopathy; EDTA, ethylenediaminetetraacetic acid; ITP, immune (idiopathic) thrombocytopenia purpura; TMA, thrombotic microangiopathies.
[a]Genes involved in inherited disorders are mentioned in *italics*.

in response to decreased platelet levels. Therefore, disorders with increased platelet consumption have a higher-than-normal MPV, though not as much as seen in inherited platelet disorders (*Br J Haematol.* 2013;162:112-119). Impaired production of platelets due to drug toxicity or bone marrow infiltration may cause low MPV values. Agranular platelets or pale platelets can be seen in states with consistently ongoing platelet activation, leading to "exhausted" granules, such as patients with cardiac devices, on cardiopulmonary bypass, or in DIC. Rarely, these abnormalities may be EDTA-induced and serve as a source of preanalytical error (*Clin Lab Haematol.* 2005;27:336-334).

Acquired von Willebrand Syndrome

Acquired von Willebrand syndrome (aVWS) occurs in the setting of prolonged and extreme thrombocytosis, typically seen in MPN-associated thrombocytosis, or in situations of abnormal high sheer blood flow. In these scenarios, elevated platelet numbers and activity cause increased binding and unraveling of ultra-large vWF molecules, leading to their cleavage by ADAMTS13. This results in a steady consumption of normal vWF, ultimately leading to a bleeding phenotype. This is also seen in Heyde syndrome (aortic stenosis causing aVWS when associated with gastrointestinal arteriovenous malformations), left ventricular assist devices, and extracorporeal membrane oxygenation due to nonphysiologic blood flow. Laboratory examination shows low vWF antigen activity (measured by either ristocetin or GP1b binding) and loss of high-molecule-weight forms on multimer analysis. Treatment strategies focus on cytoreduction for MPN-associated aVWS, with the addition of low-dose aspirin, or correction of underlying stenotic/flow physiology. Additionally, replacement of vWF with either recombinant forms (ie, Vonvendi) or plasma-derived vWF (ie, Humate-P), in combination with factor VIII.

IV. INHERITED DISORDERS OF PLATELET NUMBER, MORPHOLOGY, AND FUNCTION

To date, nearly 50 genes have been identified that are involved in megakaryocytic development and implicated in clinical thrombocytopenia or platelet dysfunction (*Blood.* 2022;139:3264-3277). Inherited causes of thrombocytopenia can be identified by their association with syndromic conditions, such as thrombocytopenia-absent radius (TAR) syndrome. With increased access to genomic sequencing, mutations in known or new genes are often identified, which requires establishing definitive guidelines for interpretation and assessment of future risks (*J Thromb Haemost.* 2021;19:2127-2136). Several syndromes causing thrombocytopenia have been critical in understanding basic platelet development (*MPL* mutations in congenital amegakaryocytic thrombocytopenia causing severe neonatal thrombocytopenia) and cancer predisposition syndromes (*ETV6*, *RUNX1*, and *GATA1* germline mutations causing mild to moderate thrombocytopenia). Based on the functional changes, patients may develop a combination of abnormalities in platelet number, microscopic appearance, and function. Most function disorders that do not affect platelet counts also do not affect platelet size. In storage pool disorders, the generation, formation, or release of signaling vesicles are abnormal (see Table 4.3-5); these disorders result in either hypogranular or agranular platelets. Signaling disorders manifest through altered posttranslational processing, expression, and changes in the ability of platelet receptors to adequately regulate their activation and binding to ligands. While the effect on platelet aggregation is beyond the scope of this chapter, these disorders can

TABLE 4.3-5 Storage Pool Disorders Causing Platelet Defects

Disease	Gene (Inheritance)	Mechanism	Findings
Hermansky-Pudlak syndrome	AP3B1 (AR) AP3D1 (AR) BLOC1S3 (AR) BLOC1S6 (AR) DTNBP1 (AR) HPS1 (AR) HPS3 (AR) HPS4 (AR) HPS5 (AR) HPS6 (AR)	Absence of dense granules due to deficiencies in intracellular trafficking	Normal size and count Bleeding phenotype Hypogranular platelets on smear Reduced number of dense granules identified by electron microscopy Albinism
Chediak-Higashi syndrome	LYST (AR)	Reduced number of dense granules	Normal size and count Bleeding phenotype Oculocutaneous albinism Recurrent pyogenic infections Giant intracellular granules in their neutrophils
Gray platelet syndrome	NBEAL2 (AR)	Absent α-granules	Macrothrombocytopenia Bleeding phenotype Increased plasma B-12
Familial platelet disorder with predisposition to AML	RUNX1 (AD)	Reduced number of platelet dense or α-granules Reduced MYH10 expression in megakaryocytes, persistence in platelets	Thrombocytopenia ~40% lifetime risk for developing a hematologic malignancy

AD, autosomal dominant; AML, acute myeloid leukemia; AR, autosomal recessive.

result in abnormal platelets. For example, Bernard-Soulier syndrome, type 2B vWD, and platelet-type vWD syndrome result in large to giant platelets accompanied by thrombocytopenia.

Features of select platelet receptor and receptor signaling disorders are summarized in Table 4.3-6. Defects in structural or cytoskeletal components include

TABLE 4.3-6 Platelet Receptor and Receptor Signaling Defects

Disease	Gene (Inheritance)	Mechanism	Findings
von Willebrand disease, type 2B	*VWF* (AD)	Increased binding of vWF to platelet receptor GP1b leading to increased vWF-platelet clearance Reduced aggregation response to ristocetin but increased with low dose	Macrothrombocytopenia Thrombocytopenia worsened with DDAVP
Bernard-Soulier syndrome	*GP1BA*, *GP1BB* and *GP9* (AR/AD)	Reduced GP1b/V/IX complex expression leading to loss of vWF binding Reduced aggregation response to ristocetin	Macrothrombocytopenia Homozygous AR more severe than AD mutations Neonatal bleeding phenotype
Scott syndrome	*ANO6* (AR)	Reduced calcium-dependent signaling and phosphatidylserine exposure to support coagulation proteases	Normal count and size Bleeding phenotype
Leukocyte integrin adhesion deficiency, type III	*FERMT3* (AR)	Absent platelet aggregation in response to all stimuli, except ristocetin (Glanzmann thrombasthenia-like)	Normal count and size Bleeding phenotype Normal integrin IIb/IIIa receptor levels
Glanzmann thrombasthenia	*ITGA2B* (AR)	Absent aggregation to all agonists except ristocetin. Abnormal integrin IIb does not bind IIIa and leads to degradation in the ER	Normal count and size Severe bleeding diathesis Lack of GPIIb/IIIa surface expression

AD, autosomal dominant; AR, autosomal recessive; ER, endoplasmic reticulum; vWF, von Willebrand factor.

MYH9-related disorders arising from mutations in the gene encoding nonmuscle myosin heavy chain IIA, which result in thrombocytopenia with platelet macrocytosis and cytoplasmic inclusions in neutrophils (Dohle-like bodes). Wiskott-Aldrich syndrome is caused by variants in the *WAS* gene, resulting in small platelets and low platelet count.

SUGGESTED READINGS

Gulati G, Uppal G, Gong J. Unreliable automated complete blood count results: causes, recognition, and resolution. *Ann Lab Med*. 2022;42(5):515-530.

Pecci A, Balduini CL. Inherited thrombocytopenias: an updated guide for clinicians. *Blood Rev*. 2021;48:100784.

Robier C. Platelet morphology. *J Lab Med*. 2020;44(5):231-239.

Rose SR, Petersen NJ, Gardner TJ, Hamill RJ, Trautner BW. Etiology of thrombocytosis in a general medicine population: analysis of 801 cases with emphasis on infectious causes. *J Clin Med Res*. 2012;4(6):415.

Sulai NH, Tefferi A. Why does my patient have thrombocytosis? *Hematol Oncol Clin North Am*. 2012;26(2):285-301.

Bone marrow

5.1 Bone Marrow Abnormalities in Systemic Conditions

Callie Torres, Brooj Abro, and Anjum Hassan

There are many non-neoplastic conditions that cause bone marrow abnormalities including infections, storage disorders, autoimmune diseases, and other systemic diseases. These disorders can result in changes in marrow cellularity and morphology, granuloma formation, fibrosis, necrosis, atrophy, and hemophagocytosis. It is important to recognize pertinent marrow changes in patients with systemic conditions as it may help to diagnose underlying etiologies and/or further guide treatment.

I. BACTERIAL INFECTIONS

Bacterial infections can lead to nonspecific changes such as left shift and granulocytic hyperplasia. In immunocompromised patients, more pronounced changes may be present. Bacterial infections that may result in granuloma formation include tuberculosis, rickettsiosis, Whipple disease, Q fever, and other tick-borne infections (see Table 5.1-1).

Tuberculosis

There are several mycobacterial species that can cause morphologic changes in the bone marrow, but the most predominant are *Mycobacterium tuberculosis* and *Mycobacterium avium-intracellulare* (MAI). Infection with either species may cause epithelioid granulomas (e-Figure 5.1-1), with occasional central, caseous necrosis. While granulomas are more prevalent in immunocompromised individuals, they may also be present in immunocompetent patients. Granulomas may contain interspersed lymphocytes and be located near bony trabeculae. In severely immunosuppressed patients, distinct granulomas may not be seen, instead loose histiocytic aggregates may form. In MAI infections, histiocytes containing organisms may appear granular or cloudy. A periodic acid-Schiff (PAS) or Ziehl-Neelsen stain can aid in identification of the organisms (e-Figure 5.1-2).

Q Fever

Q fever is caused by infection with the gram-negative bacterium *Coxiella burnetii* and is characteristically associated with the formation of lipogranulomas (also referred to as ring/fibrin ring or donut granulomas) that can be found in the bone marrow and liver (*Lancet*. 2006;367:679-688). Lipogranulomas consist of epithelioid histiocytes

TABLE 5.1-1 Etiologies of Granuloma Formation in the Bone Marrow

Viral	Bacterial
Epstein-Barr virus	Brucella
Cytomegalovirus	Bartonella
Hepatitis C	Syphilis
HIV	Typhoid
Herpes simplex	Tularemia
	Borrelia
Malignancy	Mycoplasma
Hodgkin lymphoma	Toxoplasmosis
MALT lymphoma	Whipple disease
Multiple myeloma	Tuberculosis
Acute lymphoblastic leukemia	
Acute myeloid leukemia	**Medication**
Hairy cell leukemia	NSAIDs
Chronic myelogenous leukemia	Chemotherapy
Lung cancer	Procainamide
Colon cancer	Sulfonamide
Ovarian cancer	Phenytoin
Sarcomas	Methyldopa
	Allopurinol
Fungal	Bacillus Calmette Guérin
Histoplasma	Steroids
Cryptococcosis	
Coccidioides	**Parasitic**
Aspergillus	Leishmaniasis
Blastomycosis	Malaria

MALT, mucosa-associated lymphoid tissue; NSAID, nonsteroidal anti-inflammatory drug.

and lymphocytes encircling a central lipid vacuole, creating the appearance of a donut ring. Although lipogranulomas are most commonly associated with Q fever, it is important to note that they may also be present in other infections including Epstein-Barr virus (EBV), cytomegalovirus (CMV), and leishmaniasis.

Whipple Disease

Whipple disease is a bacterial infection caused by *Tropheryma whipplei*. It commonly involves the gastrointestinal tract; however, organisms can also be present within the bone marrow, spleen, and lymph nodes (*Br J Haematol*. 2001;112:677). The organism, which is often rod or sickle shaped, can be highlighted by PAS stain and may be present both within and outside of macrophages. Other nonspecific findings include the presence of noncaseating granulomas and increased marrow cellularity.

Tick-Borne Diseases

Tick-borne illnesses such as anaplasmosis, ehrlichiosis, and rickettsioses may manifest changes in the bone marrow such as granuloma formation, dysplastic features, and hemophagocytosis. Anaplasmosis is caused by the intracellular gram-negative organism *Anaplasma phagocytophilum*. It infects myeloid cells and has been shown to cause dyserythropoiesis and dysmegakaryopoiesis, leading to peripheral cytopenias (*J Clin Exp Hematop.* 2017;56:160). Ehrlichiosis, caused by *E. chaffeensis* and *E. ewingii* species, is an intracellular bacterium that primarily infects neutrophils and monocytes. Like anaplasmosis, ehrlichiosis can cause cytopenia and dysplastic changes. Although rare, morula have been identified in bone marrow samples (*Hum Pathol.* 1993;24:391). Rickettsioses such as *Rickettsia rickettsii*, *R. prowazekii*, and *R. typhi* may also cause cytopenias, and granuloma formation in the bone marrow and formation of lipogranulomas have also been reported. Anaplasmosis, ehrlichiosis, and the rickettsioses have all been shown to cause hemophagocytic lymphohistiocytosis (HLH), which will be discussed in a later section of this chapter.

Syphilis

Syphilis, a sexually transmitted infection caused by the bacterium *Treponema pallidum*, may cause nonspecific findings in the bone marrow such as lymphoid aggregates, non-necrotizing granulomas, and hemophagocytosis. It has also been shown to cause HLH (*Eur J Pediatr.* 1999;158:553).

II. PARASITIC AND PROTOZOAL INFECTIONS

Although parasitic infections more commonly manifest in the peripheral blood, there are several organisms that may be present within the bone marrow. Granulomas, changes in cellularity, and necrosis may be the only findings in some infections, while in others identification of the organism itself may be possible.

Leishmaniasis

Leishmaniasis, caused by *Leishmania* species, is an intracellular protozoan parasite. It most commonly infects the skin, but cases of visceral leishmaniasis may affect the bone marrow. Identification of bone marrow involvement by organisms is a vital component in making the diagnosis of visceral spread. Characteristic amastigotes, termed Leishman-Donovan bodies (LDBs), may be present within monocytes/histiocytes. To distinguish LDBs from other inclusions, a nucleus and a smaller rodlike kinetoplast should be visualized. Intracellular amastigotes may be difficult to distinguish from other infections like tuberculosis, cryptococcosis, and brucellosis, thus visualization of the kinetoplast is essential. Special stains such as Grocott methenamine silver (GMS) and PAS will be negative in leishmaniasis. A Giemsa stain may also help to visualize the nucleus and kinetoplast. Other less specific findings may include hypercellular marrow, dyspoiesis, plasmacytosis, granulomas, hemophagocytosis, fibrosis, lymphoid aggregates, and necrosis.

Trypanosomiasis

Trypanosomiasis is caused by *Trypanosoma* species including *T. brucei gambiense*, *T. b. brucei*, *T. b. rhodesiense*, and *T. b. cruzi*. Trypanosomes are a group of parasitic flagellate protozoa that are commonly seen in peripheral blood. However, the presence of trypomastigotes and amastigotes in the bone marrow of immunocompromised patients has been reported.

Toxoplasmosis

Toxoplasmosis is an infection caused by the parasite *Toxoplasma gondii*. In immunocompetent individuals, granulomas may be the only finding present. However, in immunocompromised patients, tachyzoites (also called trophozoites) may be present. Tachyzoites are oblong shaped and contain a single large nucleus. Cysts containing bradyzoites may less commonly be seen. PAS can be performed in which staining will be positive in bradyzoite cysts but negative in tachyzoites.

Malaria

Malaria is a febrile illness caused by *Plasmodium* (including *P. vivax* and *P. falciparum*) parasites. Organisms are usually identified on peripheral blood smears. During infection, bone marrow is commonly hypercellular with macrophage proliferation, hemophagocytosis, and dyserythropoiesis (*J Infect Dis*. 2022;225:1274). During acute attacks, gametocytes, rings, and schizonts may be present. As part of their survival, malaria digests hemoglobin, which releases free heme. Free heme is toxic to cells, and thus it is converted into an insoluble crystal form called hemozoin (also called malaria pigment). Hemozoin can be seen on hematoxylin and eosin (H&E) where it appears as black-brown pigment within red blood cells (RBCs).

Babesiosis

Like malaria, babesiosis is an intraerythrocytic parasite. On peripheral smear, the intraerythrocytic ring is similar to that seen in malaria. However, characteristic tetrads, also called Maltese crosses, may be seen. Babesiosis commonly leads to dyserythropoiesis, thrombocytopenia, subsequent anemia, and has been reported to cause secondary HLH in several case studies (*Ann Clin Microbiol Antimicrob*. 2017;16:6).

Filariasis

Filariasis is caused by infections by nematodes such as *Wuchereria bancrofti*, *Loa loa*, and *Brugia malayi*. Infection causes eosinophilia and circulating microfilariae can be seen in peripheral blood. Although it is uncommon, microfilariae may also be observed in the bone marrow. The length, presence or absence of a sheath, and tail appearance can help classify the type of microfilariae.

III. FUNGAL INFECTIONS

Disseminated fungal infections are more prevalent in immunocompromised patients or in special circumstances such as chemotherapy, total parenteral nutrition, or use of broad-spectrum antibiotics. Prudent examination of peripheral blood and bone marrow, along with the use of special stains such as GMS and PAS, is key to establishing a diagnosis. However, the use of other techniques, such as molecular testing, is required for speciation. In general, fungal infections are associated with the formation of granulomas in the bone marrow.

Coccidioidomycosis and Paracoccidioidomycosis

Coccidioides immitis is a fungal infection endemic to the western United States and Mexico. In disseminated cases the organism may be present in the bone marrow. It has a unique morphology consisting of a large spherule (10-80 μm) containing smaller endospores (2-5 μm). The spherules of endospores are commonly located within granulomas or lymphoid aggregates. Eosinophilia may also be present. A similar dimorphic fungus, *Paracoccidioides brasiliensis*, is endemic in Mexico and South America. Granulomas, lymphoid aggregates, and giant cells may be present in the bone marrow during infection. Both *Coccidioides* and *Paracoccidioides* can be highlighted with a GMS or PAS stain.

Cryptococcosis

In patients with HIV, cryptococcosis is one of the most common fungal infections. It is caused by the fungus *Cryptococcus neoformans*, which is easy to identify due to its characteristic thick capsule. However, one should not use size to help establish the diagnosis of cryptococcosis as it may vary from 3 to 15 μm. Patients with bone marrow involvement by *Cryptococcus* commonly have pancytopenia and granulomas may be present. A Wright stain will highlight fungal elements on aspirate, while PAS, mucicarmine, and GMS will be positive in tissue.

Aspergillosis

Aspergillosis, caused by *Aspergillus fumigatus*, most commonly infects the sinopulmonary tract. However, the bone marrow may be involved in immunocompromised individuals or via anatomic barrier disruption such as after trauma or surgery. Organisms, which are 2.5 to 8.0 μm in size and have characteristic 45° angle branching, may be highlighted with GMS stain. Areas of frank necrosis may be present. In non-necrotic areas, granulomas and increased macrophages may be seen.

Histoplasmosis

Endemic to the Ohio River valley, *Histoplasma capsulatum* is a dimorphic fungus that consists of small budding yeast forms. The helmet-shaped yeasts are usually present within neutrophils and macrophages. They are uniformly small, measuring only 2 to 5 μm. Granulomas and hemophagocytosis may also be present. Fungal elements may be better seen on Giemsa, GMS, and PAS staining.

Blastomycosis

Blastomycosis is caused by the dimorphic fungus *Blastomyces dermatitidis*, which is endemic to the Ohio and Mississippi River valleys. Although it typically infects the skin and respiratory tract, bone marrow involvement can occur, even in immunocompetent individuals. The organisms of size 40 μm have pathognomonic broad-based budding and can be highlighted by a GMS stain.

Mucormycosis

Mucormycosis is a particularly deadly infection caused by angioinvasive fungal species in the order Mucorales. The fungus commonly infects the sinonasal tract and lungs but can disseminate to involve the bone marrow. Morphologically, it has wide ribbon-like filaments that branch at 90° without septae.

III. VIRAL INFECTIONS

HIV/AIDS

HIV/AIDS involvement of the bone marrow is termed HIV myelopathy, and nearly all patients with HIV/AIDS will have changes in their bone marrow. Bone marrow findings may depend on the patient's current viral status, medication use, concurrent infection, etc. A myriad of different manifestations may be seen in HIV myelopathy, although most changes are nonspecific. More common changes include granulomas and/or collections of histiocytes, hypercellular bone marrow, lymphoid aggregates, increased plasma cells, increased fibrosis, and even gelatinous transformation of marrow.

The megakaryocytic cell line is particularly affected by HIV/AIDS as the virus can directly infect the cells. As a result, dyspoietic changes such as small and/or clustered megakaryocytes, large forms, abnormal lobation, and increase in number may be present. Perhaps the most pathognomonic sign of HIV myelopathy is seeing naked megakaryocytes, in which cells are stripped leaving only nuclei remaining. This finding has been reported in over half of patients with HIV myelopathy (*Afr J Med Med Sci*. 2006;35 suppl:85). Other less specific findings can include granulocytes with Pelger-Huet anomalies, myeloid and erythroid cells with vacuolation, and plasma cell inclusions (such as Dutcher or Russell bodies).

One of the reasons bone marrow examination may be necessary in patients with HIV/AIDS is to elucidate a cause of cytopenia, which is a common occurrence. Cytopenia(s) may be due to infection, hematologic neoplasms, medication side effect, or the virus itself (*Hematol Transfus Cell Ther*. 2022;44:542).

Parvovirus B19

Parvovirus B19 is a DNA virus that infects RBC precursors. In patients with underlying disorders associated with a decreased RBC life span (such as hereditary spherocytosis), infection can lead to severe anemia due to RBC aplasia. Bone marrow biopsy during acute infection can show unique and somewhat specific findings of large pronormoblasts with ground glass intranuclear viral inclusions. These are sometimes called lantern cells, due to the shape of the inclusion appearing like a lantern. Immunohistochemistry for the virus can be performed to confirm that the viral inclusions are due to parvovirus and not another viral entity.

Epstein-Barr Virus

EBV is a double-stranded DNA virus that causes infectious mononucleosis. Although it is commonly associated with large, atypical lymphocytes (Downey cells) in peripheral blood, changes may also be present in the bone marrow. During acute infection, lymphocytosis and an increase in myeloid to erythroid ratio may be seen. Granulomas or hemophagocytosis may be present. One possible complication of EBV infection is chronic active EBV infection in which the viral replication is uncontrolled and EBV-infected cells proliferate. During this time, the bone marrow will show infiltrates of infected T or natural killer (NK) cells. Immunohistochemistry or in situ hybridization for EBV will highlight the infected cells.

Cytomegalovirus

CMV is a double-stranded DNA virus that also causes mononucleosis. While infection is commonly mild for immunocompetent individuals, it can affect hematopoiesis in immunocompromised patients. CMV infects monocytes, macrophages, and T cells. In the bone marrow, there may be nonspecific findings such as lymphocytosis, granulomas, and left shifted myelopoiesis. Immunostaining for the virus can help highlight infected cells, although only approximately 30% of cases will have the viral inclusions. A CD15 immunostain can also highlight infected cells.

COVID-19

Although bone marrow findings during acute COVID infection are still being investigated, studies have shown increase in cellularity of the bone marrow, megakaryocytic hyperplasia, myeloid left shift, and hemophagocytosis (*Am J Clin Pathol.* 2021;155:627).

IV. LIPID STORAGE DISORDERS

Lipid storage disorders, which occur due to enzyme defects in lipid metabolism pathway, lead to buildup of different substances that can be seen in the bone marrow. There are a wide variety of storage disorders (Table 5.1-2), but three of the most common are Gaucher, Niemann-Pick, and Fabry disease.

Gaucher

Gaucher disease is an autosomal recessive disorder caused by mutations in beta-glucosylceramidase, which leads to accumulation of glucocerebroside. The pathognomonic Gaucher cells are histiocytes with wrinkled tissue paper cytoplasm that stain positive for PAS and Tartrate-resistant acid phosphatase (TRAP or TRAPase). Additionally, Gaucher disease has been associated with B-cell neoplasms and amyloidosis.

Niemann-Pick

Niemann-Pick disease is an autosomal recessive disorder caused by mutations in *SMPD1*, *NPC1*, or *NPC2*, which leads to a sphingomyelinase deficiency. In the bone marrow, histiocytes filled with many vacuoles, termed foam cells, are often present. Sea-blue histiocytes can also occur, which appear blue due to cytoplasmic

TABLE 5.1-2 Storage Disorders With Marrow Involvement

Gaucher disease
Niemann-Pick disease
Fabry disease
Mucolipidosis
Cystinosis
Tay-Sachs disease
Gangliosidosis
Alpha mannosidosis
Fucosidosis
Faber disease
Acid lipase deficiency
Sialic acid storage disease
Sandhoff disease
Tangier disease

accumulation of PAS-positive sphingomyelin. It is important to note that sea-blue histiocytes are a nonspecific finding and may also be present in other storage disorders.

Fabry Disease

Fabry disease is an X-linked disease caused by mutations in alpha-galactosidase A, which leads to accumulation of ceramide trihexoside (CTH). Fabry disease is another storage disorder that can cause sea-blue histiocytes. The granules can be highlighted with a Sudan Black B or PAS stain.

V. OTHER SYSTEMIC CONDITIONS

Hemophagocytic Lymphohistiocytosis

HLH is a potentially fatal group of disorders caused by a defective and uncontrolled immune response. HLH is divided into two categories, primary and secondary. Primary, also termed familial HLH, is due to genetic mutations, while secondary, also called acquired, is due to a myriad of conditions such as infection, malignancy, and autoimmune diseases (Table 5.1-3).

Primary HLH can be inherited or occur sporadically. Common mutations include *PRF1*, *UNC13D*, *MUNC12-4*, *STX11*, *RAB27*, *STXBP2*. Primary HLH may also be associated with underlying immunodeficiency syndromes, such as Chediak-Higashi or X-linked lymphoproliferative syndrome.

When secondary HLH occurs due to rheumatologic or autoimmune disorders, it is also called macrophage activation syndrome (MAS). HLH/MAS has a strong association with systemic juvenile arthritis (SJIA), but has also been associated with

TABLE 5.1-3 Infectious Etiologies Associated With Hemophagocytic Lymphohistiocytosis (HLH)

Viral	Bacterial
Epstein-Barr virus	Brucella
Cytomegalovirus	Rickettsia
Hepatitis	Leptospira
HIV	Tuberculosis
Parvovirus	Anaplasma
Herpes simplex	Salmonella
Varicella-zoster	Ehrlichia
Measles	Syphilis
Human herpesvirus 8	Typhoid
Influenza virus	Other gram-negative bacteria
Parasitic	**Fungal**
Leishmaniasis	Histoplasma
Malaria	Candida
Babesia	Mucor

other disorders such as systemic lupus erythematosus (SLE). Malignancy-associated HLH most commonly occurs with hematopoietic malignancies such as T/NK-cell lymphoma, B-cell lymphomas, and plasma cell myeloma. It can also occur in conjunction with solid tumors such as thymomas or germ cell tumors. A broad number of infectious agents are associated with secondary HLH.

Clinically, HLH commonly presents with fever, fatigue, myalgia, hepatosplenomegaly, coagulopathy, and lymphadenopathy. Diagnosis requires mutation involving one of the genes associated with HLH or at least five of the eight following criteria (*Pediatr Blood Cancer*. 2007;48:124):

- Fever
- Splenomegaly
- Cytopenia affecting more than two cell lines: hemoglobin less than 90 g/L, platelets less than 100×10^9/L, neutrophils less than 1.0×10^9/L
- Hypertriglyceridemia and/or hypofibrinogenemia: fasting triglycerides 3.0 mmol/L or more (ie, ≥265 mg/dL), fibrinogen 1.5 g/L or less
- Hemophagocytosis in bone marrow or spleen or lymph nodes
- Decreased or absent NK-cell activity (according to local laboratory reference)
- Ferritin 500 μg/L or more
- Soluble CD25 (ie, soluble interleukin [IL]-2 receptor) 2,400 U/m or more

Aspirate smear is commonly hypocellular and may demonstrate hemophagocytosis, ingestion of hematologic cells by macrophages (e-Figure 5.1-3). Macrophages otherwise appear normal in morphology. The most common cells to be phagocytosed are erythrocytes. The bone marrow core may also be hypocellular with fibrosis, plasmacytosis, and hemophagocytosis. If infection-associated HLH is suspected, immunohistochemical or in situ hybridization for studies for EBV or other etiologies can be considered.

Amyloidosis

Amyloid, consisting of abnormally folded proteins, can deposit in the wall of vessels and interstitium of bone marrow. Both primary amyloidosis and amyloid deposition secondary to myeloma may involve the bone marrow. The eosinophilic material can also appear as pink to purple globules on aspirate. Special stains such as PAS, crystal violet, thioflavin T, and Congo red can be performed to confirm the presence of amyloid. Amyloid stained with thioflavin and Congo red will demonstrate birefringence under polarization.

Autoimmune Diseases and Collagen Vascular Disorders

In general, collagen vascular disorders present with several nonspecific findings in the bone marrow including lymphoid aggregates, granulomas, sea-blue histiocytes, and megaloblastic erythroid changes. Bony abnormalities such as osteosclerosis or osteopenia may also be present. Bone marrow cellularity is highly variable.

SLE is associated with cytopenias including anemia, thrombocytopenia, and leukopenia. Marrow findings include increased marrow fibrosis, lymphoplasmacytic infiltration, and hemophagocytosis. The erythroid lineage may show dysplastic changes including nuclear budding, multinucleation, and abnormal nuclear contours. Small immature megakaryocytes may also be seen (*Am J Hematol*. 2006;81:590).

Rheumatoid arthritis can cause large granular lymphocytosis (LGL) and is also associated with LGL leukemia. Immune thrombocytopenia (idiopathic thrombocytopenic purpura [ITP]), which leads to the destruction of platelets via antibodies, causes an increased number of small megakaryocytes. Additionally, rosette-like formations consisting of megakaryocytes surrounded by lymphocytes can rarely occur with ITP.

Autoimmune myelofibrosis commonly results in an acellular aspirate. The bone marrow core will generally appear normal apart from fibrosis. In the early stages, fibrosis may not be identifiable in H&E. Use of a reticulin stain can help to highlight early fibrosis while trichrome will highlight advanced stage fibrosis.

SUGGESTED READINGS

Diebold J, Molina T, Camilleri-Broët S, Le Tourneau A, Audouin J. Bone marrow manifestations of infections and systemic diseases observed in bone marrow trephine biopsy review. *Histopathology.* 2000;37(3):199-211.

O'Malley DP, Smith L, Fedoriw Y. Benign causes of bone marrow abnormalities including infections, storage diseases, systemic disorders, and stromal changes. In: Hsi ED, ed. *Foundations in Diagnostic Pathology, Hematopathology.* 3rd ed. Elsevier; 2018.

5.2 Bone Marrow Failure Syndromes

Ying-Chen Claire Hou and Julie Ann Neidich

Bone marrow failure (BMF) is caused by ineffective hematopoiesis of the bone marrow and is attributed to either acquired or inherited causes. BMF commonly manifests as pancytopenia in the peripheral blood. Differentiating inherited bone marrow failure syndromes (IBMFS) from acquired aplastic anemia (AA) is important for accurate diagnosis, disease-specific management, surveillance, and risk evaluation of relatives. IBMFS include Fanconi anemia (FA), dyskeratosis congenita (DC), Diamond-Blackfan anemia (DBA), and Shwachman-Diamond syndrome (SDS), which are frequently observed in children, constituting roughly 25% to 30% of constitutional/inherited bone marrow aplasia cases.

I. ACQUIRED CAUSES OF BONE MARROW FAILURE

Aplastic Anemia

Acquired AA is characterized by peripheral blood pancytopenia and hypocellular bone marrow. Anemia and thrombocytopenia are the most frequent manifestations, and neutropenia is less common. Hepatosplenomegaly and lymphadenopathy are typically not observed. Most patients are diagnosed between 10 and 25 years of age with presentations of bleeding tendency, fatigue, and infection. The incidence of AA is estimated at 1 to 2 cases per million population per year in the United States. The incidence rate is two or three times higher in Asia (*Haematologica.* 2008;93:518-523). Most acquired AA occurs without any identifiable causes. Autoimmune disorders or environmental factors, including infections, drugs, chemicals, or nutrition deficiency, have been linked to acquired AA as etiologies. Immunosuppressive therapy and hematopoietic stem cell transplantation (HSCT) are treatment options for patients with AA (*Pediatr Clin North Am*. 2013;60:1311-1336).

II. INHERITED BONE MARROW FAILURE SYNDROMES

Fanconi Anemia

- **Clinical Features**
  FA is the most common IBMFS. The hallmark of FA pathogenesis is defective homologous recombination of double-stranded DNA repair pathways in response to alkylating agents or cytotoxic drugs. FA is characterized by physical abnormalities, progressive BMF, and an increased risk of cancer. Physical abnormalities, including short stature, abnormal skin pigmentation (hypo- and hyperpigmentation or café-au-lait spots), and skeletal malformations of the upper and/or lower limbs, are commonly observed in patients with FA. Microcephaly, microphthalmia, genitourinary tract anomalies, endocrine disorders, and hypogonadism are also observed. Approximately 60% of patients with FA were reported to have at least one physical abnormality (*Blood Rev*. 2010;24:101-122).

  The prevalence of FA is estimated from 1 in 100,000 to 250,000 births and has been observed in all races. Populations, including Ashkenazi Jews, Afrikaners, northern Europeans, sub-Saharan Blacks, and Spanish Gypsies, with founder variants have increased carrier frequencies. The ratio of males to females is 1:1.2 (Fanconi anemia. In: *GeneReviews*. 2002 [Updated 2021]). The age of onset of BMF for patients with FA is highly variable, and the median age at diagnosis was 6.5 years (*Blood Rev*. 2010;24:101-122). BMF has been reported in 80% of patients with FA, and the cumulative incidence was 90% by age 40. Head and neck, skin, and genitourinary tract cancers are common in patients with FA (*Blood*. 101;4:1249-1256).

- **Histologic Features**
  The bone marrow of FA patients usually shows hypocellularity for age depending on the stage of the disease, and dyserythropoiesis in more than 90% of patients (*Blood*. 1994;84:1650-1655). In the early stages, bone marrow might be normocellular. With disease progression, bone marrow becomes hypocellular, indistinguishable from AA. FA-related myelodysplastic syndromes (MDS) are associated with an increase in blasts and the presence of dysgranulopoiesis (*Am J Clin Pathol*. 2010;133:92-100).

- **Diagnosis and Genetic Testing**
  The chromosomal breakage test is the diagnostic testing method for FA. Clinical diagnosis of FA is established when lymphocytes treated with diepoxybutane (DEB) and mitomycin C (MMC) show increased chromosomal breakage and radial forms on cytogenetic testing (Fanconi anemia. In: *GeneReviews*. 2002 [Updated 2021]). FA is inherited in an autosomal recessive pattern and rarely inherited in an X-linked recessive pattern. FA is caused by pathogenic variants in one of 23 FA-associated genes that encode proteins involved in DNA damage response (Table 5.2-1) (*Exp Hematol*. 2022;105:18-21). Patients with FA with *FANCA* pathogenic variants are the most commonly observed (60%). Patients with FA with *FANCC* and *FANCG* variants are the next most common, consisting of 15% and 10%, respectively (Fanconi anemia. In: *GeneReviews*. 2002 [Updated 2021]). Therefore, sequencing analysis of *FANCA*, which detects missense, nonsense, splice site variants, and small intragenic deletions/insertions, can be performed first. Gene-specific deletion and duplication analysis can be performed to detect exon and whole-gene deletions

TABLE 5.2-1 Inherited Bone Marrow Failure Syndromes

	Fanconi Anemia	Dyskeratosis Congenita	Diamond-Blackfan Anemia	Shwachman-Diamond Syndrome
Age of onset, median (range)	6.5 y (birth to 64 y)	14 y (birth to 79 y)	3 mo (birth to 87 y)	2 wk (birth to 39 y)
Genes	BRCA1, BRCA2, BRIP1, ERCC4, FAAP100, FANCA, FANCB, FANCC, FANCD2, FANCE, FANCF, FANCG, FANCI, FANCL, FANCM, PALB2, RAD51C, REV7, RFWD3, SLX4, UBE2T, XRCC2	ACD, CTC1, DKC1, NAF1, NHP2, NOP10, PARN, POT1, RPA1, RTEL1, STN1, TERC, TERT, TINF2, WRAP53, ZCCHC8	GATA1, RPL5, RPL9, RPL11, RPL15, RPL18, RPL26, RPL27, RPL31, RPL35, RPL35A, RPS7, RPS10, RPS15A, RPS17, RPS19, RPS24, RPS26, RPS27, RPS28, RPS29, TSR2	DNAJC21, EFL1, SBDS, SRP54
Prevalence	1:100,000-250,000	800-1,000 individuals	1:150,000	1:200,000
Inheritance	AR and X-linked recessive	AD, AR, and X-linked recessive	AD	AR
Diagnostic test	Increased chromosome breakage with DEB or MMC; gene sequencing	Decreased telomere length by flow cytometry, FISH, gene sequencing	Increased fetal hemoglobin and erythrocyte adenosine deaminase activity, gene sequencing	Decreased pancreatic enzymes (trypsinogen and isoamylase), gene sequencing

AD, autosomal dominant; AR, autosomal recessive; DEB, diepoxybutane; FISH, fluorescence in situ hybridization; MMC, mitomycin C.

or duplications. A multigene panel test that includes 23 FA-associated genes may be considered if single-gene testing does not detect *FANCA* pathogenic variants. Exome or genome sequencing may be considered if single-gene or multigene panel testing does not provide a molecular diagnosis in an individual with FA features.

- **Prognosis and Treatment**
  For patients with FA, the relative risk for acute myeloid leukemia (AML) is approximately 500-fold, and the relative risk for solid tumors is 500- to 700-fold higher than in the general population. The use of oral androgens has been shown to improve blood counts. Life expectancy for FA ranges from birth to 64 years, and the median age of survival is 39 years (*Blood Rev.* 2010;24:101-122). For the hematologic manifestations, HSCT is the only curative therapy. Management by a multidisciplinary team is recommended.

Dyskeratosis Congenita

- **Clinical Features**
  The phenotype spectrum of DC and telomere biology disorders is broad, ranging from children with multisystem disorders to adults with one or two DC features. The hallmark of DC pathogenesis is defective telomere maintenance, and patients with DC have very short telomere length. DC affects many parts of the body and is characterized by a triad of abnormal-shaped fingernails and toenails, changes in skin pigmentation of the upper chest and/or neck, and oral leukoplakia (Dyskeratosis congenita and related telomere biology disorders. In: *GeneReviews*. 2009 [Updated 2022]).

  The prevalence of DC is not known, and approximately 800 to 1,000 cases have been reported (Dyskeratosis congenita and related telomere biology disorders. In: *GeneReviews*. 2009 [Updated 2022]). The ratio of males to females is 1.8:1. The median age at diagnosis is 14 years (*Blood Rev.* 2010;24:101-122). Patients with DC also have an increased risk for progressive BMF, MDS, AML, solid tumors (head/neck squamous cell cancer or anogenital adenocarcinoma), and pulmonary fibrosis. Dysplastic nails are observed in nearly all patients with DC. The cumulative incidence of BMF in patients with DC is 45% by age 40. Severe subtypes of DC with multisystem disorders include Hoyeraal-Hreidarsson (HH) syndrome, Revesz syndrome (RS), and Coats plus syndrome (*Hematol Oncol Clin North Am.* 2009;23:215-231).

- **Histologic Features**
  The bone marrow of patients with DC typically exhibits hypocellularity correlated with the severity of BMF (*Haematologica*. 2012;97:353-359). Features of dysplasia in one or more lineages are often present (*Hematology Am Soc Hematol Educ Program*. 2011;2011:480-486).

- **Diagnosis and Genetic Testing**
  Telomere length measurement can be performed by multicolor flow cytometry fluorescence in situ hybridization (flow-FISH). When comparing telomere length between patients with DC and unaffected relatives, less than the 1st percentile for age in lymphocyte subsets had a sensitivity of 97% and specificity of 91%, and 85% positive predictive value (*Haematologica*. 2012;97:353-359). Abnormally short telomeres (<1st percentile for age) in four out of six leukocyte subsets, excluding granulocytes, are correlated with the diagnosis of DC (*Hematol Oncol Clin North Am.* 2009;23:215-231). DC is inherited in an X-linked recessive, autosomal dominant, or autosomal recessive pattern. DC is caused by pathogenic variants in one of 16 telomere biology pathway genes that encode proteins involved in telomere maintenance (Table 5.2-1). A multigene panel test that includes 16 DC-associated

genes is likely to detect the pathogenic variants in patients with DC features. Exome or genome sequencing may be considered if multigene panel testing does not provide a molecular diagnosis in patients with DC features. Approximately 20% of individuals with DC features did not have identifiable pathogenic variants after multigene panel testing (*Hematol Oncol Clin North Am.* 2009;23:215-231).

- **Prognosis and Treatment**
Morbidity is typically caused by BMF, cancer, and/or lung complications due to fibrosis. The cumulative incidence of MDS and AML is 20% by age 50 and of solid tumors is 20% by age 65. Life expectancy ranges from infancy to late adulthood, and the median age of survival is 51 years (*Blood Rev.* 2010;24:101-122). HSCT and lung transplantation are the only current therapeutic options for BMF and pulmonary fibrosis, respectively, but are complicated by numerous comorbidities (*Expert Rev Hematol.* 2019;12:1037-1052).

Diamond-Blackfan Anemia

- **Clinical Features**
DBA is a clinically and genetically heterogeneous BMF disorder caused by defective ribosome biogenesis, known as ribosomopathies. The clinical features of DBA include macrocytic anemia, physical abnormalities, growth deficiency, and predisposition to cancer. The hematologic phenotype ranges from mild anemia to severe fetal anemia resulting in nonimmune hydrops fetalis. Approximately 50% of patients with DBA have at least one physical abnormality, including craniofacial features, upper limb anomalies, genitourinary malformations, and heart defects.

  The median age at diagnosis for patients with DBA is 3 months. The prevalence of DBA is estimated at 1:150,000 with both sexes equally affected, and the incidence is consistent across ethnicities (*Br J Haematol.* 2008;142:859-856). DBA is associated with an increased risk of AML, osteosarcoma, colon cancer, lung cancer, or cervical cancer (Diamond-Blackfan anemia. In: *GeneReviews.* 2009 [Updated 2021]).

- **Histologic Features**
The bone marrow of patients with DBA is usually normocellular for age. Erythroid precursors are absent or sparsely distributed in a few small clusters consisting of proerythroblasts, lacking maturing/matured erythroid cells. Mild dysplastic changes are often observed. Granulopoiesis and megakaryopoiesis are usually preserved, and lymphocytes are frequently increased (*Br J Haematol.* 2008;142:859-856).

- **Diagnosis and Genetic Testing**
The clinical diagnosis of DBA is established with the following features: macrocytic anemia with onset before age 1 year, no other significant cytopenias, reticulocytopenia, and normal marrow cellularity with a paucity of erythroid precursors. Elevated fetal hemoglobin and erythrocyte adenosine deaminase activity are supporting criteria for the diagnosis of DBA. DBA is inherited in an X-linked recessive and autosomal dominant manner and is caused by pathogenic variant(s) in one of 22 DBA-associated genes that encode ribosomal proteins (Table 5.2-1). Approximately 25% of patients with DBA have a pathogenic variant in the *RPS19* gene. A multigene panel test that includes 22 DBA-associated genes can be used for the clinical diagnosis of DBA. Exome or genome sequencing may be considered if multigene panel testing does not provide a molecular diagnosis in patients with DBA features. Approximately 20% of patients with DBA do not have identifiable pathogenic variants after multigene panel testing (Diamond-Blackfan anemia. In: *GeneReviews.* 2009 [Updated 2021]).

- **Prognosis and Treatment**
  Patients with DBA have an increased risk of lung, colon, and cervical cancer compared to the general population. In patients with DBA, the cumulative incidence of severe BMF is 50% by age 70, and of solid tumors is 50% by age 70. Life expectancy ranges from infancy to late adulthood, and the median age of survival is 67 years (*Haematologica*. 2018;103:30-39). Corticosteroids and red blood cell transfusions are the main treatment for anemia in patients with DBA. For patients with DBA who are transfusion-dependent or develop other cytopenias, HSCT is recommended and is the only curative therapy. Management by a multidisciplinary team is recommended (Diamond-Blackfan anemia. In: *GeneReviews*. 2009 [Updated 2021]).

Shwachman-Diamond Syndrome

- **Clinical Features**
  SDS is a multisystem disease, involving the bone marrow, pancreas, skeleton, and other organs. The clinical features of SDS include BMF, exocrine pancreatic dysfunction, and predisposition to MDS/AML. Intermittent or persistent neutropenia is the most common hematologic manifestation and is often observed in the neonatal period. Exocrine pancreatic dysfunction is usually observed within the first year of life with manifestations of malabsorption, steatorrhea, and failure to thrive. Skeletal, cardiac, neurocognitive, gastrointestinal, and immune systems are also affected in patients with SDS (*Ann N Y Acad Sci*. 2011;1242:40-55).

  The prevalence of SDS is estimated at 1:200,000 and the ratio of males to females is 1:1.3. The median age at diagnosis for patients with SDS was 2 weeks (*Blood Rev*. 2010;24:101-122). The cumulative incidence of BMF is 40% by age 50. The cumulative incidence of MDS/AML is approximately 20% by age 20 and 36% by age 30 (*Haematologica*. 2012;97:1312-1319).

- **Histologic Features**
  The bone marrow of patients with SDS typically exhibits hypocellularity for age or variable cellularity. In patients with SDS, mild dyshematopoiesis is commonly observed. Multilineage dysplasia is less common and may indicate malignant transformation (*Ann N Y Acad Sci*. 2011;1242:40-55).

- **Diagnosis and Genetic Testing**
  Hematologic abnormalities and exocrine pancreas dysfunction are criteria for the clinical diagnosis of SDS. Hematologic abnormalities include intermittent or persistent neutropenia, cytopenias of other blood cell lineages, or BMF. Reduced levels of pancreatic enzymes, including serum trypsinogen, serum isoamylase, and fecal elastase, are the hallmark of SDS (*Ann N Y Acad Sci*. 2011;1242:40-55). SDS is inherited in an autosomal recessive or autosomal dominant manner. Identification of biallelic pathogenic variants in *DNAJC21*, *EFL1*, and *SBDS* or a heterozygous pathogenic variant in *SRP54* is used to establish the molecular diagnosis of SDS. Targeted analysis of three common *SBDS* pathogenic variants, including c.183_184delinsCT, c.258+2T>C, or c.[183_184delinsCT; c.258+2T>C] resulting from gene conversion with *SBDSP*, can be performed first. The targeted analysis provides molecular diagnosis in 62% of affected patients with SDS. Parental testing is essential to determine *in cis* or *in trans* configuration for the complex allele, c.[183_184delinsCT; c.258+2T>C]. A multigene panel testing that includes four SDS-associated genes is likely to detect the pathogenic variants in patients with SDS features (Table 5.2-1). Exome or genome sequencing may also be considered if single or multigene panel testing does not provide a molecular diagnosis. Approximately 10% of patients with

SDS features did not have identifiable pathogenic variants from molecular testing (Shwachman-Diamond syndrome. In: *GeneReviews*. 2008 [Updated 2018]).
- **Prognosis and Treatment**
  Life expectancy ranges from infancy to late adulthood, and the median age of survival is 41 years (*Blood Rev*. 2010;24:101-122). Oral pancreatic enzyme treatment and fat-soluble vitamin supplementation for pancreatic dysfunction are employed in patients with SDS, and usually, the clinical response is excellent. Transfusions can be considered for anemia and/or thrombocytopenia. HSCT can be considered for the treatment of severe pancytopenia, MDS, or AML (*Ann N Y Acad Sci*. 2011;1242:40-55).

SUGGESTED READINGS

Mehta PA, Ebens C. Fanconi anemia. In: Adam MP, Everman DB, Mirzaa GM, et al, eds. *GeneReviews* [Internet]. University of Washington, Seattle; 2002 (Updated 2021). https://www.ncbi.nlm.nih.gov/books/NBK1401/

Nelson A, Myers K. Shwachman-Diamond syndrome. In: Adam MP, Everman DB, Mirzaa GM, et al, eds. *GeneReviews* [Internet]. University of Washington, Seattle; 2008 (Updated 2018). https://www.ncbi.nlm.nih.gov/books/NBK1756/

Savage SA, Niewisch MR. Dyskeratosis congenita and related telomere biology disorders. In: Adam MP, Everman DB, Mirzaa GM, et al, eds. *GeneReviews* [Internet]. University of Washington, Seattle; 2009 (Updated 2022). https://www.ncbi.nlm.nih.gov/books/NBK22301/

Lymph node

6.1: Reactive Lymphoid Hyperplasia and Benign Noninfectious Lymphadenopathies

Krithika Shenoy, Ekaterina Menshikova, Carina A. Dehner, and Brooj Abro

Reactive/nonneoplastic conditions can manifest with lymphadenopathy, and some benign entities mimic lymphoma. It is crucial to recognize the features of nonneoplastic causes of lymphadenopathy to avoid misdiagnosis of lymphoma. Several nonneoplastic causes of lymphadenopathy are also now included in the WHO-HAEM5 to facilitate the differential diagnosis of lymphoma and highlight potential pitfalls and nonneoplastic mimickers (see Table 6.1-1). This chapter discusses common and important causes of nonneoplastic and noninfectious lymphadenopathies. Infectious lymphadenopathies are discussed in Chapter 6.2.

I. REACTIVE LYMPHOID HYPERPLASIA PATTERNS

Reactive lymphoid hyperplasia (RLH) refers to a benign enlargement of lymphoid tissue from an expansion of one or more cellular compartments. It is a nonspecific response to a variety of intrinsic and environmental stimuli. Based on the predominant lymphoid compartment involved, RLH is divided into four main histologic patterns: follicular, interfollicular/paracortical, sinusoidal, and diffuse. A combination of one or more of these architectural patterns may be present in most cases. Evaluation of morphology in combination with clinical history and laboratory findings can help determine an underlying etiology. See Table 6.1-2 for a list of differential diagnoses based on the underlying histologic pattern (*Mod Pathol.* 2013;26(suppl 1):S88-S96; *Semin Diagn Pathol.* 2018;35:4-19).

- **Florid follicular hyperplasia**
  Follicular hyperplasia (FH) is the most frequently encountered pattern of RLH. It can occur at any age but is more frequent in children and young adults. Various infectious, autoimmune, and inflammatory conditions can cause florid follicular hyperplasia (FFH). The location of lymph node involvement and associated symptoms may suggest an underlying etiology. Histologically, FFH can mimic follicular lymphoma (FL). However, certain features help distinguish FFH from FL (Table 6.1-3 and e-Figure 6.1-1).
- **Paracortical hyperplasia**
  Reactive paracortical hyperplasia (PH) is characterized by benign expansion of the paracortical areas and represents a predominantly T-cell response to drugs, pollutants, viral infections, or vaccines. It affects mostly children and young adults and

TABLE 6.1-1 Nonneoplastic/Tumor-like Lesions Included in the WHO-HAEM5

Tumor-like lesions with B-cell predominance
- Reactive B-cell-rich proliferations that can mimic lymphoma
  - Florid follicular hyperplasia
  - Progressive transformation of germinal centers
  - Systemic lupus erythematosus
  - Sjogren's syndrome
  - Lymphoma-like lesions of the female genital tract
  - Rectal tonsil
  - Marginal zone hyperplasia
  - Infectious mononucleosis lymphadenitis
  - Cytomegalovirus lymphadenitis
  - Indolent B-lymphoblastic proliferation
- IgG4-related disease
- Unicentric Castleman disease
- Idiopathic multicentric Castleman disease
- KSHV/HHV8-associated multicentric Castleman disease

Tumor-like lesions with T-cell predominance
- Kikuchi-Fujimoto disease
- Autoimmune lymphoproliferative syndrome
- Indolent T-lymphoblastic proliferation

HHV8, human herpesvirus 8; IgG4, immunoglobulin G subclass 4; KSHV, Kaposi's sarcoma-associated herpesvirus.

presents as localized or generalized lymphadenopathy with or without constitutional symptoms. On histologic evaluation, the paracortex is expanded. The nodal architecture may be distorted but is not effaced. Paracortical areas demonstrate a mixture of small lymphocytes, larger lymphocytes, or immunoblasts with intermixed dendritic cells and histiocytes, imparting a mottled or "moth-eaten" appearance at low power. Significant cytologic atypia is absent. Occasionally, Hodgkin Reed-Sternberg (HRS)-like cells may be present. Vascularity may be increased with prominent high endothelial venules. PH can mimic T-cell lymphomas (TCLs). Helpful features that distinguish PH from TCLs include normal T-cell antigen expression and lack of effacement of nodal architecture. Clinical history and serologic studies may help identify the underlying cause of reactive PH.

- **Marginal zone hyperplasia**
Marginal zone (MZ) is usually prominent in the spleen but is not as readily identified in normal lymph nodes. In some cases of RLH, MZ can be prominent in the lymph nodes. In marginal zone hyperplasia (MZH), the expanded MZ comprises memory B cells with abundant cytoplasm, which gives it a pale appearance. The MZ B cells express pan B-cell markers and BCL2 but lack CD5 and CD10. In reactive MZH, the nodal architecture is preserved. Pediatric MZH may

TABLE 6.1-2 Pattern-Based Classification of Reactive Lymphoid Hyperplasia

Follicular pattern

- Reactive follicular hyperplasia
- Progressive transformation of germinal centers
- Castleman disease, hyaline-vascular type
- Autoimmune lymphadenopathies (eg, RA, SLE, SS)
- IgG4-related disease—types I, II, IV
- Kimura disease
- Infectious: toxoplasmosis, syphilis, HIV

Interfollicular, paracortical, and mixed patterns

- Reactive paracortical hyperplasia
- Dermatopathic lymphadenitis
- Kikuchi-Fujimoto disease
- Drug-associated lymphadenitis
- IgG4-related disease—type III
- Viral: EBV, CMV, HSV
- Castleman disease, plasma cell type

Sinus pattern

- Reactive sinus histiocytosis
- Monocytoid B-cell hyperplasia
- Sinus histiocytosis with massive lymphadenopathy (Rosai-Dorfman disease)
- Vascular transformation of sinuses

Diffuse pattern

- Various drugs and infections

CMV, cytomegalovirus; EBV, Epstein-Barr virus; HSV, herpes simplex virus; IgG4, immunoglobulin G subclass 4; RA, rheumatoid arthritis; SLE, systemic lupus erythematosus; SS, Sjogren's syndrome.

TABLE 6.1-3 Florid Follicular Hyperplasia (FFH) Versus Follicular Lymphoma (FL)

FFH	FL
Follicles are well-spaced.	High density of back-to-back follicles
A heterogeneous population of cells, including tangible body macrophages	Variable mixture of centrocytes and centroblasts. Tingible body macrophages are usually absent.
Moderate-to-high Ki-67	Usually low-to-moderate Ki-67
BCL2 is negative in reactive, secondary follicles.	BCL2 is usually positive in neoplastic follicles.

demonstrate monotypic immunoglobulin light chain expression without clonal immunoglobulin gene rearrangements (*Blood.* 2004;104:3343-3348). MZH should be distinguished from MZ lymphoma, which usually effaces or distorts the nodal architecture.

- **Sinus hyperplasia**

  Reactive sinus hyperplasia (SH) or benign expansion of lymph node sinuses can result from sinus histiocytosis, monocytoid B-cell hyperplasia, and vascular transformation of sinuses. Sinus histiocytosis is a common nonspecific reactive change in which lymph node sinuses become filled and expanded by histiocytes. The lymph node architecture is preserved. Histiocytes are confined within the sinuses and have a bland appearance consisting of oval or indented nuclei with indistinct nucleoli. Monocytoid B-cell hyperplasia in the sinuses can be seen in various inflammatory and infectious conditions, particularly in HIV and toxoplasmosis. The sinuses are expanded by mature B cells with abundant cytoplasm. Vascular transformation of sinuses is a benign entity also known as nodal angiomatosis. Endothelial cells proliferate and form complex networks of anastomosing capillary-like channels within nodal sinuses. It is usually an incidental finding most often seen in intra-abdominal lymph nodes.

II. DERMATOPATHIC LYMPHADENOPATHY

Dermatopathic lymphadenopathy (DL) is characterized by PH and usually manifests in skin-draining lymph nodes in chronic dermatologic disorders. DL can be associated with benign and neoplastic skin conditions, including chronic inflammatory dermatoses, mycosis fungoides, melanoma, squamous cell carcinoma, Kaposi sarcoma, and other chronic skin disorders/neoplasms. However, about half of the patients with DL do not have any dermatologic manifestations (*Mod Pathol.* 2020;33:1104-1121). Axillary and inguinal lymph nodes are the most common sites of involvement. If a lymph node is not enlarged, the term "dermatopathic changes" can be used.

On histologic examination, DL shows preserved lymph node architecture with paracortical expansion by a mixture of lymphocytes, interdigitating dendritic cells (IDCs), langerhans cells (LCs), and histiocytes with abundant eosinophilic cytoplasm resulting in irregular pale areas (e-Figure 6.1-2). IDCs and LCs show similar features on histology; both have ill-defined cell borders, pale cytoplasm, and elongated nuclei with linear grooves. Phagocytic cells may contain melanin and, less often, hemosiderin, grossly showing as a distinct pigmented rim underneath the lymph node capsule. Paracortical eosinophils are present in up to half of the cases (*Mod Pathol.* 2020;33:1104-1121). In later stages, paracortical expansion may be more confluent, compressing the follicles, and prominent plasmacytosis and immunoblast proliferation may be present.

In most cases, ancillary stains or tests are not required. Differential diagnosis includes LC histiocytosis, which causes at least partial architectural distortion, and the neoplastic cells are positive for S100, CD1a, and langerin (CD207). Early involvement by mycosis fungoides (MF) can look very similar to DL and is difficult to distinguish. Immunohistochemical studies for T-cell markers, flow cytometry, and TCR gene rearrangement studies may be helpful when MF is suspected.

III. INDOLENT B- AND T-LYMPHOBLASTIC PROLIFERATIONS

Indolent B- and T-lymphoblastic proliferations (IB-LBP and IT-LBP) are nonmalignant entities that may mimic malignancy. The key characteristic of these proliferations is their indolent clinical behavior.

- **Indolent B-lymphoblastic proliferations**
  IB-LBP, also known as hematogone hyperplasia, is a reactive immature B-cell proliferation that can mimic B-lymphoblastic lymphoma. IB-LBP is most frequently encountered in children. The lymph node is otherwise reactive appearing. The immature B cells are scattered individually or in small clusters within the paracortex and sinuses, are usually small, and show variable expression of TdT and B-cell markers. In contrast, B-lymphoblastic lymphoma shows larger cells, often in sheets effacing the nodal architecture, with a uniform expression of TdT and B-cell markers (*Am J Clin Pathol*. 2002;118:248-254).
- **Indolent T-lymphoblastic proliferation**
  IT-LBP is a reactive, non-clonal proliferation of immature T cells in lymph nodes or other extra-thymic tissues. It may be associated with neoplastic and nonneoplastic disorders, including autoimmune diseases, Castleman disease (CD), nodal TFH (T follicular helper cell) lymphoma, angioimmunoblastic type, and other tumors (*Int J Lab Hematol*. 2022;44:700-711). Histologic examination shows clusters or sheets of immature lymphoid cells without tissue destruction. The cells in IT-LBP are usually small, with minimal cytologic atypia, and show normal antigen expression pattern of precursor thymocytes (positive for TdT, CD3, other T-cell markers, and often double CD4 and CD8$^+$) and lack clonal TCR gene rearrangements (*Adv Anat Pathol*. 2013;20:137-140). In contrast, neoplastic cells of T-lymphoblastic lymphoma show cytologic atypia, aberrant antigen expression, and loss of T-cell markers and clonal TCR gene rearrangements.

IV. RECTAL TONSIL

Rectal tonsil, or rectal lymphoid polyp, is an uncommon reactive proliferation of unknown etiology characterized by localized lymphoid hyperplasia in the rectum. On endoscopy, it presents as a sessile or polypoid lesion. Histologically, rectal tonsil comprises a dense lymphoid infiltrate in the lamina propria or submucosa and shows features of RLH. FH with expanded germinal centers is typical (*World J Gastroenterol*. 2015;21:2563-2567). Differential diagnosis includes low-grade B-cell lymphomas. Immunophenotypic and clonality studies can be performed when there is suspicion of lymphoma.

V. LYMPHOMA-LIKE LESIONS OF THE FEMALE GENITAL TRACT

Florid lymphoid hyperplasia of the lower female genital tract, also known as pseudolymphoma or lymphoma-like lesion (LLL), is characterized by reactive B-cell-rich lymphoid proliferations that can mimic lymphoma. Etiology is unclear, but associations with infectious agents such as Epstein-Barr virus (EBV) have been reported (*Int J Gynecol Pathol*. 2022;41:459-469). The most common location is the cervix. Clinically, LLL is asymptomatic or can present as vaginal bleeding. Some patients are discovered to have LLL on follow-up of an abnormal pap smear (*Ann Diagn Pathol*. 2012;16:21-28). A pelvic exam may reveal ulceration or erosion. Histologically, these lesions usually show a superficial band-like polymorphous infiltrate of small lymphocytes, plasma cells (PCs), neutrophils, and scattered large cells. The large cells are usually intermixed within the polymorphous infiltrate and do not form diffuse sheets. Cytologically, they may resemble centroblasts, immunoblasts, or mimic HRS cells (*Ann Diagn Pathol*. 2012;16:21-28). Other common findings include the presence of reactive lymphoid follicles and ulceration of superficial epithelium. LLL can mimic diffuse large B-cell lymphoma and MZ lymphoma, making it challenging to distinguish from lymphoma, particularly on small biopsies. The presence of monoclonal *IGH/IGK* gene rearrangement is not uncommon, which can be misleading. The diagnosis requires clinicopathologic correlation. These lesions are benign and do not show clinical signs and symptoms of lymphoma.

VI. PROGRESSIVE TRANSFORMATION OF GERMINAL CENTERS

Progressive Transformation of Germinal Centers (PTGC) is typically an incidental finding in reactive lymph nodes and is often discovered in children and young adults. Patients are generally asymptomatic or present with localized lymphadenopathy, usually involving the cervical lymph nodes. Axillary and inguinal lymph node groups can also be involved. In PTGC nodules, the mantle zones are typically prominent and thickened. Small lymphocytes from the mantle zone "invade" and eventually disrupt the structure of the germinal center (e-Figure 6.1-3). Five immuno-architectural patterns have been described, ranging from thickened or scalloped mantle zones to complete obliteration of the germinal centers (*Hum Pathol*. 2015;46:1655-1661). PTGC can also be associated with lymphoma and coexist with nodular lymphocyte predominant Hodgkin lymphoma (NLPHL). Early involvement by NLPHL may be difficult to exclude in small biopsies, and excisional biopsies should be performed if there is concern for lymphoma. Unlike NLPHL, neoplastic lymphocyte predominant (LP) cells are absent in reactive lymph nodes with PTGC. Other differential diagnoses include FL (floral pattern) and IgG4 (immunoglobulin G subclass 4)-related disease. Although PTGC can be associated with lymphoma, the presence of PTGC on its own in otherwise reactive lymph nodes is not a risk factor for lymphoma (*Pediatr Blood Cancer*. 2013;60:26-30).

VII. KIKUCHI-FUJIMOTO DISEASE

Kikuchi-Fujimoto disease (KFD) is a rare necrotizing lymphadenitis of unknown etiology. Although the prevalence is higher in Asian countries, cases have been reported worldwide (*World J Clin Cases*. 2023;11:3664-3679). KFD most commonly affects young adults (<40 years of age) with a female preponderance (*Am J Clin Pathol*. 2004;122:141-152). Patients usually present with unilateral tender lymphadenopathy and may have systemic symptoms such as fever, fatigue, and respiratory symptoms (similar to viral illness). Skin involvement presenting as a rash is common. Posterior cervical lymph nodes are most commonly involved.

Characteristic histologic findings include the presence of pale, irregular/wedge-shaped foci in the paracortex composed of a variable mixture of lymphocytes, immunoblasts, plasmacytoid dendritic cells, histiocytes, necrotic and karyorrhectic debris (e-Figure 6.1-4). Neutrophils and eosinophils are absent, which provides clues to the diagnosis. The histologic findings evolve in three phases:

- **Proliferative phase:** characterized by the proliferation of plasmacytoid dendritic cells, histiocytes with crescent-shaped (C-shaped) nuclei, and scattered

immunoblasts. Necrosis and karyorrhectic debris are minimal. A purely proliferative phase is uncommon.
- **Necrotic phase:** most common phase encountered in biopsies. In addition to the proliferative phase findings, patchy necrotic areas are present.
- **Xanthomatous phase:** accumulation of foamy histiocytes

The necrotic phase of KFD overlaps with systemic lupus erythematosus (SLE)-associated lymphadenitis (*Am J Case Rep.* 2020;21:e922784). The diagnosis of KFD requires the integration of clinical and pathologic findings. Other etiologies (autoimmune conditions such as SLE, infections, lymphomas) should be excluded. KFD is a self-limited illness and usually spontaneously resolves within a few months. Patients may need symptomatic treatment.

VIII. KIMURA DISEASE

Kimura disease (KD) is a rare inflammatory disorder of unknown etiology that mainly affects individuals of Asian descent with a male predominance. Sporadic cases have been reported in other populations. KD usually involves the head and neck region; subcutaneous tissue, salivary glands, and lymph nodes may be involved. Patients usually present with mass-like growth in the head and neck region and localized lymphadenopathy. Systemic symptoms are uncommon. Laboratory evaluation shows peripheral blood eosinophilia ($>0.5 \times 10^9$/L) and elevated serum IgE levels (*Am J Surg Pathol.* 2004;28:505-513).

Morphologic findings (e-Figure 6.1-5) include FH with hyperplastic germinal centers and prominent mantle zones, eosinophilia, and eosinophilic microabscesses, a characteristic finding. PCs, mast cells, and Warthin-Finkeldey-type giant cells are also commonly present. Thin-walled capillaries may be prominent in the paracortex. Hyaline proteinaceous material (IgE deposits) can be seen within the germinal centers. Advanced cases may show marked capsular fibrosis and obliteration of subcapsular sinuses (*Am J Surg Pathol.* 2004;28:505-513). IgE immunohistochemistry/immunofluorescence highlights IgE deposits in the germinal centers.

Treatment options include surgical resection, radiation therapy, and steroid therapy. The prognosis is excellent; however, recurrences are common. The main differential diagnosis is angiolymphoid hyperplasia with eosinophilia (ALHE), also known as epitheloid hemangioma. The following features of ALHE differ from KD: more common in Caucasians and women, the lesion is localized to the skin, and lymph nodes are not involved.

IX. IMMUNOGLOBULIN G4-RELATED DISEASE ASSOCIATED LYMPHADENOPATHY

Immunoglobulin G4-related disease associated lymphadenopathy (IgG4-LAD) refers to lymph node enlargement associated with IgG4-related disease (IgG4-RD); in some cases, lymphadenopathy may be the only manifestation at initial presentation. IgG4-RD is an uncommon immune-mediated disorder characterized by sclerosis and lymphoplasmacytic infiltrate rich in IgG4+ PCs in affected organs, elevated serum IgG4 levels, and variable clinical presentation depending on the organs/sites involved. It is more common in individuals of Asian descent with a male predominance. The diagnostic criteria of IgG-RD are summarized in Table 6.1-4.

TABLE 6.1-4	WHO-HAEM5 Diagnostic Criteria for IgG4-Related Disease and Associated Lymphadenopathy

IgG4-RD-associated lymphadenopathy
Essential

- Extranodal IgG4-RD[a] (see diagnostic criteria of IgG4-RD discussed below)
- Polytypic IgG4+ plasma cells >400/mm^2, and IgG4/IgG >40%
- Exclusion of other entities that mimic IgG4-RD (see below)

Desirable

- IgG4+ plasma cells and eosinophils in fibrotic and/or interfollicular zone of lymph node

IgG4-RD in extranodal sites
Essential

- Lymphoplasmacytic infiltrate with increased IgG4+ plasma cells and IgG4/IgG ratio >40%
- Storiform fibrosis
- Exclusion of other entities that mimic IgG4-RD (see below)

Desirable

- Obliterative phlebitis
- Clinically compatible features: IgG4-RD in other body sites, elevated serum IgG4, and response to steroids/rituximab

Entities that mimic IgG4-RD

- Autoimmune conditions: ANCA-associated vasculitis and rheumatoid arthritis
- Multicentric Castleman disease
- Inflammatory myofibroblastic tumor
- Syphilis and other chronic infections
- Hyper IL-6 syndrome
- Rosai-Dorfman disease
- Lymphomas
- Plasma cell neoplasia

ANCA, antineutrophil cytoplasmic antibodies; IgG4-RD, immunoglobulin G4-related disease associated lymphadenopathy; IL-6, interleukin-6.
[a]In some cases, lymphadenopathy may be the initial manifestation, and diagnosis of extranodal disease is established later. Based on the WHO Classification of Tumours Editorial Board. Haematolymphoid tumours [Internet]. Lyon (France): International Agency for Research on Cancer; 2024 (WHO classification of tumours series, 5th ed.; vol. 11). Available from: https://tumourclassification.iarc.who.int/chapters/63.

Clinical Features

Lymphadenopathy is often painless and incidentally discovered on clinical examination or imaging. The most common sites of IgG4-LAD include mediastinal, cervical, axillary, and abdominal. Four clinical phenotypes of IgG4-RD have been described: (1) pancreatic-hepatobiliary disease, (2) retroperitoneal fibrosis and aortitis, (3) disease limited to the head and neck, and (4) head and neck disease with systemic involvement (pattern consistent with Mikulicz syndrome) (*Ann Rheum Dis.* 2019;78:406-412). Lab tests show elevated IgG4 levels (>135 mg/dL), although this finding is not specific to IgG4-RD. Increased IgE levels, hypergammaglobulinemia, and peripheral blood eosinophilia may be present.

Morphology and Immunohistochemistry

Characteristic findings of IgG4-RD include dense lymphoplasmacytic infiltrate with increased IgG4+ PCs (>100 per high power field) and IgG4/IgG ratio (>40%), storiform fibrosis, and obliterative phlebitis. Not all these features are present in all organs/sites involved. Lymph nodes may show nonspecific features (e-Figure 6.1-6), and it should be noted that the presence of increased IgG4+ PCs alone is insufficient for diagnosing IgG4-RD. Increased IgG4+ PCs can be seen in other conditions.

Five histologic patterns of IgG4-LAD have been described: type I (multicentric Castleman-like), type II (FH), type III (PH), type IV (PTGC-like), and type V (inflammatory pseudotumorlike) (*Adv Anat Pathol.* 2010;17:303-332). All these patterns show increased IgG4+ PCs. Types I-IV show nonspecific reactive features as suggested by their names. Features of type V are more specific, such as storiform fibrosis, which is less common in other inflammatory conditions.

Prognosis and Treatment

Corticosteroids are the first-line treatment, and most patients respond. Rituximab and surgery may be beneficial for some patients. The disease may recur after treatment.

Differential Diagnosis

The differential diagnosis is broad and includes other inflammatory conditions. B-cell lymphomas with plasmacytic differentiation, such as MZ lymphoma, may also show increased IgG4+ PCs. The diagnosis of IgG4-RD requires the integration of clinical, radiologic, histologic, and immunophenotypic findings.

X. CASTLEMAN DISEASE

CD encompasses a group of heterogeneous lymphoproliferative disorders with overlapping histologic findings and variable clinical presentation, treatment, and outcomes. CD primarily involves lymph nodes. Two main histologic patterns have been described: hyaline-vascular (HV) and mixed/PC type. The clinical subtypes include unicentric and multicentric Castleman diseases (UCD and MCD). The latter is classified into HHV8 (human herpesvirus 8)-associated MCD (discussed in Chapter 19.9) and idiopathic multicentric Castleman disease (iMCD).

a. **Histologic patterns and immunophenotypic features**
   - **Hyaline vascular:** Lymph nodes demonstrate architectural distortion from follicular and interfollicular abnormalities (e-Figure 6.1-7): FH with variable degrees of germinal center atrophy and hyalinization, two or more germinal centers per follicle ("twinning"), prominent mantle zones arranged in concentric rings ("onion skin"), prominent follicular dendritic cell (FDC) meshwork proliferation, interfollicular proliferation of vessels and penetration of germinal centers by sclerosed vessels. FDCs and stromal cells can show abnormal or dysplastic morphology. Aggregates of plasmacytoid dendritic cells may be present. Obliteration of sinuses is common. The lymph node capsule often shows thickening, and fibrotic bands may be present within the nodal tissue.

- **Mixed/plasma cell:** The nodal architecture is mostly preserved. Interfollicular expansion by large clusters or sheets of mature PCs and vascular proliferation are typical findings. Germinal centers with features of the HV variant may be present.
- **Immunophenotype:** Both morphologic types demonstrate polyclonal B cells and T cells do not show aberrant immunophenotype. Markers for B, T, and PCs and FDC meshworks help highlight the overall architecture and can help exclude lymphoma. PCs usually express polytypic immunoglobulin light chains; however, in PC variant and HHV8-positive CD, PCs may have monotypic cytoplasmic immunoglobulin. All cases demonstrating PC pattern should be stained for HHV8.

b. **Unicentric Castleman disease**

UCD is a benign lymphoproliferative disorder that involves one or more lymph nodes within one nodal group at the same anatomic site. The most commonly affected locations are mediastinal, cervical, abdominal, and retroperitoneal lymph nodes. Rare cases of extranodal involvement have been reported (*Urol Case Rep.* 2021;40:101876). The disease may have an asymptomatic clinical course or present with manifestations related to mass effect. Systemic symptoms are uncommon, and lab tests are usually normal. Most cases display HV morphology (*Blood.* 2020;135:1353-1364). Mixed/PC morphology is less common, and it is important to exclude MCD carefully in such cases. UCD does not show clonal *IGH* or *TCR* gene rearrangements (*Mod Pathol.* 2014;27:823-831). Complete surgical resection is the gold standard treatment for UCD and is usually curative (*Ann Surg.* 2012;255:677-684). The diagnostic criteria are summarized in Table 6.1-5.

c. **Idiopathic multicentric Castleman disease**

iMCD is a complex disease, and the diagnosis requires the integration of clinical history, imaging, histologic features, and other lab findings. iMCD is HHV8 negative by definition, involves two or more lymph node sites, and is associated with systemic inflammatory symptoms and organ dysfunction related to hypercytokinemia. Signs and symptoms at presentation include B-symptoms, hepatosplenomegaly, renal dysfunction, effusions, cytopenia(s), and elevated inflammatory markers such as CRP (C-reactive protein), ESR (erythrocyte sedimentation rate), and cytokines (*Blood.* 2017;129(12):1646-1657).

Two clinical subtypes have been described: (1) iMCD-TAFRO (**t**hrombocytopenia, **a**nasarca, **f**ever/inflammatory symptoms, **r**enal dysfunction/bone marrow reticulin fibrosis, **o**rganomegaly) and (2) iMCD-NOS (not otherwise specified). iMCD-NOS is associated with thrombocytosis and hypergammaglobulinemia, and in contrast, patients with iMDC-TAFRO have thrombocytopenia and normal immunoglobulin levels. The diagnostic criteria are summarized in Table 6.1-5.

iMCD frequently demonstrates mixed-type histopathologic features, exhibiting HV and PC morphology. iMCD-TAFRO is a more aggressive disease with worse clinical outcomes compared to iMCD-NOS (*Ann Hematol.* 2022;101:485-490; *Blood.* 2020;135:1353-1364). Treatment options include IL-6 (interleukin-6) inhibitors (first-line therapy), steroids, and other agents.

XI. AUTOIMMUNE DISEASE-ASSOCIATED LYMPHADENOPATHY

Autoimmune diseases can cause lymphadenopathy. The lymph nodes generally show reactive proliferation/hyperplasia of various cellular compartments with overall preserved architecture. In some cases, an atypical lymphoid proliferation may be present, mimicking a B-cell lymphoma or TCL.

TABLE 6.1-5 WHO-HAEM5 Diagnostic Criteria for Castleman Disease

Unicentric Castleman disease
Essential
- Involvement of a single lymph node or multiple lymph nodes in a single lymph node station, requiring clinical/radiographic correlation

Hyaline-vascular subtype
- Hyaline-vascular follicles
- Fibrotic and hypervascular stroma with sinus compression

Mixed/plasmacytic subtype
- Dense, interfollicular sheets of plasma cells extending to the cortex
- Polytypic, or rarely monotypic, plasmacytosis
- Variably sized lymphoid follicles, including some with regressive changes

Idiopathic multicentric Castleman disease
Essential
- Enlarged lymph nodes in >2 sites
- Lymph node morphology showing Grade 2 or 3 regressed germinal centers[a] or plasmacytosis
- Clinicopathologic correlation is required and other etiologies should be excluded.

[a]Grading is discussed in Fajgenbaum DC, Uldrick TS, Bagg A, et al. International, evidence-based consensus diagnostic criteria for HHV-8-negative/idiopathic multicentric Castleman disease. *Blood*. 2017;129(12):1646-1657. Based on the WHO Classification of Tumours Editorial Board. Haematolymphoid tumours [Internet]. Lyon (France): International Agency for Research on Cancer; 2024 (WHO classification of tumours series, 5th ed.; vol. 11). Available from: https://tumourclassification.iarc.who.int/chapters/63.

- **Sarcoidosis lymphadenopathy:** Sarcoidosis is a multisystem chronic inflammatory disease characterized by granulomatous inflammation. Any site may be involved; lungs and hilar lymph nodes are the most common sites. Well-formed, non-necrotizing epithelioid granulomas are present in all involved tissues (e-Figure 6.1-8). Lymph nodes show partial or complete effacement of architecture by multiple granulomas. The granulomas comprise epithelioid histiocytes, lymphocytes, PCs, and multinucleated giant cells of Langhans type.
- **SLE-associated lymphadenopathy:** SLE is an autoimmune disease that affects multiple organ systems, and lymphadenopathy is common. Lymphadenitis associated with acute SLE shows features overlapping with KFD. In some cases, hematoxylin bodies (extracellular aggregates of amorphous eosinophilic necrotic material) are present, and this finding helps differentiate SLE from KFD. Hematoxylin bodies stain positive for periodic acid-Schiff (PAS). Lymphadenopathy associated with chronic SLE shows variable features overlapping with other autoimmune and inflammatory conditions. FH, plasma cell hyperplasia (PCH), plasmacytosis, immunoblast proliferation, and Castleman-like features may be present.

- **Rheumatoid arthritis (RA)-associated lymphadenopathy:** RA is an autoimmune disorder that most commonly affects joints. Lymphadenopathy is observed in a subset of patients and usually involves lymph nodes draining involved joints. RA-associated lymphadenopathy typically shows marked FH, hyperplastic germinal centers with a "starry sky" appearance, interfollicular plasmacytosis, immunoblast proliferation, and vascular proliferation. Amorphous eosinophilic deposits (PAS+) are present in some cases. Foci of necrosis and granulomas may be present.
- **Autoimmune lymphoproliferative syndrome (ALPS):** ALPS is caused by FAS pathway mutations leading to defective lymphocyte apoptosis and chronic lymphoproliferation mimicking lymphoma. ALPS usually affects children, and common clinical findings include lymphadenopathy, hepatosplenomegaly, cytopenia(s), other autoimmune manifestations, and increased CD4 and CD8 negative/double negative αβ-T cells (DNTs) in nodal and extranodal sites including blood. Lymph nodes show FH, paracortical expansion by DNTs (pale zones on low power), plasmacytosis, PTGC, and Castleman-like changes. The DNTs are positive for cytotoxic markers. Bone marrow also shows increased DNTs in most cases. The diagnosis requires the presence of chronic lymphadenopathy and/or splenomegaly, αβ DNTs in the blood, and detection of *FAS*, *FASLG*, *CASP8*, *FADD*, or *CASP10* mutation (WHO-HAEM5).

SUGGESTED READINGS

Fajgenbaum DC, Uldrick TS, Bagg A, et al. International, evidence-based consensus diagnostic criteria for HHV-8-negative/idiopathic multicentric Castleman disease. *Blood.* 2017;129(12):1646-1657.

Medeiros LJ. *Ioachim's Lymph Node Pathology.* 5th ed. Wolters Kluwer Health; 2021.

Tzankov A, Dirnhofer S. A pattern-based approach to reactive lymphadenopathies. *Semin Diagn Pathol.* 2018;35(1):4-19.

Weiss LM, O'Malley D. Benign lymphadenopathies. *Mod Pathol.* 2013;26(suppl 1):S88-S96.

WHO Classification of Tumours Editorial Board. Haematolymphoid tumours [Internet]. Lyon (France): International Agency for Research on Cancer; 2024 [cited 2024 06 22]. (WHO classification of tumours series, 5th ed.; vol. 11). https://tumourclassification.iarc.who.int/chapters/63

6.2 Infectious Lymphadenopathies

Ekaterina Menshikova, Anne L. Chen, and Brooj Abro

Infectious lymphadenopathies have varying histologic features depending on the pathogen. Salient features of select infectious lymphadenopathies, including HIV- and Epstein-Barr virus (EBV)-associated lymphadenitis, are discussed further. HIV and EBV infection are also commonly associated with lymphoid malignancies, and excluding lymphoma may be an important consideration in these cases. Etiologies by morphologic patterns and features of various infectious lymphadenopathies (clinical features, histologic findings, and ancillary tests) are summarized in Tables 6.2-1, 6.2-2, 6.2-3, and 6.2-4.

TABLE 6.2-1 Morphologic Patterns and Associated Etiologies

Histologic Pattern	Etiology
Granulomas	Mycobacterial infection, fungal infection, lymphogranuloma venereum, cat scratch disease, yersinia lymphadenitis, sarcoidosis, lymphomas (especially Hodgkin and T-cell lymphoma), Crohn disease
Necrosis without granulomas	HSV, SLE, Kawasaki disease, Kikuchi histiocytic necrotizing lymphadenitis, necrotic high-grade malignancy
Follicular hyperplasia	Toxoplasma lymphadenitis, autoimmune disease, Kimura disease, HIV, Castleman disease
Fibrotic capsule	Syphilis, Hodgkin lymphoma, HIV, Castleman disease
Paracortical expansion with immunoblasts	EBV, CMV, HSV, post-vaccination reaction, drug-induced reaction, dermatopathic lymphadenitis

CMV, cytomegalovirus; EBV, Epstein-Barr virus; HSV, herpes simplex virus; SLE, systemic lupus erythematosus.

TABLE 6.2-2 Clinical Features of Common Infectious Lymphadenopathies

Etiology/Disease	Presentation	Common Site(s) of Involvement
Mycobacterium tuberculosis lymphadenitis	Multiple, painless enlarged lymph nodes	Head and neck
Cat scratch disease caused by *Bartonella henselae*	Clinical history of cat scratch; may have fever and malaise	Regional lymphadenopathy around arms; skin lesion at site of cat scratch
Syphilitic lymphadenitis	Painless lymphadenopathy as part of primary or secondary syphilis. Secondary infection may have rash, sore throat, and/or B symptoms.	Primary syphilis: regional lymph node(s) near site of inoculation about 1 wk after infection and may persist for months. Secondary syphilis: 4-10 wk after initial infection, generalized lymphadenopathy
Infectious mononucleosis	Fever, pharyngitis, fatigue	Anterior and posterior neck
Toxoplasma lymphadenitis	Clinical history of cat exposure; asymptomatic lymphadenopathy most common	Head and neck, especially posterior cervical, inframammary

TABLE 6.2-2 Clinical Features of Common Infectious Lymphadenopathies (*continued*)

Etiology/Disease	Presentation	Common Site(s) of Involvement
Herpes simplex lymphadenitis	Clinical history of HSV infection; reactivation due to immunosuppression/malignancy; association with CLL	Inguinal or femoral; regional at site of exposure
Atypical mycobacterial lymphadenitis	Painless lymphadenopathy in children or immunocompromised adults	Head and neck
Bacillary angiomatosis	Affects immunocompromised patients; exposure to cat scratches and human louse; cat exposure less common than cat scratch disease	Regional lymphadenopathy
Lymphogranuloma venereum due to *Chlamydia trachomatis*	Sexually transmitted; malaise, fever; strong association with HIV; symptoms more prominent in men	Inguinal lymph nodes
Histoplasma lymphadenitis	Exposure to bird and bat droppings in midwestern United States, Central America, South America; immunocompromised more likely to have symptomatic pneumonitis	Lung and abdomen
CMV lymphadenitis	Asymptomatic in immunocompetent; if immunocompromised, may have pneumonitis, encephalitis, retinitis	Cervical lymph nodes
HIV lymphadenitis	About half of patients are asymptomatic; idiopathic lymph node enlargement of at least 3 mo	Diffuse lymphadenopathy

CLL, chronic lymphocytic leukemia; CMV, cytomegalovirus; HSV, herpes simplex virus.

TABLE 6.2-3 Morphology of Common Infectious Lymphadenopathies

Etiology	Classic Histology
Mycobacterium tuberculosis lymphadenitis	Caseating granulomas
Cat scratch disease caused by *Bartonella henselae*	Stellate, necrotizing granulomas at advanced stage; follicular hyperplasia, necrosis, and neutrophilia in subcapsular sinus at early stage
Syphilitic lymphadenitis	Capsular fibrosis and thickening, follicular hyperplasia and plasmacytosis
EBV lymphadenitis (infectious mononucleosis)	Paracortical expansion with immunoblast hyperplasia that may resemble Hodgkin lymphoma. There may also be follicular hyperplasia.
Toxoplasma lymphadenitis	Triad of epithelioid histiocytes, sinuses expanded by monocytoid B cells, and florid follicular hyperplasia
Herpes simplex lymphadenitis	Patchy interfollicular necrosis; sinusoidal monocytoid B cells; infected cells show multinucleation, intranuclear inclusions.
Atypical mycobacterial lymphadenitis	Sheets of foamy macrophages
Bacillary angiomatosis	Nodular proliferation of small vessels in a lymph node
Lymphogranuloma venereum due to *Chlamydia trachomatis*	Stellate, necrotizing granulomas
Histoplasma lymphadenitis	Necrotizing granulomas
CMV lymphadenitis	Paracortical expansion with immunoblasts, follicular hyperplasia, and monocytoid B-cell aggregates. Cytomegalic cells with "owl's eye" inclusions may be present.
HIV lymphadenitis	A progressive spectrum of changes beginning with dramatic follicular hyperplasia, followed by follicular involution and atrophy, follicular lysis, Castleman-like features, capsular fibrosis, increased plasma cells, and histiocytes; the final stage is lymphocyte depletion without visible follicles with the main cell types being histiocytes and small blood vessels.

CMV, cytomegalovirus; EBV, Epstein-Barr virus.

TABLE 6.2-4 Ancillary Tests for Common Infectious Lymphadenopathies

Etiology	Ancillary Testing
Mycobacterium tuberculosis lymphadenitis	Acid-fast stains—the best place to look for organisms is in caseating necrosis.
	Other lab tests: skin test, interferon-gamma, culture, PCR
Cat scratch disease caused by *Bartonella henselae*	Warthin-Starry stain can be done but is difficult to interpret due to the high background and patchy organism distribution. IHC for *B. henselae* is available; PCR-based tests can also detect organisms in tissue.
	Other lab tests: serology
Syphilitic lymphadenitis	IHC for *Treponema* is available.
	Non-treponemal and treponemal serologic tests can be performed to confirm diagnosis.
EBV lymphadenitis (IM)	EBER ISH is positive. IHC can be performed to exclude lymphomas (HRS-like cells in IM are positive for CD45 and CD30 and negative for CD15).
	Other lab tests: Monospot, serology
Toxoplasma lymphadenitis	IHC- and PCR-based tests can be performed on tissue; however, they may not detect organisms in immunocompetent patients.
	Other lab tests: serology
Herpes simplex lymphadenitis	IHC is available for HSV I and II.
	Other lab tests: serology
Atypical mycobacterial lymphadenitis	Acid-fast stains and PCR-based tests can detect organisms in tissue.
	Other lab tests: culture
Bacillary angiomatosis	IHC and PCR to *B. henselae*
Lymphogranuloma venereum due to *Chlamydia trachomatis*	Giemsa, Warthin-Starry, and Brown-Hopps-Gram stains, but high background
	Other lab tests: PCR of swabs or urine
Histoplasma lymphadenitis	GMS and PAS stains can highlight yeast forms in tissue.
	Other lab tests: culture, serology, antigen tests (urine or blood)
CMV lymphadenitis	IHC stain for CMV; the infected cells may be positive for CD15 and negative for CD45.
HIV lymphadenitis	P24 IHC can detect HIV in tissues. Clinical confirmatory testing is required to establish the diagnosis.

CMV, cytomegalovirus; EBER, EBV-encoded RNA; EBV, Epstein-Barr virus; GMS, Grocott methenamine silver; HRS, Hodgkin Reed-Sternberg; HSV, herpes simplex virus; IHC, immunohistochemistry; IM, infectious mononucleosis; ISH, in situ hybridization; PAS, periodic acid–Schiff; PCR, polymerase chain reaction.

I. VIRAL LYMPHADENITIS

HIV Lymphadenitis

There are two strains of HIV: HIV-1, which is the predominant strain globally, and HIV-2, which is mainly confined to Africa. HIV-1 is a retrovirus transmitted through contact with an infected person's blood and bodily fluids. A lymph node biopsy may be performed in patients with unexplained lymphadenopathy, and subsequent workup may lead to the diagnosis of HIV-associated lymphadenitis. Patients with known HIV infection may also get a lymph node biopsy to rule out lymphoma.

Clinical Features

Three clinical stages of HIV infection have been recognized: acute, chronic/asymptomatic, and AIDS. In acute HIV infection, patients usually present with flu-like symptoms, which can last for a few weeks. The chronic phase is characterized by immune dysregulation and suppression. Patients may remain asymptomatic for a long period of time. With progressive decline in CD4 count and immune suppression, patients with HIV develop AIDS and frequently present with opportunistic infections at this stage. Lymphadenopathy in a patient with HIV may be due to HIV itself and various other etiologies including reactive/inflammatory processes such as immune reconstitution syndrome, opportunistic infections, and malignancy (*AJR Am J Roentgenol.* 2021;216:526-533). HIV-associated lymphadenitis is asymptomatic in many patients.

Morphology

Various morphologic patterns have been described in HIV-associated lymphadenitis (*Hum Pathol.* 1989;20:579-587). The patterns usually correspond to various stages of HIV infection. Pattern A is usually seen at the acute stage, and patterns B and C are typically associated with chronic infection.

- **Florid follicular hyperplasia (pattern A):** Lymph nodes show large confluent follicles, hyperplastic germinal centers with increased apoptosis, tingible body macrophages, and attenuated mantle zones (e-Figure 6.2-1). Follicle lysis with associated hemorrhage may be present. Interfollicular areas may show increased monocytoid B cells. Scattered Warthin-Finkeldey type multinucleated giant cells may be present (e-Figure 6.2-2).
- **Mixed pattern (pattern B):** This pattern is characterized by areas with follicular hyperplasia and follicular involution, features mimicking hyaline vascular Castleman disease (e-Figure 6.2-3). Areas with follicular involution show small, atrophic follicles, and hyalinization may be present. Interfollicular areas show lymphocyte depletion, increased histiocytes and plasma cells, and vascular proliferation, which may be prominent.
- **Lymphocyte depletion (pattern C):** Distorted nodal architecture with prominent vascular proliferation, fibrosis, atrophic burned-out follicles, and predominance of histiocytes and plasma cells.

Ancillary Tests

The morphologic features described earlier may give clues to an underlying HIV infection. However, the diagnosis of HIV requires serologic testing. P24 immunohistochemistry (IHC) has been demonstrated to detect HIV infection in tissues (*Histopathology.* 2010;56(4):530-541). Special stains for infectious organisms (Grocott methenamine silver [GMS], acid-fast bacilli [AFB], Fite) can be performed on tissue sections to evaluate for other superimposed infections. Flow cytometry and IHC studies can be helpful in ruling out lymphoproliferative disorders.

Differential Diagnosis

Given its variable morphologic patterns that can overlap with several infectious and inflammatory conditions, HIV-associated lymphadenitis has a broad differential diagnosis. In acute HIV lymphadenitis, the morphologic features (pattern A) overlap with other viral infections. In the chronic phase (patterns B and C), the morphology overlaps with Castleman disease and chronic lymphadenitis. The appropriate clinical context is required to diagnose HIV-associated lymphadenitis.

Epstein-Barr Virus Lymphadenitis

EBV is a ubiquitous herpesvirus (also known as human herpesvirus 4). EBV is transmitted through direct contact with human secretions, primarily via exposure to saliva. In acute EBV infection, EBV infects and replicates in B cells, resulting in B-cell proliferation and production of antibodies against EBV. Subsequently, a cellular response mediated by T cells (mainly natural killer [NK] and CD8+ T cells) develops to clear the infection. After the resolution of acute infection, EBV remains latent in memory B cells throughout life (*N Engl J Med.* 2000;343:481-492).

Clinical Features

EBV exposure and primary infection in young children are usually asymptomatic. In older children and adults, it may manifest as a self-limited acute illness known as infectious mononucleosis (IM). IM often begins with nonspecific symptoms of low-grade fever and fatigue, and subsequently, other symptoms may develop, including lymphadenopathy, pharyngitis, tonsillar exudates, and hepatosplenomegaly. The classic triad of fever, tonsillar pharyngitis, and lymphadenopathy is often present; however, atypical presentation is frequent and, in rare cases, may simulate lymphoma.

Morphology

Lymph nodes in EBV lymphadenitis demonstrate a mixed pattern of lymphoid hyperplasia, including prominent paracortical expansion with varying degrees of follicular hyperplasia, which can lead to distorted architecture. Immunoblasts, variably sized lymphocytes, plasma cells, and histiocytes are seen within the paracortex, often imparting a "moth-eaten" appearance. Immunoblast hyperplasia is prominent, and some larger forms may mimic Hodgkin Reed-Sternberg (HRS) cells (e-Figure 6.2-4). HRS-like cells are more frequently seen in tonsils than in lymph nodes. Sheets of immunoblasts may mimic diffuse large B-cell lymphoma (DLBCL). Follicles typically display prominent hyperplastic germinal centers with increased numbers of tingible body macrophages and frequent mitoses. Foci of necrosis are common.

Ancillary Tests

- **Immunohistochemistry and in situ hybridization (ISH) studies**
  IHC studies may be performed to evaluate the distribution of B and T cells and exclude the possibility of lymphoma. Although the lymphoid architecture may be distorted, CD20 and CD3 usually demonstrate the preservation of B- and T-cell compartments (B cells are most prominent in the follicles, and T cells are

predominant in the paracortical regions). The immunoblasts are usually positive for CD20, PAX5, CD30, MUM1, OCT-2, BOB-1, CD45 (variable) and negative for CD15. CD30-positive T-immunoblasts may also be present.

ISH for EBV-encoded RNA (EBER) highlights numerous EBV-positive small to large lymphocytes (mostly immunoblasts). EBER-positive cells' proportions vary among cases (*J Mol Diagn.* 2002;4(1):37-43).
- **Other laboratory tests**
  - Complete blood count (CBC) and peripheral smear examination: The most common finding on CBC is lymphocytosis, although some patients may have mild neutropenia and thrombocytopenia. Blood smear demonstrates atypical lymphocytes, also known as Downey cells: they represent activated CD8-positive T lymphocytes with larger cell size, moderate to abundant cytoplasm, which tends to be indented by surrounding red blood cells, and nucleoli.
  - Monospot test: The Monospot test is a latex agglutination test that utilizes equine erythrocytes to test for nonspecific heterophile antibodies produced in response to EBV infection.
  - Serologic tests: Detection of EBV-specific antibodies is the gold standard for the diagnosis of IM. Primary infection is diagnosed in the absence of antibodies to Epstein-Barr nuclear antigen (EBNA; nuclear antigen) with immunoglobulin (Ig) M against the Epstein-Barr viral capsid antigen (anti-VCA IgM) or rising levels of anti-VCA IgG.
  - Molecular tests: Detection of EBV DNA with polymerase chain reaction (PCR) techniques can be performed on blood or tissue samples. PCR tests are also useful for EBV DNA quantification.

Differential Diagnosis

Since EBV infection may lead to severe symptoms with generalized lymphadenopathy clinically mimicking lymphoma and demonstrate atypical large cells on lymph node or tonsillar biopsy, the differential diagnosis includes classic Hodgkin lymphoma (CHL), anaplastic large cell lymphoma, and DLBCL. Other virus-induced lymphadenitis, particularly cytomegalovirus (CMV) lymphadenitis, may show similar morphologic features in lymph nodes. IHC, ISH, and serologic studies are helpful to establish the diagnosis and exclude other causes.

Cytomegalovirus Lymphadenitis

CMV is a double-stranded DNA virus that belongs to the Herpesviridae family (also known as human herpesvirus 5). CMV is transmitted via exposure to infected blood and body fluids. Primary CMV infection is more common in children. After primary infection, the virus may integrate into the host genome and remain latent for many years. Secondary CMV infection may result from reactivation in settings of immune deficiency/dysfunction (IDD). In immunocompetent patients, CMV infection may be asymptomatic or manifest with IM-like symptoms. Patients with IDD are at increased risk of severe CMV infection, particularly patients with HIV and transplant recipients. In patients with HIV, disseminated CMV infection is considered an AIDS-defining illness. Disseminated CMV infection can present with widespread lymphadenopathy raising concern for lymphoma.

In CMV lymphadenitis, lymph nodes show histologic features similar to those seen in EBV and other viral infections. Examination of the blood smear may reveal reactive lymphocytes (similar to EBV infection). The nonspecific histologic features on lymph node sections include follicular and paracortical hyperplasia (e-Figure 6.2-5), frequent immunoblasts, intermixed plasma cells, histiocytes, and aggregates of monocytoid B cells. CMV-infected cytomegalic cells with large nuclei and characteristic "owl's eye" nuclear inclusions (e-Figure 6.2-6A) may be present, which can provide clues to the diagnosis. These cells are usually few and often found in areas with monocytoid B-cell hyperplasia. CMV IHC and ISH studies can detect CMV-infected cells in tissue (e-Figure 6.2-6B).

The differential diagnosis includes EBV and other viral infections. CMV-infected cells may mimic HRS cells, possibly raising concern for CHL. IHC studies can be performed to rule out CHL.

II. BACTERIAL LYMPHADENITIS

Cat Scratch Disease

Cat scratch disease (CSD) is caused by *Bartonella henselae*, with cats serving as a natural reservoir. Inoculation of *B. henselae* from a cat scratch or bite can lead to erythematous papule at the site of the injury and the subsequent development of regional tender lymphadenopathy. Suppuration of affected lymph node(s) occurs in some cases. The disease is usually self-limited and resolves spontaneously. In immunocompromised patients, disseminated disease can occur.

Early morphologic changes include follicular hyperplasia with hyperplastic germinal centers containing increased tingible body macrophages, sinus hyperplasia, small subcapsular abscesses containing eosinophilic necrotic material admixed with neutrophils, and karyorrhectic debris. Clusters of monocytoid cells can be seen in sinuses and interfollicular areas. As the disease progresses, clusters of neutrophils extend from the subcapsular sinus into the cortex and medulla. At the advanced stage, stellate necrotizing granulomas consisting of central necrosis, abundant neutrophils, and a rim of histiocytes are the characteristic features of CSD (e-Figure 6.2-7). Bacilli can be visualized by Warthin-Starry stain or IHC and are more easily detected in the early stage. Serology and PCR studies can be performed to confirm the diagnosis.

Differential diagnosis includes suppurative lymphadenitis, tuberculous lymphadenitis, fungal lymphadenitis, Kikuchi-Fujimoto disease, lymphogranuloma venereum, and tularemia.

Syphilitic Lymphadenitis

Syphilis is a sexually transmitted disease caused by *Treponema pallidum*, a gram-negative spirochete. It can also be transmitted in utero from mother to fetus. Without treatment, syphilis progresses through three stages. The primary stage is characterized by a painless ulcer—a chancre—with the spread of treponemas to regional lymph nodes causing lymphadenopathy. In weeks to a few months from the initial localized infection, secondary syphilis manifests with systemic symptoms, including skin rash and generalized lymphadenopathy. Approximately 30% of untreated patients develop tertiary syphilis with destructive gummatous lesions, cardiovascular and neurologic disease.

Syphilitic or luetic lymphadenitis is caused by the persistence of *Treponema* in the lymph nodes, leading to constant antigenic stimulation and resulting in lymphoid hyperplasia. Inguinal lymph nodes are most commonly affected at the primary stage, and diffuse lymphadenopathy can be present at the secondary stage.

Histologic findings on lymph node sections include thickening of capsule due to fibrosis, expansion of paracortex with lymphoplasmacytic infiltrate, follicular hyperplasia, vasculitis with perivascular cuffs of plasma cells and lymphocytes. Plasmacytosis is usually prominent, and aggregates of plasma cells can also be seen within the capsule and pericapsular areas. While these findings are not entirely specific, their simultaneous presence raises suspicion of syphilis. *T. pallidum* IHC, silver stain, and PCR studies can be used to identify spirochetes in tissue sections. Serologic tests are usually performed to confirm the diagnosis.

The differential diagnosis includes other infectious and inflammatory conditions that can cause follicular hyperplasia and plasmacytosis, including autoimmune disease–associated lymphadenopathy, IgG4 disease–related lymphadenopathy, inflammatory pseudotumor of lymph nodes, other infectious organisms such as herpes simplex virus (HSV), mycobacteria, and chlamydia.

Mycobacterial Lymphadenitis

Mycobacterial lymphadenitis may be caused by *Mycobacterium tuberculosis* (MTB; tuberculous lymphadenitis) or nontuberculous mycobacteria.

- **Tuberculous lymphadenitis:** MTB infection can cause tuberculosis (TB) and lymphadenitis. MTB infection is more prevalent in developing countries and is spread via inhalation of aerosolized droplets from patients with active TB.

  MTB lymphadenitis usually occurs in children and young adults following primary infection. Lymph nodes of the head and neck are commonly affected (also known as scrofula), and patients usually present with nontender cervical lymphadenopathy. Histologic examination demonstrates necrotizing granulomatous inflammation: areas of central necrosis surrounded by epithelioid histiocytes, Langhans-type giant cells, lymphocytes, plasma cells, and fibroblasts at the periphery. The necrosis is caseous and appears as eosinophilic amorphous material without cellular debris, and neutrophils are usually absent (caseating granulomas) (e-Figure 6.2-8). Granulomas tend to coalesce. Follicular hyperplasia can be seen in areas uninvolved by necrotizing granulomas. Special stains for AFB (Fite-Faraco, Ziehl-Neelsen, Kinyoun) and fluorescent stains (auramine-rhodamine) can detect AFB in tissue sections. Tuberculous bacilli can be difficult to find and tend to be located in necrotic areas. PCR-based tests and culture studies can be performed to confirm the diagnosis.

- **Nontuberculous lymphadenitis:** *M. avium complex* (MAC) is the most common cause of nontuberculous lymphadenitis. Other mycobacteria species that do not cause TB or leprosy can also cause nontuberculous lymphadenitis. MAC lymphadenitis is more common in children and immunocompromised patients and typically affects anterior cervical lymph nodes. Morphologic findings include chronic granulomatous inflammation, suppurative inflammation, and sheets of foamy histiocytes effacing the nodal architecture (e-Figure 6.2-9A). Caseous necrosis is usually not present. Bacilli can be identified by acid-fast stains (e-Figure 6.2-9B).

- ***Mycobacterium leprae* lymphadenitis:** Leprosy, caused by *M. leprae* or *M. lepromatosis*, can also affect lymph nodes. The Ridley-Jopling classification divides leprosy into six categories based on the spectrum of the disease's clinical and pathologic features. Of these, there are two main categories: tuberculoid and lepromatous leprosy, which represent opposite ends of the disease spectrum.

a. **Tuberculoid leprosy:** Lymph nodes show non-necrotizing granulomas with epithelioid histiocytes and Langhans-type giant cells (resembling granulomas in sarcoidosis). Bacilli are rare.
b. **Lepromatous leprosy:** Lymph nodes show accumulation of large pale rounded histiocytes, also called lepra cells or Virchow cells, in the paracortex without granuloma formation and with minimal or no necrosis. Acid-fast stains can demonstrate large clusters of mycobacteria (globi) within the cytoplasm of foamy histiocytes.

III. OTHER INFECTIOUS LYMPHADENITIS

Toxoplasma Lymphadenitis

Toxoplasma gondii is an intracellular protozoan that can invade various cell types. Humans are intermediate hosts and can be infected by ingesting oocysts from the environment (contaminated soil, feline feces), consuming infected undercooked meat, organ transplantation from infected donors, and vertical transmission (congenital toxoplasmosis). In most immunocompetent individuals, the infection is asymptomatic; however, some may develop acute disease with painless lymphadenopathy. Immunocompromised patients can develop severe disseminated infection.

Posterior cervical lymph nodes are the most commonly affected site in toxoplasmosis with bilateral symmetrical nontender enlargement. Histologic features of toxoplasma lymphadenitis include the classic triad of florid follicular hyperplasia, clusters of epithelioid histiocytes (microgranuloma), and dilated sinuses with monocytoid B-cell hyperplasia (e-Figure 6.2-10). This triad is pathognomonic of toxoplasma lymphadenitis; however, the features are not entirely specific. One of the characteristic features is the encroachment of germinal centers by epithelioid histiocytes. The epithelioid histiocytes in toxoplasmosis typically do not form organized granulomas, and necrosis and giant cells are usually absent. Although *Toxoplasma* organisms (tachyzoites) may be seen in tissues, they are rarely visualized in immunocompetent patients. Toxoplasma IHC may detect organisms in immunocompromised patients.

The diagnosis requires confirmation by serologic testing. The differential diagnosis is broad and includes HIV lymphadenitis, leishmania lymphadenitis, Rosai-Dorfman disease, nodular lymphocyte-predominant Hodgkin lymphoma, lymphoepithelioid variant of peripheral T-cell lymphoma, and histiocytic disorders.

Histoplasma Lymphadenitis

Histoplasma capsulatum is a dimorphic fungus, endemic to Ohio and Mississippi River Valleys. Transmission occurs via spore inhalation from soil contaminated with bird and bat droppings. *H. capsulatum* infection may be asymptomatic in immunocompetent patients or manifest with acute pulmonary disease. Disseminated infection occurs in immunocompromised patients. Symptoms of disseminated infection often include fever, pancytopenia, and hepatosplenomegaly.

Histologic evaluation of the lymph nodes often shows necrotizing granulomas surrounded by epithelioid histiocytes and giant cells. Granulomas are less prominent in patients with immunodeficiency. In some cases, sheets of histiocytes may be present without the formation of distinct granulomas. In tissues, *H. capsulatum* exists in yeast forms and does not have a capsule.

The yeast forms can be detected by GMS or periodic acid–Schiff (PAS) stains within necrotic areas and inside histiocytes and giant cells (e-Figure 6.2-11). *H. capsulatum* infection can be confirmed clinically by performing antigen tests.

Differential diagnoses include sarcoidosis, tuberculosis, other fungal lymphadenitis, Langerhans cell histiocytosis, and Kikuchi-Fujimoto disease.

SUGGESTED READINGS

Cualing HD, Bhargava P, Sandin RL. *Non-neoplastic Hematopathology and Infections.* John Wiley & Sons, Inc; 2012.

Medeiros LJ. *Ioachim's Lymph Node Pathology.* 5th ed. Wolters Kluwer Health; 2021.

Medeiros LJ, Miranda RN. *Lymph Nodes and Extranodal Lymphomas.* Elsevier; 2018.

Weiss L. *Lymph Nodes.* Cambridge University Press; 2008.

7 Spleen

7.1 Nonneoplastic Disorders of the Spleen

John D. Pfeifer, Brooj Abro, and Anjum Hassan

I. CONGENITAL ANOMALIES

- **Accessory spleen**
  Alternatively termed "spleniculi," these are most commonly located in the splenic hilum, tail of the pancreas, and the gastrohepatic ligament (*N Engl J Med.* 1981;304:11) and are found in up to one-third of autopsy cases. In most cases, only one accessory spleen is present, although two or more accessory spleens are not uncommon. They share the same histologic and pathologic features as the native spleen (e-Figure 7.1-1). Accessory spleens are clinically significant in patients requiring splenectomy for hypersplenism.
- **Asplenia**
  The most common causes of asplenia are trauma, infarction, and surgery. Congenital asplenia, most often inherited in an autosomal dominant pattern, is quite rare; it is associated with heterotaxy syndromes, although it can occur in isolation. Regardless of the cause, asplenia shows the clinical features of hyposplenism.
- **Splenic gonadal fusion**
  This congenital abnormality results from the fusion of the gonadal mesoderm of the left urogenital fold with the splenic anlage, and manifests in the pediatric age group with a male-to-female ratio of 20:1. The more common continuous form is characterized by a continuous cord of fibrous or splenic tissue between the ectopic mass and the normal spleen, while the less common discontinuous form shows no connection between the spleen and the mass. Cryptorchidism, micrognathia, and limb defects are often associated with the continuous form.

II. SPLENIC TRAUMA

- **Splenic rupture**
  Splenic rupture is classified as either spontaneous or delayed. Spontaneous rupture, more common in males, is usually related to infarction, tumors, lymphoma, leukemia, or thrombocytopenia. Delayed rupture (defined as occurring more than 7 days after injury) is thought to arise from evolving contusions. Histologically, a ruptured spleen shows subcapsular hemorrhage and reactive white pulp changes.

- **Splenosis**
  Splenosis refers to splenic implants or regrowth of splenic tissue after trauma or surgical splenectomy and is thought to arise from seeding and/or hematogenous spread of splenic tissue. When associated with trauma, the most common location is the abdominal cavity, but splenosis has been reported at virtually all anatomic sites, including the brain (*Am J Surg Pathol*. 1998;22:894). Usually a benign incidental finding, its clinical importance lies in its potential to mimic neoplastic and nonneoplastic splenic lesions.

III. SPLENOMEGALY

The spleen often becomes enlarged due to infectious causes or congestive states (Table 7.1-1). Red pulp congestion is the most common finding in such cases.

IV. DISORDERS OF SPLENIC FUNCTION

- **Hypersplenism**
  Hypersplenism refers to the destruction of one or more blood cell lines by the spleen (*Eur J Gastroenterol Hepatol*. 2001;13:317). It is the most important indication for

TABLE 7.1-1 Conditions Associated With Splenomegaly

I. Infection
   a. Infectious endocarditis
   b. Infectious mononucleosis
   c. Tuberculosis
   d. Histoplasmosis
   e. Syphilis
   f. Parasitic infections (eg, malaria)
   g. Cytomegalovirus
II. Congestive states
   a. Cirrhosis
   b. Splenic vein thrombosis
   c. Heart failure
III. Hematologic malignancy
   a. Non-Hodgkin lymphoma
   b. Hodgkin lymphoma
   c. Myeloproliferative disorders
   d. Multiple myeloma
IV. Immune-related conditions
   a. Rheumatoid arthritis
   b. Systemic lupus erythematosus
   c. Storage disorders (eg, Gaucher disease)

Adapted from Kumar V, Abbas AK, Aster JC. *Robbins & Cotran Pathologic Basis of Disease*. 9th ed. Saunders; 2014.

TABLE 7.1-2 Disorders Associated With Hypersplenism

I. Abnormal sequestration of intrinsically defective blood cells in a normal spleen
  a. Congenital disorders of erythrocytes
     (Hereditary spherocytosis, elliptocytosis; hemoglobinopathies, eg, sickle cell disease, unstable hemoglobins)
  b. Acquired disorders of erythrocytes
     (Autoimmune hemolytic anemias, malaria, babesiosis)
  c. Autoimmune thrombocytopenia and/or neutropenia

II. Abnormal spleen causing sequestration of normal blood cells
  a. Disorders of the monocyte/macrophage system
     (Chronic congestion, storage diseases, parasitic infections, Langerhans cell histiocytosis, etc)
  b. Malignant infiltrative disorders
     (Leukemias, lymphomas, plasma cell dyscrasias, metastatic carcinoma)
  c. Extramedullary hematopoiesis
     (Severe hemolytic states, chronic idiopathic myelofibrosis)
  d. Chronic infections, for example, tuberculosis, brucellosis
  e. Vascular/stromal abnormalities
     (Vascular tumors, peliosis, splenic cysts, hamartomas)

III. Miscellaneous conditions
  a. Hyperthyroidism
  b. Hypogammaglobulinemia
  c. Progressive multifocal leukoencephalopathy

---

elective splenectomy. Diagnostic criteria for hypersplenism include cytopenia(s) of one or more blood cell lines, bone marrow hyperplasia, splenomegaly, and correction of the cytopenia(s) following splenectomy. Of the many possible etiologies (Table 7.1-2), congenital disorders such as hereditary spherocytosis (e-Figure 7.1-2), infiltrative disorders such as leukemias and lymphomas, and autoimmune disorders are the most common.

- **Hyposplenism**

  Hyposplenism refers to any deficiency (including the absence) of a functioning spleen, and though it has a variety of etiologies, it is most often due to splenectomy. Peripheral blood smear examination can inform the diagnosis; findings suggesting hyposplenism can occur in any blood cell line, including erythrocytes (Howell-Jolly bodies [e-Figure 7.1-3], poikilocytosis with target cells, acanthocytes, and nucleated red blood cells), platelets (thrombocytosis), and leukocytes (lymphocytosis or monocytosis and eosinophilia). Other causes of hyposplenism include congenital hypoplasia (most commonly due to sickle cell disease [e-Figure 7.1-4]), infiltrative disorders, and old age (Table 7.1-3).

  Regardless of the cause of hyposplenism, the most important consequence is increased susceptibility to infection by encapsulated bacteria, most commonly *Streptococcus pneumoniae*.

TABLE 7.1-3 Disorders Associated With Hyposplenism

I. Congenital
  a. Asplenia
  b. Hypoplasia
  c. Immunodeficiency disorders
II. Acquired
  a. Splenectomy
  b. Acquired atrophy and/or infarction
    1. Sickle cell disease
    2. Vascular disorders (vasculitides, thromboembolic conditions)
    3. Essential thrombocythemia
    4. Malabsorption syndromes
    5. Autoimmune diseases
    6. Irradiation
    7. Cytotoxic chemotherapy
    8. Chronic alcoholism
    9. Hypopituitarism
  c. Functional asplenia with normal-sized or enlarged spleen
    1. Infiltration by leukemia, lymphoma, multiple myeloma, mastocytosis
    2. Early (splenomegalic) sickle cell disease
    3. Amyloidosis
    4. Sarcoidosis
    5. Benign and malignant vascular tumors
    6. Malabsorption syndromes
  d. Depressed immune function
    1. AIDS
    2. Status post
      a. Irradiation
      b. Cytotoxic chemotherapy
      c. Immunosuppressive agents, including corticosteroids
    3. Endocrine disorders
      a. Hypothyroidism
      b. Hypopituitarism
      c. Diabetes mellitus
    4. Chronic alcoholism

V. REACTIVE SPLENIC DISORDERS

These can be divided into diffuse and localized processes. Diffuse disease entities include reactive lymphoid hyperplasia (e-Figure 7.1-5), follicular hyperplasia, and disorders such as Castleman disease. Localized disease includes granulomatous disorders and infectious processes. Regardless of the etiology, most reactive disorders present with splenomegaly.

- **Diffuse Reactive Processes**
  Reactive lymphoid hyperplasia in the spleen may occur with or without germinal center formation. Non–germinal center hyperplasia is often associated with viral infections, especially herpes simplex virus and Epstein-Barr virus (e-Figure 7.1-5), which explains the common occurrence of splenomegaly in patients with infectious mononucleosis.

  Reactive lymphoid hyperplasia with germinal center formation (e-Figure 7.1-5) is commonly referred to as "follicular" hyperplasia. It is the most common pattern of lymphoid hyperplasia in the spleen and is seen in both acute and chronic immune reactions. Follicular hyperplasia is frequently observed in bacterial infections, often as an incidental finding. In fact, splenomegaly is characteristic of subacute bacterial endocarditis.
- **Focal Reactive Processes**
- **Granulomas.** The most common form of a focal benign process is granulomatous inflammation, ranging from lipogranulomatous inflammation (of unknown etiology) to caseating or noncaseating granulomatous inflammation. Caseating granulomas are primarily due to infectious disease, most commonly *Brucella* species, tuberculosis, and fungal infection; however, they are also seen in X-linked chronic granulomatous disease. Noncaseating granulomatous disease is most frequently associated with sarcoidosis (e-Figure 7.1-6). For most granulomas in the spleen, no known etiology can be found (*Arch Pathol Lab Med.* 1974;98:261).
- **Abscesses.** Splenic abscesses are usually caused by hematogenous seeding of infectious pathogens from another site. As at other sites, the abscesses are typically well circumscribed with a central region of necrotic and fibrinopurulent debris surrounded by a white fibrous wall. The most common bacterial pathogens are *Staphylococcus aureus*, *Streptococcus* species, and, in patients with sickle cell disease, *Salmonella* species. The most common pathogens in the rare fungal abscesses are *Candida* species, *Aspergillus* species, and *Cryptococcus* species.
- **Infarcts.** The spleen is a frequent site of systemic emboli, which commonly arise from cardiac valve lesions or mural thrombi. Infarcts are usually wedge shaped with a hemorrhagic to pale-tan to fibrotic appearance depending on the age of the lesion (e-Figure 7.1-7).

  Non–wedge-shaped infarcts arise in a variety of intrinsic hematopoietic and non-hematopoietic processes. Essential thrombocythemia and chronic idiopathic myelofibrosis are the most frequently associated hematopoietic disorders; less common causes include paroxysmal nocturnal hemoglobinuria, sickle cell disease, and aplastic anemia. Among non-hematopoietic etiologies, vasculitides (polyarteritis nodosa, thrombotic thrombocytopenic purpura [TTP]/immune thrombocytopenic purpura [ITP] associated, etc) and splenic artery aneurysms are common causes.

VI. STORAGE DISEASES COMMONLY INVOLVING THE SPLEEN

Lysosomal storage diseases are the most common metabolic diseases that involve the spleen. In general, the morphologic features of splenic involvement generally develop in infancy or childhood and are similar to those in the bone marrow.

- **Gaucher Disease**
  Gaucher disease is the most common lysosomal storage disease and is due to a deficiency of glucocerebrosidase that has an autosomal recessive pattern of inheritance. The spleen is usually diffusely enlarged, and microscopic examination shows that it is filled with histiocytes that have eccentric nuclei and an abundance of blue-gray foamy cytoplasm with a texture that resembles tissue paper, histiocytes that are classically referred to as Gaucher cells. The differential diagnosis includes other lysosomal storage diseases (especially Niemann-Pick disease) and a variety of hematologic malignancies that can show Gaucher-like cells.
- **Niemann-Pick Disease**
  This very rare lysosomal storage disease (which occurs in approximately 1/120,000 live births) has an autosomal recessive pattern of inheritance and is due to a deficiency of either acid sphingomyelinase (types A and B) or Niemann-Pick C proteins (types C and D). In addition to typing based on the specific enzyme deficiency, the disease is also divided into five categories based on clinical features (type IA, IS, IC, IIS, and IIC). Clinical types IA and IS typically show massive splenomegaly (up to 10 times the normal size). Regardless of the disease type, the red pulp is characteristically diffusely expanded by foamy macrophages laden with sphingomyelin that are small and uniform and, because of an accumulation of lipid droplets, resemble small mulberries.
- **Mucopolysaccharidoses**
  These progressive diseases are caused by a lack of effective processing of glycosaminoglycan and have an autosomal recessive pattern of inheritance, except for Hunter syndrome, which has an X-linked recessive pattern. Hepatosplenomegaly is common in this group of diseases, and microscopically, the spleen demonstrates plump vacuolated histiocytes.
- **Others**
  A wide range of other metabolic diseases involves the spleen, of which the most notable is perhaps Tay-Sachs disease, caused by hexosaminidase A deficiency that results in the accumulation of GM2 ganglioside in the heart, liver, and spleen, which microscopically characteristically manifests as an accumulation of plump vacuolated histiocytes.

7.2 Non-hematopoietic Tumors and Tumor-Like Lesions of the Spleen

Safee Faraz Ahmed and John D. Pfeifer

I. VASCULAR TUMORS

- **Benign**
  1. **Littoral Cell Angioma.** This is a rare benign splenic vascular tumor that originates from littoral cells, which are specialized cells lining the splenic red pulp sinuses that have a dual endothelial and histiocytic differentiation. An association with malignancies at other sites has been described (*Histopathology*.

2016;69:762-774). Grossly, the tumor is characterized by multiple spongy, cystic nodules. Microscopically, there is proliferation of tortuous, anastomosing, cystic, blood-filled vascular channels, often with papillary projections and marked sloughing of the endothelial cells. Immunohistochemically, the endothelial cells have a distinct hybrid endothelial-histiocytic phenotype, with expression of the endothelial marker CD31 (but not CD34) and the histiocytic markers CD68 and CD163. The differential diagnosis includes splenic littoral cell hemangioendothelioma, angiosarcoma, hamartoma, and Kaposi sarcoma.

2. **Splenic Hamartoma.** This rare benign tumor is mostly found incidentally or at autopsy. It affects all age groups; however, it is mostly seen in the elderly population. Microscopically, it is characterized by disorganized slit-like vascular channels lined by plump endothelial cells and entrapped adipocytes. The endothelial cells lining the vascular channels are positive for CD8, CD31, CD34, and vimentin; it is the CD8 immunopositivity of the vascular endothelium that distinguishes splenic hamartoma from other vascular lesions of the spleen.

3. **Sclerosing Angiomatoid Nodular Transformation (SANT) of the Spleen.** This rare benign lesion of the spleen primarily affects middle-aged adults and has a female predominance. Histologically, the lesion is characterized by multiple angiomatoid nodules with slit-like vascular spaces lined by plump endothelial cells, surrounded by sclerotic stroma and exhibiting a lymphoplasmacytic/myofibroblastic response (e-Figure 7.2-1). SANT endothelium has a characteristic immunoprofile: CD31 and CD8 positive but CD34 negative in the sinusoids, CD34 and CD31 positive but CD8 negative in capillaries, and CD31 positive but CD34 and CD8 negative in the veins, all with variable CD68 expression (*Arch Pathol Lab Med.* 2013;137:1309-1312). The lesion does not recur after splenectomy. The differential diagnosis includes lymphomas with lymphoplasmacytic differentiation.

4. **Peliosis.** Microscopically, this rare lesion is characterized by multiple ectatic blood-filled cystic spaces with or without an endothelial lining, usually adjacent to the periarteriolar lymphoid sheath (PALS) and follicles. While the etiology is unknown, it apparently has more than one pathway of development since it may be associated with infection, malignancies (especially lymphomas and leukemias), and chemotherapy (*Forensic Sci Int.* 2005;149:25-33). Most patients are asymptomatic, although very rarely a patient can present with spontaneous rupture of the spleen, particularly in patients with carcinomatosis or chronic leukemia, or in the posttransplantation setting. The differential diagnoses include hemangiomas and involvement of the spleen in hairy cell leukemia.

5. **Hemangioma.** This benign vascular proliferation is a frequent incidental finding in splenectomy specimens (e-Figure 7.2-2). The endothelial cells are immunopositive for CD31, CD34, and von Willebrand factor (vWF), but immunonegative for CD21, CD68, and CD8.

6. **Lymphangioma.** This rare slow-growing benign neoplasm is often seen in children with congenital malformations of the lymphatic system or lymphangiomatosis syndromes. It is characterized by enlarged, cystic spaces, lined by flat endothelial cells, with eosinophilic lymphatic fluid within septations.

- **Intermediate**
  1. **Kaposi Sarcoma.** Linked to human herpesvirus 8 (HHV-8) infections typically in patients with HIV/AIDS, Kaposi sarcoma must be included in the differential diagnosis of any splenic vascular neoplasm. The tumor has a characteristic

immunophenotypic profile in that it is positive for the vascular markers CD31, CD34, ERG, and D-240 and is also positive for HHV-8.
    2. **Epstein-Barr Virus (EBV)+ Inflammatory Follicular Dendritic Cell Sarcoma.** This tumor is unique to the spleen and liver and is associated with EBV. It is a fibroinflammatory process distinct from inflammatory pseudotumor (*Appl Cancer Res.* 2017;37:45; *Int J Surg Pathol.* 2021;29:443-446).
- **Malignant**
    1. **Hemangioendothelioma**. This rare malignant vascular tumor occurs mostly in middle-aged adults with an equal male-to-female distribution. Microscopically, the bland tumor cells have low-grade nuclear features and a low mitotic rate. Endothelial differentiation is evident by the formation of intracytoplasmic lumina (that produces a signet ring cell appearance), but distinct vascular channels are not prominent. Hemangioendothelioma harbors a set of characteristic translocations that form the *WWTR1-CAMTA1* fusion gene (most common) or the *YAP1-TFE3* fusion gene. The tumor cells express CD31 and CD34, as well as proteins resulting from the involved characteristic translocation. Since the tumor can be solid, the differential diagnosis includes spindle cell sarcomas and angiosarcoma.
    2. **Primary Splenic Angiosarcoma**. This highly aggressive neoplasm carries a poor prognosis. Microscopically, it is characterized by plump, pleomorphic, and mitotically active endothelial cells with significant nuclear atypia that form irregular anastomosing vascular channels in the splenic sinusoids. A solid pattern is often seen in poorly differentiated cases. Primary splenic angiosarcoma is immunopositive for CD31, CD34, ERG, and AE1/AE3 (the latter in epithelioid angiosarcoma); D2-40 positivity suggests focal lymphatic differentiation in the tumor.

II. PSEUDONEOPLASTIC LESIONS

- **Splenic Cyst**. These are one of the most common benign lesions of the spleen. They occur predominantly in males, typically in the third decade, and are classically designated as either primary or secondary. Primary cysts account for approximately 20% of cases and are unilocular. Microscopically, they have a firm fibrous wall lined by mesothelial cells or squamous epithelium (although the epithelium can become denuded over time and thus resemble a secondary cyst). Primary cysts are subdivided into parasitic types (usually attributed to *Echinococcus* species and easily identified by the parasite scolices) and nonparasitic types (thought to arise from congenital inclusions of capsule mesothelium). Symptomatic cases require complete resection to avoid recurrence. Secondary cysts, responsible for approximately 80% of cases, are also unilocular and usually associated with a history of abdominal trauma (e-Figure 7.2-3). Microscopically, they are thin walled and demonstrate a complete absence of an epithelial or mesothelioma lining. They usually do not recur even if only partially excised.
- **Inflammatory Pseudotumor.** This extremely rare reactive process is comprised of inflammatory cells, myofibroblastic stroma, and epithelioid cells (e-Figure 7.2-4). Although the etiology is unknown, injury from prolonged chronic inflammation is thought to play a role. Some splenic inflammatory pseudotumors are associated with EBV and HHV-8 infection. The differential diagnosis includes inflammatory pseudotumor-like follicular dendritic cell sarcoma (IPT-FDCS) and lymphomas with lymphoplasmacytic differentiation.

- **Post-chemotherapy Histiocyte-Rich Pseudotumor of Spleen.** As the name indicates, the tumor is associated with prior chemoradiation in patients receiving treatment for lymphomas or solid tumors, and is characterized by a florid reparative response (*Am J Surg Pathol.* 2021;45:160-168). It is slow growing, but on imaging appears metabolically active. Microscopically, the lesion has a xanthogranulomatous appearance, abundant lipid-laden macrophages, giant cells, and an inflammatory infiltrate; necrosis is often present in the background. Diagnosis is challenging as the lesion can resemble recurrent or relapsed disease, as well as a variety of other neoplasms.

III. METASTATIC TUMORS

A variety of carcinomas and sarcomas can metastasize to the spleen, although the lack of afferent lymphatics renders the spleen generally less amenable to metastatic disease. Metastases therefore commonly arise in the setting of widely disseminated disease. The most common metastatic tumors are breast, lung, colorectal, and ovarian carcinomas, as well as melanoma (*Arch Pathol Lab Med.* 2007;131:965). Sarcomas involving the spleen tend to be of dendritic/histiocytic or vascular lineage.

IV. OTHER NEOPLASMS

Benign fibromas, osteomas, and chondromas occur rarely in the spleen. Rare cases of splenic angiomyolipoma have even been described.

SECTION III
Neoplastic

PART 1: Myeloid Neoplasms

8. Overview and Classification of Myeloid Neoplasms

Lianqun Qiu and Cecilia CS Yeung

The classification of myeloid neoplasms (MNs) was primarily based on the WHO-HAEM4R published in 2016 (*Blood*. 2016;127:2375-2390). The recent major advances in understanding the molecular pathogenesis of MNs prompted the updates in the classification of MNs in the WHO-HAEM5 and the International Consensus Classification (ICC) (*Leukemia*. 2022;36:1703-1719; *Blood*. 2022;140:1200-1228). The definition, classification, and diagnostic criteria of many myeloid entities have been refined with improved understanding of morphology, integration of new genetic findings, and emphasis on actionable therapeutic and prognostic biomarkers. This chapter summarizes the key changes in the new classification schemes and highlights the differences between the two classifications for a wide variety of MNs. A flowchart and algorithm outlining the diagnostic workup for MNs are illustrated in Figure 8.1.

I. OVERVIEW OF CHANGES IN MYELOPROLIFERATIVE NEOPLASMS

The major categories of myeloproliferative neoplasms (MPNs) remain unchanged in both the WHO-HAEM5 and the ICC (Table 8.1) from the WHO-HAEM4R. Diagnostic evaluation continues to rely on the integration of clinical, molecular, and morphologic features (Figure 8.1).

In chronic myeloid leukemia (CML), the WHO-HAEM5 has proposed the consolidation of a three-phase scheme into chronic phase (CP) and blast phase (BP) in the era of tyrosine kinase inhibitors (TKI). Accelerated phase (AP) is omitted in favor of an emphasis on high-risk features associated with CP, progression and resistance to TKI, stemming from *ABL1* kinase mutations, additional cytogenetic abnormalities (ACAs), and development of BP as key disease attributes. In contrast, the ICC has retained the category of AP (CML-AP) and refined the criteria to emphasize the presence or acquisition of major route ACAs at diagnosis or on treatment as the hallmark of CML-AP. The diagnostic criteria for BP are similar in the WHO-HAEM5 and ICC, with the

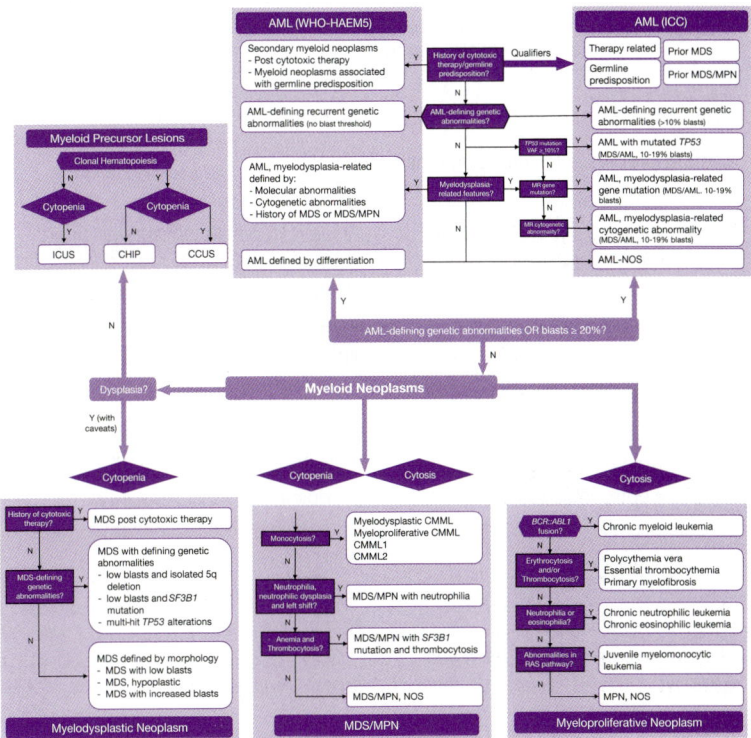

Figure 8.1. **Flow chart for diagnosis of major categories of myeloid neoplasms using morphology and/or genetic-focused algorithms.** The classification is based on the WHO-HAEM5 for MDS, MPN, and MDS/MPN, and both WHO-HAEM5 and ICC for AML and related precursor neoplasms. Y (with caveats)—Caveats mean the ICC does not require morphologic dysplasia in the presence of MDS-defining genetic abnormalities defined by del(5q), *SF3B1* or *TP53* (multihit or biallelic) mutations, −7/del(7q), or complex karyotype. Y, yes; N, no; AML, acute myeloid leukemia; CCUS, clonal cytopenia of undetermined significance; CHIP, clonal hematopoiesis of indeterminate potential; CMML, chronic myelomonocytic leukemia; ICUS, idiopathic cytopenia(s) of unknown significance; MDS, myelodysplastic syndrome/neoplasm; MPN, myeloproliferative neoplasm; MR, myelodysplasia related; NOS, not otherwise specified.

exception of lymphoblast assessment. The optimal cutoff for lymphoblasts is not specified in the WHO-HAEM5, whereas morphologically apparent lymphoblasts (>5%) are proposed in the ICC to prompt further laboratory and genetic studies.

Only minor changes have been proposed in diagnostic criteria for the classical *BCR::ABL1*-negative MPN subtypes including polycythemia vera (PV), essential thrombocythemia (ET), and primary myelofibrosis (PMF). The integration of molecular findings with bone marrow (BM) morphology and blood counts remains the cornerstone of diagnosis. Both classifications emphasize the importance of accurate identification of MPN-associated driver mutations by highly sensitive single target polymerase chain reaction (PCR)-based detection or multitarget panel/next generation sequencing (NGS) assays with a minimal sensitivity of variant allele frequency (VAF) of 1%.

TABLE 8.1 Comparison of Myeloid Neoplasm Classifications in WHO-HAEM5 and ICC

WHO-HAEM5	2022 ICC
Myeloid precursor lesions/clonal hematopoiesis	
Clonal hematopoiesis	Clonal hematopoiesis
Clonal cytopenias of undetermined significance	Clonal cytopenias of undetermined significance
	Paroxysmal nocturnal hemoglobinuria
	VEXAS syndrome
	Aplastic anemia with somatic mutation(s)
Myeloproliferative neoplasms (MPN)	
Chronic myeloid leukemia	Chronic myeloid leukemia
(Accelerated phase is omitted)	(Accelerated phase is retained)
Chronic neutrophilic leukemia	Chronic neutrophilic leukemia
Chronic eosinophilic leukemia	Chronic eosinophilic leukemia, NOS
Polycythemia vera	Polycythemia vera
Essential thrombocythemia	Essential thrombocythemia
Primary myelofibrosis	Primary myelofibrosis
Juvenile myelomonocytic leukemia	
MPN, NOS	MPN, unclassifiable
Mastocytosis	
Cutaneous mastocytosis	Cutaneous mastocytosis
Systemic mastocytosis (SM)	• Systemic mastocytosis
• Bone marrow mastocytosis	• Indolent SM (includes bone marrow mastocytosis)
• Indolent SM	
• Smoldering SM	• Smoldering SM
• Aggressive SM	• Aggressive SM
• Mast cell leukemia	• Mast cell leukemia
• SM with an associated hematologic neoplasm (SM-AHN)	• ***SM with an associated myeloid neoplasm (SM-AMN)***
Mast cell sarcoma	Mast cell sarcoma
Extracutaneous mastocytoma	
Myelodysplastic neoplasms (MDS)	
MDS with defining genetic abnormalities	
MDS with low blasts and isolated 5q deletion	Myelodysplastic syndrome (MDS) with del(5q)
MDS with low blasts and *SF3B1* mutation	MDS with mutated *SF3B1*
MDS with biallelic *TP53* inactivation	MDS with mutated *TP53*

TABLE 8.1	Comparison of Myeloid Neoplasm Classifications in WHO-HAEM5 and ICC (*continued*)

WHO-HAEM5	2022 ICC
MDS, morphologically defined	
MDS with low blasts	MDS, not otherwise specified (MDS, NOS)
	• MDS, NOS, without dysplasia
	• MDS, NOS with SLD
	• MDS-NOS with MLD
MDS, hypoplastic	
• MDS with increased blasts	MDS with excess blasts
• MDS-IB1	
• MDS-IB2	
• ***MDS with IB and fibrosis (MDS-f)***	
	MDS/AML[a]
	• With myelodysplasia-related cytogenetic abnormalities
	• With myelodysplasia-related gene mutations
	• NOS
	• With mutated *TP53*
MDS of childhood	
Childhood (c) MDS with low blasts	
• cMDS-LB, hypocellular	
• cMDS-LB, NOS	
Childhood MDS with increased blasts	
Pediatric and/or germline mutation-associated disorders	
	JMML
	JMML-like neoplasms
	Noonan syndrome—associated myeloproliferative disorder
	Refractory cytopenia of childhood
	Hematologic neoplasms with germline predisposition
MDS/MPN neoplasms	
Chronic myelomonocytic leukemia (CMML)	Chronic myelomonocytic leukemia
• ***Myelodysplastic CMML***	• CMML-1
• ***Myeloproliferative CMML***	• CMML-2
	• (CMML-0 is eliminated)

(*continued*)

TABLE 8.1	Comparison of Myeloid Neoplasm Classifications in WHO-HAEM5 and ICC (*continued*)

WHO-HAEM5	2022 ICC
• CMML-1	
• CMML-2	
• (CMML-0 is eliminated)	
	Clonal monocytosis of undetermined significance (CMUS)
	Clonal cytopenia with monocytosis of undetermined significance
Myelodysplastic/myeloproliferative neoplasm with neutrophilia	Atypical chronic myeloid leukemia
Myelodysplastic/myeloproliferative neoplasm with *SF3B1* mutation and thrombocytosis	Myelodysplastic/myeloproliferative neoplasm with *SF3B1* mutation and thrombocytosis
	Myelodysplastic/myeloproliferative neoplasm with ring sideroblasts and thrombocytosis, NOS
Myelodysplastic/myeloproliferative neoplasm, NOS	Myelodysplastic/myeloproliferative neoplasm, NOS
Acute myeloid leukemia (AML) with defining genetic abnormalities	
Acute promyelocytic leukemia (APL) with *PML::RARA* fusion	APL with *PML::RARA* fusion
	APL with other *RARA* rearrangement
AML with *RUNX1::RUNX1T1* fusion	AML with *RUNX1::RUNX1T1* fusion
AML with *CBFB::MYH11* fusion	AML with *CBFB::MYH11* fusion
AML with *DEK::NUP214* fusion	AML with *DEK::NUP214* fusion
AML with *RBM15::MRTFA* fusion	
AML with *BCR::ABL1* fusion	AML with *BCR::ABL1*
AML with *KMT2A* rearrangement	AML with *MLLT3::KMT2A* fusion
AML with *MECOM* rearrangement	AML with *GATA2::MECOM(EVI1)*
	AML with other *MECOM* rearrangement
AML with *NUP98* rearrangement	
AML with *NPM1* mutation	AML with *NPM1* mutation
AML with *CEBPA* mutation	**AML with in-frame bZIP *CEBPA* mutation**
AML, myelodysplasia related[b,c]	AML and MDS/AML with myelodysplasia-related gene mutations[b]
	AML with myelodysplasia-related cytogenetic abnormalities[d]
	AML with mutated *TP53*

TABLE 8.1	Comparison of Myeloid Neoplasm Classifications in WHO-HAEM5 and ICC (*continued*)

WHO-HAEM5	2022 ICC
AML with other defined genetic alterations	AML with other rare recurring translocations

AML, defined by differentiation

AML with minimal differentiation	AML, NOS
AML without maturation	
AML with maturation	
Acute basophilic leukemia	
Acute myelomonocytic leukemia	
Acute monocytic leukemia	
Acute erythroid leukemia	
Acute megakaryoblastic leukemia	
Myeloid sarcoma	Myeloid sarcoma

Myeloid neoplasms, secondary

Myeloid neoplasms and proliferations associated with antecedent or predisposing conditions

Myeloid neoplasms post-cytotoxic therapy	
Myeloid neoplasms associated with germline predisposition	
Myeloid proliferations associated with Down syndrome	Myeloid proliferations associated with Down syndrome

Myeloid/lymphoid neoplasms (M/LN) with eosinophilia and defining gene rearrangement

M/LN with *PDGFRA* rearrangement	M/LN with *PDGFRA* rearrangement
M/LN with *PDGFRB* rearrangement	M/LN with *PDGFRB* rearrangement
M/LN with *FGFR1* rearrangement	M/LN with *FGFR1* rearrangement
M/LN with *JAK2* rearrangement	M/LN with *JAK2* rearrangement
M/LN with *FLT3* rearrangement	M/LN with *FLT3* rearrangement
M/LN with *ETV6::ABL1* fusion	M/LN with *ETV6::ABL1* fusion
M/LN with other tyrosine kinase gene fusions	

Acute leukemias of mixed or ambiguous lineage

Acute leukemia of ambiguous lineage (ALAL) with defining genetic abnormalities

MPAL with *BCR::ABL1* fusion	Mixed-phenotype acute leukemia (MPAL) with *BCR::ABL1*
MPAL with *KMT2A* rearrangement	MPAL with t(v;11q23.3); *KMT2A*-rearranged

(*continued*)

TABLE 8.1	Comparison of Myeloid Neoplasm Classifications in WHO-HAEM5 and ICC (*continued*)

WHO-HAEM5	2022 ICC
Acute leukemia of ambiguous lineage with other defined genetic alterations	MPAL with *ZNF384* rearrangement
• MPAL with *ZNF384* rearrangement	MPAL with *BCL11B* activation
• ALAL with *BCL11B* rearrangement	
Acute leukemia of ambiguous lineage, immunophenotypically defined	
MPAL, B/myeloid	B/myeloid MPAL
MPAL, T/myeloid	T/myeloid MPAL
MPAL, rare types	B/T/myeloid MPAL
	B/T MPAL
Acute undifferentiated leukemia (AUL)	Acute undifferentiated leukemia
ALAL, NOS	ALAL, NOS

bZIP, basic leucine zipper; cMDS-LB, childhood myelodysplastic neoplasm with low blasts; IB, increased blasts; JMML, juvenile myelomonocytic leukemia; MLD, multilineage dysplasia; SLD, single lineage dysplasia; VEXAS, vacuoles, E1 enzyme, X-linked, autoinflammatory, somatic syndrome.
Modified from the WHO-HAEM5 and the 2022 International Consensus Classification (ICC). New entities and entities that are different between the two classifications are set in bold italics.
[a]Per the ICC, diagnostic qualifiers that can be applied after any MDS or MDS/AML entity include (1) therapy related; and/or (2) germline mutation or syndrome.
[b]Myelodysplasia-related genes are defined by somatic mutations in *ASXL1, BCOR, EZH2, RUNX1* (ICC), *SF3B1, SRSF2, STAG2, U2AF1,* or *ZRSR2.*
[c]Per the WHO-HAEM5, myelodysplasia-related cytogenetic abnormalities are defined by detecting a complex karyotype (≥3 abnormalities), 5q deletion or loss of 5q due to unbalanced translocation, monosomy 7, 7q deletion, or loss of 7q due to unbalanced translocation, 11q deletion, 12p deletion or loss of 12p due to unbalanced translocation, monosomy 13 or 13q deletion, 17p deletion or loss of 17p due to unbalanced translocation, isochromosome 17q, and/or idic(X)(q13).
[d]Per the ICC, myelodysplasia-related cytogenetic abnormalities are defined by detecting a complex karyotype (≥3 unrelated clonal chromosomal abnormalities in the absence of other class-defining recurring genetic abnormalities), del(5q)/t(5q)/add(5q), −7/del(7q), +8, del(12p)/t(12p)/add(12p), i(17q), −17/add(17p) or del(17p), del(20q), and/or idic(X)(q13) clonal abnormalities.

Chronic neutrophilic leukemia (CNL) is a rare *BCR::ABL1*-negative MPN characterized by sustained peripheral blood (PB) neutrophilia, BM neutrophilic granulocyte proliferation, hepatosplenomegaly, and *CSF3R* mutations in more than 60% of cases. The ICC suggests lowering the key diagnostic threshold for leukocytosis from 25 or more to 13 or more $\times 10^9$/L in cases with *CSF3R* T618I or other activating *CSF3R* mutation, to reflect the critical role of *CSF3R* signaling in leukemogenesis.

Several changes to the diagnostic criteria for chronic eosinophilic leukemia (CEL) are introduced in the WHO-HAEM5, including a reduced time interval to 4 weeks for qualifying as sustained hypereosinophilia, evidence of clonality and abnormal BM morphology, and elimination of the requirement for increased blasts. The qualifier "not otherwise specified" has been omitted from the name in the WHO-HAEM5. In contrast, the ICC has retained requirements for a minimal 6-month duration and increased blasts but has similarly introduced abnormal BM histopathology into the diagnostic criteria, to improve the distinction between CEL and entities such as idiopathic hypereosinophilic syndrome and hypereosinophilia of unknown significance.

Both the WHO and ICC have retained the category of MPN, unclassifiable (MPN-U), and the name has been updated to MPN-NOS (MPN, not otherwise specified) in the WHO-HAEM5. The category is reserved for cases with clinicopathologic features of MPN that lack diagnostic criteria of a specific MPN but show features that overlap across distinct MPN subtypes.

Juvenile myelomonocytic leukemia (JMML) is now categorized as a hematopoietic stem cell-derived MPN of early childhood with RAS pathway activation in the WHO-HAEM5, where approximately 90% of cases are associated with germline pathogenic gene variants. The diagnostic criteria have been modified to reflect the molecular pathogenesis to underscore the absence of bona fide myelodysplastic neoplasia and the importance of the genetic background in risk stratification and therapeutic approaches. In contrast, the ICC has moved JMML under the category of "pediatric disorders and/or germline mutation-associated disorders" and divided it into two genetically and clinically distinct subtypes based on the mutation profile in the canonical RAS pathway. Clonal disease that phenotypically mimics JMML but does not harbor any of the RAS pathway mutations is classified as JMML-like neoplasm. Noonan syndrome–associated myeloproliferative disorder in its severe form is also included as a JMML mimicker.

II. OVERVIEW OF MYELOID PRECURSOR LESIONS

Myeloid precursor lesions have been formally included for the first time in the WHO-HAEM5 and ICC. Mutation-driven clonal hematopoiesis (CH) underlies several associated entities. Clonality is identified by somatic mutations, with deep sequencing being the preferred detection modality over exome or genome sequencing.

Myeloid precursor lesions without unexplained cytopenia include CH, age-related clonal hematopoiesis (ARCH), and clonal hematopoiesis of indeterminate potential (CHIP). ARCH has been employed to refer to CH in association with aging; however, ARCH does not have a defined specific gene alteration or quantitative criteria. In contrast, the term CHIP was coined to denote the presence of somatic mutations in MN driver genes and requires a VAF of 2% or more (≥4% for X-linked gene mutations in genetic males with one X chromosome) in an otherwise healthy individual. The ICC has introduced non-myelodysplasia (myelodysplastic syndrome [MDS])-defining clonal cytogenetic aberration as alternative evidence of clonality in patients lacking a MN or unexplained cytopenia. CHIP is rare in people under 40 years of age, and the incidence increases with age, affecting 10% to 40% of older individuals after 65 years. The most commonly affected genes are *DNMT3A*, *TET2*, and *ASXL1* (DTAs), with a median VAF of 10%, associated with an increased risk of developing myeloid neoplasia (*Virchows Arch.* 2023;482:39-51).

CHIP detected in individuals with unexplained cytopenia(s) has been officially defined as clonal cytopenia of undetermined significance (CCUS). Definitions for cytopenia(s) have been standardized and harmonized for both myeloid precursor lesions and MNs in the WHO-HAEM5 and ICC. The duration of cytopenia(s) must be at least 4 months or longer. In the absence of evidence of clonality, sustained unexplained cytopenia(s) are referred to as idiopathic cytopenia(s) of unknown significance (ICUS). In general, the risk of progression from CCUS to MDS and acute myeloid leukemia (AML) is very low but increases with the size of the clonal population, the number of somatic alterations, and the presence of specific gene mutations.

Aside from CCUS, the ICC has introduced several unique clonal cytopenic syndromes including aplastic anemia (AA) with somatic mutation(s), paroxysmal nocturnal hemoglobinuria (PNH), and VEXAS (vacuoles, E1 enzyme, X-linked, autoinflammatory, somatic) syndrome. Over one-third of patients with AA display CH, with the most commonly affected genes (*BCOR*, *BCORL1*, and *PIGA*) being different from those of CCUS. PNH and VEXAS are each associated with unique mutations. It is recommended to separate VEXAS from MDS given its unique multisystem features and extremely low incidence of progression to AML (*Virchows Arch*. 2023;482:39-51).

CCUS and other premalignant clonal cytopenia(s) are distinguished from MDS by lack of dysplasia or increased blasts on PB and BM examination. Therefore, the diagnosis of CCUS requires a BM sample for morphologic, molecular, and cytogenetic examination to confirm the absence of diagnostic features of any defined myeloid neoplasms. Conversely, the presence of significant dysplasia, excess blasts, and/or an MDS-defining genetic abnormality separates MDS from these non-MDS clonal cytopenias.

III. OVERVIEW OF CHANGES IN MYELODYSPLASTIC SYNDROME

The WHO-HAEM5 introduces myelodysplastic neoplasm (MDS) to replace myelodysplastic syndrome to harmonize terminology with MPN. Both the WHO-HAEM5 and ICC have refined the definition of MDS and grouped cases as having defining genetic abnormalities or those defined by morphology. The category of MDS unclassifiable has been eliminated in the WHO-HAEM5 and ICC.

Of MDS-defining genetic abnormalities, the list has been updated to include del(5q), multihit or biallelic *TP53* mutation, or *SF3B1* mutation (at VAF of ≥10%, per the ICC). The WHO-HAEM5 recommends 15% or more ring sideroblasts to be interchangeable with *SF3B1* mutation. The ICC has additionally recognized −7/del(7q) or complex karyotype as MDS-defining genetic abnormalities to permit a diagnosis of MDS, NOS without dysplasia. In both classifications, MDS with mutated *TP53* requires two or more distinct *TP53* mutations, or a single *TP53* mutation with *TP53* copy loss, or copy-neutral loss of heterozygosity (cnLOH). The ICC also requires a VAF of greater than 10% for each *TP53* mutation and has accepted a VAF of greater than 50% or a complex karyotype as alternative evidence for lacking any residual wild-type P53 protein. Of note, the presence of *SF3B1* or a single *TP53* mutation (not multihit) does not per se override the diagnosis of MDS-5q, where MDS-bi*TP53* supersedes the other two.

The morphologically defined MDS subgroup includes entities of MDS with low blasts and increased blasts. The WHO-HAEM5 has introduced a new subtype of hypoplastic MDS (MDS-h) defined by age-adjusted marrow cellularity 25% or less to cover a minority of cases that can resemble AA and/or PNH. Single-lineage and multi-lineage dysplasia subtypes are retained in ICC (in the category of MDS, NOS) but removed in the WHO-HAEM5.

While the WHO-HAEM5 acknowledges the softened boundary between MDS and AML, the blast threshold to separate MDS from AML remains unchanged (<20% blasts) from the WHO-HAEM4R, with exception for AML-defining genetic alterations that lead to rapid disease progression even if they present initially with less than 20% blasts. In contrast, the ICC proposes to classify AML-defining genetic alterations with less than 10% blast as MDS and introduced a new MDS/AML entity that encompasses cases with 10% to 19% blasts in the PB and/or BM to acknowledge the biologic continuum between MDS and AML, and to overcome imprecision in blast enumeration. Of note, the entity MDS/AML does not apply to pediatric patients (<18 years), and the blast thresholds for MDS with excess blasts (MDS-EB) have remained at 5% to 19% in BM and 2% to 19% in PB.

Childhood MDS is biologically distinct from that seen in adults. The WHO-HAEM5 proposes to use the term childhood MDS with low blasts to replace the former term "refractory cytopenia of childhood (RCC)". Childhood MDS with low blasts includes two subtypes: (1) childhood MDS with low blasts, hypocellular, and (2) childhood MDS with low blasts, NOS.

IV. OVERVIEW OF CHANGES IN MYELODYSPLASTIC SYNDROMES/MYELOPROLIFERATIVE NEOPLASMS

The myelodysplastic syndromes/myeloproliferative neoplasms (MDS/MPN) category comprises a heterogeneous group of MNs characterized by overlapping pathologic and molecular features of MDS and MPN, often manifesting clinically with both cytopenias and cytoses (Figure 8.1). Both the WHO-HAEM5 and ICC have introduced major revisions in the diagnostic criteria of CMML (chronic myelomonocytic leukemia) and terminology changes for other MDS/MPN types.

The diagnostic criteria of CMML in both classifications have incorporated revised prerequisites and supporting criteria. The cutoff for absolute monocytosis as one prerequisite criterion is lowered from 1.0×10^9/L to 0.5×10^9/L in PB to incorporate cases formerly referred to as oligomonocytic CMML. Abnormal partitioning of peripheral blood monocyte subsets is introduced as a new supporting criterion, with patients with CMML demonstrating an expansion (>94%) of classical monocytes ($CD14^+/CD16^-$) in the absence of reactive conditions. In cases when absolute monocytosis is low, the detection of clonal cytogenetic or molecular abnormalities and the documentation of dysplasia in at least one lineage are required. Based on the white blood cell (WBC) count and morphologic features, CMML is subtyped into myelodysplastic CMML (MD-CMML) and myeloproliferative CMML (MP-CMML). Based on the percentage of blasts and blast equivalents, CMML is subgrouped into CMML-1 and CMML-2 (CMML-1: <5% blasts in the PB or <10% in the BM; CMML-2: 5%-19% blasts in the PB or 10%-19% in the BM). CMML-0 has been eliminated.

For unexplained clonal monocytosis in the absence of BM morphologic findings of CMML, the ICC introduces an independent entity, namely clonal monocytosis of undetermined significance (CMUS), as a precursor condition to CMML, analogous to CCUS. In cases of cytopenia, the disorder is renamed clonal cytopenia and monocytosis of undetermined significance (CCMUS).

Atypical chronic myeloid leukemia (aCML), *BCR::ABL1* negative, has been replaced with a new terminology, MDS/MPN with neutrophilia in the WHO-HAEM5, while ICC has kept the original name but dropped the notation of "*BCR::ABL1*." The change highlights the MDS/MPN nature of the disease and avoids potential confusion with both CML and other Philadelphia-negative disorders. The ICC requires the presence of cytopenia(s) and specifies that hypereosinophilia is incompatible with this entity.

Both the WHO-HAEM5 and the ICC have redefined MDS/MPN with ring sideroblasts and thrombocytosis (MDS/MPN-RS-T) and renamed it MDS/MPN with *SF3B1* mutation and thrombocytosis. Both thrombocytosis and anemia must be present at the time of initial diagnosis. The ICC requires *SF3B1* mutation to be greater than 10% of VAF with identification of ring sideroblasts no longer needed. In cases with wild-type *SF3B1* and 15% or more of ring sideroblasts, the term MDS/MPN-RS-T has been retained in both classifications but designated as "MDS/MPN-RS-T, NOS" in the ICC.

MDS/MPN, unclassifiable is now termed MDS/MPN, not otherwise specified (MDS/MPN, NOS) in both the WHO-HAEM5 and the ICC. It remains a diagnosis of exclusion. The ICC has introduced a new provisional sub-entity, namely MDS/MPN with isolated isochromosome (17q) [MDS/MPN with i(17q)]. It is unclear whether this is a distinct entity or falls within the spectrum of aCML, with which it shares a similar genomic signature.

V. OVERVIEW OF ACUTE MYELOID LEUKEMIA AND RELATED PRECURSOR NEOPLASMS

Both the WHO-HAEM5 and the ICC have re-envisioned the AML classification to incorporate major breakthroughs in genetics over the past years with an emphasis on leukemogenesis, clinical management, and prognostic impact. One major change is to separate AML with defining genetic abnormalities from AML defined by differentiation. The term of AML, NOS is eliminated in the WHO-HAEM5 classification.

Under AML defined by genetic changes, the WHO-HAEM5 has simplified AML with *KMT2A*, *MECOM*, and *NUP98* rearrangements to incorporate various partner fusion genes and introduced several new entities with specific cytogenetic features (Table 8.1). The ICC has retained AML with *MLLT3::KMT2A* and AML with inv(3) or t(3;3), and introduced new entities of acute promyelocytic leukemia (APL) with other *RARA* rearrangements and AML with other *KMT2A* and *MECOM* rearrangements as AML-defining genetic alterations to encompass variable fusion partners that may lead to rapid disease progression and have an adverse impact on clinical management and prognosis. A new entity of AML, with other defined genetic alterations or other rare recurring translocations, has been introduced into the WHO-HAEM5 and ICC, respectively, as a landing spot for new and uncommon AML subtypes that may (or may not) become defined types in future editions of the classification. AML defined by mutations includes AML with *NPM1* and AML with *CEBPA*. The WHO-HAEM5 recommends refining this entity to include both biallelic (bi*CEBPA*) and single mutations in the basic leucine zipper (bZIP) region (smbZIP-*CEBPA*) of the gene, whereas the ICC only recognizes in-frame bZIP *CEBPA* mutation without the necessity for biallelic mutations.

The prior category of AML with myelodysplasia-related changes (AML-MRC) in the WHO-HAEM4R is now renamed as AML, myelodysplasia related (AML-MR) in the WHO-HAEM5 with several updates. MDS-defining specific cytogenetic and molecular abnormalities have been specified and introduced into the diagnostic criteria, irrespective of arising de novo or following a known history of MDS or MDS/MPN. Morphologic dysplasia alone is no longer required as a diagnostic premise. Similarly, the ICC has eliminated the category of AML-MRC while retaining a category of AML-MR cytogenetic abnormalities and has introduced new categories of AML with mutated *TP53* and AML-MR gene mutations. In contrast to the WHO-HAEM5, the ICC does not consider a documented MDS or MDS/MPN history as required for diagnosis of AML-MR but rather uses it as a diagnostic qualifier. Both classifications have abandoned the previous stand-alone category of AML with *RUNX1* mutation, and these cases are now included under AML-MR or AML with MR gene mutation.

In the ICC, AML with mutated *TP53* is recognized as a separate entity within the group of MNs with mutated *TP53*. *TP53* mutations define a distinctly aggressive AML category that can present either de novo as the progression of MDS or as a therapy-related disease. As pure erythroid leukemia is typically associated with *TP53* mutations, these cases are now classified within the category of AML with *TP53* mutations in the ICC. Different from the requirement for *multihit TP53 mutations* in the diagnosis of MDS with mutated *TP53*, any pathogenic *TP53* mutation with a VAF of greater than 10% is sufficient for diagnoses of AML and MDS/AML with mutated *TP53*.

The ICC has retained AML, NOS for cases lacking defining genetic abnormalities, while this family of AML cases will continue to be classified based on differentiation in the WHO-HAEM5. A comprehensive framework of differentiation markers and criteria has been updated and harmonized with those of mixed-phenotype acute leukemia (MPAL) and early T-precursor lymphoblastic leukemia/lymphoma. Of note, the previously pure erythroid leukemia is now renamed as acute erythroid leukemia (AEL) in the WHO-HAEM5, and the central role of biallelic *TP53* mutation in this aggressive AML type has been underscored. The diagnosis of AEL supersedes AML-MR in the WHO-HAEM5.

The hierarchy of disease categories follows in the order of recurring translocations, AML-defining somatic mutations, myelodysplasia-related gene mutations, followed by myelodysplasia-related cytogenetic abnormalities, and AML by differentiation (Figure 8.1).

The ICC has additionally proposed to apply diagnostic qualifiers as disease attributes to relevant myeloid neoplasia: therapy related, progressing from MDS, progressing from MDS/MPN, and germline predisposition mutation or syndrome. Using this approach, the prior stand-alone categories of therapy-related MNs and AML-MRC are eliminated in the ICC.

Both the ICC and the WHO-HAEM5 have adopted a framework for a molecular-based classification and separated acute leukemia of ambiguous lineage (ALAL)/MPAL defined by genetic abnormalities from those defined by traditional immunophenotyping. Two new genetically defined subtypes, MPAL with *ZNF384* rearrangement and ALAL/MPAL with *BCL11B* rearrangement/activation, are introduced and included under the new entity of ALAL with other defined genetic alteration in the WHO-HAEM5. In cases of bilineal MPAL that have immature populations of two or more lineages, the WHO-HAEM5 suggests measuring leukemic cells in aggregation to meet the quantity criteria, whereas the ICC requires the small aberrant clones to be greater than 5% as a diagnostic criterion. In cases with aberrant clones representing less than 5% of all analyzed events, the ICC suggests a diagnosis based on the major leukemic population with a descriptive modifier.

VI. OVERVIEW OF SECONDARY MYELOID NEOPLASMS

MNs that arise secondary to exposure to cytotoxic therapy or germline predisposition are grouped in this category. In the WHO-HAEM5, MN post-cytotoxic therapy is used to replace MN therapy related. Exposure to PARP1 [poly (ADP-ribose) polymerase 1] inhibitors is added as a qualifying criterion, and methotrexate has been excluded. The ICC has eliminated this category and suggested the use of diagnostic qualifiers under respective specific categories.

MNs associated with germline predisposition are now classified using a formulaic approach that couples the myeloid disease phenotype with the predisposing germline genotype, for example, AML with germline pathogenic variants in *RUNX1* in the WHO-HAEM5. In contrast, the ICC has modified the category from "myeloid neoplasms" to "hematologic neoplasms" with germline predisposition to reflect the fact that many genes predispose to both myeloid and lymphoid malignancies. Myeloid proliferations associated with Down syndrome (specifically, transient abnormal myelopoiesis [TAM] and myeloid leukemia of Down syndrome) in the WHO-HAEM4R are now included in this category. Newly recognized germline mutations (*SAMD9, SAMD9L,* and *TP53*) have been added.

In addition, the ICC has introduced a new category to encompass pediatric disorders and/or germline mutation-associated disorders unified by their unique and overlapping genetic features. With respect to the category of RCC, the diagnostic criteria have been updated in the ICC. The ICC emphasizes that while some RCC cases are associated with acquired somatic mutations or cytogenetic abnormalities, others result from the progression of germline predisposition disorders to BM failure or frank MDS.

VII. OVERVIEW OF CHANGES IN MYELOID/LYMPHOID NEOPLASMS WITH EOSINOPHILIA AND GENE REARRANGEMENTS

Both classifications have renamed myeloid/lymphoid neoplasms with eosinophilia (M/LN-eo) and gene rearrangement to myeloid/lymphoid neoplasms with eosinophilia and tyrosine kinase gene fusions (M/LN-TK or M/LN-eo-TK) to emphasize the unifying feature of rearrangements involving genes encoding specific tyrosine kinases that result in constitutive action of the kinase domain (*Am J Hematol.* 2023;98:1286-1306). M/LN-eo with *JAK2* rearrangement is now accepted as a formal member of this category, along with the new additions of ETV*6*::ABL*1* or *FLT3* rearrangements. The WHO-HAEM5 has additionally introduced a new scalable genetic framework under MLN-TK with other defined tyrosine kinase fusions to include other less common defined genetic alterations involving tyrosine kinase genes. A diagnosis of MLN-TK supersedes other myeloid and lymphoid types, as well as systemic mastocytosis (SM).

IX. OVERVIEW OF CHANGES IN MASTOCYTOSIS

While most diagnostic criteria for SM have remained unchanged, several criteria have been refined. Both classifications have introduced new minor diagnostic criteria to include CD30 expression and *KIT* mutation other than D816V with subsequent ligand-independent *KIT* activation. In the case of hereditary α-tryptasemia, the WHO-HAEM5 recommends that adjusted basal serum tryptase levels should be used.

The framework of subclassification remains unchanged in the two classifications. Bone marrow mastocytosis (BMM) is now accepted as a new SM subtype in the WHO-HAEM5, whereas it is considered as a clinicopathologic variant of indolent SM in the ICC to recognize its unique clinicopathologic features characterized by absence of skin lesions, absence of B findings, and a basal serum tryptase level below 125 ng/mL (*Am J Hematol.* 2023;98:1286-1306). The ICC has also modified the subtype of SM with an associated hematologic neoplasm (SM-AHN) to SM with an associated myeloid neoplasm (AMN) to indicate the nature of the associated malignancy and allow appropriate risk stratification and management. Well-differentiated systemic mastocytosis (WDSM) as a morphologic pattern that can occur in any SM subtype has been introduced into the two classifications. The criteria for assessing disease burden (B- and C-findings) have undergone minor refinements as well.

X. OVERVIEW OF PLASMACYTOID DENDRITIC CELL NEOPLASM

The WHO-HAEM5 has introduced a new disease category to recognize the presence of mature plasmacytoid dendritic cell proliferation (MPDCP) in association with MNs. The most common associated MNs are CMML followed by AML, MDS, and MPN. Clonal MPDCP in MP-CMML has been associated with activating RAS pathway mutations (*Leukemia.* 2019;33:2466-2480). Clonal proliferation of pDCs in patients with AML (pDC-AML) shares the same mutational landscape as the AML blasts and frequently arises in association with *RUNX1* mutations. The diagnosis requires the presence of specific morphologic and immunophenotypic criteria to distinguish it from blastic plasmacytoid dendritic cell neoplasm (BPDCN).

SUGGESTED READINGS

Arber DA, Orazi A, Hasserjian RP, et al. International Consensus Classification of myeloid neoplasms and acute leukemias: integrating morphologic, clinical, and genomic data. *Blood.* 2022;140(11):1200-1228.

Hasserjian RP, Orazi A, Orfao A, Rozman M, Wang SA. The International Consensus Classification of myelodysplastic syndromes and related entities. *Virchows Arch.* 2023;482(1):39-51.

Khoury JD, Solary E, Abla O, et al. The 5th edition of the World Health Organization classification of haematolymphoid tumours: myeloid and histiocytic/dendritic neoplasms. *Leukemia.* 2022;36(7):1703-1719.

Swerdlow SH, Campo E, Pileri SA, et al. The 2016 revision of the World Health Organization classification of lymphoid neoplasms. *Blood.* 2016;127(20):2375-2390.

Wang SA, Orazi A, Gotlib J, et al. The International Consensus Classification of eosinophilic disorders and systemic mastocytosis. *Am J Hematol.* 2023;98(8):1286-1306.

9. Myeloproliferative Neoplasms

Frido K. Bruehl and Shiyong Li

Myeloproliferative neoplasms (MPNs) are a group of myeloid malignancies characterized by clonal expansion of one or more hematopoietic lineages leading to peripheral cytosis. Blasts may be slightly increased in the bone marrow and are occasionally seen in the peripheral blood. Dysplasia is usually absent. The age-adjusted bone marrow cellularity is increased in most MPNs. Other clinical and laboratory findings may include hepatosplenomegaly, hyperviscosity, elevated serum lactate dehydrogenase (LDH) level, and hyperuricemia. Nevertheless, MPNs are frequently asymptomatic and discovered incidentally on a routine complete blood count (CBC) workup. Precise classification of MPNs is challenging in the early stages because of overlapping morphologic features between the different entities and potential reactive mimickers. While progression to acute leukemia does occur, patients with MPNs have seen improvements in survival since the discovery of a few well-characterized and targetable genetic abnormalities. It is important to recognize and distinguish between the various MPNs because they have different propensity for transformation and require different treatment regimens and clinical follow-ups.

I. CHRONIC MYELOID LEUKEMIA

Chronic myeloid leukemia (CML) is one of the most common MPNs and is characterized by an overproduction of maturing myeloid precursors. The estimated annual incidence rate is 1 to 2 per 100,000 adults, with a slight male predominance (male/female ratio of 1.2-1.7) and a median age of 56 years at diagnosis in Western countries (*Blood Rev.* 2020;42:100706). Patients are frequently asymptomatic or present with signs and symptoms related to blood, bone marrow, and extramedullary infiltration by the maturing granulocytic precursors, such as fatigue, weight loss, and hepatosplenomegaly. If untreated, CML progresses from a chronic phase (CP) to an accelerated phase (AP), to a terminal blast phase (BP). Rare patients may present in an advanced disease stage without a recognized preceding CP. With the advent of tyrosine kinase inhibitors (TKIs), the prognosis for CML has significantly improved; high rates of complete hematologic, cytogenetic, and molecular responses are typically achieved, leading to prolonged survival and even the possibility of treatment-free remission in some cases.

Morphologic and Immunophenotypic Features

Peripheral blood typically shows marked leukocytosis (ranging from 12 to 1,000 k/μL, median of 100 k/μL) with a myelocyte "bulge" (myelocytes increased out of proportion to what can be seen in patients with reactive leukocytosis), basophilia, and thrombocytosis (e-Figure 9.1-1). Granulocytes do not display significant dysplasia, and toxic granulation is uncommon. Monocytosis, eosinophilia, erythrocytosis, nucleated red blood cells, and circulating blasts can occur but should not constitute a prominent finding. Thrombocytopenia is rare in CP and should raise suspicion of presentation at an advanced stage.

The bone marrow is markedly hypercellular (approaching 100% cellularity) in all disease phases (e-Figures 9.1-2 to 9.1-5). In CP, there is granulocytic predominance with complete maturation but without significant granulocytic dysplasia and less than 5% blasts, reflecting the peripheral blood morphology. Basophils and eosinophils are usually easily identified in bone marrow aspirates. Erythroid precursors are typically decreased and lack dysplasia. Megakaryocytes are quantitatively normal or increased, and show characteristically small and hyposegmented forms ("dwarf" megakaryocytes). Other features that can be observed include pseudo-Gaucher cells and the so-called "sea-blue" histiocytes, both reflecting the increased cell turnover and their origin from the abnormal myeloid clone. Reticulin fibrosis is not a typical feature of CP and may represent a feature of progression, although its significance has been deemphasized in the TKI era.

BP CML is characterized by 20% or more myeloid blasts in the blood or bone marrow, or the presence of an extramedullary proliferation of blasts. The presence of increased lymphoblasts (even if <10%) in peripheral blood or bone marrow should raise suspicion of lymphoblastic transformation, although the WHO has not designated a precise cutoff level. The International Consensus Classification (ICC) has suggested more than 5% as a threshold warranting further laboratory and genetic workup.

Immunophenotyping is usually not required for the primary diagnosis of CP CML, but it may be helpful to corroborate the percentage of blasts identified by morphology. While blasts in CP usually display a normal myeloid phenotype with variable expression of myeloperoxidase (MPO) and myeloid lineage-associated markers (CD13, CD33, CD117), aberrant expression of CD7 and CD56 may be seen. Immunophenotyping plays a more important role in BP CML to assess the lineage of blast cell populations, particularly emerging lymphoblasts.

Genetic Features

The Philadelphia chromosome (Ph) t(9;22)(q34;q11) or *BCR::ABL1* gene fusion is the hallmark and a major diagnostic criterion of CML. The classic Ph juxtaposes the breakpoint cluster region gene (*BCR*) at chromosome 22q11 with the Abelson tyrosine kinase gene (*ABL*) 1 at chromosome 9q34. The resultant functional *BCR::ABL1* fusion gene on derivative chromosome 22 leads to a constitutive activation of ABL1 tyrosine kinase producing a consistent clinical, laboratory, and bone marrow morphology. While *BCR::ABL1* gene fusion defines CML, it is not unique to the disease and itself exists in variable forms across diseases; in CML, BCR::ABL1 is typically of the 210 kDa (p210) form, compared with the 190 kDa (p190) form in B-lymphoblastic leukemia/lymphoma. The p230 (230 kDa) form of BCR::ABL1 is less frequently identified in CML; such cases show a predominance of mature neutrophils rather than immature granulocytes. Cases of CML with p190 have been associated with monocytosis. In rare cases, variant translocations exist that cannot be readily identified by routine cytogenetic karyotyping; in such instances, FISH (fluorescence in situ hybridization) and PCR (polymerase chain reaction) are paramount.

Diagnosis and Differential Diagnosis

In the appropriate clinical and laboratory setting, the diagnosis of CML is established based on the detection of the *BCR::ABL1* gene fusion through cytogenetic and molecular testing methods (see Table 9.1). The differential diagnosis of CP CML includes reactive leukocytosis and various other myeloid neoplasms, such as *BCR::ABL1*-negative MPNs, MDS (myelodysplastic neoplasm)/MPNs, and myeloid/lymphoid neoplasms with tyrosine kinase gene fusions. Reactive leukocytosis typically

TABLE 9.1 WHO-HAEM5 Diagnostic Criteria for CML

Chronic phase

1. Peripheral blood leukocytosis
and
2. Detection of Ph and/or *BCR::ABL1* gene fusion by cytogenetic and molecular genetic methods
and/or
3. Bone marrow examination

Chronic phase with high-risk features[a]

At diagnosis

1. High European treatment and outcome study long-term survival (ELTS) score[b]
2. 10%-19% myeloid blasts in the blood and bone marrow
3. ≥20% basophils in the peripheral blood
4. ACAs in Ph-positive cells, including 2nd Ph, isochromosome 17q, monosomy 7, 3q26.2 rearrangements, and complex karyotype
5. Clusters of dysplastic megakaryocytes with associated significant reticulin and collagen fibrosis

Emerging on treatment

1. Failure to achieve a complete hematologic response to the first TKI
2. Any hematologic, cytogenetic, or molecular indications of resistance to two sequential TKIs
3. Development of new ACAs
4. Occurrence of compound mutations in the *BCR::ABL1* gene fusion during TKI therapy

Blast phase

1. ≥20% myeloid blasts in the blood and bone marrow
or
2. Presence of an extramedullary proliferation of blasts
or
3. Presence of increased lymphoblasts in the blood and bone marrow (even if <10%)[c]

ACA, additional chromosomal abnormality; CML, chronic myeloid leukemia; Ph, Philadelphia chromosome; TKI, tyrosine kinase inhibitor.
[a]Equivalent to accelerated phase (AP) of CML in ICC 2022.
[b]Calculated based on age, spleen size, platelet, and peripheral blood blast counts.
[c]The optimal cutoff for lymphoblasts and the significance of low-level B lymphoblasts remain unclear and require additional studies. The ICC 2022 states that the presence of morphologically apparent lymphoblasts, even if less than 5% of cells, warrants consideration of lymphoblastic phase.
Based on the WHO Classification of Tumours Editorial Board. Haematolymphoid tumours [Internet]. Lyon (France): International Agency for Research on Cancer; 2024 (WHO classification of tumours series, 5th ed.; vol. 11). Available from: https://tumourclassification.iarc.who.int/chapters/63.

shows toxic granulation of neutrophils and lacks a myelocyte "bulge," basophilia, and hypolobated megakaryocytes in the bone marrow. MDS/MPN shows more pronounced dysplastic changes and monocytosis with cytopenia, while myeloid/lymphoid neoplasm with tyrosine kinase gene fusion frequently has prominent eosinophilia. Regardless, the presence of a *BCR::ABL1* gene fusion excludes the diagnosis of these morphologic mimickers. BP CML should be distinguished from *de novo* acute myeloid and lymphoblastic leukemias based on clinical history, presentation, and the genomic profile of the leukemic blasts.

Prognosis and Treatment

In the past, the initial CP was invariably succeeded by a transition into advanced disease phases due to the continued and unmitigated proliferation of the malignant clone, resulting in the inevitable accumulation of additional genetic abnormalities. A number of clinical, laboratory, and pathologic features have traditionally been used to designate progression of CML from CP to AP, including clinical and hematologic unresponsiveness to TKI therapy, 20% or more basophilia, 10% or more bone marrow or peripheral blood blasts, and additional cytogenetic abnormalities (ACAs) at diagnosis or during therapy. In the TKI era, these high-risk features have in practice mostly been replaced by monitoring of the *BCR::ABL1* fusion transcript levels and molecular testing for TKI-resistance mutations in *BCR::ABL1*, based on which clinical management is primarily directed. To this end, the WHO-HAEM5 has removed AP from the classification and focuses on the distinction of CP from BP (Table 9.1).

The development of TKIs directed at the causative BCR::ABL1 fusion protein has led to improved survival and high rates of complete hematologic, cytogenetic, and molecular responses. Monitoring of the *BCR::ABL1* transcript is performed by real-time quantitative or digital droplet PCR and measured on a standardized scale, in which 100% is defined as the quantity of *BCR::ABL1* transcripts at diagnosis. A 3-fold reduction at 12 months is defined as a major molecular response to TKIs. Molecular remission is usually achieved, and when prolonged, TKI therapy may be stopped in carefully selected individuals. In the event of suboptimal response to TKIs or molecular relapse, ABL1 kinase domain mutational testing is standard of care, and effective second- and third-generation TKIs are available (*J Natl Compr Canc Netw*. 2020;18:1385-1415). Rarely, bone marrow biopsies may be performed during therapy, and normalization of the abnormal bone marrow features, including cellularity, myeloid to erythroid (ME) ratio, and megakaryocyte morphology, is expected. Transplantation plays a minor role in the frontline therapy of CML but has utility in patients with TKI resistance, in advanced-stage CML, and in children with CML.

II. POLYCYTHEMIA VERA

Polycythemia vera (PV) is characterized by elevated hemoglobin and hematocrit due to an unencumbered red blood cell production. The annual incidence is in the range of 0.5 to 4 per 100,000 persons, with a slight male predominance (male/female ratio of 1.5), and a median age of 60 years at diagnosis. Approximately one-third of patients are asymptomatic at diagnosis. Signs and symptoms are related to hyperviscosity within small blood vessels and venous thrombosis, such as paresthesias, visual impairment, headache, and abdominal pain. Gastric ulcer and intestinal hemorrhage, hepatosplenomegaly, gout, and aquagenic pruritus are also frequently reported. While phlebotomy and low-dose aspirin are still a mainstay of primary therapy, the identification of the JAK2 (Janus kinase 2) pathway has led to the development of specific JAK2 inhibitors that have expanded treatment options and improved the overall outcomes of the disease. The WHO-HAEM5 recognizes and defines two disease phases: polycythemic and post-polycythemic ("spent phase") PV (also known as post-PV myelofibrosis).

Morphologic and Immunophenotypic Features

Peripheral blood erythrocytosis is usually normochromic and normocytic. Mild neutrophilia, monocytosis, and basophilia may be seen. Thrombocytosis is present in half of cases, either as part of the clonal process or if hemorrhage-related iron-deficiency masks the usual PV phenotype; in such cases, careful attention to the bone marrow morphology allows distinction from *JAK2*-mutated essential thrombocythemia (ET). Prominent poikilocytosis, left shift, or circulating blasts are not typically a feature of PV in the early phases of the disease and should raise concern for post-PV myelofibrosis in a patient with a history of PV.

The bone marrow in PV in polycythemic phase is hypercellular in more than 80% of cases with a characteristic increase in all three cell lines (panmyelosis, e-Figures 9.2-1 and 9.2-2). The ME ratio is frequently skewed toward erythroid predominance, although this is by no means an absolute requirement. Dysplasia is absent, and blasts should not be increased. The megakaryocytes may show loose clusters and a spectrum of sizes and cytologic features. Staghorn-like nuclei, as seen in ET, are usually present. A mild increase in reticulin fibrosis, while rare, constitutes a diagnostic pitfall warranting consideration of and distinction from the prefibrotic phase of primary myelofibrosis (PMF). Iron stores are usually decreased or absent. Progression to post-PV myelofibrosis is characterized by moderate to marked myelofibrosis (e-Figures 9.2-3 and 9.2-4, reticulin fibrosis grade MF-2 to MF-3); in addition, erythropoiesis decreases, the bone marrow cellularity becomes variable, and immature bone marrow precursors slightly increase (typically <10%). Osteosclerosis and intrasinusoidal hematopoiesis with increasingly atypical megakaryocytes also develop in post-PV myelofibrosis. If blasts in the peripheral blood or bone marrow exceed 10%, PV is considered to have entered an AP, and blasts 20% or more constitute transformation to the overt BP of PV.

The role of immunophenotyping in PV diagnosis is limited. Evaluation of erythroid precursors and megakaryocytes may be aided by CD71 or E-cadherin and CD61 or CD42b staining, respectively. CD34 staining should demonstrate no increase in CD34 positive blasts but may highlight expanded sinuses filled with hematopoietic precursors (though this can be readily identified in H&E [hematoxylin and eosin]-stained sections).

Genetic Features

The *JAK2* V617F hotspot mutation in exon 14 is detected in more than 95% of PV cases; functionally similar but nonrecurrent *JAK2* exon 12 mutations are identified in most of the remaining patients. The *JAK2* V617F mutation leads to the constitutive activation of the JAK-STAT (signal transducer and activator of transcription) signaling pathway, leading to unregulated red blood cell production and increased red blood cell mass. In addition to *JAK2* mutations, mutations in the calreticulin (*CALR*) and myeloproliferative leukemia virus (*MPL*) genes are found in some PV cases, albeit very infrequently, and their testing is usually not required in cases clinically suspected to represent PV. Patients with *JAK2* exon 12 mutation are typically younger, have higher red blood cell indices, and lower white blood cell (WBC) counts than patients with *JAK2* V617F; however, both groups of patients have similar clinical outcomes. The presence of one or more concurrent "adverse variant/mutations" in *ASXL1*, *SRSF2*, *IDH1/2*, or *RUNX1* is an independent adverse prognostic indicator in PV. Cytogenetic abnormalities (which do not include the Ph chromosome) are present in 20% of cases at the time of diagnosis and frequently include trisomy 8 and 9, or del(20q); their incidence increases with progression.

Diagnosis and Differential Diagnosis

All three major or the first two major plus the minor criterion are required for a diagnosis of PV (Table 9.2). A diagnosis of post-PV myelofibrosis relies on a separate set of diagnostic criteria (Table 9.3). PV should be distinguished from reactive and hereditary erythrocytosis; the former is the result of high serum erythropoietin (EPO) level seen in smokers, endurance athletes, or patients with EPO-secreting neoplasms, while the latter is seen in patients with high-oxygen affinity hemoglobinopathies or germline EPO receptor (*EPOR*) mutations. The differential diagnosis from other *BCR::ABL1*-negative MPNs requires clinical history and careful morphologic evaluation. For example, ET usually has a normocellular marrow with large hyperlobated megakaryocytes while PMF has more atypical megakaryocytes with dense clusters and significant marrow fibrosis. In the absence of prior history, post-PV myelofibrosis may be indistinguishable from PMF.

Prognosis and Treatment

The median survival in PV is approximately 14 years, lower than in age-matched control groups. Thrombotic events are the major cause of mortality and morbidity.

TABLE 9.2 WHO-HAEM5 Diagnostic Criteria for PV

All major criteria or the first two major criteria plus the minor criterion

Major criteria:

1. Elevated hemoglobin concentration (>16.5 g/dL in men, >16.0 g/dL in women)
   or
   Elevated hematocrit (>49% in men, >48% in women)
   or
   Increased red blood cell mass (>25% above mean normal predicted value)[a]

2. Bone marrow biopsy showing age-adjusted hypercellularity with trilineage growth (panmyelosis), including prominent erythroid, granulocytic, and megakaryocytic proliferation with pleomorphic, mature megakaryocytes (differences in size)

3. Presence of *JAK2* V617F or *JAK2* exon 12 mutation

Minor criterion:

1. Subnormal serum erythropoietin level

PV, polycythemia vera.
[a]Increased red blood cell mass (>25% above mean normal predicted value) remains one of the major criteria in ICC 2022 but not required in WHO-HAEM5.
Based on the WHO Classification of Tumours Editorial Board. Haematolymphoid tumours [Internet]. Lyon (France): International Agency for Research on Cancer; 2024 (WHO classification of tumours series, 5th ed.; vol. 11). Available from: https://tumourclassification.iarc.who.int/chapters/63.

TABLE 9.3 WHO-HAEM5 Diagnostic Criteria for Post-PV Myelofibrosis

Both required criteria plus two additional criteria

Required criteria:
1. Previously established diagnosis of PV
2. Bone marrow fibrosis of grades 2-3 of 3

Additional criteria:
1. Anemia (ie, below the reference range for given age, sex, and altitude considerations)
   or
   Sustained loss of requirement of either phlebotomy (in the absence of cytoreductive therapy) or cytoreductive treatment for erythrocytosis
2. Leukoerythroblastosis
3. Increase in palpable splenomegaly of >5 cm from baseline or the development of a newly palpable splenomegaly
4. Development of any 2 (or all 3) of the following constitutional symptoms: >10% weight loss in 6 months, night sweats, unexplained fever (>37.5 °C)

PV, polycythemia vera.
Diagnostic criteria are the same in ICC 2022.
Based on the WHO Classification of Tumours Editorial Board. Haematolymphoid tumours [Internet]. Lyon (France): International Agency for Research on Cancer; 2024 (WHO classification of tumours series, 5th ed.; vol. 11). Available from: https://tumourclassification.iarc.who.int/chapters/63.

Advanced age, leukocytosis, thrombotic events, adverse mutations, a high *JAK2* mutation allelic burden, and an abnormal karyotype are poor prognostic indicators in PV. Post-PV myelofibrosis occurs in 10% to 15% of patients with PV over 10 years. Transformation to secondary acute myeloid leukemia (AML) is a rare event, occurring in less than 10% of patients 20 years from diagnosis, and follows an aggressive clinical course with a median survival of 4 months.

The goal of therapy is alleviation of symptoms and prevention of thrombosis. Some patients with low-risk disease may only require close clinical observation. Phlebotomy remains the mainstay of low- and high-risk disease for patients with an elevated hematocrit. Aspirin likewise is critical to control thrombosis but requires careful consideration in a subset of patients with acquired von Willebrand syndrome and propensity for hemorrhage. Cytoreductive therapies include first-line hydroxyurea and second-line drugs such as interferon-α and busulfan. *JAK2* inhibitor ruxolitinib is reserved for cytoreductive therapy-resistant PV or post-PV myelofibrosis.

III. PRIMARY MYELOFIBROSIS

PMF is the least common MPN with an annual incidence rate of approximately 0.5 cases per 100,000 and more frequently affects older males (*Blood Rev.* 2020;42:100706). It is characterized by impaired hematopoiesis due to clonal proliferation of granulocytes and megakaryocytes with a gradual increase in bone marrow reticulin and collagen fibrosis produced by reactive fibroblasts. The natural disease course of PMF follows two clinical and pathologic stages: a prefibrotic/early and overt

TABLE 9.4 — WHO-HAEM5 Diagnostic Criteria for Prefibrotic/Early and Overt Fibrotic PMF

All major criteria plus one minor criterion

Major criteria:

1. Megakaryocytic proliferation and atypia, with reticulin fibrosis of grade <2 of 3 (**grades 2-3 of 3 for overt fibrotic stage**), accompanied by increased age-adjusted bone marrow cellularity, granulocytic proliferation, and (often) decreased erythropoiesis
2. WHO criteria for *BCR::ABL1*-positive CML, PV, ET, MDS, or other myeloid neoplasms are not met.
3. *JAK2*, *CALR*, or *MPL* mutation or presence of another clonal marker (eg, *ASXL1*, *EZH2*, *TET2*, *IDH1*, *IDH2*, *SRSF2*, and *SF3B1* mutations) or absence of reactive bone marrow reticulin fibrosis

Minor criteria:

1. Anemia not attributed to a comorbid condition
2. Leukocytosis ≥11 k/µL
3. Palpable splenomegaly
4. LDH level above the upper limit of the institutional reference range
5. **Leukoerythroblastosis (for overt fibrotic stage)**

Diagnostic criteria are the same in ICC 2022.
CML, chronic myeloid leukemia; ET, essential thrombocythemia; LDH, lactate dehydrogenase; MDS, myelodysplastic neoplasm; PMF, primary myelofibrosis; PV, polycythemia vera; WHO, World Health Organization.
Based on the WHO Classification of Tumours Editorial Board. Haematolymphoid tumours [Internet]. Lyon (France): International Agency for Research on Cancer; 2024 (WHO classification of tumours series, 5th ed.; vol. 11). Available from: https://tumourclassification.iarc.who.int/chapters/63.

fibrotic phase (Table 9.4). In the prefibrotic phase, thrombocytosis is common and disease manifestations are minimal but may include mild splenomegaly. Transition to the fibrotic stage is marked by elevated LDH level, cytopenias, leukoerythroblastosis, and extensive organomegaly as a result of extramedullary hematopoiesis. In addition, hyperuricemia due to high cell turnover, with all its associated effects, and hemorrhagic or thrombotic events may occur. Compared to other MPNs, PMF carries an overall worse prognosis and requires more aggressive therapy including bone marrow transplantation.

Morphologic and Immunophenotypic Features

Peripheral blood often shows only nonspecific CBC changes including, most commonly, moderate thrombocytosis during the prefibrotic/early phase of PMF (e-Figure 9.3-1). In the overt fibrotic phase, peripheral blood findings are distinctively characteristic: Leukoerythroblastosis is the hallmark of PMF; interestingly, the circulating blast percentage can be inversely correlated with the bone marrow blast count; circulating megakaryocytes and atypical platelets may be observed; and erythrocytes take on the characteristic teardrop shape (dacrocytes).

The bone marrow in prefibrotic/early PMF shows hypercellularity with increased and left-shifted granulopoiesis and abnormal megakaryopoiesis (e-Figure 9.3-2). Fibrosis is absent (MF-0) or minimal (MF-1). Reproducible morphologic findings of megakaryocytes include nuclear pleomorphism with dark chromatin, frequent mitotic figures, cloudlike and bulbous nuclei, variable nuclear sizes, and dense clusters. Sheets of megakaryocytes can be seen but are more common in the overt fibrotic PMF (e-Figure 9.3-3). Blasts are not increased in prefibrotic/early PMF and are less than 10% in fibrotic PMF. Immature cells may be focally increased and should be assessed across the whole biopsy, as the cellularity and distribution in fibrotic PMF may be highly variable, with alternating areas of residual hypercellularity and progressive fibrosis being common during the transition. Myelofibrosis should be repeatedly assessed using a semiquantitative grading scheme (Table 9.5) during the disease course as it correlates with the clinical course and therapeutic response. In later phases of fibrotic PMF, hematopoiesis in the bone marrow is markedly reduced or absent, and frequently restricted to dilated sinusoids (e-Figure 9.3-4). Neoangiogenesis is common, along with osteosclerosis and lymphoid aggregates. In patients with a previous diagnosis of PMF, increased monocytes, increased clusters of blasts, or a blast count between 10% and 19% indicates an AP of PMF. The cutoff for PMF in the BP is 20%.

Immunophenotyping by flow cytometry (FC) is of limited utility as the bone marrow aspirate is typically a "dry tap." Immunohistochemical staining for CD34 can be useful in the enumeration of blasts in the bone marrow biopsy. In addition, CD34 staining helps highlight neoangiogenesis and can also help detect extramedullary hematopoiesis in unusual locations along with CD61 for megakaryocytes. CD34 and other myeloid markers should always be considered in the advanced stages of the disease when unusual nodular and mononuclear aggregates are encountered to rule out the possibility of myeloid sarcoma. Reticulin staining is necessary to document the degree of reticulin fibrosis. If moderate to marked reticulin fibrosis is present (MF-2/MF-3), it is recommended to assess the degree of collagen fibrosis by trichrome staining (Table 9.5).

TABLE 9.5 Morphologic Assessment of Bone Marrow Fibrosis According to the European Consensus on Grading Marrow Fibrosis (ECGMF) Semiquantitative Grading Scheme (see Suggested Readings)

Grade	Definition
MF-0	No increase in reticulin fibers. Identical to normal bone marrow reticulin fibers
MF-1	Mild increase in reticulin fibers with focal increased crossing-over and density
MF-2[a]	Moderate increase in reticulin fibers with extensive crossing-over of thickened reticulin fibers and reticulin bundles associated with focal osteosclerosis
MF-3[a]	Extensive, coarse, and thickened bundles of reticulin fibers with osteosclerosis

[a]Trichrome staining to assess for collagen fibrosis is recommended in cases with MF-2 or MF-3 reticulin fibrosis.

Genetic Features

PMF is a more genetically diverse disease than CML and PV; nevertheless, more than 90% of cases carry mutually exclusive mutations in the three genes with the commonly encountered driver mutations: approximately 50% show a *JAK2* V617F mutation, approximately 30% *CALR*, and approximately 8% *MPL* mutations. Approximately 12% are "triple negative," but whole exome sequencing has revealed underlying gain-of-function mutations and reduced the number of true "triple-negative" cases. Concurrent somatic mutations in genes involved in splicing, such as *SRSF2, SF3B1, U2AF1, ZRSR2*, chromatin structure regulation (*EZH2*), epigenetic modulation (*IDH1/2*), and cellular signaling, such as *CBL, KRAS, NRAS, STAG2*, and *TP53*, are more commonly observed in PMF compared to other MPNs, particularly in advanced stages of PMF. Mutations in *EZH2, IDH1, IDH2, SRSF2, U2AF1, ASXL1*, and *TP53* are associated with poor outcomes in PMF. Cytogenetic abnormalities occur in approximately 40% of PMF cases and are important to define adverse risk categories: a complex karyotype, +8, −7/del(7q), i(17), inv(3), −5/del(5q), del(12q), or rearrangement of 11q23 (*MLL/KMT2A*).

Diagnosis and Differential Diagnosis

In a patient with appropriate laboratory and clinical findings, the diagnosis of PMF relies on the demonstration of the characteristic bone marrow morphologic changes, evidence of clonality, and exclusion of other MPNs (Table 9.4).

The differential diagnosis of PMF includes reactive or secondary marrow fibrosis and other myeloid neoplasms with marrow fibrosis. In autoimmune myelofibrosis, the bone marrow is typically hypercellular, with lymphoid aggregates in almost all cases. Reticulin fibrosis is less pronounced (MF-1 to MF-2). Leukoerythroblastosis is not prominent in the blood. *JAK2, MPL*, and *CALR* driver mutations are absent. Other secondary cause of marrow fibrosis includes chronic osteomyelitis and involvement by mastocytosis, classic Hodgkin lymphoma or non-Hodgkin lymphoma, and metastatic disease.

Morphologic assessment, with correlation with clinical and other laboratory data, is of paramount importance in the differential diagnosis between prefibrotic PMF and ET, as PMF has a markedly worse clinical prognosis, with many patients with high-risk disease undergoing primary transplantation. No single morphologic feature is pathognomonic or distinctive, but scrupulous assessment of the pathologic findings allows for a reasonable distinction between the two entities (Table 9.6). In the fibrotic phase of PMF, distinction from post-PV or post-ET myelofibrosis is impossible without a previous diagnosis due to overlapping clinical, morphologic, and molecular characteristics.

MDS and MDS/MPN may show fibrosis; they typically display more pronounced morphologic dysplasia and a lesser extent of megakaryocyte hyperplasia than PMF. However, substantial morphologic overlap may exist, including shared *JAK2* mutations in up to 20% of MDS and MDS/MPN cases.

Prognosis and Treatment

The progression to overt fibrotic PMF from prefibrotic/early PMF occurs in 20% to 30% of patients at 5 years from diagnosis. Secondary AML occurs in 10% to 15% of patients with PMF at 5 years and is associated with poor treatment response and dismal outcomes. High-risk genetic features are strongly associated with transformation to secondary AML and are similar to those seen in AML arising from MDS or MDS/MPN (*Blood Adv*. 2019;3:3700-3708).

TABLE 9.6 Morphologic Features Aiding in the Distinction Between ET and Prefibrotic/Early PMF

Prefibrotic/Early PMF	ET
Overall bone marrow appearance	
Hypercellular	Normocellular
Decreased storage iron	Normal storage iron
Commonly lymphoid aggregates (~30%)	Rarely lymphoid aggregates
Variable osteosclerosis	Osteosclerosis absent
Granulopoiesis	
Increased (ME ratio >4:1)	Normal (ME ratio 1.5-4:1)
Left-shifted granulopoiesis	No left shift
Megakaryopoiesis	
Pleomorphic and of variable sizes	Increased, markedly enlarged megakaryocytes
Frequent hyperchromatic nuclei, bulbous, and cloudlike nuclei	Megakaryocyte emperipolesis
Dense clusters with atypical perisinusoidal or paratrabecular location	Frequent platelet clumps on aspirate
	Loose clusters

None of the above features are pathognomonic or can serve as definitive evidence of either prefibrotic/early PMF or ET.
ET, essential thrombocythemia; ME, myeloid to erythroid; PMF, primary myelofibrosis.

The prognosis of patients with PMF varies depending on a number of factors. Firstly, survival in PMF is influenced by the specific driver mutation present. Patients with *CALR*, *MPL*, or *JAK2* mutations have median survivals of 16, 10, or 6 years, respectively. In contrast, those with "triple-negative" PMF have a median survival of 2.3 years (*Blood*. 2014;124:2507-2513). Secondly, the timing of the diagnosis, and particularly early recognition, may be important to allow for early treatment intervention. Third, the international prognostic scoring system utilizes patient-specific factors such as age, hemoglobin concentration, WBC and platelet counts, presence of circulating blasts, transfusion dependence, and constitutional symptoms, as well as karyotype, to produce an adverse risk score for prognostication and treatment decisions. Transplantation is the first-line therapy for patients with adequate performance status but *JAK2* inhibitors are available and, while not curative, are associated with significant clinical improvement and reversal of bone marrow fibrosis.

IV. ESSENTIAL THROMBOCYTHEMIA

ET is characterized by a clonal proliferation of hyperlobated megakaryocytes in the bone marrow resulting in blood thrombocytosis. The annual incidence of ET is 1.5 per 100,000, similar to that of PV and CML. The median age at diagnosis of ET is in the second half of the sixth decade. Unlike other MPNs, there is a female predominance (male/female ratio of 0.5). An interesting observation is the increasing incidence in the recent past, while other MPNs have held a steady incidence rate (*Blood Rev.* 2020;42:100706). Patients are typically asymptomatic in more than 50% of cases. When symptoms occur, they are either due to occlusive/thrombotic events or hemorrhage. When bleeding occurs, mucosal sites are most frequently affected; thrombosis can involve major veins and arteries, but transient ischemic attacks and other symptoms secondary to disruptions in microvascular circulation do occur. Leukocytosis and erythrocytosis, elevated serum LDH, and a leukoerythroblastic blood picture are typically not features of ET. Splenic macrophages in the red pulp are responsible for the platelet sequestration that may lead to splenomegaly. Hepatosplenomegaly may develop in later disease stages. The WHO-HAEM5 recognizes and defines two disease phases: essential thrombocythemic and post-ET myelofibrosis (Tables 9.7 and 9.8).

Morphologic and Immunophenotypic Features

The CBC shows an increased number of platelets. On peripheral blood smears, thrombocytosis may result in platelet clumps, platelet satellitism (surrounding WBC), or simply an increased quantity of thrombocytes, frequently exhibiting anisocytosis (increased platelet size distribution), and atypically large platelets.

Morphologic evaluation of bone marrow aspirates is frequently complicated by large platelet aggregates, offering another clue to the diagnosis but sometimes hindering the microscopic examination of aspirate smears. Megakaryocytes are markedly enlarged with ample amounts of cytoplasm, beyond what is typically seen in other MPNs (e-Figures 9.4-1 and 9.4-2). Hyperlobation of nuclei is easily recognized when

---

TABLE 9.7   WHO-HAEM5 Diagnostic Criteria for ET

All four major criteria or the first three major criteria plus one minor criterion

Major criteria

1. Platelet count ≥450 k/μL

2. Bone marrow biopsy showing normocellular bone marrow with megakaryocytic proliferation with increased number of enlarged, mature megakaryocytes with hyperlobulated staghorn-like nuclei without significant clustering. No significant increase in left-shifted neutrophilic granulopoiesis, or erythropoiesis, and no or rarely minimal increase in reticulin fibrosis (MF-1)

3. WHO criteria for *BCR::ABL1*-positive CML, PV, PMF, or other myeloid neoplasm are not met.

4. *JAK2*, *CALR*, or *MPL* mutation

Minor criteria

1. Presence of another marker of clonality

2. Absence of reactive thrombocytosis

CML, chronic myeloid leukemia; ET, essential thrombocythemia; PMF, primary myelofibrosis; PV, polycythemia vera; WHO, World Health Organization.
Diagnostic criteria are the same in ICC 2022.
Based on the WHO Classification of Tumours Editorial Board. Haematolymphoid tumours [Internet]. Lyon (France): International Agency for Research on Cancer; 2024 (WHO classification of tumours series, 5th ed.; vol. 11). Available from: https://tumourclassification.iarc.who.int/chapters/63.

TABLE 9.8 — WHO-HAEM5 Diagnostic Criteria for Post-ET Myelofibrosis

Both required criteria plus two additional criteria

Required criteria
1. Previous diagnosis of ET
2. Bone marrow fibrosis of grade MF-2 or MF-3

Additional criteria:
1. Anemia (ie, below the reference range for given age, sex, and altitude considerations) and a >2 g/dL decrease from baseline hemoglobin level
2. Leukoerythroblastosis
3. Increase in palpable splenomegaly of >5 cm from baseline or the development of a newly palpable splenomegaly
4. Elevated LDH level above the reference range
5. Development of any 2 (or all 3) of the following constitutional symptoms:
>10% weight loss in 6 months, night sweats, unexplained fever (>37.5 °C)

ET, essential thrombocythemia; LDH, lactate dehydrogenase.
Diagnostic criteria are the same in ICC 2022.
Based on the *WHO Classification of Tumours Editorial Board. Haematolymphoid Tumours* [Internet]. Lyon (France): International Agency for Research on Cancer; 2024 (WHO classification of tumours series, 5th ed.; vol. 11). Available from: https://tumourclassification.iarc.who.int/chapters/63.

enough megakaryocytes are available for evaluation in the bone marrow aspirate, and this finding is reproducible in an adequate bone marrow core biopsy or aspirate clot section specimen. Dense clusters, or atypical paratrabecular location of megakaryocytes, should not be a prominent finding. The myeloid and erythroid lineages should be unremarkable or mildly increased. The age-adjusted bone marrow cellularity should be normal or mildly increased at most.

Reticulin staining is necessary to document a lack of reticulin fibrosis, which may be minimally increased in a subset of cases. Immunophenotyping by FC or immunohistochemical stains is not necessary for establishing a diagnosis of ET.

Genetic Features

While approximately 90% of patients harbor a mutation in either *JAK2* (55%), *CALR* (35%), or *MPL* (5%), the remaining cases are referred to as "triple-negative" ET, analogous to the other MPNs. A subset of "triple-negative" ET shows underlying germline mutations in *JAK2*, *CALR*, *MPL*, or the thrombopoietin gene or thrombopoietin receptor gene, but in most patients with "triple-negative" mutations, the causative molecular abnormality remains unknown. Interestingly, most patients with *CALR* or triple-negative mutations are diagnosed at a younger age. Secondary chromosomal abnormalities are seen in less than 10% of cases, most frequently involve trisomy 8 or del(20q), and are of uncertain clinical significance.

Diagnosis and Differential Diagnosis

The diagnostic criteria focus on the presence of thrombocytosis (≥450 k/μL), characteristics of bone marrow morphology, a marker of clonality, and the exclusion of other MPNs (Table 9.7). In the absence of a clonal marker, excluding a secondary cause of thrombocytosis, such as iron deficiency, is essential before diagnosing ET. The differential diagnosis between ET and prefibrotic/early PMF has been discussed earlier (see Table 9.6). "Masked" PV may mimic ET, but the EPO level is subnormal. MDS with del(5q) may have mild thrombocytosis in less than 50% of cases; anemia and morphologic dysplasia are typically present in contrast to ET. MDS/MPN with *SF3B1* mutation and thrombocytosis, by definition, harbors the diagnostic *SF3B1* mutation, which is absent in ET.

Prognosis and Treatment

The risk for the development of post-ET myelofibrosis appears to be half of that of post-PV myelofibrosis. Once secondary myelofibrosis develops, the overall survival appears to be slightly favorable compared to PMF, with a slightly lower risk of developing a subsequent BP than PMF. Transformation to acute leukemia is rare in ET, occurring in less than 5% of cases; it can occur directly from the classic phase of ET or via post-ET myelofibrosis. In a subset of cases, transformation may result from the cytotoxic therapy for ET (*Blood Adv*. 2019;3:3700-3708).

Patients with ET typically experience a slowly progressing clinical course. The 5-year mortality rate is 12%, and the estimated median survival is 15 to 20 years, which approaches normal life expectancy for older adults diagnosed with ET. The primary clinical challenge is the risk of thromboembolic events, and key risk factors include older age, leukocytosis, and a history of prior thromboses. Transformation to BP is relatively uncommon, occurring in 5% of patients over a span of 15 years. Better distinction from prefibrotic/early PMF has allowed the recognition of the superior clinical course of ET compared to PMF. Development of post-ET myelofibrosis has a cumulative incidence rate of approximately 10% over a decade. The main objective of treatment is to reduce platelet counts to prevent symptoms associated with hyperviscosity and platelet dysfunction resulting in bleeding and thrombosis. Patients are stratified according to the level of thrombocytosis and other factors; patients with very low-risk disease may be observed or only require aspirin, while those with higher-risk disease require additional cytoreductive therapy and systemic anticoagulation (*Am J Hematol*. 2020;95:1599-1613). *CALR* mutations are associated with an overall better clinical course, while additional mutations in *TP53, SH2B3, IDH2, U2AF1, SRSF2, SF3B1, EZH2*, or *RUNX1* constitute "adverse mutations" independent of age and negatively affect the risk of progression/transformation.

V. JUVENILE MYELOMONOCYTIC LEUKEMIA

Juvenile myelomonocytic leukemia (JMML) is a rare myeloid neoplasm that occurs in young children before the age of 5 and is defined by the presence of a mutation in one of the *RAS* pathway genes, oversensitizing the hematopoietic precursors to granulocyte colony-stimulating factor (G-CSF). Affected patients have somatic or predisposing germline mutations, and clonal cell proliferation is usually restricted to the granulocytic and monocytic lineages. Persistent monocytosis, anemia, and thrombocytopenia are the prototypic peripheral blood findings. The typical clinical setting is that of a young child with hepatosplenomegaly, occasionally with skin lesions, and in up to 25% of cases in the context of neurofibromatosis, casitas B-lineage lymphoma (CBL) syndrome, or Noonan syndrome. The bone marrow shows hypercellularity with granulocytic predominance and decreased megakaryocytes; the component of blasts or promonocytes is always less than 20% in peripheral blood and bone marrow.

When all clinical and laboratory criteria are fulfilled (in a patient without neurofibromatosis 1), and genetic studies are unavailable, additional laboratory findings may be used to arrive at a diagnosis of JMML (Table 9.9). The prognosis of JMML largely depends on the underlying genetics of a particular case, ranging from spontaneous resolution in patients with Noonan or CBL syndrome, to transient or mild myeloproliferative disease in patients with somatic *KRAS* or *NRAS* mutations, to rapidly fatal disease in patients with somatic *PTPN11* mutations or neurofibromatosis 1.

Morphologic and Immunophenotypic Features

Peripheral blood smears show leukocytosis with left shift and monocytosis, including atypical monocytes, but always fewer than 20% monoblasts and promonocytes. Presence of increased immature monocytes and blasts 20% or more, or Auer rods, rules out JMML. Anemia and thrombocytopenia are usually present, as are circulating myeloid and erythroid precursors.

The bone marrow is hypercellular, and granulocytic precursors predominate, with a variable increase in monocytic precursors (to a lesser degree than in the peripheral

---

TABLE 9.9 WHO-HAEM5 Diagnostic Criteria for JMML

Criteria from both categories must be met.

Clinical, hematologic, and laboratory criteria (all five are required)

1. Peripheral blood monocyte count ≥1,000/μL
2. Blasts and promonocytes ≤20% (in peripheral blood and bone marrow)
3. Clinical evidence of organ involvement, most commonly splenomegaly
4. No Ph chromosome or *BCR::ABL1* gene fusion
5. No *KMT2A* (*MLL*) gene rearrangement

Genetic criteria (any one criterion will suffice)[a]

1. Conal somatic mutation in *PTPN11, KRAS,* or *NRAS*
2. Clonal somatic or germline mutation, or loss of heterozygosity in *NF1* (including compound heterozygosity)
3. Clonal somatic or germline mutation, or loss of heterozygosity in *CBL* (including compound heterozygosity)
4. Clonal noncanonical *RAS* pathway pathogenic mutations or gene fusions resulting in activation of tyrosine kinase genes upstream of the RAS pathways

---

JMML, juvenile myelomonocytic leukemia; Ph, Philadelphia chromosome.
JMML is classified under the category of pediatric disorders and germline mutation-associated disorders in ICC 2022 with similar diagnostic criteria.
[a]Cases that do not fulfill the genetic criteria (or when genetic testing is unavailable) may fulfill the diagnostic criteria if there is evidence of ≥ 2 of the following in addition to the five required clinical, hematologic, and laboratory criteria: increased hemoglobin F for age, myeloid and erythroid precursor cells in peripheral blood, hypersensitivity of myeloid progenitors to G(M)-CSF, or thrombocytopenia with hypercellular marrow and decreased megakaryocytes.
Based on the WHO Classification of Tumours Editorial Board. Haematolymphoid tumours [Internet]. Lyon (France): International Agency for Research on Cancer; 2024 (WHO classification of tumours series, 5th ed.; vol. 11). Available from: https://tumourclassification.iarc.who.int/chapters/63.

blood, e-Figures 9.5-1 and 9.5-2). Erythroid predominance is rarely reported. Megakaryocytes are virtually always decreased. Dysplasia is typically not prominent, although dysgranulopoiesis and atypical megakaryocytes may be observed in later stages of the disease, particularly in cases with monosomy 7.

In most cases, leukemic cells infiltrate the red pulp of the spleen and portal tracts and sinusoids of the liver, leading to hepatosplenomegaly. The skin shows a dermal peri-adnexal and perivascular myelomonocytic infiltrate, and the lungs show a bronchial and peribronchial myelomonocytic infiltrate. Lymph nodes, if involved, show sinusoidal and interfollicular infiltrates.

Immunohistochemical staining for CD11b, CD14, CD68, or lysozyme may be helpful in the identification of the myelomonocytic infiltrate. MPO may also be useful in granulocytic predominant extramedullary infiltrates.

Genetic Features

Approximately 25% of cases of JMML have an underlying germline disposition syndrome, including neurofibromatosis 1 (*NF1*), Noonan syndrome (*PTPN11*), or CBL syndrome. Patients with somatic *PTPN11* mutations account for most (35%) of JMML cases; somatic mutations in *NRAS* or *KRAS* occur in another 25% of patients. Together, mutations in these five canonical *RAS* pathway genes account for more than 90% of cases. The presence of secondary mutations usually portends a more aggressive disease course. In up to 25% of patients, additional alterations of chromosome 7 are detected, and these cases display somewhat distinct clinicopathologic features. However, most cases show a normal karyotype (65%); an additional 10% show other nonrecurrent cytogenetic abnormalities. Fewer than 10% of cases, particularly those in older individuals, show kinase fusions upstream of the *RAS* pathway (including *ALK*, *ROS1*, *PDGFRA*) or noncanonical *RAS* pathway mutations in *RRAS* or *RRAS2*. The ICC 2022 classification names those disorders with clinical and pathologic features of JMML but without canonical *RAS* pathway (or *RRAS*) mutations "JMML-like" disorders.

Diagnosis and Differential Diagnosis

The diagnosis of JMML is based on clinical, hematologic, and laboratory criteria with evidence of clonality. In the absence of clonality or when genetic testing is unavailable, JMML can still be diagnosed based on additional clinical and laboratory findings (Table 9.9). The differential diagnosis of JMML is broad, including reactive and neoplastic diseases. Cytomegalovirus, Epstein-Barr virus, human herpes virus 6, and parvovirus B19 may mimic JMML but lack the genetic findings of JMML. Importantly, patients not infrequently present with JMML and additional concomitant infections. Patients with *RAS*-associated lymphoproliferative disorder (RALD) harbor somatic mutations in *NRAS* or *KRAS* and clinically demonstrate splenomegaly, lymphadenopathy, hypergammaglobulinemia, and autoimmunity with laboratory findings including monocytosis, hypergammaglobulinemia, and hypercellular bone marrow. The overlap with JMML and reports of transformation to JMML has led to the hypothesis that RALD and JMML represent a phenotypic spectrum of the same disease. Pediatric MDS can harbor *RAS/MAPK* pathway mutations in up to 40% of cases, making its distinction from JMML difficult. Meticulous evaluation of the bone marrow and peripheral blood findings is required for the distinction from JMML. AML, CML, and myeloid/lymphoid neoplasms with tyrosine kinase gene fusions can occur in children and need to be excluded for precise management.

Prognosis and Treatment

The prognosis of JMML is variable. Management depends, in large part, on the underlying genetic cause of the disease and may range from a watch-and-wait approach to mild chemotherapy to urgent stem cell transplantation.

VI. OTHER MYELOPROLIFERATIVE NEOPLASMS

Chronic neutrophilic leukemia (CNL) and chronic eosinophilic leukemia (CEL) are included in the category of MPNs and occur very infrequently. CNL is characterized by increased mature neutrophils in the blood and bone marrow and is genetically associated with an activating mutation in the colony-stimulating factor 3 receptor (CSF3R; the G-CSF receptor). Except for the close association with *CSF3R* mutation, the overall mutational spectrum of CNL is similar to myeloid neoplasms in the MDS/MPN spectrum. Unlike the WHO-HAEM5, the ICC lowered the threshold of neutrophilia required for a diagnosis to 13 k/µL or more (Table 9.10). Due to its rarity, comprehensive studies regarding its clinical presentation, prognosis, and effective treatment modalities are limited.

CEL is a rare but frequently suspected MPN; the diagnosis requires stringent exclusion of other myeloid or lymphoid neoplasms and secondary causes of eosinophilia (Table 9.11). Patients with CEL have a poor prognosis and present with highly variable symptoms affecting multiple organ systems secondary to eosinophil infiltration and eosinophil degranulation. Idiopathic hypereosinophilic syndrome is clinically and

TABLE 9.10 WHO-HAEM5 Diagnostic Criteria for CNL

All five criteria must be met.

1. Peripheral blood: neutrophilia (≥25 k/µL, with ≥80% segmented, non-dysplastic neutrophils and bands). Circulating blasts are rare. Monocyte count <10% or <1 k/µL[a]

2. Hypercellular bone marrow. Increased granulocytes with normal maturation and without left shift. Myeloid blasts constitute <10% in the bone marrow.

3. Not meeting WHO criteria for another MPN

4. No *PDGFRA*, *PDGFRB*, or *FGFR1* rearrangement and no *PCM1::JAK2* fusion

5. *CSF3R* T618I or another *CSF3R* activating mutation
   or
   Persistent neutrophilia (≥3 months), splenomegaly, and no identifiable cause of reactive neutrophilia including absence of a plasma cell neoplasm or, if a plasma cell neoplasm is present, demonstration of clonality of myeloid cells by cytogenetic or molecular studies

CNL, chronic neutrophilic leukemia; MPN, myeloproliferative neoplasm; WHO, World Health Organization.
[a]ICC requires a WBC count of more than 13 k/µL and requires a blast count of less than 20% in blood and bone marrow. If 10% to 19% blasts are identified, the diagnosis qualifier CNL in the "accelerated phase" is used.
Based on the WHO Classification of Tumours International Agency for Research on Cancer; 2024 (WHO classification of tumours series, 5th ed.; vol. 11). Available from: https://tumourclassification.iarc.who.int/chapters/63.

TABLE 9.11 WHO-HAEM5 Diagnostic Criteria for CEL

All five criteria must be met.

1. Peripheral blood: eosinophilia (≥ ~1.5 k/µL) for 4 weeks and <20% blasts
2. Bone marrow: megakaryocytic and erythroid dysplasia and <20% blasts[a]
3. Not meeting WHO criteria for another MPN, CMML, or mastocytosis[b]
4. No *PDGFRA*, *PDGFRB*, or *FGFR1* rearrangement and no *PCM1::JAK2*, *ETV6::JAK2*, or *BCR::JAK2* fusion
5. There is a clonal cytogenetic or molecular abnormality.[c]

CEL, chronic eosinophilic leukemia; CMML, chronic myelomonocytic leukemia; MPN, myeloproliferative neoplasm; WHO, World Health Organization.
[a]ICC requires hypercellularity and dysplastic megakaryocytes with or without dysplastic features in other lineages. Alternatively, the criterion for abnormal bone marrow findings in the ICC may be fulfilled by increased blasts 5% or more in the bone marrow and 2% or more in the peripheral blood.
[b]Specifically mentioned as an exclusion criterion in the ICC 2022. An important caveat is that CEL may present as a systemic mastocytosis-associated hematologic neoplasm.
[c]Because clonal molecular genetic abnormalities occur in a minority of patients without eosinophilia and the absence of hematologic abnormalities (clonal hematopoiesis of indeterminate potential), all possible causes of secondary eosinophilia must be excluded before making a diagnosis of CEL.
Based on the WHO Classification of Tumours Editorial Board. Haematolymphoid tumours [Internet]. Lyon (France): International Agency for Research on Cancer; 2024 (WHO classification of tumours series, 5th ed.; vol. 11). Available from: https://tumourclassification.iarc.who.int/chapters/63.

pathologically similar but distinct from CEL, but it has historically not always been possible to distinguish between the two. To this end, the diagnosis of CEL received several refinements and updates to the diagnostic criteria in the WHO-HAEM5: morphologic dysplasia affecting megakaryopoiesis or erythropoiesis is a new requirement; demonstration of clonality is essential and can no longer be substituted by demonstration of increased circulating or bone marrow blasts; the time requirement for eosinophilia was lowered to 4 weeks (from 6 months).

Cases that do not fit into any specific MPN class remain in MPN, not otherwise specified (MPN-NOS), termed MPN, unclassifiable (MPN-U) in the ICC 2022.

SUGGESTED READINGS

CML

Hidalgo-López JE, Kanagal-Shamanna R, Quesada AE, et al. Bone marrow core biopsy in 508 consecutive patients with chronic myeloid leukemia: assessment of potential value. *Cancer.* 2018;124(19):3849-3855. doi:10.1002/cncr.31663

Soverini S, Bavaro L, De Benedittis C, et al. Prospective assessment of NGS-detectable mutations in CML patients with nonoptimal response: the NEXT-in-CML study [published correction appears in *Blood.* 2022;139(10):1601]. *Blood.* 2020;135(8):534-541. doi:10.1182/blood.2019002969

Thiele J, Kvasnicka HM, Facchetti F, Franco V, van der Walt J, Orazi A. European consensus on grading bone marrow fibrosis and assessment of cellularity. *Haematologica.* 2005;90(8):1128-1132.

PV

Tefferi A, Vannucchi AM, Barbui T. Polycythemia vera: historical oversights, diagnostic details, and therapeutic views. *Leukemia*. 2021;35(12):3339-3351. doi:10.1038/s41375-021-01401-3

PMF

Guglielmelli P, Pacilli A, Rotunno G, et al. Presentation and outcome of patients with 2016 WHO diagnosis of prefibrotic and overt primary myelofibrosis. *Blood*. 2017;129(24):3227-3236. doi:10.1182/blood-2017-01-761999

Mudireddy M, Gangat N, Hanson CA, Ketterling RP, Pardanani A, Tefferi A. Validation of the WHO-defined 20% circulating blasts threshold for diagnosis of leukemic transformation in primary myelofibrosis. *Blood Cancer J*. 2018;8(6):57. doi:10.1038/s41408-018-0095-2

ET

Kamiunten A, Shide K, Kameda T, et al. Early/prefibrotic primary myelofibrosis in patients who were initially diagnosed with essential thrombocythemia. *Int J Hematol*. 2018;108(4):411-415. doi:10.1007/s12185-018-2495-2

Tefferi A, Mudireddy M, Mannelli F, et al. Blast phase myeloproliferative neoplasm: Mayo-AGIMM study of 410 patients from two separate cohorts. *Leukemia*. 2018;32(5):1200-1210. doi:10.1038/s41375-018-0019-y

Other MPNs

Kelemen K, Saft L, Craig FE, et al. Eosinophilia/hypereosinophilia in the setting of reactive and idiopathic causes, well-defined myeloid or lymphoid leukemias, or germline disorders. *Am J Clin Pathol*. 2021;155(2):179-210. doi:10.1093/ajcp/aqaa244

Szuber N, Finke CM, Lasho TL, et al. CSF3R-mutated chronic neutrophilic leukemia: long-term outcome in 19 consecutive patients and risk model for survival. *Blood Cancer J*. 2018;8(2):21. doi:10.1038/s41408-018-0058-7

Wang SA, Hasserjian RP, Tam W, et al. Bone marrow morphology is a strong discriminator between chronic eosinophilic leukemia, not otherwise specified and reactive idiopathic hypereosinophilic syndrome. *Haematologica*. 2017;102(8):1352-1360. doi:10.3324/haematol.2017.165340

10. Myeloid Precursor Lesions and Myelodysplastic Syndromes/Neoplasms
Alnoor and George Deeb

I. MYELOID PRECURSOR LESIONS

Clonal Hematopoiesis of Indeterminate Potential

Clonal hematopoiesis (CH) is a clonal proliferation of somatically mutated hematopoietic stem cells that increases with advancing age (age-related CH), and is associated with increased risk of hematologic neoplasms and nonneoplastic disorders such as cardiovascular disease (*N Engl J Med.* 2014;371(26):2477-2487; *N Engl J Med.* 2014;371(26):2488-2498). Encompassed within CH is clonal hematopoiesis of indeterminate potential (CHIP) that is defined as clonal proliferation of hematopoietic stem cells harboring somatic mutations that are usually seen in association with myeloid neoplasms, with variant allele frequency (VAF) of more than 2% (≥4% if X-linked mutated genes in male patient), and without cytopenia, dysplasia, or myeloid or nonmyeloid neoplasms. The somatic mutations detected most involved the epigenetic regulator genes (*DNMT3A*, *TET2*, and *ASXL1* [DTA]) (*Blood.* 2015;126(1):9-16; World Health Organization 5th edition [WHO-HAEM5] = *Leukemia.* 2022;36(7):1703-1719; International Consensus Classification [ICC] = *Blood.* 2022;140(11):1200-1228; *NEJM Evid.* 2023;2(5):10). CHIP has a prolonged natural course with very low clinical risk of developing hematologic neoplasm at a rate of 0.5% to 1% per year (*Blood.* 2015;126(1):9-16).

Clonal Cytopenia of Undetermined Significance

Clonal cytopenia of undetermined significance (CCUS) is defined as CHIP associated with persistent cytopenia (for 4 months or longer) without identifiable etiology ("unexplained cytopenia") affecting one or more hematopoietic cell lineages, and with no diagnostic criteria of a specific myeloid neoplastic entity (WHO-HAEM5; ICC). CCUS is distinguished from myelodysplastic syndrome/neoplasm (MDS) by lacking significant dysplasia (dysplasia if present affecting <10% of one of the hematopoietic lineages) or increased blasts (MDS-IB). CCUS carries a higher risk of evolving to overt MDS than CHIP with several factors that may contribute to such clinical course including the burden of clonal proliferation (the VAF), the number of concurrent driver mutations, and the presence of certain mutated genes designated as high risk including *FLT3*, *IDH1*, *IDH2*, *JAK2*, *RUNX1*, *SF3B1*, *SRSF2*, and *ZRSR2* (*Hematology Am Soc Hematol Educ Program.* 2021;2021(1):399-404; *NEJM Evid.* 2023;2(5):10; see also clonal hematopoiesis risk score [CHRS], calculator at: www.chrsapp.com).

- Of note, idiopathic cytopenia of undetermined (unknown) significance (ICUS) is defined as persistent unexplained cytopenia lacking diagnostic features of MDS and

evident clonality and may evolve into myeloid or nonmyeloid (eg, lymphoid) neoplasm (*Oncotarget*. 2017;8(43):73483-73500; *Pathobiology.* 2019;86(1):30-38).
- Also, it is of interest to mention herein that idiopathic dysplasia of undetermined (unknown) significance (IDUS) may exhibit morphologic dysplasia like that seen in MDS but without cytopenia or MDS-defining molecular or cytogenetic abnormalities. IDUS carries the potential of being a temporary designation that would be explained or replaced by a specific entity during the clinical follow-up (*Pathobiology*. 2019;86(1):30-38).

A comparative summary of CHIP, CCUS, and MDS is listed in Table 10.1.

II. MYELODYSPLASTIC NEOPLASMS

MDSs are a heterogeneous group of chronic myeloid neoplasms with less than 20% blasts and no detectable genetic abnormalities that define certain subtypes of acute myeloid leukemias (AMLs) as recognized by WHO-HAEM5. MDSs are characterized by clonal hematopoietic stem cell proliferation associated with ineffective hematopoiesis resulting in persistent cytopenia and increased risk of transformation to AML (*N Engl J Med*. 2009;361(19):1872-1885; *N Engl J Med*. 2020;383(14):1358-1374). The etiologies and pathophysiology of MDS are multifactorial and encompass aging-related factors, acquired somatic genetic abnormalities, epigenetic alteration, environmental factors (eg, exposure to solvents or benzene), cytotoxic chemotherapy, proinflammatory and activation of innate immune responses, immune-modulated ineffective hematopoiesis, microenvironment immune dysregulation and increased inflammatory cytokines (*Leukemia*. 2021;35(8):2182-2198; *Blood Rev*. 2023;60:101072), and germline predisposition (*Blood*. 2022;140(24):2533-2548). MDS is typically a neoplasm

TABLE 10.1 A Comparative Summary of CHIP, CCUS, and MDS

	CHIP	CCUS	MDS
Cytopenia	Absent	Present	Present
Dysplasia	Absent	Minimal but <10%	Present (>10%)[a]
Blasts (%)	<5	<5	Variable
Clonality	Present[b]	Present[b]	Present
VAF cut off	2% (>4% if X-linked gene in male)	2% (>4% if X-linked gene in male)	None

CCUS, clonal cytopenia of undetermined significance; CHIP, clonal hematopoiesis of indeterminate potential; ICC, International Consensus Classification; MDS, myelodysplastic syndrome; VAF, variant allele frequency; WHO-HAEM5, World Health Organization 5th edition.
[a]Dysplasia is required in the absence of other MDS-defining features including increased blasts in peripheral blood or bone marrow and the presence of MDS-defining cytogenetic aberrations.
[b]Somatic mutations identified in myeloid neoplasm driver genes. No MDS-defining genetic abnormalities such as *SF3B1* mutation (VAF >10%, based on ICC), multihit (VAF >10%, based on ICC), or biallelic (based on WHO-HAEM5) *TP53* mutation/inactivation, or del(q5), del(7q), −7, or complex karyotype (based on ICC).

affecting older adults with a median age of 70 years at diagnosis, and increased incidence with 65 years of age and older (*JAMA*. 2022;328(9):872-880). Except for MDS with deletion chromosome 5q (-5q) that is more common in females, the incidence of these neoplasms is higher in male patients (*Leukemia*. 2011;25(1):110-120; *Leukemia*. 2021;35(8):2182-2198; *Blood Cancer J*. 2022;12(9):132). It is less common for MDS to affect younger patient population, and when it occurs in patients under 50 years of age, a germline predisposition may be investigated (*Hematol Oncol Clin North Am*. 2020;34(2):333-356).

Diagnostic Criteria

The diagnosis of MDS requires persistent cytopenia (neutropenia, anemia, and/or thrombocytopenia) for at least 4 months or longer that could not be explained by non-MDS hematologic neoplasm or nonneoplastic conditions (unexplained cytopenia), in addition to an overt morphologic dysplasia affecting 10% or more of granulocytic, erythroid, or megakaryocytic lineages (WHO-HAEM5). Of note, such an extent of dysplasia is not always required in certain subtypes of MDS with related or defining genetic abnormalities (*Oncotarget*. 2017;8(43):73483-73500) or "MDS not otherwise specified (NOS) without dysplasia" as designated by the ICC (see Table 10.4 for MDS classification). The histomorphologic findings (eg, megakaryocytic dysplasia in core biopsy, clusters of abnormally localized immature precursors [ALIPs]), abnormal multiparameter flow cytometry (MFC) findings, and/or genetic mutations detected by molecular diagnostics including next-generation sequencing (NGS) could also provide supportive evidence to increase the diagnostic confidence or suggest MDS diagnosis in the absence of the required level of morphologic dysplasia or defining genetic abnormalities (*Oncotarget*. 2017;8(43):73483-73500). Therefore, a comprehensive multidisciplinary approach is needed to establish the diagnosis and classification of MDS by correlating the clinical, laboratory, hematologic, morphologic, immunophenotypic (by MFC and/or immunohistochemistry, IHC), and genetic findings. The data points provided by pathologists usually include microscopic assessment of the presence and extent of morphologic dysplasia, visual enumeration of blasts and the presence of Auer rods, the presence and percentage of ring sideroblasts, and the exclusion of non-MDS conditions that may result in or contribute to the cytopenia and/or dysplasia (eg, other myeloid or nonmyeloid neoplasms; autoimmune connective tissue diseases; systemic inflammatory disease; nutritional deficiencies such as that of vitamins B_{12}, folate, and copper; toxins such as alcohol; colony stimulating therapy including erythropoietin; among others) (*Oncotarget*. 2017;8(43):73483-73500; WHO-HAEM5).

Laboratory Hematology Features

The presence of cytopenia (anemia, neutropenia, and/or thrombocytopenia) is a prerequisite criterion for the diagnosis of MDS; however, the laboratory hematology values that determine cytopenia could be varied between patients and the reference ranges of different laboratories. The following are accepted as cutoffs for defining cytopenias that were standardized across CCUS, MDS, and MDS/myeloproliferative neoplasms (MPNs): hemoglobin (Hb) less than 13 g/dL (males) and less than 12 g/dL (females), absolute neutrophil count (ANC) less than 1.8×10^9/L, and platelet count of less than 150×10^9/L (*Blood*. 2016;128(16):2096-2097; WHO-HAEM5; ICC). Of note, cytopenia levels mildly above the aforementioned may still be diagnostic of MDS in the appropriate clinicopathologic context along with the presence of other collaborative definite morphologic and genetic findings of MDS (*Blood.* 2016;128(16):2096-2097). It is noteworthy that lower cutoffs are adopted by the Revised International Prognostic Scoring System (IPSS-R) for prognostic purposes: Hb less than 10 g/dL, ANC less than 0.8×10^9/L, and platelet count less than 100×10^9/L (*Blood.* 2012;120(12):2454-2465). Of note, if laboratory hematology findings of cytosis such as monocytosis, eosinophilia, and thrombocytosis are present, other non-MDS entities of myeloid neoplasms should be considered in the differential diagnosis. The following may represent practical examples: considering chronic myelomonocytic leukemia (CMML) if there are relative monocytosis of 10% or more of white blood cells (WBCs) and absolute monocytosis of 0.5×10^9/L or more (see Chapter 11), eosinophilia-associated disorders such as systemic mastocytosis or myeloid/lymphoid neoplasms with eosinophilia and tyrosine kinase gene fusions if there is eosinophilia (see Chapters 14 and 15), and MDS/MPN with *SF3B1* mutation and thrombocytosis (see Chapter 11) if there is thrombocytosis with platelet count more than 450×10^9/L (except in patients with MDS with low blasts [MDS-LB] and 5q deletion) (WHO-HAEM5 and ICC).

Morphologic Features
- **Blasts**

Blasts in MDS are less than 20% out of 200 WBC or 500 nucleated cells counted in adequate blood and bone marrow aspirate smears, respectively (*Blood.* 2009;114(5):937-951). The conventional blasts are medium-to-large mononuclear cells with round or mildly irregular nuclei with high nuclear-to-cytoplasm ratio (N/C), evenly distributed fine chromatin, one or more prominent nucleoli, scant cytoplasm with no (agranular blasts) or few azurophilic granules (granular blasts), and lack lineage-associated morphologic features except when harboring Auer rods that imply myeloid lineage (*Haematologica.* 2008;93(11):1712-1717). Other types of blasts include megakaryoblasts, proerythroblast, and monoblasts/promonocytes (blast equivalents). The first two may require immunophenotypic studies for precise lineage characterization. The blasts should be enumerated via microscopic assessment, and this could not be replaced by MFC assessing the CD34-positive blasts due to variable blood dilution of the analyzed sample and processing-related issues such as lysing of the erythroid cells (*Blood.* 2009;114(5):937-951).
- **Dysplasia**

The term "dysplasia" has been used to describe the abnormal cytomorphologic features affecting the myeloid cells seen in blood and bone marrow samples from patients with MDS (*Oncologist.* 1997;2(6):389-401). These abnormalities, which are critical to establishing the morphologic diagnosis of MDS, are assessed principally based on the bone marrow aspirate smears, and to a lesser extent the bone marrow core biopsy tissue sections. Selected dysplastic changes are listed in Table 10.2 and example photomicrographs of dysplasia affecting the erythroid, granulocytic, and megakaryocytic lineages are shown in e-Figures 10.1-1A-C, 10.1-1D, and 10.1-1E and F, respectively.
  - **Peripheral blood**

  The Wright-Giemsa-stained peripheral blood smear provides critical diagnostic information including essential screening for the presence of circulating blasts and

TABLE 10.2 Examples of Morphologic Dysplastic Changes

Cell Lineage	Cell Morphology
Erythroid	Abnormal nuclear contours and nuclear budding
	Multinucleation
	Internuclear bridging
	Pyknotic nuclei and karyorrhexis
	Megaloblastoid changes
	Ring sideroblasts
Granulocytic	Hyposegmentation (pseudo-Pelger-Huët)
	Hypogranulation
Megakaryocytic	Hypolobated megakaryocytes
	Megakaryocytes with separated nuclei
	Micromegakaryocytes

References: WHO-HAEM5-Table 1 #36674, Accessed March 1, 2024; *Oncologist.* 1997;2(6):389-401; *Ann Hematol.* 2005;84(7):429-433; *Pathobiology.* 2007;74(2):97-114.

the presence or absence of Auer rods. It is recommended that 200 cells are counted whenever possible in peripheral blood smear when myeloid neoplasm especially MDS is of consideration (*Blood.* 2009;114(5):937-951). The presence of blast equivalents (eg, promonocytes), principally those encountered in the context of CMML, should alert to such. In addition, various dysplastic features could be seen that are not specific or diagnostic by themselves of MDS, such as neutrophils with hyposegmentation (pseudo-Pelger-Huët) and hypogranulation, red blood cells with anisopoikilocytosis (including elliptocytosis), basophilic stippling, macrocytosis, and platelets with abnormal granulation (*Oncologist.* 1997;2(6):389-401; *Clin Lab Med.* 2023;43(4):577-596).

- **Bone marrow aspirate**
Blast count is very critical for the diagnosis and classification of MDS; however, this may be challenging especially when dysplasia is profound, making it difficult to discriminate blasts from dysplastic granulocytic precursors. At least 500 cell count is recommended when evaluating for myeloid neoplasm, especially if there is coexistent erythroid hyperplasia (at least 100 non-erythroid cells should be included in total cell count in this instance) (*Ann Hematol.* 2005;84(7):429-433). The blasts that are counted include conventional myeloblasts with or without Auer rods and megakaryoblasts. Blast equivalents (essentially promonocytes), if present, are counted in the context of CMML and should raise the attention to such diagnosis. Erythroblasts (proerythroblast) are counted only if acute erythroid leukemia is being entertained. Although benign B-precursors (hematogones), lymphoblast-like forms, are usually decreased in MDS, they could be seen in a portion of low-grade disease (*Cytometry B Clin Cytom.* 2020;98(1):36-42) and should not be included in the blast count if noted. As previously mentioned, dysplasia affecting at least one myeloid lineage is the hallmark of

morphologic diagnosis of MDS; however, the assessment of dysplasia requires standardization of the defining criteria and professional expertise to improve the interobserver concordance (*Ann Hematol.* 2005;84(7):429-433; *Leuk Res.* 2018;69:54-59). In addition, dysplastic features are not specific for MDS and could be seen in non-neoplastic conditions such as nutritional deficiency (e.g., vitamin B12 and folate deficiency), infection, and drug/toxin exposure (e.g., cytotoxic chemotherapy, alcohol, heavy metal, zinc toxicity), and in non-MDS neoplasms such as MDS/MPN, primary myelofibrosis, and large granular lymphocyte leukemia, among others (*Clin Lab Med.* 2023;43(4):577-596). Of note, cytoplasmic vacuolization affecting early granulocytic and erythroid cells could be seen in MDS but also in nonclonal (eg, copper deficiency) or somatic clonal (eg, VEXAS syndrome, vacuoles, E1 enzyme, X-linked, autoinflammatory, somatic) conditions (*Eur J Haematol.* 2023;110(6):633-638). In this regard, the presence of dysmyelopoiesis associated with vacuolization in VEXAS syndrome is inadequate per se to establish the diagnosis of associated MDS (*Expert Rev Hematol.* 2023;16(7):495-499). Also, of interest, atypical megakaryocytes including variably sized forms with separate nuclei, hypolobated forms, and micromegakaryocytes could be seen in bone marrow samples from patients with findings associated with *GATA2* and *RUNX1* germline mutations (*Hematol Oncol Clin North Am.* 2018;32(4):713-728; *Pediatr Dev Pathol.* 2019;22(4):315-328).

Iron-stained aspirate smear (adequately representative smear with marrow particles should be chosen for staining with Prussian blue iron stain) is needed to assess the presence of stainable iron and the frequency of ring sideroblasts if present. The latter are nucleated erythroid precursors with at least five iron granules surrounding one-third of their nuclei (e-Figure 10.1-1C) (*Haematologica.* 2008;93(11):1712-1717). Of note, ring sideroblasts could be seen in nonneoplastic conditions such as exposure to alcohol and copper deficiency (*Clin Lab Med.* 2023;43(4):577-596).

- **Trephine core biopsy**

The bone marrow core biopsy (BM Bx) could be critically helpful if the aspirate is inadequate. It is usually stained with hematoxylin-and-eosin (H&E) for routine assessment. The BM Bx is ideal to assess cellularity that is usually increased for age (hypercellular) in patients with MDS due to ineffective hematopoiesis except for a subset of patients with hypocellular marrow (eg, MDS, hypoplastic [MDS-h] as designated by the WHO-HAEM5). In this setting, the differential may also include aplastic anemia (*Curr Hematol Malig Rep.* 2012;7(4):310-320). Other MDS-related features that could be seen in BM Bx include disorganized hematopoiesis with ALIP (*Clin Lab Med.* 2023;43(4):577-596) and atypical cytomorphology and topographic distribution of megakaryocytes (*Expert Rev Hematol.* 2023;16(7):495-499). In addition, the BM Bx could be useful to elucidate space-occupying lesions, infiltrative processes, or lymphoid aggregates (eg, metastatic solid tumor, lymphoma, granulomas, among others). The core biopsy is also ideal for assessing the extracellular matrix such as reticulin deposition (utilizing reticulin special stain) that could be increased in certain types of MDS, notably, the subtype designated as MDS with fibrosis (MDS-f) that is usually also associated with increased blasts (WHO-HAEM5).

Immunophenotypic Features
- **Multiparameter flow cytometry**

The modern diagnostic workup of hematologic neoplasms has integrated two principal types of phenotypic assessment: morphologic (microscopic) and MFC (physical light scatter properties and immunophenotypic characteristics of the hematolymphoid cells). The utility of MFC in the assessment of MDS has been thoroughly addressed in the medical literature, proposed as co-criterion for the diagnosis of MDS by the international working group (*Oncotarget*. 2017;8(43):73483-73500) and recommended at initial evaluation by the National Comprehensive Cancer Network (NCCN, guidelines Version 1. 2024, MDS, Accessed March 3, 2024). MFC was shown to be capable of estimating the frequencies of myeloid and B-lymphoid (hematogones) progenitors, determining the lineage of the blasts of interest, assessing the immunophenotypic aberrations of myeloid progenitors and progenies including granulocytic cells and monocytes and their distorted maturation, assessing the distorted light scatter properties of maturing granulocytic cells, and detecting non-MDS neoplasia that may be a major or minor contributing etiology to the cytopenia being investigated (eg, large granular lymphocytic leukemia, plasma cell myeloma, among others). The neoplastic cells in MDS exhibit a wide spectrum of abnormal antigen expression patterns such as asynchronous maturation and/or aberrant (lineage infidelity) expression of markers (*Cytometry B Clin Cytom*. 2023;104(1):27-50). Several scoring systems had been studied to aid in predicting the diagnosis of MDS based on MFC findings including the prototype scoring system "Ogata score" (*Haematologica*. 2009;94(8):1066-1074). Ogata score essentially includes assessing the following parameters: the frequency (%) of CD34+ myeloblasts of all nucleated cells, the frequency (%) of benign B-precursors (hematogones) of all CD34+ cells, CD45 expression on CD34+ myeloblasts, and side scatter value of CD10− granulocytic cells. However, standardization of MFC, including preanalytical and analytical processes such as sample collection, transportation time, assay design, and sample processing, is needed for reproducible outcome (*Cancers (Basel)*. 2022;14(3):473; *Cytometry B Clin Cytom*. 2023;104(1):15-26; *Cytometry B Clin Cytom*. 2023;104(1):27-50; *Cytometry B Clin Cytom*. 2023;104(1):51-65). Of note, caution must be taken when interpreting certain MFC light scatter and immunophenotypic alterations that may not be strictly specific for MDS including analytical (eg, altered the granulocytes' CD11b/CD13 maturation pattern due to aged sample) or related to non-MDS conditions (eg, infection, granulocyte–colony stimulating factor therapy, autoimmune diseases, bone marrow regeneration, and HIV infection) (*Leuk Res*. 2008;32(2):215-224; *Haematologica*. 2009;94(8): 1124-1134; *Cancer*. 2010;116(19):4549-4563).

The following are selected MFC abnormalities that are variably associated with MDS (*Haematologica*. 2009;94(8):1066-1074; *Haematologica*. 2009;94(8): 1124-1134; *Leukemia*. 2012;26(7):1730-1741; *Leukemia*. 2014;28:1793-1798; *Cytometry B Clin Cytom*. 2020;98(1):36-42; *Cytometry B Clin Cytom*. 2023;104(1): 27-50; *Expert Rev Hematol*. 2023;16(12):1049-1062).

Myeloid Progenitors

1. Increased frequency of CD34-positive blasts (>3% highly correlated with MDS) (*Cytometry B Clin Cytom*. 2023;104(1):27-50)

2. Altered expression of maturation markers CD13, CD33, CD38, and/or CD117
3. Aberrant expression of CD5, CD7, and/or CD56 T/NK-cell markers, and various other markers such as CD10, CD11b, CD15, and/or CD36

Lymphoid Progenitors

Decreased frequency of B-lymphoid precursors (hematogones) that could be still seen in subset of MDS especially those with low-risk cytogenetic abnormalities (*Haematologica*. 2009;94(8):1066-1074; *Cytometry B Clin Cytom*. 2020;98(1):36-42).

Maturing Granulocytic Cells

1. Decreased side scatter or decreased expression of CD45 (Ogata score)
2. Abnormal maturation patterns (CD11b/CD13, CD16/CD13, and CD10/CD15)
3. Diminished or lack of CD10 on mature neutrophils and aberrant expression of CD56

Monocytes

Altered expression of human leukocyte antigen (HLA)-DR, CD11b, CD13, CD14, CD33, and/or CD36 and aberrant expression of CD56

Erythroid Cells

1. Decreased or increased CD117-positive erythroid subset (early erythroid cells)
2. Altered expression (decreased or increased) of CD71 and CD105
3. Increased coefficient of variation (CV) of CD36 or CD71 expression

Megakaryocytes

They are not routinely assessed by MFC.

- **Immunohistochemistry (IHC)**
  IHC performed on BM Bx and/or aspirate clot sections during the workup of MDS may supplement the findings of an adequate aspirate or provide alternative source of diagnostically relevant data when dealing with an inadequate aspirate. A battery of IHC markers could be utilized to highlight several immunohistochemical findings in support of MDS. CD34 highlights positive blasts estimating their frequency and assessing their topographic distribution (eg, interstitially dispersed or clustering), positive megakaryocytes in increased frequency that is usually associated with MDS or MDS/myeloproliferative neoplasm (MDS/MPN), and positive endothelial cells helping in assessing increased angiogenesis (*Leuk Res*. 2007;31(12):1609-1616; *Am J Clin Pathol*. 2020;154(1):5-14). CD117 highlights myeloblasts (alternative to CD34), early erythroid cells, and mast cells (*Leuk Res*. 2007;31(12):1609-1616; *Oncotarget*. 2017;8(43):73483-73500; *Mod Pathol*. 2018 May;31(5):705-717). Terminal deoxynucleotidyl transferase (TdT) usually known to highlight subset of hematogones (early stage), and shown to be positive in a portion of myeloblasts in MDS and AML (*Leuk Res*. 2006;30(8):957-963; Appl Immunohistochem Mol Morphol. 2007;15(2):154-159). Myeloperoxidase (MPO) is a myeloid lineage specific marker that could help estimate the quantity of granulocytic cells and their topographic localization (*Pathobiology*. 2007;74(2):97-114). CD71, CD235a (glycophorin-A), HbA, and E-cadherin are erythroid markers with CD235a and HbA being lineage specific. CD71 is a pan-erythroid marker (highlighting early [EEP] and late erythroid precursor [LEP]), CD235a and HbA

highlight LEP more than EEP, and E-cadherin highlights EEP more than LEP (*Haematologica*. 2018;103(10):1593-1603). CD42b (glycoprotein 1ba) and CD61 (glycoprotein 3a) are megakaryocytic markers that could be useful in confirming the megakaryocytic lineage of blasts and assessing the megakaryocyte dysplastic features and topographic distribution in marrow (*Leuk Res*. 2007;31(12):1609-1616; *Pathobiology*. 2007;74(2):97-114). p53 stain shows very low expression in normal marrow due to short-lived wild-type p53 protein. When p53 is strongly expressed, it highly correlates with the presence of mutation, worse clinical outcome, and cytogenetic abnormalities and fibrosis (*Haematologica*. 2014;99(6):1041-1049; *Int J Mol Sci*. 2020;21(10):3432). Strong p53 expression is also useful to differentiate erythroid hyperplasia from clonal erythroid proliferation (acute erythroid leukemia) (*J Hematop*. 2021;14:15-22).

Genetic Features

The genetic abnormalities detected in patients with MDS are heterogeneous, reflecting the heterogeneity of the neoplasm, and encompass copy number changes (CNC), copy-neutral loss of heterozygosity/uniparental disomy (CN-LOH/UPD), less frequent genomic translocations, and more frequent mutated genes belonging to varied biologic pathways (*Blood*. 2007;110(13):4385-4395; *Best Pract Res Clin Haematol*. 2023;36(4):101512). Therefore, utilization of a combination of genetic testing methodologies is still needed to delineate the genetic profile of MDS in individual patients. These methodologies include, but are not restricted to, conventional karyotyping (CK), fluorescence in situ hybridization (FISH), molecular cytogenetics such as single-nucleotide pleomorphism array (SNP array), and next-NGS. Establishing a genetic profile of MDS is critical for diagnosis, classification, monitoring response to therapy and assessing residual disease, and following up on the disease relapse, especially that encountered post-allogeneic hematopoietic stem cell transplant and the disease progression and/or transformation to AML (*J Clin Oncol*. 2017;35(9):968-974; *Haematologica*. 2017;102(3):498-508; *Bone Marrow Transplant*. 2022;57(10):1615-1619). Deletion 5q (−5q) is the most common abnormality of those detected by CK and FISH, followed by (in order of decreased frequency) −7/7q−, +8, −18/18q, 20q−, −5, −Y, −17/17p− (including isochromosome 17q), among others; −5q and −7/7q− were reported in 15% and 11%, respectively (*Blood*. 2007;110(13):4385-4395). Other genetic abnormalities such as CN-LOH that could not be detected by CK and FISH affecting the 7q and 17p (the region of *TP53* gene) could be detected by SNP array (*Blood*. 2008;111(3):1534-1542; *Leukemia*. 2009;23(9):1605-1613; *Int J Mol Sci*. 2020;21(10):3432). There are numerous gene mutations that carry significant implications attributing to the understanding of the pathogenesis, diagnosis, classification, risk stratification, and germline predisposition to MDS in addition to being potential targeted therapy as well. These genes have been shown to represent a continuum of disease spectrum and progression from CH/CHIP to CCUS to MDS. Overall, when multiple testing modalities were utilized, most of the tested patients with MDS were found to harbor at least one mutation (about 90% of tested patients) (*Leukemia*. 2014;28(2):241-247). Initially, *TP53*, *EZH2*, *ETV6*, *RUNX1*, and *ASXL1* were shown to be associated with poor outcome in patients with MDS (*N Engl J Med*. 2011;364(26):2496-2506). Thereafter, a larger cohort of implicated genes were identified (see Table 10.3 for list of frequently encountered mutated genes and their biologic functions/pathways and associated clinical risk). Of note, some of the MDS-defining genetic abnormalities, specifically *TP53* gene abnormalities,

TABLE 10.3 Selected Frequently Mutated Genes and Their Biologic Function/Pathway and Prognostic Implication in MDS

Gene	Biologic Pathway	Prognosis
SF3B1	RNA splicing	Good[a]
SRSF2	RNA splicing	Poor
U2AF1	RNA splicing	Poor
ZRSR2	RNA splicing	Unclear
ASXL1	Epigenetic modifiers-chromatin modification	Poor
EZH2	Epigenetic modifiers-chromatin modification	Poor
DMNT3A	Epigenetic modifiers-DNA methylation	Poor
IDH2	Epigenetic modifiers-DNA methylation	Unclear
TET2	Epigenetic modifiers-DNA methylation	Unclear
RUNX1	Transcription factor	Poor
TP53	Transcription factor-tumor suppressor	Poor
NRAS	Signal transduction	Poor
STAG2	Cohesin complex	Poor

MDS, myelodysplastic syndrome.
These genes are listed due to their increased frequency in MDS (roughly about 5% or more incidence in association with MDS with the *SF3B1* gene carrying the highest incidence). There are other prognostically critical genes (such as *ETV6*, a transcription factor) that are not listed herein due to their low frequency.
The table data is based collectively on the following references (*N Engl J Med.* 2011;364(26):2496-2506; *Front Oncol.* 2022;12:989483; *Cells.* 2023;12(4):627; *NCCN*, guidelines Version 1. 2024, MDS, Accessed March 3, 2024).
[a]*SF3B1* gene mutation carries good prognosis in the absence of coexistent deletion 5q abnormalities or *RUNX1* (ICC; WHO-HAEM5; *NEJM Evid.* 2022;1(7):EVIDoa2200008; *Leukemia.* 2022;36(12):2894-2902).

require multimodalities testing to achieve the designation "biallelic inactivation" that encompasses gene mutation at the molecular level and deletions of the region containing *TP53* gene via detecting either CNC or CN-LOH (WHO-HAEM5).

Classification

The criteria for the diagnosis and classification of MDS overlap and closely interrelate except for the lineages and number of such affected by cytopenia or dysplasia that are important for diagnosis but not for classification of MDS based on WHO-HAEM5. MDS classification is based on genetic and morphologic findings. The genetic findings are those designated as "MDS-defining genetic abnormalities" including chromosome 5q deletion, *SF3B1* and *TP53* mutations, and other cytogenetic abnormalities that are critical to exclude to render the first two strata. The morphologic findings essentially are the blast counts in peripheral blood and bone marrow, the presence of Auer rods, and the histopathology of the BM Bx (specifically the cellularity and presence of fibrosis). Therefore, accurate and precise MDS classification requires a comprehensive multimodality assessment (see Table 10.4 for WHO-HAEM5 classification of MDS).

Key features of selected MDS subtypes are discussed below:

- **MDS-LB and 5q deletion**

  This subtype is unique in exhibiting characteristic demographic, clinical, and morphologic features such as more prevalence in female patients, possible association with thrombocytosis more than 450×10^9/L, and marrow hyperplastic dysmegakaryopoiesis with frequent small megakaryocytes (*Leukemia*. 2018;32(7):1493-1499). This subtype is responsive to lenalidomide therapy that induces transfusion independence and cytogenetic remission in portion of treated patients (*Blood Cancer J.* 2022;12(9):132), but eventually a resistance to such treatment may develop in association with disease progression and acquiring additional mutations that may include *TP53*, *RUNX1*, and *TET2* (*Haematologica*. 2017;102(3):498-508). It is noteworthy that the differential classification for patients presented with cytopenia, cytosis (thrombocytosis $>450 \times 10^9$/L), and dysplasia, which is usually present but not required at least by ICC, includes MDS-LB and 5q deletion (thrombocytosis usually presents in 20% of patients) (*Blood Cancer J.* 2022;12(9):132), myeloid neoplasm with 3q26 rearrangement (*MECOM* rearrangement), and MDS/MPN with *SF3B1* mutation and thrombocytosis (WHO-HAEM5). The myeloid neoplasm with 3q26, usually commonly those associated with inv(3)(q21q26)/t(3;3)(q21;q26) or other partners to *MECOM*, and is currently classified as AML with defining genetic abnormality/AML with *MECOM* rearrangement based on WHO-HAEM5.

- **MDS-LB and *SF3B1* mutation**

  SF3B1 gene belongs to the RNA-splicing family of genes that are somatically mutated in about half of patients with MDS, constitutes the most frequently mutated gene of this family, and is usually associated with ineffective dyserythropoiesis and ring sideroblasts (*Leukemia*. 2014;28(2):241-247; *Leukemia*. 2022;36(12):2894-2902). As mentioned under MDS-LB and deletion 5q, if thrombocytosis ($>450 \times 10^9$/L) is present with *SF3B1* gene mutation, MDS/MPN with *SF3B1* mutation and thrombocytosis should be excluded (WHO-HAEM5). It is an essential diagnostic criterion for this entity to be associated with low blast count according to WHO-HAEM5 (WHO-HAEM5; ICC; *Blood*. 2020;136(2):157-170). However, the potential negative effect on prognosis of this entity, independent of blast count, could be induced by the coexistence of deletion 5q and/or *RUNX1* mutation as shown by one study (*Leukemia*. 2022;36(12):2894-2902) and required to be excluded by ICC (see Table 10.4).

- **MDS with biallelic *TP53* inactivation**

  Biallelic inactivation mutation of *TP53* gene requires demonstrating biallelic abnormalities of varied combinations of gene mutations and/or gene deletions, CNC or CN-LOH, and is associated with marked dysplastic changes of marrow, increased blasts, and usually a complex karyotype (WHO-HAEM5). Therefore, acute erythroid leukemia (aka pure erythroid leukemia) that is usually associated with *TP53* mutation including biallelic inactivation pattern (*Haematologica*. 2022;107(9):2232-2237) and MDS/AML ($\geq$10% blasts per ICC) or AML with *TP53* mutation/s are included in the differential diagnosis of such entity.

- **MDS defined morphologically (not meeting criteria for MDS with defining genetic abnormalities)**

  There are two recently included MDS subtypes based on histomorphologic findings. The first is MDS-LB and hypoplastic marrow that carries a major differential with

TABLE 10.4 Classification of MDS in Adult Patients Based on WHO-HAEM5

	Blast Count and Morphologic Findings	Cytogenetic and Molecular Genetic Findings
MDS with defining genetic abnormalities (genetically defined)		
MDS with low blasts and 5q deletion[a]	<5% blasts in BM and <2% blasts in PB	5q deletion alone, or with one other abnormality other than monosomy 7 or 7q deletion. No biallelic *TP53* inactivation
MDS with low blasts and *SF3B1* mutation[a,b]	<5% blasts in BM and <2% blasts in PB	Absence of 5q deletion, monosomy 7, or complex karyotype. No biallelic *TP53* inactivation
MDS with biallelic *TP53* inactivation[b]	<20% blasts in BM and PB, and <30% erythroblasts in BM[c]	Usually complex karyotype. Two or more *TP53* mutations, or one mutation with evidence of *TP53* copy number loss or copy-neutral LOH
MDS, defined morphologically (not meeting criteria for MDS with defining genetic abnormalities)		
MDS with low blasts (MDS-LB)[d]	<5% blasts in BM and <2% blasts in PB	No defining genetic abnormalities
MDS, hypoplastic (MDS-h) (≤25% bone marrow cellularity, age adjusted)	<5% blasts in BM and <2% blasts in PB	No defining genetic abnormalities
MDS with increased blasts (MDS-IB)		
MDS-IB1	5%-9% blasts in BM or 2%-4% blasts in PB	No diagnostic criteria of MDS with biallelic *TP53* inactivation or AML

MDS-IB2	10%-19% blasts in BM or 5%-19% blasts in PB or Auer rods. No significant reticulin fibrosis
MDS-IB: MDS with fibrosis (MDS-f)	5%-19% blasts in BM or 2%-19% blasts in PB, with significant reticulin fibrosis (grade 2 or 3)

AML with defining genetic abnormalities and myeloid/lymphoid neoplasms with tyrosine kinase gene fusions, and *BCR::ABL1* translocation should be excluded.

AML, acute myeloid leukemia; BM, bone marrow; ICC, International Consensus Classification; LOH, loss of heterozygosity; MDS, myelodysplastic syndrome; PB, peripheral blood; VAF, variant allele frequency; WHO-HAEM5, World Health Organization 5th edition.

[a] Allowed except in patients with MDS with 5q deletion associated with thrombocytosis (ICC).

[b] MDS with wild-type *SF3B1* and ≥15% ring sideroblasts could be designated MDS with ring sideroblasts. *SF3B1* mutation ≥10% VAF without biallelic *TP53* inactivation or *RUNX1* mutation (according to ICC). TP53 mutation ≥10%. MDS not otherwise specified (NOS), with low blast count, without dysplasia, with monosomy 7, 7q deletion, or complex karyotype, and no biallelic *TP53* inactivation or *SF3B1* mutation (≥10% VAF) (according to ICC).

[c] Increased erythroblasts in marrow should alert to investigate acute erythroid leukemia.

[d] MDS-LB could be optionally divided into MDS-LB with single or multilineage (two or more lineages) dysplasia.

References: WHO-HAEM5 (Solary E, Khoury JD, Campbell P. Myelodysplastic neoplasms. 5th ed. International Agency for Research on Cancer; 2022. Accessed March 1, 2024-Modified from WHO-HAEM5 Table #36675.; *Blood.* 2022;140(11):1200-1228; *Am J Hematol.* 2023;98(3):481-492).

AA and could be favored over such by the presence of morphologic dysplasia essentially affecting the myeloid and/or the megakaryocytic lineages, and clonal genetic abnormalities (WHO-HAEM5; *Cancers (Basel)*. 2021;13(1):132). The other entity is MDS-IB and fibrosis that is usually of grade 2-3 nature (according to WHO grading system of myelofibrosis); therefore, reticulin stain is critically needed to establish such classification. In addition, CD34 immunostain could also be of great significance to facilitate the enumeration of positive blasts especially if aspirate is inadequate due to fibrosis (dry tap) and to differentiate this entity from AML (WHO HAEM5; *Ann Lab Med*. 2022;42(3):299-305).

Clinical and Risk Stratification (Prognosis)

The evolution of MDS terminology, diagnosis, classification, and therapeutics reflects the inherent heterogeneity, varied clinical presentations and outcomes, and progression of biologic and genetic understanding of this group of neoplasms. Therefore, individualizing clinical management of adult patients with MDS requires a prognostic model that predicts clinical outcome and risk of AML transformation, and assesses the planning of personalized management. IPSS-R is one of the scoring systems established to fulfill these aims at initial diagnosis before clinical management (*Blood*. 2012;120(12):2454-2465; *Cancers (Basel)*. 2022;14(8):1941). IPSS-R incorporates prognostic parameters encompassing clinicopathologic and genetic data points including cytogenetic (principally those reflecting CNC), BM blasts, Hb level, platelet, and ANCs, and "differentiating variables" added to principally refine survival scoring values, including performance status (Eastern Cooperative Oncology Group [ECOG] score), serum ferritin, serum lactic acid dehydrogenase (LDH), serum β-2 microglobulin, and marrow fibrosis. After scoring each parameter and adjusting for age, an individual patient could be stratified in one of the five risk categories: very low, low, intermediate, high, and very high. The growing genetic data with significant clinical correlation made revising the scoring system to incorporate such data a paramount task. Hence, the development of IPSS-molecular (IPSS-M) prognostic system that incorporates the IPSS-R parameters in addition to mutational data (*NEJM Evid*. 2022;1(7):EVIDoa2200008; and a calculator available at https://www.mds-risk-model.com/).

Management

The clinical management of patients with MDS is dependent on precise diagnosis and classification and prognostic data aiming to improve patients' quality of life and survival. As cytopenia is the hallmark of MDS, related symptomatology, most significantly the anemia, has a major determinant effect on patients with MDS. The clinical management modalities vary from supportive, transfusion-based, erythropoiesis-stimulating agents (ESAs) such as epoetin alfa and darbepoetin alfa for lower-risk MDS, and hypomethylating agents, chemotherapy, and allogenic bone marrow transplant for higher-risk MDS. In addition, there are disease-type targeted therapies including the immunomodulator lenalidomide for MDS with -5q (US Food and Drug Administration [FDA] approved), luspatercept for MDS with ring sideroblasts (FDA approved), and IDH2 inhibitors for MDS with *IDH2* mutations, among others (*Leukemia*. 2021;35(8):2182-2198; *Blood Cancer J*. 2022;12(9):132; *Blood Adv*. 2023;7(11):2378-2387; *Leukemia*. 2023;37(11):2314-2318).

> **Key Points**
>
> - CHIP is characterized by the presence of genetic alterations in myeloid neoplasm–associated genes in healthy individuals without cytopenia and myeloid neoplasm. The minimum mutation VAF is more than 2% (>4% if patient is male with X-linked gene).
> - CCUS is a myeloid precursor lesion characterized by clonal cytopenia without MDS-diagnosed dysplasia or MDS-defining genetic abnormalities.
> - MDS is characterized by persistent unexplained cytopenia in one or more hematopoietic lineage and dysplasia affecting at least one lineage and/or genetic defining abnormalities including 5q deletion, *SF3B1* mutation, and biallelic inactivation of *TP53* gene. The former two exhibit a good prognosis in contrast to the poor prognosis associated with the latter.
> - Morphologically defined MDS entities include MDS with low blasts and hypoplastic marrow and MDS with increased blasts and fibrotic marrow.
>
> **Diagnostic Caveats**
>
> - Precise diagnosis and classification of MDS requires multimodality diagnostic approach.
> - Persistent unexplained cytopenia is required for MDS diagnosis in contrast to dysplasia that carry lower diagnostic weight in certain subtypes (especially those genetically defined).
> - Certain conditions such as autoimmune disease, infections, and drug therapies can show atypical morphology and mimic MDS. A detailed history with integrated genetic testing is required to distinguish reactive conditions from MDS.

SUGGESTED READINGS

Arber DA, Orazi A, Hasserjian RP, et al. International Consensus Classification of myeloid neoplasms and acute leukemias: integrating morphologic, clinical, and genomic data. *Blood*. 2022;140(11):1200-1228. doi:10.1182/blood.2022015850

Bernard E, Tuechler H, Greenberg PL, et al. Molecular international prognostic scoring system for myelodysplastic syndromes. *NEJM Evid*. 2022;1(7):EVIDoa2200008. doi:10.1056/EVIDoa2200008

Khoury JD, Solary E, Abla O, et al. The 5th edition of the World Health Organization classification of haematolymphoid tumours: myeloid and histiocytic/dendritic neoplasms. *Leukemia*. 2022;36(7):1703-1719. doi:10.1038/s41375-022-01613-1

WHO Classification of Tumours Editorial Board. Haematolymphoid tumours [Internet]. Lyon (France): International Agency for Research on Cancer; 2024 [cited 2024 Jun 20]. (WHO classification of tumours series, 5th ed.; vol. 11). Available from: https://tumourclassification.iarc.who.int/chapters/63

11 Myelodysplastic/Myeloproliferative Neoplasms

Linsheng Zhang

Myelodysplastic/myeloproliferative neoplasms (MDS/MPN) represent a group of myeloid neoplasms characterized by overlapping features of both MDS and MPN. This chapter discusses the four categories of MDS/MPN with distinct morphologic and molecular genetic features recognized by the WHO-HAEM5 and differences in International Consensus Classification (ICC).

I. CHRONIC MYELOMONOCYTIC LEUKEMIA

Chronic myelomonocytic leukemia (CMML) is the prototypical and most prevalent subtype of MDS/MPN characterized by persistent unexplained peripheral blood (PB) monocytosis ($\geq 0.5 \times 10^9$/L and $\geq 10\%$ of leukocytes) and dysplastic changes in one or more of the three lineages of hematopoietic components, usually associated with cytopenia(s) in at least one lineage of blood cells. While conventional karyotyping infrequently detects chromosomal abnormalities in CMML, gene mutations are frequently observed. The incidence of CMML ranges from 0.35 to 0.51 per 100,000 population, increases with age (median age 71-76 years), is higher in males, and lower in Blacks and Asian/Pacific islanders (*Br J Haematol.* 2021;192(3):474-483; *Leuk Lymphoma.* 2017;58(7):1648-1654). Although some cases of CMML may progress from preceding MDS, monocytosis present in other myeloid neoplasms is excluded from CMML diagnosis (*Leukemia.* 2022;36(7):1703-1719).

The diagnostic criteria for CMML and its subgroups are summarized in Table 11.1.

TABLE 11.1 WHO-HAEM5 Diagnostic Criteria and Subcategories of CMML

Required Criteria

1. Persistent absolute ($\geq 0.5 \times 10^9$/L) and relative ($\geq 10\%$) peripheral blood monocytosis.
2. Blasts constitute <20% of the cells in the peripheral blood and bone marrow.[a]
3. Not meeting diagnostic criteria of chronic myeloid leukemia or other myeloproliferative neoplasms.[b]
4. Not meeting diagnostic criteria of myeloid/lymphoid neoplasms with eosinophilia and defining gene rearrangements (eg, *PDGFRA, PDGFRB, FGFR1,* or *JAK2*).[c]

Supporting Criteria

1. Dysplasia involving ≥ 1 myeloid lineages.[d]
2. Acquired clonal cytogenetic or molecular abnormality.[e]
3. Abnormal partitioning of peripheral blood monocyte subsets.[f]

TABLE 11.1	WHO-HAEM5 Diagnostic Criteria and Subcategories of CMML *(continued)*

Criteria for diagnosis:
- All required criteria must be met.[g]
- When monocytes $\geq 1 \times 10^9$/L: at least one supporting criterion is present.
- If monocytosis is $< 1 \times 10^9$/L: both supporting criteria 1 and 2 must be met.[h]

Subtypes: based on PB white blood cell count (WBC)	Subgroups: based on (blast + promonocytes)%
• Myelodysplastic CMML (MD-CMML): WBC $< 13 \times 10^9$/L	• CMML-1: $< 5\%$ in PB and/or $< 10\%$ in BM
• Myeloproliferative CMML (MP-CMML): WBC $\geq 13 \times 10^9$/L	• CMML-2: 6%-19% in PB and/or 10%-19% in BM

BM, bone marrow; CMML, chronic myelomonocytic leukemia; PB, peripheral blood.
[a]Blasts include myeloblasts, monoblasts, and promonocytes.
[b]Myeloproliferative neoplasms (MPN) can be associated with monocytosis at presentation or during the course of the disease, mimicking CMML. A documented history of MPN excludes CMML. A high burden of MPN-associated mutations (in *JAK2*, *CALR*, or *MPL*) supports MPN with monocytosis rather than CMML.
[c]Myeloid/lymphoid neoplasms with eosinophilia and defining gene rearrangements should be specifically excluded in cases with eosinophilia.
[d]Morphologic dysplasia should be present in $\geq 10\%$ of hematopoietic cells in the bone marrow. Per International Consensus Classification (ICC), ineffective hematopoiesis leading to cytopenia is a more reliable feature of dysplasia than morphologic features.
[e,f]See details in text.
[g]Cytopenia is a criterion required for CMML by the ICC.
[h]Based on ICC, if monocytosis $\geq 0.5 \times 10^9$/L and only supporting criterion 2 is met (no dysplasia or increased blasts), the case is diagnosed as clonal monocytosis of undetermined significance (CMUS).
Based on the WHO Classification of Tumours Editorial Board. Haematolymphoid tumours [Internet]. Lyon (France): International Agency for Research on Cancer; 2024 (WHO classification of tumours series, 5th ed.; vol. 11). Available from: https://tumourclassification.iarc.who.int/chapters/63.

Clinical Features

- **Clinical presentation:** Symptoms are associated with cytopenia and/or organ infiltration due to monocytosis and leukocytosis. Variable fatigue due to anemia, susceptibility to infection due to leukopenia and white cell dysfunction, easy bruising, and bleeding associated with thrombocytopenia and platelet dysfunction are often observed in patients with myelodysplastic CMML (MD-CMML, see Table 11.1). In contrast, hypercatabolic symptoms, such as weight loss, fever, night sweats, bone pain, and splenomegaly, are more frequently observed in myeloproliferative CMML (MP-CMML). Some early evolving CMML cases may not have cytopenia, and the diagnosis is based on evidence of clonal myeloid proliferation; these patients are usually asymptomatic.
- **Sites of involvement:** Blood and bone marrow (BM) are always involved, with increased monocytes. Extramedullary infiltrates may be seen in the spleen, skin, lymph nodes, and rarely in other sites.

Morphology

- **Peripheral blood:** Mature monocytes are increased, usually $\geq 1.0 \times 10^9/L$, and frequently show atypical features, such as abnormal nuclear lobulation, condensed chromatin, deeply basophilic cytoplasm, and prominent granulation. Variable numbers of immature monocytes are frequently observed. Red blood cells may show variable anisopoikilocytosis and/or macrocytosis. Nucleated red blood cells and large platelets may also be present (e-Figure 11.1A).
- **Bone marrow:** Most cases have hypercellular BM with an increased myeloid to erythroid ratio. Normocellularity or hypocellularity is rarely observed. Variable dysgranulopoiesis is more frequent in patients with MD-CMML. Dyserythropoiesis and dysmegakaryopoiesis may or may not be present. In most cases, monocytic cell numbers increase with left-shift maturation. It may be difficult to distinguish monocytes from dysplastic granulocytes (e-Figure 11.1B); nonspecific esterase cytochemistry staining of BM aspirate smears or touch preparations can be used to assist the enumeration of monocytic cells when necessary. Focal and mild reticulin fibrosis is not uncommon. Rare cases can display moderate to severe fibrosis at the initial diagnosis, usually seen in MP-CMML.
- **Blasts**: Myelomonocytic blasts, including myeloblasts, monoblasts, and promonocytes, account for <20% of blood leukocytes and nucleated BM cells. Based on the percentage of blasts, CMML is further categorized into CMML-1 and CMML-2 (see Table 11.1).
- **Extramedullary sites:** Splenic infiltration presents as red pulp expansion by myelomonocytic precursors accompanied by variable numbers of nucleated red cells and megakaryocytes. Proliferation of foamy histiocytes in the marginal zone of the splenic white pulp has also been reported. When involving the lymph nodes, extramedullary hematopoiesis partially distorts or completely effaces the lymphoid architecture and frequently shows left-shifted myelomonocytic proliferation with a variable increase in blasts. Cutaneous manifestations range from mild dermal perivascular to extensive myelomonocytic infiltration, which is frequently associated with abnormal infiltration of plasmacytoid dendritic cells (pDC). Body cavity effusion with a predominance of myelomonocytic cells is occasionally observed, with or without a significant increase in blasts.
- **Associated pDC proliferation:** Nodular proliferation of mature pDC is associated with 10% to 20% of CMML, present in BM or extramedullary sites, particularly in the skin. Notably, pDC proliferation has been found to be clonal and related to CMML.

Immunophenotype

- **Monocytic population:** Blood monocytes comprise three subsets: (1) classical: CD14(+)/CD16(−), (2) intermediate: CD14(+)/CD16(+), and (3) nonclassical: CD14(low)/CD16(+). CMML shows a characteristic increase in classical monocytes (>94%), distinct from reactive monocytosis and other hematologic neoplasms, including MDS and other MDS/MPN (*Blood*. 2015;125(23):3618-3626). However, in patients with concurrent autoimmune disorders or other inflammatory conditions, monocyte subsets are altered, and their diagnostic utility is limited. Mature monocytes may exhibit aberrant overexpression of CD56 and decreased expression of CD14, CD15, CD16, CD36, and CD64.
- **Blasts:** Aberrant phenotype of myeloblasts are frequently detected by flow cytometry (FC), including increased intensity of CD13, CD34, CD117, and CD123;

decreased CD38 expression; aberrant expression of CD2, CD5, CD7, CD19, and CD56; and asynchronous expression of CD15 and CD64. Immunohistochemistry has limited utility for CMML, except for the enumeration of blasts in BM tissue sections.

Genetic Features

- **Cytogenetics:** Cytogenetic abnormalities, including trisomy 8, monosomy 7 or del(7q), loss of chromosome Y, trisomy 21, and rarely complex karyotype, are only seen in 23% to 34% of CMML cases and are not specific. Trisomy 8, −7/del(7q), and complex karyotypes are considered high risk (*Blood*. 2016;128(10):1408-1417).
- **Molecular genetics:** Over 90% of patients exhibited one or more mutations, affected genes include those involved in cytosine methylation (*TET2, DNMT3A, IDH1,* and *IDH2*), histone modification (*ASXL1* and *EZH2*), nucleosome assembly (*SETBP1* and *RUNX1*), RNA splicing (*SRSF2, SF3B1, U2AF1,* and *ZRSR2*), and signaling pathways (*NRAS, KRAS, CBL, PTPN11, JAK2, FLT3,* and *CSF3R*). *TP53* mutations are characteristically rare. Concurrent mutations in *TET2* and *SRSF2* appear to be highly specific to CMML (*Haematologica*. 2015;100(9):1117-1130).

Prognosis and Treatment

The median overall survival is 2 to 3 years with a 15% to 30% risk of transformation to acute myeloid leukemia (AML). Poor prognostic factors include cytopenia, cytosis, high blast percentage, high-risk cytogenetic abnormalities, and somatic mutations in *ASXL1, RUNX1, NRAS,* and *SETBP1* (*Blood*. 2016;128(10):1408-1417; *Blood*. 2013;121(15):3005-3015). Additional prognostic parameters include increased serum lactate dehydrogenase, splenomegaly, extramedullary presentation, high β2-microglobulin, elevated thymidine kinase, lymphocytosis and the number of somatic mutations.

The only curative option for CMML is allogeneic hematopoietic stem cell transplantation (alloHSCT). *ASXL1* and/or *NRAS* mutations appear to be factors that may affect alloHSCT outcomes. Treatment of patients ineligible for alloHSCT aims at normalizing the blood cell counts when no poor prognostic factors are present. Hypomethylating agents (HMAs) are the preferred treatment option in the presence of excessive blasts and other poor prognostic factors. Predictive parameters for the response to HMA are lacking.

Differential Diagnosis

The differential diagnosis of CMML includes reactive monocytosis and neoplastic monocytosis associated with other myeloid neoplasms. Persistent monocytosis with no specific primary etiology over 3 to 6 months with morphologic features of dysplasia in the blood and marrow cells makes reactive monocytosis unlikely. Acute myelomonocytic leukemia can present with the same morphologic features as CMML in PB. Therefore, a CMML diagnosis should not be rendered without BM examination. Other myeloid neoplasms defined by molecular genetic abnormalities frequently showing monocytosis include myeloid/lymphoid neoplasms with eosinophilia and defining gene rearrangements, *BCR::ABL1*-positive (especially p190 variant) or negative MPN. Whether *NPM1* mutation defines AML remains controversial. The presence of *NPM1* mutations in cases that otherwise meet the criteria of CMML would be classified as AML with mutated *NPM1* according to the WHO-HAEM5; however, according to ICC (*Blood.* 2022;140(11):1200-1228), AML with mutated *NPM1* requires PB or BM blasts ≥10%. Cases meeting the diagnostic criteria for CMML that developed after radiation or cytotoxic chemotherapy and cases occurring concurrently with systemic mastocytosis are discussed in other chapters. Notably, patients with a prior history of MPN developing monocytosis are considered to have disease progression, but MDS cases progressing with monocytosis are diagnosed as CMML.

> ### Key Points
> - CMML is characterized by blood monocytosis ($\geq 0.5 \times 10^9$/L and ≥10% of leukocytes) with dysplasia in blood and bone marrow cells, often presenting as cytopenia(s).
> - Monocytosis can be seen in other well-defined myeloid neoplasms; these should not be classified as CMML.
> - Based on the WBC at a threshold of 13×10^9/L, CMML are divided into two subtypes: myelodysplastic (MD-CMML) and myeloproliferative (MP-CMML); two subgroups (CMML-1 and CMML-2) are established based on the blood and/or bone marrow blast percentage.
>
> **Diagnostic Caveats**
> - Other myeloid neoplasms, including MDS, MPN, and AML defined by genetic abnormalities can present with monocytosis. A complete molecular genetic workup is required to rule out these diagnoses.
> - Monocytic cells show more mature features in blood in cases of acute myelomonocytic leukemia. A diagnosis of CMML should not be rendered without a bone marrow examination.
> - Although some mutation combinations (such as concurrent mutations in *TET2* and *SRSF2*) are more characteristic of CMML, mutation profiles of CMML largely overlap with MDS and other MDS/MPN.

II. MYELODYSPLASTIC/MYELOPROLIFERATIVE NEOPLASM WITH NEUTROPHILIA

Myelodysplastic/myeloproliferative neoplasm with neutrophilia (MDS/MPN-N), a name changed from the previous "atypical chronic myeloid leukemia," is characterized by granulocytic proliferation with dysplasia and persistent left-shifted neutrophilia in the blood. The morphologic features resemble those of *BCR::ABL1* positive chronic myeloid leukemia (CML), with additional marked dysgranulopoiesis and lack of *BCR::ABL1* fusion. MDS/MPN-N is a rare disease with an estimated incidence of 1 to 2 cases per 100 CML and medium age at diagnosis of over 70 years. Male to female ratio is 1 to 2:1 (*Blood.* 2014;123(17):2645-2651).

The diagnostic criteria for MDS/MPN-N are summarized in Table 11.2.

Clinical Features

Patients usually present with symptoms related to anemia (fatigue) and thrombocytopenia (bleeding tendency) and are found to have leukocytosis. Presentations related to neutrophilia, such as splenomegaly and hepatomegaly, may also develop in the later stages.

TABLE 11.2 WHO-HAEM5 Diagnostic Criteria for MDS/MPN-N

Essential Criteria

1. PB leukocytosis ≥13 × 10^9/L, with neutrophilia and ≥10% circulating immature myeloid cells, as well as neutrophilic dysplasia.[b]
2. BM hypercellularity with granulocytic hyperplasia and dysplasia, with or without megakaryocytic and erythroid dysplasia.
3. Blasts <20% of PB leukocytes and BM nucleated cells.
4. Not meeting diagnostic criteria for:
   1. myeloproliferative neoplasms, BCR::ABL1 fusion positive or negative by molecular and genetic studies[c]
   2. myeloid/lymphoid neoplasms with eosinophilia and defining gene rearrangement
   3. CMML
   4. MDS/MPN with SF3B1 mutation and thrombocytosis

Desirable Criteria[a]

1. Detection of *SETBP1* and/or *ETNK1* mutations
2. Absence of mutations in *JAK2, CALR, MPL,* and *CSF3R*

While WHO-HAEM5 changed the diagnosing name, ICC still uses the original name "atypical chronic myeloid leukemia" for this subtype of MDS/MPN.
BM, bone marrow; CMML, chronic myelomonocytic leukemia; MDS/MPN, myelodysplastic/myeloproliferative neoplasms; PB, peripheral blood.
[a]Presence of *JAK2, CALR, MPL,* and *CSF3R* mutations should prompt complete clinical and laboratory evaluations to exclude MPN.
[b]Per International Consensus Classification (ICC), cytopenia is required and is considered a reliable surrogate of dysplasia. ICC also requires eosinophils <10% of leukocytes.
[c]Detection of *BCR::ABL1* fusion may require all available methodologies, including cytogenetics, fluorescence in situ hybridization (FISH), and polymerase chain reaction (PCR) or sequencing-based assays to exclude cryptic rearrangements and/or alternate transcripts.
Based on the WHO Classification of Tumours Editorial Board. Haematolymphoid tumours [Internet]. Lyon (France): International Agency for Research on Cancer; 2024 (WHO classification of tumours series, 5th ed.; vol. 11). Available from: https://tumourclassification.iarc.who.int/chapters/63.

Morphology

- **Peripheral blood:** White blood cell (WBC) count ≥13 × 10^9/L with predominance of neutrophils displaying dysplastic features and circulating immature neutrophilic granulocytes (promyelocytes, myelocytes, and metamyelocytes) ≥10% (e-Figure 11.2A), while blasts are usually <5% and monocytes <10% of leukocytes. Basophils may be mildly increased, usually <2%. Red blood cell and platelet counts frequently decrease and may show dysplastic features.

- **Bone marrow:** Hypercellular with increased myeloid to erythroid ratio (frequently >10:1, e-Figure 11.2B). Dysplastic features, including cytoplasmic hypogranulation, nuclear hyposegmentation (pseudo-Pelger-Huët nuclei), hypersegmentation, condensed chromatin, and nuclear projections, are present in ≥10% of granulocytes. Blasts comprise <20% of nucleated cells, and large aggregates and sheets of blasts should not be present. Dyserythropoiesis is a common finding. The number of megakaryocytes is variable and can decrease; megakaryocytes are frequently dysplastic with hypolobated and unilobed nuclei, and small megakaryocytes and micromegakaryocytes are common. Mild fibrosis can occur; however, severe fibrosis is rare.

Immunophenotype

Myeloblasts may show mild aberrancy, but there are no specific immunophenotypic abnormalities. Immunohistochemical staining for CD34 can be used to confirm the blast percentage, and monocyte markers can be used to exclude CMML.

Genetic Features

- **Cytogenetics:** Nonspecific abnormal karyotypes, the most common abnormalities including trisomy 8 and del(20q), are detected in 30% to 40% of cases. Isochromosome 17q [i(17q)] has been reported. By definition, the presence of t(9;22);*BCR::ABL1* fusion excludes the diagnosis of MDS/MPN-N.
- **Molecular genetics:** Gene mutations occur in most cases, with a median mutation burden of 2 to 4 per case. *SETBP1* and/or *ETNK1* mutations, which are less common in other myeloid neoplasms, support a diagnosis of MDS/MPN-N. The other mutations largely overlap with other MDS/MPN and are frequently seen in clonal hematopoiesis, involving *ASXL1* (60%-80%), *TET2* (30%-40%), and/or *DNMT3A* (<10%), as well as genes involved in RNA splicing (*SRSF2, SF3B1, U2AF1,* and *ZRSR2*), signaling pathways (eg, *CBL, JAK2, NF1,* and *NRAS*), transcription factors (*CUX1, GATA2,* and *RUNX1*), and chromosomal separation regulators (eg, *STAG2*).

Prognosis and Treatment

The median survival time ranges from 14 to 29 months. Disease progression often presents as BM failure, and approximately 20% to 40% of cases transform to AML. Poor prognostic factors include older age, female gender, high WBC count (>50 × 10^9/L), anemia, and thrombocytopenia. Increased percentage of BM blasts (>5%) and marked dyserythropoiesis have been reported to be predictive of leukemic transformation (*Blood.* 2014;123(17):2645-2651; *Haematologica.* 2006;91(11):1566-1568). Currently, specific treatments for MDS/MPN-N are lacking. Most patients require supportive care for cytopenia or cytoreduction for leukocytosis. AlloHSCT improves outcomes in younger patients (*Blood.* 2017;129(7):838-845).

Differential Diagnosis

The major differential diagnoses include *BCR::ABL1* positive CML, chronic neutrophilic leukemia (CNL), and CMML. Molecular genetic studies can provide definitive evidence of *BCR::ABL1* fusion and may reveal a mutation profile specific to CNL, such as *CSF3R* mutation, as well as other distinct abnormalities inconsistent with MDS/MPN-N. Of note, routine cytogenetic tests may not always reveal t(9;22);*BCR::ABL1* rearrangement, and polymerase chain reaction (PCR) or RNA sequencing–based methods may be required to identify all CML cases. If the monocyte percentage exceeds 10% of PB leukocytes, the case should be classified as CMML.

Key Points

- MDS/MPN-N is characterized by blood neutrophilia, circulation of immature neutrophilic granulocytes, and bone marrow granulocytic hyperplasia with dysplasia.
- The morphologic features of MDS/MPN-N are essentially the same as chronic myeloid leukemia, but by definition *BCR::ABL1* fusion is absent.
- Other myeloid neoplasms occasionally can present with features similar to MDS/MPN-N including myeloid/lymphoid neoplasms with eosinophilia and defining gene rearrangement, CMML and MDS/MPN with *SF3B1* mutation and thrombocytosis.

Diagnostic Caveats

- CML with cryptic *BCR::ABL1* rearrangement may be missed by routinely available cytogenetic tests.
- *SETBP1* and/or *ETNK1* mutations are more frequently seen in MDS/MPN-N but are not entirely specific for the diagnosis.
- Presence of *JAK2*, *CALR*, *MPL*, and *CSF3R* suggests a diagnosis of MPN instead of MDS/MPN-N.

III. MYELODYSPLASTIC/MYELOPROLIFERATIVE NEOPLASM WITH *SF3B1* MUTATION AND THROMBOCYTOSIS

Myelodysplastic/myeloproliferative neoplasm with *SF3B1* mutation and thrombocytosis (MDS/MPN-*SF3B1*-T), a diagnosis evolved from morphology-defined MDS/MPN with ring sideroblasts and thrombocytosis (MDS/MPN-RS-T), is a myeloid neoplasm with myelodysplasia, characterized by anemia, *SF3B1* mutation, with or without the presence of ring sideroblasts, and myeloproliferative features represented by thrombocytosis. Although the exact incidence is unknown, MDS/MPN-*SF3B1*-T is rare. The median age at diagnosis is approximately 70 years, and slightly more females are affected in the reported cases (*Blood Cancer J.* 2022;12(2):26; *Haematologica*. 2012;97(7):1036-1041).

The diagnostic criteria for MDS/MPN-*SF3B1*-T are summarized in Table 11.3.

Clinical Features

The clinical presentation is associated with anemia (eg, fatigue), thrombocytosis, leukocytosis, as well as splenomegaly and thrombotic events.

Morphology

- **Peripheral blood:** Red blood cells are decreased with anisopoikilocytosis and are frequently macrocytic. The WBC count and differential counts are normal in most cases, but can be increased. Blasts are either rare or absent. The platelet count is $\geq 450 \times 10^9$/L, with variable sizes, ranging from tiny to giant platelets, but hypogranular platelets are uncommon.
- **Bone marrow:** Usually hypercellular with dysplastic erythroid and megakaryocytic hyperplasia. By iron stain, ring sideroblasts are present at $\geq 15\%$ in most cases. The morphologic features of megakaryocytes are usually similar to those seen in *BCR::ABL1*-negative MPN; however, dysplastic features in granulocytes and megakaryocytes, as well as fibrosis, may be identified in some cases. Blasts are usually <5% of marrow nucleated cells.

TABLE 11.3 WHO-HAEM5 Diagnostic Criteria for MDS/MPN-*SF3B1*-T

Peripheral blood:
- Anemia (Hb <13 g/dL in males and <12 g/dL in females)
- Thrombocytosis (platelet count over 450×10^9/L)
- No or very rare blast cells

Bone marrow:
- Dysplasia, especially dyserythropoiesis (ring sideroblasts usually present)

Molecular analyses not performed (or results not available):	Molecular analyses performed on PB or BM:
• Ring sideroblasts ≥15%[a]	• *SF3B1* heterozygous mutation[a] • Concurrent *JAK2* V617F or, in the absence of *JAK2* V617F, mutation in other myeloproliferative genes such as *MPL* or *CALR*

Excluding the following diagnosis[b]:
- Therapy-related myeloid neoplasms
- MDS with isolated del(5q)
- Myeloid neoplasms with a double-hit *TP53* alteration
- Myeloid neoplasms with t(3;3)(q21.3;q26.2) or inv(3)(q21.3q26.2)
- Presence of a disease-defining gene fusion such as *BCR::ABL1*

BM, bone marrow; MDS, myelodysplastic neoplasm; PB, peripheral blood.
[a] In the absence of the *SF3B1* mutation, a diagnosis of MDS/MPN-*SF3B1*-T can still be rendered if ring sideroblasts are present in ≥15% of marrow nucleated red cells. However, according to the International Consensus Classification (ICC), these cases should be diagnosed as MDS/MPN-RS-T, NOS.
[b] Cases that initially present as MDS-*SF3B1* (with ring sideroblasts) and later develop thrombocytosis (usually upon acquisition of a *JAK2*, *MPL*, or *CALR* mutation) may be classified as MDS/MPN-*SF3B1*-T. However, per the ICC, these cases are considered thrombocytotic progression of MDS-*SF3B1*.
Based on the WHO Classification of Tumours Editorial Board. Haematolymphoid tumours [Internet]. Lyon (France): International Agency for Research on Cancer; 2024 (WHO classification of tumours series, 5th ed.; vol. 11). Available from: https://tumourclassification.iarc.who.int/chapters/63.

- **Extramedullary sites:** If involved, presents as neoplastic extramedullary hematopoiesis similar to that of MPNs.

Immunophenotype

No specific immunophenotypic features are observed. CD34-positive myeloblasts may show an aberrant phenotype by FC, as observed in other myeloid neoplasms.

Genetic Features

Cytogenetic abnormalities are detected in approximately 15% of patients; however, there are no specific abnormalities characteristic of MDS/MPN-*SF3B1*-T (*Blood Cancer J.* 2022;12(2):26). By definition, an *SF3B1* mutation, most frequently p.K700E, p.H662Q, or p.K666R, is present when molecular tests are performed. Concurrent *JAK2* p.V617F mutation is present in ~50% of cases. The profile of other mutations is similar to that of MDS and MPN, involving *TET2, ASXL1, DNMD3A, SETBP1, SRSF2, U2AF1, ZRSR2, EZH2, IDH2, ETV6, RUNX1, CBL, CALR,* and *MPL*.

Prognosis and Treatment

No formal treatment guidelines have been established for MDS/MPN-*SF3B1*-T. Current treatment approaches primarily involve blood transfusion and the use of erythropoiesis-stimulating agents to manage anemia. Cytoreductive agents, such as hydroxyurea, may be administered to reduce thrombocytosis, whereas antiplatelet agents are employed to mitigate the risk of thrombotic events. The effectiveness of novel drugs, including lenalidomide and HMAs, is currently under investigation.

MDS/MPN-*SF3B1*-T has a relatively favorable prognosis compared to other MDS/MPN types, with a reported median overall survival of 76 to 128 months. Unfavorable factors include anemia with hemoglobin ≤10 g/dL and an abnormal karyotype. Presence of *ASXL1* and/or *SETBP1* mutations may be prognostic. Concurrent *JAK2* mutation has been associated with better prognosis (*Blood Cancer J.* 2022;12(2):26; *Leukemia.* 2013;27(9):1826-1831; *Leuk Lymphoma.* 2022;63(1):199-204; *Blood.* 2020;136(16):1851-1862; *Am J Hematol.* 2016;91(5):492-498).

Differential Diagnosis

Nonclonal conditions and otherwise defined myeloid neoplasms with ring sideroblasts and thrombocytosis should be excluded. Reactive thrombocytosis with concurrent anemia is not rare and should be ruled out based on the clinical history and molecular tests. When similar clinical and morphologic features are present, other myeloid neoplasms (see Table 11.3) can only be excluded by relevant molecular genetic studies.

Key Points

- MDS/MPN-*SF3B1*-T is characterized by anemia, thrombocytosis, the presence of ring sideroblasts, and/or *SF3B1* mutation.
- Defined by blood cell count changes and *SF3B1* mutation, myelodysplasia and ring sideroblasts are usually present but not required for the diagnosis of MDS/MPN-*SF3B1*-T.

Diagnostic Caveats

- When molecular tests for *SF3B1* mutation are not available or negative, bone marrow ring sideroblasts ≥15% can be used as a surrogate for diagnosis per WHO-HAEM5; however, cases without *SF3B1* mutation are classified as MDS/MPN-RS-T, NOS by the ICC.
- Anemia, thrombocytosis, and ring sideroblasts can be seen in other myeloid neoplasms. Presence of disease-defining genetic abnormalities rules out MDS/MPN-*SF3B1*-T. Therefore, a relatively extensive molecular genetic workup is required before rendering the diagnosis of MDS/MPN-*SF3B1*-T.

IV. MYELODYSPLASTIC/MYELOPROLIFERATIVE NEOPLASM, NOS

Myelodysplastic/myeloproliferative neoplasm, not otherwise specified or unclassifiable (MDS/MPN-NOS) is a group of rare myeloid neoplasms characterized by a combination of dysplastic and proliferative features that do not meet the criteria for other defined MDS/MPN entities. ICC considers cytopenia, a reliable presentation of ineffective hematopoiesis resulting from dysplasia, to be required for the diagnosis of MDS/MPN-NOS. It represents a small percentage of all MDS/MPN cases; however, its true incidence is challenging to determine because of the difficulty in diagnosing overlapping neoplasms. MDS/MPN-NOS may be the second most common type of MDS/MPN. The median age at diagnosis is approximately 70 years. It is slightly more frequent in males.

There are no specific clinical manifestations of MDS/MPN-NOS. Patients usually present with symptoms from cytopenia due to ineffective hematopoiesis, including fatigue, dyspnea, infections, and bleeding, as well as presentations from cytosis due to myeloproliferation such as weight loss, night sweats, splenomegaly, and thromboembolic complications.

MDS/MPN-NOS affects PB, BM, and in some cases, extramedullary tissues such as the spleen and liver. Blood cell counts show both cytosis, most frequently leukocytosis, followed by thrombocytosis, and cytopenia, most commonly anemia, followed by thrombocytopenia, and rarely neutropenia. BM is hypercellular with hyperplasia and dysplasia in at least one hematopoietic lineage. Elevated lactate dehydrogenase levels and BM fibrosis may also be seen.

Approximately 50% of MDS/MPN-NOS cases exhibit abnormal karyotypes with common abnormalities including trisomy 8, monosomy 7/del(7q), del(20q), and monosomal or complex karyotypes. The WHO-HAEM5 does not recognize MDS/MPN with isolated i(17q) as a separate category, but ICC has added MDS/MPN with isolated i(17q) as a new provisional subentity under the diagnostic umbrella of MDS/MPN-NOS. The presence of mutations in genes such as *TET2, NRAS, RUNX1, CBL, SETBP1*, and *ASXL1* is frequently detected and desirable to establish a diagnosis. *TP53* mutations occur in 10% to 15% of cases (*Int J Hematol*. 2015;101(3):229-242). Genetic profiling is required to exclude other myeloid neoplasms, including MDS/MPN-*SF3B1*-T. Cases with combined del(5q) and *JAK2* p.V617F mutation are currently classified as MDS with isolated del(5q), rather than being included in the MDS/MPN-NOS category. The presence of double or multiple hit *TP53* mutations should also exclude MDS/MPN-NOS, although the classification of these cases is not consistent between the WHO-HAEM5 and ICC.

Limited information is available regarding the prognosis of MDS/MPN-NOS, but previous studies have demonstrated poor outcomes, with median overall survival ranging from 12 to 24 months. The prognostic scoring systems commonly used for MDS do not adequately represent this type of myeloid neoplasm. Similar to other MDS/MPNs, treatment for MDS/MPN-NOS is guided by symptoms and blood cell counts (*Curr Opin Hematol*. 2014;21(2):131-140).

SUGGESTED READINGS

Arber DA, Orazi A, Hasserjian RP, et al. International Consensus Classification of myeloid neoplasms and acute leukemias: integrating morphologic, clinical, and genomic data. *Blood*. 2022;*140*(11):1200-1228.

Czader M, Orazi A. Myelodysplastic/Myeloproliferative neoplasms and related diseases. In: Orazi A, Foucar K, Knowles D, Weiss LM. *Knowles Neoplastic Hematopathology*. 3rd ed. Lippincott Williams & Wilkins; 2014:1140-1156.

Khoury JD, Solary E, Abla O, et al. The 5th edition of the World Health Organization classification of haematolymphoid tumours: myeloid and histiocytic/dendritic neoplasms. *Leukemia*. 2022;36(7):1703-1719.

Palomo L, Meggendorfer M, Hutter S, et al. Molecular landscape and clonal architecture of adult myelodysplastic/myeloproliferative neoplasms. *Blood*. 2020;*136*(16):1851-1862.

Tiu RV, Sekeres MA. Making sense of the myelodysplastic/myeloproliferative neoplasms overlap syndromes. *Curr Opin Hematol*. 2014;*21*(2):131-140.

12. Acute Myeloid Leukemia

Jiannan Li, Jephne (Tianjiao) Wang, Brooj Abro, and Michael C. Horwath

I. ACUTE MYELOID LEUKEMIA: INTRODUCTION AND OVERVIEW

Acute myeloid leukemia (AML) is an aggressive myeloid neoplasm in which an imbalance of maturation and proliferation results in an overabundance of myeloblasts in the blood or bone marrow (e-Figures 12.1-1 and 12.1-2). Proliferating immature cells impair the development of normal hematopoiesis, leading to cytopenias, immune compromise, severe infections, and death (*Lancet*. 2018;392:593-606). AML is the most common type of acute leukemia in adults, with 20,380 estimated new cases in the United States in 2023, accounting for 1.0% of all new cancer cases (Cancer Stat Facts, NCI SEER Program, https://seer.cancer.gov/statfacts/html/amyl.html). AML is slightly more common among men than women, and approximately 0.5% of the population will be affected at some point during their lifetime (NCI SEER Program, https://seer.cancer.gov/). While AML can occur at any age, the risk increases in the elderly, with a median age at diagnosis of 68 years (*Blood Rev*. 2019;36:70-87).

Clinical Presentation

The hampered production of normal blood cells due to leukemic infiltration of the bone marrow can cause patients to experience various symptoms, including anemia, recurrent infections, fever, easy bruising, excessive bleeding, and bone pain. Depending on the degree of anemia, patients may present with generalized weakness, fatigue, shortness of breath, and pallor. Physical examination can reveal splenomegaly and hepatomegaly, while lymphadenopathy is rare. Disseminated intravascular coagulation (DIC) can occur in AML patients. Sometimes, proliferating blasts can form an extramedullary mass (see "Myeloid Sarcoma" section) or cause a skin rash due to infiltration of leukemic cells.

Some AML cases are considered "secondary" in that they progress from underlying myelodysplastic syndrome (MDS) and MDS/myeloproliferative neoplasm (MPN), are associated with an underlying germline genetic lesion, or arise in the setting of prior cytotoxic therapy for an unrelated disease. Diagnostic considerations for the latter two categories are discussed in Chapter 13. Blast-phase MPN is sometimes called "secondary AML" but has separate diagnostic and clinical considerations, as discussed in Chapter 9.

Morphology

AML is a disease characterized by the proliferation of immature myeloid cells (e-Figures 12.1-1 and 12.1-2), with or without maturing neoplastic cells. The finding of 20% or more myeloblasts or blast equivalents in the blood or bone marrow aspirate by smear morphology is generally diagnostic for AML if a few specific diagnoses, such as blast-phase chronic myeloid leukemia (CML) and Down syndrome (DS)-associated myeloid proliferations, can be excluded. The 20% blast cutoff may be lowered if specific genetic associations are present. Myeloblasts should be differentiated from other immature cells by morphology (eg, fine chromatin, nucleoli, presence of cytoplasmic granules) and immunophenotype. Auer rods are crystallized cytoplasmic inclusions that are highly specific to neoplastic myeloid differentiation but are only identified in a subset of AML cases (e-Figure 12.2-1). Blast equivalents for AML diagnosis include abnormal promyelocytes in acute promyelocytic leukemia (APL), monoblasts and promonocytes in cases with monocytic differentiation, and megakaryoblasts in cases with megakaryocytic differentiation. The acute erythroid leukemia subtype has separate criteria (see "Acute Myeloid Leukemia Defined by Differentiation" section-). AML marrow is usually hypercellular, and maturing neoplastic cells may show atypical/dysplastic features.

Cytochemistry and Immunophenotype

Traditional cytochemistry takes advantage of the expression of lineage-specific enzymes, which result in cellular staining when an appropriate substrate is applied. While often replaced by immunohistochemistry (IHC) in the United States, cytochemistry remains an inexpensive and often effective tool for lineage determination. Myeloperoxidase (MPO), which can also be assessed by immunophenotyping, is the single most defining and specific marker for myeloid/granulocytic differentiation. However, it is commonly weak or negative in AML with monocytic or minimal differentiation. Sudan Black B (SBB) and chloroacetate esterase (CAE) also demonstrate myeloid/granulocytic differentiation. Monocytic differentiation is characterized by positivity for nonspecific esterase (NSE, also called naphthyl butyrate esterase/NBE).

Flow cytometric (FC) immunophenotyping and, to a lesser extent, IHC are central for establishing bona fide myeloblast (or equivalent) differentiation. One common caveat is that in cases with monocytic differentiation, promonocytes and more mature atypical monocytes may not be separable by immunophenotype. Immunophenotyping is also used in AML subcategorization (as in the WHO-HAEM5 differentiation-defined categories) and may suggest the presence of specific genetic lesions. Immunophenotypic markers that distinguish myeloid lineages and maturation patterns are useful in the workup and diagnosis of AML (Table 12.1). In addition to establishing AML diagnosis, initial immunophenotyping aids in follow-up and minimal residual disease (MRD) detection and may guide antigen-targeted treatments (ie, anti-CD33 therapy).

Follow-Up Marrow Assessment

In addition to AML diagnosis, morphologic assessment of bone marrow is also important for evaluating treatment response. According to the National Comprehensive Cancer Network (NCCN) guidelines (https://www.nccn.org/professionals/physician_gls/pdf/aml.pdf), some induction protocols for AML include an early or "nadir" bone marrow biopsy corresponding to the expected period of hypocellularity prior to marrow recovery, often biopsied at days 14 to 21. An appropriate response to treatment is indicated by marrow hypoplasia, defined as less than 20% total cellularity, of which less than 5% is blasts. The cutoff of less than 5% blasts in the bone marrow is also used for morphologic assessment after induction, with the following definitions (based on European LeukemiaNet [ELN] and NCCN guidelines):

- **Morphologic leukemia-free state (MLFS):** Requires less than 5% blasts in the marrow, the absence of extramedullary disease, and (depending on guidelines) the absence of circulating blasts and/or Auer rods.

TABLE 12.1 Immunophenotypic Markers for Characterization of Myeloid Lineages

Cell Populations/Lineages	Markers
Blast/precursors	CD34, CD117, HLA-DR
Myeloid (blasts + mature)	CD13, CD33, MPO (weak/negative in monocytic), CD43 (nonspecific)
Myeloid maturation (both granulocytes and monocytes)	CD11b, CD64 (bright in monocytes), CD65
Granulocytic maturation	CD15, CD10 (late), CD16 (late)
Monocytic maturation	CD4, CD11c (bright), CD14, CD36, CD68, CD163, Lysozyme
Megakaryocytic	CD36, CD41, CD61, CD42a, CD42b
Erythroid	CD235/glycophorin-A, CD71, CD36, E-cadherin
Common aberrant markers	CD56, CD7

- **Complete remission,** also called **complete response (CR):** Requires MLFS plus hematologic recovery: transfusion independence, neutrophil count more than 1 K/μL, and platelet count more than 100 K/μL.
- **CR with incomplete hematologic recovery (CRi):** Otherwise meeting CR criteria but with persistent neutropenia (<1 K/μL) and/or thrombocytopenia (<100 K/μL).
- **First complete remission (CR1):** Refers to CR achieved after primary induction therapy (generally one or two chemotherapy cycles).

Morphologic CR does not imply the elimination of the leukemic clone. MRD testing by FC and/or molecular assays should also be performed after induction and with follow-up monitoring. In general, MRD testing by FC for AML utilizes a myeloid-targeted antibody panel with an assessment of a large number of events (on the order of 10^6) for adequate sensitivity. The ELN recommends acquiring 5×10^5 or more CD45+ cells with 100 or more cells in the blast compartment (*Blood.* 2021;138:2753-2767).

Genetic Features

AML is caused by a range of cytogenetic lesions and mutations that alter cellular differentiation and promote proliferation and survival. Cytogenetic and molecular testing is important for the diagnosis, subclassification, prognosis, and treatment of AML; lists of suggested genetic lesions to screen can be found in professional guidelines (*Blood.* 2022;140:1345-1377; *Am J Hematol.* 2023;98:502-526). Genetic studies are also important for tracking MRD or recurrence after treatment. In addition to the AML-subtype-defining and myelodysplasia-related genetic lesions (including *TP53*) described later in this chapter, important mutations include:

- ***FLT3:*** FMS-like tyrosine kinase 3 (FLT3) signaling promotes hematopoietic cell survival and proliferation. Activating mutations of *FLT3* occur in about 30% of

AML and come in two main types: internal tandem duplication (ITD) in the juxtamembrane domain, and mutation of the tyrosine kinase domain (TKD). *FLT3*-ITD was traditionally a poor prognostic indicator in AML, with its effect on prognosis somewhat dependent on the specific AML subtype and the wild-type-to-mutant allele ratio. Currently, FLT3 inhibitors (eg, midostaurin, gilteritinib) are indicated for the treatment of both FLT3-ITD and *FLT3*-TKD AMLs and have improved the prognosis of *FLT3*-ITD AMLs. However, *FLT3*-ITD remains an adverse indicator in some subtypes of AML.

- ***IDH1/IDH2*:** Activating mutations in the isocitrate dehydrogenase enzymes IDH1 and IDH2 result in disruption of epigenetic regulation, and IDH mutation occurs in 15% to 20% of AML. Identification of IDH mutations is of increasing therapeutic significance due to the development of selective IDH1 and IDH2 inhibitors.
- ***DNMT3A*, *TET2*, and *ASXL1* ("DTA") mutations:** The three DTA mutations are common early events in clonal hematopoiesis and can be found in a wide range of precursor and malignant myeloid neoplasms, including AML. *ASXL1* is also a qualifying mutation for acute myeloid leukemia, myelodysplasia related (AML-MR) by WHO-HAEM5 and International Consensus Classification (ICC)-2022 criteria, and is an adverse prognostic indicator by the ELN 2022 risk classification. Of note, molecular persistence of DTA mutations after AML treatment does not imply treatment failure, as they may persist in underlying clonal hematopoiesis.

Prognosis and Treatment

Treatment

AML treatment guidelines incorporating genetics and patient characteristics are provided by professional groups such as the ELN and the US-based NCCN. Therapy for AML commonly incorporates the following steps:

- **Induction therapy** is the initial treatment aiming to achieve CR1. For decades, 7 days of cytarabine with an anthracycline such as daunorubicin for the first 3 days ("7+3") has been the mainstay of high-intensity/standard induction. Older and nonmedically fit patients receive lower-intensity therapy. Recently, alternate regimens such as those incorporating the B-cell lymphoma (BCL)-2 inhibitor venetoclax or the liposomal cytarabine + daunorubicin preparation CPX-351 have shown benefit for various high-risk and nonmedically fit patient groups. Induction may also incorporate targeted therapy such as FLT3 inhibitors.
- **Consolidation therapy** follows induction to help prevent relapse. Depending on risk stratification and availability of a donor, consolidation may include chemotherapy alone or high-dose myeloablative chemotherapy followed by auto-hematopoietic stem cell transplantation (HSCT) or allo-HSCT. Allo-HSCT provides an anti-leukemic "graft vs. tumor" effect and generally provides the greatest chance of long-term remission, but carries the risk of graft-versus-host disease (GVHD).
- **Maintenance** may include additional lower-dose chemotherapy or targeted therapy, along with monitoring for recurrence.
- **Salvage therapy** is used for patients with relapsed or treatment-refractory AML, and often incorporates newer therapeutics and/or clinical trial regimens.

The last decade has seen a revolution in AML treatment options, with US Food and Drug Administration (FDA) approval of 11 new therapeutics or drug combinations since 2017 (and many more currently in clinical trials). Many new agents target AML-specific signaling pathways or antigens (*Am J Hematol.* 2023;98:502-526).

Prognosis

AML as a whole carries a relatively poor prognosis. Advances in therapy have improved the outcomes for younger adult patients, with 2-year overall survival of 43.5% to 78.6% for patients 60 years of age or younger in a recent 2000 to 2018 cohort study. However, prognosis in older patients, who constitute the majority of new cases, remains low, with a 2-year overall survival rate of only 15.8% among patients above 60 years (*Leuk Res Rep.* 2020;14:100206). Across all age groups, the 5-year overall survival of AML is approximately 30%, and AML comprises approximately 2% of all cancer deaths in the United States (2017-2019 data, NCI SEER Program, https://seer.cancer.gov/).

II. CLASSIFICATION OF ACUTE MYELOID LEUKEMIA: WORLD HEALTH ORGANIZATION AND INTERNATIONAL CONSENSUS CLASSIFICATION

The diagnosis and classification of AML require comprehensive evaluation and integration of clinical, pathologic, cytogenetic, and molecular findings. The WHO revised 4th edition (WHO-HAEM4R) emphasized the biologic and clinical importance of genetics over phenotype in its genetically defined diagnostic categories, of which three (*RUNX1-RUNX1T1*, *CBFB-MYH11*, *PML-RARA*) could be diagnosed with less than 20% blasts. Significant updates have been made in the recent new classifications: WHO-HAEM5 and ICC. Both systems updated the WHO-HAEM4R with additional genetic categories, and lowered the 20% blast cutoff for most genetic categories (removing a definite cutoff in WHO-HAEM5, and requiring 10% or more in ICC). ICC makes additional changes to the WHO framework with the introduction of MDS/AML for MDS cases with 10% to 19% blasts, and the use of "diagnostic qualifiers" for secondary AMLs. Key changes and differences are summarized in Table 12.2. Of note, the ICC criteria specify that AML listed higher in their diagnostic table generally take diagnostic precedence over those lower in the table (Table 12.3 is arranged in ICC-2022 descending order).

TABLE 12.2 Summary of Major Diagnostic Differences in the Classification of AML

	WHO 5th Edition (HAEM5)	ICC-2022
Diagnostic blast % in blood or bone marrow	• Most genetically defined AML categories have no specific blast cutoff (see Table 12.2). • For remaining categories, ≥**20%** blasts required.	• Most genetically defined AML categories require ≥**10% blasts** (see Table 12.2). • For remaining categories, ≥**20%** blasts required for AML, and introduces "**MDS/AML**" for cases with **10%-19%** blasts.

TABLE 12.2 Summary of Major Diagnostic Differences in the Classification of AML (*continued*)

	WHO 5th Edition (HAEM5)	**ICC-2022**
Secondary AMLs	• MN post-cytotoxic therapy (MN-pCT) takes precedence over most AML diagnoses, but should be combined with MN subclassification. • Progression from MDS or MDS/MPN is an AML-MR criteria. • Myeloid neoplasm with germline predisposition (MN-GP) form parallel diagnostic categories, which should be combined with MN subclassification.	Introduces "diagnostic qualifiers" applied to any AML, MDS/AML, or MDS diagnosis that meets criteria for: • Therapy related • Progressing from MDS • Progression from MDS/MPN • Germline predisposition
MDS-related AML	**AML, myelodysplasia related:** Requires one or more of: • Prior history of MDS or MDS/MPN • MDS-related cytogenetic abnormality • MDS-related gene mutation	**Two categories:** • AML and MDS/AML with MDS-related cytogenetic abnormalities • AML and MDS/AML with MDS-related gene mutations "Progressing from MDS" and "Progressing from MDS/MPN" are diagnostic qualifiers.
AML-"NOS"	**AML defined by differentiation:** • Subclassify by differentiation.	**AML-NOS and MDS/AML-NOS:** • Describing differentiation is optional.
Differences related to specific mutations	• *TP53* mutation does not define an AML subtype (but does for MDS). • **AML with *CEBPA* mutation:** requires either biallelic *or* bZIP mutation, and ≥20% blasts. • ***RUNX1*** mutation removed as a diagnosis-defining mutation.	• Introduces **AML and MDS/AML with mutated *TP53*** (requiring ≥10% VAF) • **AML with in-frame bZIP *CEBPA* mutation:** requires in-frame bZIP mutation, ≥10% blasts. • ***RUNX1*** mutation included in AML with MDS-related gene mutations.

AML, acute myeloid leukemia; AML-MR, AML myelodysplasia related; AML-NOS, AML-not otherwise specified; ICC, International Consensus Classification; MDS, myelodysplastic syndrome; MPN, myeloproliferative neoplasm; MN, myeloid neoplasm; WHO-HAEM5, 5th edition of the World Health Organization.

TABLE 12.3 AML Types and Blast Requirements by Diagnostic System

WHO-HAEM5 Diagnosis	Blasts Required	ICC-2022 Diagnosis	Blasts Required
APL with *PML::RARA* fusion (subtype: APL with variant *RARA* fusion)	NA	APL with t(15;17)(q24.1;q21.2)/ *PML::RARA*	≥10%
		APL with other *RARA* rearrangements	≥10%
AML with *RUNX1::RUNX1T1* fusion	NA	AML with t(8;21)(q22;q22.1)/ *RUNX1::RUNX1T1*	≥10%
AML with *CBFB::MYH11* fusion	NA	AML with inv(16)(p13.1q22) or t(16;16)(p13.1;q22)/ *CBFB::MYH11*	≥10%
AML with *KMT2A* rearrangement	NA	AML with t(9;11)(p21.3;q23.3)/ *MLLT3::KMT2A*	≥10%
		AML with other *KMT2A* rearrangements	≥10%
AML with *DEK::NUP214* fusion	NA	AML with t(6;9)(p22.3;q34.1)/ *DEK::NUP214*	≥10%
AML with *MECOM* rearrangement	NA	AML with inv(3)(q21.3q26.2) or t(3;3)(q21.3;q26.2)/ *GATA2; MECOM(EVI1)*	≥10%
		AML with other MECOM rearrangements	≥10%
AML with *RBM15::MRTFA* fusion	NA	*Included under "AML with other rare recurring translocations"*	
AML with *NUP98* rearrangement	NA	*Included under "AML with other rare recurring translocations"*	
AML with other defined genetic alterations	≥20%	AML with other rare recurring translocations	≥10%
AML with *BCR::ABL1* fusion	>20%	AML with t(9;22)(q34.1;q11.2)/ *BCR::ABL1*	**≥20%**

TABLE 12.3 AML Types and Blast Requirements by Diagnostic System (*continued*)

WHO-HAEM5 Diagnosis	Blasts Required	ICC-2022 Diagnosis	Blasts Required
AML with *NPM1* mutation	NA	AML with mutated NPM1	≥10%
AML with *CEBPA* mutation [biallelic or bZIP]	**≥20%**	AML with in-frame bZIP *CEBPA* mutations	≥10%
TP53 mutation is not AML-subtype-defining		AML and MDS/AML with mutated *TP53*	AML: ≥20% MDS/AML: 10%-19%
AML, myelodysplasia related (*Defined by prior MDS or MDS/MPN, specific cytogenetics, or specific mutations*)	≥20%	AML and MDS/AML with myelodysplasia-related gene mutations	AML: ≥20% MDS/AML: 10%-19%
		AML and MDS/AML with myelodysplasia-related cytogenetic abnormalities	AML: ≥20% MDS/AML: 10%-19%
AML defined by differentiation (subclassify by phenotype)	≥20%	AML and MDS/AML-not otherwise specified (NOS)	AML: ≥20% MDS/AML: 10%-19%

AML, acute myeloid leukemia; APL, acute promyelocytic leukemia; ICC, International Consensus Classification; MDS, myelodysplastic syndrome; MPN, myeloproliferative neoplasm; WHO-HAEM5, 5th edition of the World Health Organization.

III. ACUTE MYELOID LEUKEMIA WITH DEFINING GENETIC ABNORMALITIES

AML is a group of heterogeneous diseases characterized by recurrent genetic abnormalities. In WHO-HAEM4R, the diagnosis of AML required the detection of at least 20% blasts in the bone marrow. There were two important exceptions to the requirement: (1) AMLs with *RUNX1::RUNX1T1*, *CBFB::MYH11*, and *PML::RARA* fusion genes were classified as AML regardless of the percentage of blasts, and (2) acute erythroid leukemia was characterized by neoplastic proliferation of immature cells in the erythroid lineage comprising more than 80% of the bone marrow cells, of which at least 30% of this population are proerythroblasts.

In the recent classifications, additional genetically defined disease types now qualify for the diagnosis of AML without the 20% blast cutoff (Table 12.3). In fact, AML with *BCR::ABL1* and AML with *CEBPA* mutations are the only two types with a defined genetic abnormality (not including AML-MR) that require 20% or more blasts for diagnosis by the WHO-HAEM5 criteria. As a general principle, the diagnosis of AML with defining genetic abnormalities takes diagnostic precedence over other AML categories.

The clinical features, morphology, immunophenotype, and prognosis of the major genetically defined AML subtypes are summarized further and in Table 12.4. Occasional cases with more than one subtype-defining genetic abnormality can present diagnostic challenges, require careful referral to the diagnostic criteria, and likely warrant a comment in the pathology report on the genetics.

- **APL with *PML::RARA*:** APL is a favorable prognosis subtype of AML with distinctive phenotype, clinical features, and management. It accounts for 5% to 8% of AML cases and most commonly presents in young and middle-aged patients. Because of abrupt onset with a high incidence of DIC, and the availability of an effective specific treatment with all-trans retinoic acid (ATRA), prompt diagnosis is essential.

  APL typically has the *PML::RARA* fusion resulting from the t(15;17)(q22;q21) translocation. Less commonly, APL results from the fusion of *RARA* with a different partner; these cases can be classified as "APL with variant *RARA* fusion" per WHO-HAEM5 and include *NUMA1::RARA* and *NPM1::RARA* (which are sensitive to ATRA) and *ZBTB16::RARA* and *STAT5B::RARA* (which are resistant to ATRA). The ICC criteria similarly splits APL into "APL with t(15;17)(q24.1;q21.2)/*PML::RARA*" and "APL with other *RARA* rearrangements."

  The neoplastic cells in APL are predominantly abnormal promyelocytes, counted as blast equivalents, and classically show bilobed nuclei ("butterfly cells"). In the more common "hypergranular" variant, the cytoplasm contains abundant dark granules and/or Auer rods, there is corresponding high side scatter on FC, and the initial presentation is frequently pancytopenia with relatively few circulating APL cells (e-Figures 12.2-1 to 12.2-3). In the "hypogranular" or "microgranular" variant, granules and Auer rods are inconspicuous, bilobed blasts are often present (e-Figure 12.2-2), and presentation tends to be more overtly leukemic. Both variants usually share immunophenotypic features with normal promyelocytes, including expression of CD13, CD33, and CD117, but dim/absent CD34 and HLA-DR. However, a similar immunophenotype can also be seen in some non-APL cases of AML, especially AML with mutated *NPM1*.

  APL generally has an excellent prognosis if treated promptly. A cutoff of peripheral white blood cell (WBC) of 10×10^9/L or more at diagnosis defines a higher-risk subset. Non–high-risk cases are usually treated with ATRA and arsenic trioxide (ATO) alone, while high-risk cases benefit from the addition of conventional AML chemotherapeutics. ATRA induces maturation of APL cells, and in a minority of cases treatment is complicated by "differentiation syndrome," a systemic inflammatory response associated with cytokine production and peripheral migration by maturing neoplastic cells (*Cancers* (*Basel*). 2023;15:4767).

- **AML with *RUNX1::RUNX1T1*:** This is one of the two classic favorable prognosis "core binding factor" (CBF) AML subtypes. It is defined by fusion of *RUNX1* (formerly *CBFA*) with *RUNX1T1* (formerly *ETO*), usually t(8;21)(q22;q22.1). The usual morphology is large blasts with perinuclear hof, salmon-colored granules, and occasional thin Auer rods. The immunophenotype generally shows myeloblast markers with the characteristic addition of aberrant B-lineage markers (CD19, cCD79a, and/or PAX5) and variably CD56 and/or CD15. Maturing but dysplastic neoplastic granulocytes are often present as well.

TABLE 12.4 Clinical and Phenotypic Characteristics of AML With Defining Genetic Abnormalities

AML Subtype	Clinical Features	Usual Morphology	Usual Immunophenotype
Favorable Prognosis			
AML with *PML::RARA*, t(15;17)	Coagulopathy/DIC, normal/low WBC (hypergranular variant); or high WBC (hypogranular variant)	Abnormal promyelocytes with abundant granules and/or Auer rods (few granules/rods in hypogranular variant)	CD13+ (heterogeneous), CD33+ (bright), CD117+, HLA-DR–, CD34–. High side scatter in usual (hypergranular) variant
AML with *RUNX1::RUNX1T1*, t(8;21)	Can present with extramedullary disease (MS)	Blasts with long slender Auer rods, abnormal salmon-colored granulations	CD13+, CD33 (weak), MPO+, CD19+, cCD79a+, CD34+, CD56+/–, CD15+/–
AML with *CBFB::MYH11*, t(16;16)/inv(16)[a]	Can present with extramedullary disease (MS)	Myelomonocytic; may also have atypical eosinophils with large basophilic granules	Blasts CD13+, CD33+, MPO+; monocytic component CD4+, CD14+, CD11b+, CD11c+, CD64+, CD36+, Lysozyme+
AML with *NPM1* mutation[b]	About 30% of adult AML. Occasionally extramedullary	Blasts with cup-like nuclear indentations; often myelomonocytic or monocytic, +/– dysplasia	CD33+, CD117+, CD123+, CD13+/weak, CD34–/+, HLA-DR+/–, MPO+/– monocytic markers +/–
AML with *CEBPA* mutation (biallelic or bZIP)	Subset having germline mutation	May or may not show maturation, dysplasia common	CD7+/–, CD13+, CD15+, CD33+, CD34+, HLA-DR+
Intermediate Prognosis			
AML with *KMT2A* rearrangement,[c] t(9;11) most common	Frequently occurs in children	Variable, often with monocytic features, sometimes megakaryoblastic	Variable: CD13+/–, CD34+/–, CD117+/–, usually CD4+, CD33+, CD65+, usually + other monocytic markers

(continued)

TABLE 12.4 Clinical and Phenotypic Characteristics of AML With Defining Genetic Abnormalities (*continued*)

AML Subtype	Clinical Features	Usual Morphology	Usual Immunophenotype
AML with *RBM15::MRTFA*, t(1;22)[c]	Infants and young children; hepatosplenomegaly	Megakaryoblastic	CD41+, CD42b+, and/or CD61+. CD13+, CD33+, CD34−, HLA-DR−, MPO−
Poor Prognosis			
AML with *DEK::NUP214*, t(6;9)	Pancytopenia	Multilineage dysplasia, sometimes basophilia	CD13+, CD33+, CD38+, MPO+, HLA-DR+, CD117+, CD123+, CD7+/−, CD34+/−, TdT+/−
AML with *BCR::ABL1*, t(9;22)	Leukocytosis, mostly adults; no preceding CML	Nonspecific blast morphology, sometimes monocytic differentiation	CD13+, CD33+, CD34+, HLA-DR+, CD117+, CD7+/−, CD19+/−, TdT+/−
AML with *MECOM* rearrangement, inv(3)/t(3;3) most common	Normal/elevated platelet count, cytopenias	Multilineage dysplasia, including marked dysmegakaryopoiesis	CD13+, CD33+, CD38+, HLA-DR+, CD34+, CD117+, CD7+/−, CD41/CD61+/−
AML with *NUP98* rearrangement	Rare, pediatric > adult, thrombocytopenia	Variable, including myeloblasts w/o differentiation, monocytic, megakaryoblastic, erythroid	Variable by differentiation; blasts most commonly CD13+, CD33+, MPO+, CD117+, CD34+, HLA-DR+

AML, acute myeloid leukemia; CML, chronic myeloid leukemia; DIC, disseminated intravascular coagulation; MS, myeloid sarcoma; WBC, white blood cell.
[a]The prognosis is worse with *KIT* mutation.
[b]The prognosis is worse when there is concurrent *FLT3*-ITD.
[c]The prognosis is variable.

- **AML with *CBFB::MYH11*:** This is the other classic "CBF" AML subtype with a favorable prognosis. The defining *CBFB::MYH11* fusion usually results from inv(16)(p13.1q22) or less frequently t(16;16). This is a relatively subtle abnormality on classic karyotype, with fluorescence in situ hybridization (FISH) and reverse transcriptase–polymerase chain reaction (RT-PCR) having greater sensitivity. AML with *CBFB::MYH11* usually carries a myelomonocytic phenotype, with several abnormal populations corresponding to different myeloid sublineages: an immature population of myeloblasts; a more mature promonocyte-like population; and abnormal maturing eosinophils that may contain large, purple granules (so-called "baso-eos" or "harlequin cells"). See e-Figures 12.2-4 and 12.2-5. Extramedullary disease (myeloid sarcoma [MS]) is relatively frequent.
- **AML with *DEK::NUP214* fusion:** This is a rare AML subtype in both children and adults associated with poor prognosis. It is defined by the *DEK::NUP214* fusion, usually resulting from the translocation t(6;9)(p22.3;q34.1). Most cases also carry *FLT3*-ITD. Morphology is nonspecific but usually shows multilineage dysplasia and blasts with granulocytic maturation or myelomonocytic features. Some cases also have basophilia.
- **AML with *KMT2A* rearrangement:** This is an AML subtype with greater frequency in the pediatric population and variable prognosis. It is defined by a translocation involving *KMT2A*, most commonly *KMT2A::MLLT3* t(9;11)(p21.3;q23.3). ICC criteria split this category into "AML with t(9;11)(p21.3;q23.3)/*MLLT3::KMT2A*" and "AML with other *KMT2A* rearrangements." *KMT2A* rearrangement is usually associated with monocytic/monoblastic differentiation, but can have other phenotypes, including megakaryoblastic differentiation. *KMT2A* was formerly known as *MLL* for "mixed lineage leukemia," and rearrangements of this gene are also found in cases of mixed-phenotype acute leukemia and B-cell acute lymphoblastic leukemia (B-ALL).
- **AML with *MECOM* rearrangement:** This AML type occurs mostly in adults and has a poor prognosis. It is defined by rearrangement of *MECOM (EVI1)*, most commonly *GATA2::MECOM*/inv(3)(q21.3;q26.2) or t(3;3). ICC criteria split this category into cases with the usual *GATA2::MECOM* and AML with other *MECOM* rearrangements. Blasts show variable myeloid or myelomonocytic differentiation with frequent aberrant CD7; a subset of cases have megakaryoblastic differentiation. Background dysplasia is common, including the characteristic finding (although not entirely sensitive or specific) of abundant small hypolobated megakaryocytes (see e-Figures 12.2-6 to 12.2-9). Peripheral blood is frequently pancytopenic with few blasts, but may show leukocytosis and/or thrombocytosis.
- **AML with *RBM15::MRTFA* fusion:** This rare AML subtype occurs mostly in infants, frequently presents with cytopenia and marked organomegaly, and has an intermediate/variable prognosis. AML with *RMB15::MRTFA* t(1;22)(p13.3;q13.1) usually shows a megakaryocytic phenotype with megakaryoblasts, micromegakaryocytes, and marrow fibrosis. The morphologic differential often includes other acute megakaryocyte leukemias (AMKLs) arising in young children such as myeloid leukemia of Down syndrome (DS-ML). AML with *RBM15::MRTFA* is included in the ICC under the bucket category "AML with other rare recurring translocations."
- **AML with *BCR::ABL1* fusion:** This is a rare subtype of de novo AML characterized by the *BCR::ABL1* fusion without underlying CML. It occurs mostly in adults and carries a poor prognosis. The classic "Philadelphia chromosome" translocation t(9;22)(q34;q11) can usually be detected, with most cases carrying the p210 major

breakpoint variant of BCR-ABL (also the most common in CML). Under both WHO-HAEM5 and ICC criteria, the diagnosis of AML with *BCR::ABL1* requires more than 20% blasts. WHO-HAEM5 also makes explicit the essential criteria of *BCR::ABL1* detection at diagnosis (not later developing in a subclone) and "lack of features of CML prior to or at diagnosis or after therapy." The morphology and immunophenotype are nonspecific, with some cases showing minimal or monocytic differentiation. Characteristic morphologic features of CML such as elevated basophils and small hypolobated megakaryocytes are usually absent.

- **AML with *NUP98* rearrangement:** This is a rare AML subtype with poor prognosis, more common in pediatric AML. It is defined by a fusion of *NUP98* on chromosome 11p15.4 with multiple possible partners, most commonly *NSD1*, *KDM5A*, or a *HOX*-family gene. Many of these translocations are cryptic (not detectable by conventional karyotype). Accompanying *FLT3*-ITD and/or *WT1* mutations are common. Morphologic and immunophenotypic findings are variable and partially dependent on the fusion partner. Especially in children, some cases show erythroid or megakaryoblastic differentiation (*Blood Adv.* 2020;4:6000-6008). ICC includes *NUP98*-rearranged AMLs under "AML with other rare recurring translocations."

- **AML with *NPM1* mutation:** Mutation of the nucleophosmin (*NPM1*) gene is the single most common subtype-defining genetic lesion in AML, occurring in approximately 30% of all de novo AML in adults and an even higher percentage of normal karyotype AML (*N Engl J Med.* 2005;352:254-266; *Blood.* 2006;107:4011-4020). Patients usually present with leukocytosis and occasionally with MS. Cases with no high-risk genetic lesions and no *FLT3*-ITD carry a good prognosis. *FLT3*-ITD somewhat worsens the prognosis of *NPM1*-mutated AML, especially in cases with high *FLT3* mutant-to-WT allelic ratio (*Blood.* 2008;111:2776-2778; *Blood.* 2013;121:2734-2738). However, the 2022 update to the widely used ELN guidelines no longer utilizes allelic ratio for risk stratification and places all *FLT3*-ITD cases (without other high-risk genetics) into the "intermediate risk" category (*Blood.* 2022;140:1345-1377).

  AML with *NPM1* mutation has variable morphology but frequently shows myelomonocytic or monocytic differentiation and sometimes background dysplasia. The finding of blasts with "cup-like" or "fish mouth" nuclear indentations is characteristic (e-Figure 12.1-1) and is usually most pronounced in cases with *FLT3*-ITD. Immunophenotypically, blasts frequently lack expression of CD34 and in some cases lack HLA-DR, which may raise the differential diagnosis of APL. Aberrant cytoplasmic localization of NPM1 protein can be detected by IHC (*Haematologica.* 2010;95:529-534).

- **AML with *CEBPA* mutation:** This is a moderately common AML subtype occurring in children and adults with a good prognosis and two notable diagnostic caveats: it retains a requirement of 20% or more blasts in WHO-HAEM5, and only a subset of *CEBPA* mutations qualify. Since 2009, double-mutant (biallelic) *CEBPA* mutations have been known to predict favorable prognosis of AML, with single-mutant/monoallelic cases having more variable behavior (*Blood.* 2009;113:3088-3091). Recent studies have shown that in-frame mutation in the bZIP domain of *CEBPA* is the major determinant of a favorable prognosis; at least one of these bZIP mutations is present in the predominance of biallelic *CEBPA* cases and a subset of monoallelic cases (*Blood.* 2022;139:87-103; *Blood Adv.* 2022;6:238-247). Double non-bZIP *CEBPA* mutations are rare and of uncertain prognostic significance. WHO-HAEM5 allows diagnosis of AML with *CEBPA* mutation either by the presence of biallelic mutations or by a single mutation in the bZIP region, while the ICC molecular criteria are more stringent with only in-frame mutations in bZIP qualifying. Of note, a subset of cases (especially biallelic mutations in younger individuals) are secondary to an underlying germline *CEBPA* variant.

Morphologically, blasts may or may not show maturation and background dysplasia is common. Immunophenotype typically shows myeloblast markers with aberrant CD15 and CD7 but without CD14 or CD56 (*Clin Cancer Res.* 2005;11:1372-1379). Diagnosis requires 20% or more blasts in bone marrow or blood per WHO-HAEM5, while ICC requires only 10% or more blasts for diagnosis of "AML with in-frame bZIP *CEBPA* mutations."

- **AML with other defined genetic alterations:** There are additional rare or recently identified genetic lesions (mostly balanced translocations) that give rise to clinically and biologically distinct subtypes of AML. In WHO-HAEM5, these are grouped under "AML with other defined genetic alterations" and include cases with *CBFA2T3::GLIS2, KAT6A::CREBBP, FUS::ERG, MNX1::ETV6,* or *NPM1::MLF1*. Similarly, the ICC includes these five translocations, *RBM15::MRTFA* and *NUP98* rearrangements, and several others under the category "AML with other rare recurring translocations." Epidemiology, phenotype, and prognosis vary by the specific translocation, with many of these entities skewing to pediatric or young adult populations. WHO-HAEM5 requires 20% or more blasts for this diagnostic category, while ICC requires only 10% or more. Additionally, in WHO-HAEM5, the diagnosis of AML-MR supersedes the diagnosis of AML with "other defined genetic alterations," while in ICC, the latter category takes diagnostic precedence over AML-MR and MDS/AML-MR categories.

IV. ACUTE MYELOID LEUKEMIA, MYELODYSPLASIA RELATED AND ACUTE MYELOID LEUKEMIA WITH MUTATED *TP53*

AML-MR as defined in WHO-HAEM5 is a myeloid neoplasm with 20% or more blasts harboring specific cytogenetic and molecular abnormalities associated with MDS. It can arise de novo or follow a known history of MDS or MDS/MPN. AML-MR is an update to the category of AML with myelodysplasia-related changes (AML-MRC) in WHO-HAEM4R, and substantially overlaps with the ICC diagnoses of AML with MDS-related cytogenetic abnormalities (AML-MRCA) and MDS-related gene mutations (AML-MRGM). ICC also introduced MDS/AML-MRCA and MDS/AML-MRGM for cases with 10% to 19% blasts; many of these cases qualify for MDS-IB2 by WHO-HAEM5 criteria. See Table 12.2 for diagnostic differences between the systems and Table 12.5 for the WHO-HAEM5 criteria. Under these systems, most other subtype-defining genetic abnormalities supersede AML-MR in diagnostic priority, while AML-MR supersedes AML-not otherwise specified (AML-NOS)/AML defined by differentiation (AML-DBD).

Clinical Features

AML-MR is a common AML subtype comprising 25% to 34% of all AML (*Genes (Basel).* 2020;11:845), although this may vary depending on the specific classification system and population studied. Incidence increases with age, with a median of about 70 years, and there is moderate male predominance (*Am J Hematol.* 2020;95:612-622). Presentation varies, but there is often severe pancytopenia. AML-MR with lower blast counts (<30%) forms a biologic and clinical continuum with MDS-IB2 (or MDS/AML), and some of these cases progress more slowly.

TABLE 12.5 Diagnostic Characteristics of AML-MR, (WHO-HAEM5)

Essential Diagnostic Criteria (WHO-HAEM5)

- History of MDS or MDS/MPN and/or detection of one or more chromosomal or molecular aberrations listed in table (see WHO-HAEM5 online Table #31404; Table 12.4 in this handbook)
- ≥20% blasts with myeloid immunophenotype in bone marrow or blood
- Criteria for other AML types with defined genetic alterations are not met.
- Not fulfilling diagnostic criteria for MN-pCT

Diagnostic Caveats

- Patients should not have a history of MPN (MPN evolving to ≥20% blasts will generally be considered blast-phase MPN).
- The diagnosis of AEL (formerly pure erythroid leukemia) supersedes AML-MR.
- Morphologic dysplasia is not specific for AML-MR and has been dropped as a diagnostic criterion for AML-MR in WHO-HAEM5.
- The WHO diagnosis of MN-pCT supersedes AML-MR (and as a general principle supersedes all AML, MDS, and MDS/MPN diagnoses). However, MN-pCT should still be subcategorized to the greatest extent feasible and a combined diagnosis rendered, that is, "AML, myelodysplasia related, post-cytotoxic therapy."

AEL, acute erythroid leukemia; AML, acute myeloid leukemia; AML-MR, acute myeloid leukemia myelodysplasia related; MDS, myelodysplastic syndrome; MN-pCT, myeloid neoplasm post-cytotoxic therapy; MPN, myeloproliferative neoplasm; WHO-HAEM5, 5th edition of the World Health Organization.

Morphology, Immunophenotype, and Genetics

Morphology is variable, but most cases show multilineage dysplasia, with a similar range of dysplastic features to those seen in MDS (see Chapter 10). Multilineage dysplasia could be used to diagnosis AML-MRC under WHO-HAEM4R, but dysplasia is also found in many genetically defined AML types and was removed as a criterion in ICC and WHO-HAEM5. By definition, blasts are increased and usually show a myeloblast phenotype including expression of CD13, MPO, CD34, CD117, and HLA-DR, with variable immunophenotypic aberrancy in blasts and maturing neoplastic cells.

Genetic changes that can be used to diagnose AML-MR and AML-MRCA/AML-MRGM are listed in Table 12.6. Cytogenetic abnormalities generally include large-segment or whole-chromosome gains or losses, rather than balanced translocations. Many of the defining cytogenetic abnormalities and mutations are also considered adverse risk indicators in AML (*Blood.* 2022;140:1345-1377). *TP53* mutation is not a qualifying mutation for AML-MR diagnosis, but is relatively common in AML-MR, is associated with P53 overexpression by IHC, and carries poor prognosis; see further discussion of *TP53*-mutated AML below.

Prognosis and Treatment

AML-MR has a worse prognosis than most other subtypes of AML. This is reflected by the fact that many of the AML-MR-defining genetic lesions also define high-risk

TABLE 12.6 Cytogenetic and Molecular Abnormalities Defining Myelodysplasia-Related AML

Qualifying genetics lesions for AML, myelodysplasia (WHO-HAEM5), AML and MDS/AML with myelodysplasia-related gene mutations, AML and MDS/AML myelodysplasia-related cytogenetic abnormalities (ICC)

Defining Cytogenetic Abnormalities

Both WHO-HAEM5 and ICC:

- **Complex karyotype (≥3 abnormalities)**[a]
- **5q deletion or loss of 5q due to unbalanced translocation**[b]
- **Monosomy 7, 7q deletion, or loss of 7q due to unbalanced translocation**[b]
- **17p deletion or loss of 17p due to unbalanced translocation**[b]
- 12p deletion or loss of 12p due to unbalanced translocation[b]
- Isochromosome 17q
- idic(X)(q13)

WHO-HAEM5 only:

- 11q deletion
- Monosomy 13 or 13q deletion

ICC only:

- Gain of 8
- 20q deletion

Defining Somatic Mutations

Both WHO-HAEM5 and ICC:

- ***ASXL1***
- ***BCOR***
- ***EZH2***
- ***SF3B1***
- ***SRSF2***
- ***STAG2***
- ***U2AF1***
- ***ZRSR2***

WHO-HAEM5 only:

None

ICC only:

RUNX1[c]

The first four listed cytogenetic abnormalities **(bold)** and all defining mutations are also considered to be adverse prognostic risk indicators for AML by ELN 2022 guidelines (*Blood*. 2022;140(12):1345-1377).

AML, acute myeloid leukemia; ELN, European LeukemiaNet; ICC, International Consensus Classification; MDS, myelodysplastic syndrome; MPN, myeloproliferative neoplasm; WHO-HAEM5, 5th edition of the World Health Organization.
[a]See WHO-HAEM5 for definition of qualifying abnormalities for complex karyotype (based on ISCN criteria). ICC-2022 specifies "≥3 unrelated clonal chromosomal abnormalities in the absence of other class defining recurring genetic abnormalities."
[b]Per the WHO-HAEM5. ICC defines as "del(5q)/t(5q)/add(5q)," "−7/del(7q)," "−17/add(17p) or del(17p)," and "del(12p)/t(12p)/add(12p)."
[c]*RUNX1* mutation previously defined a provisional AML entity in WHO-HAEM4R.

AML by clinical criteria, such as the ELN guidelines (*Blood*. 2022;140:1345-1377). An increased proportion of AML-MR patients are ineligible for high-intensity induction chemotherapy due to age or other clinical factors. Newer chemotherapy options have shown evidence for improved outcomes and are being incorporated into treatment guidelines for AML-MR, including CPX-351 or venetoclax + hypomethylating agent (*Am J Hematol*. 2023;98:502-526).

Acute Myeloid Leukemia With Mutated *TP53*

TP53 mutation is a significant indicator of adverse risk in AML. Some studies have shown an especially strong association with relapse and poor prognosis when there is biallelic inactivation of *TP53*, that is, when there is a mutation of one *TP53* allele, and an additional mutation, 17p deletion, or copy-neutral loss-of-heterozygosity affecting the second allele (*Blood Adv.* 2022;6:2847-2853; *Blood.* 2022;139:2347-2354). AML cases with *TP53* mutation frequently also have myelodysplasia-related genetic lesions, including complex karyotypes and high-risk gene mutations. *TP53* mutation is frequent in secondary AML post-cytotoxic therapy, and biallelic mutation is highly prevalent in acute erythroid leukemia (see "Acute Erythroid Leukemia" section).

Unlike WHO-HAEM4R and WHO-HAEM5, ICC includes a separate genetically defined AML category of "AML with mutated *TP53*," which requires 20% or more blasts plus any somatic *TP53* mutation with variant allele frequency (VAF) of more than 10%. This diagnosis sits below most other genetically defined AML diagnoses in the ICC hierarchy but supersedes the AML-MR and AML-NOS categories. Therefore, cases of AML-*TP53* by ICC criteria usually correspond to AML-MR (or occasionally acute erythroid leukemia [AEL]) by WHO-HAEM5 criteria. ICC also includes MDS/AML with mutated *TP53* (10%-19% blasts) and MDS with mutated *TP53* (<10% blasts), both of which partially overlap with the WHO-HAEM5 category of MDS with biallelic *TP53* inactivation.

V. ACUTE MYELOID LEUKEMIA DEFINED BY DIFFERENTIATION/ACUTE MYELOID LEUKEMIA-NOT OTHERWISE SPECIFIED

WHO-HAEM5 introduces the category of AML *defined by differentiation*, which replaces the term AML-NOS for AML types categorized by differentiation in WHO-HAEM4R. In general, only cases lacking AML-subtype-defining genetic abnormalities should receive a diagnosis of AML-DBD. ICC retains the term "AML, NOS" for cases lacking specific genetics but does not require subclassification by differentiation. In the current era of expanded genetic focus in diagnostic criteria, AML-DBD/AML-NOS is a shrinking category accounting for less than 10% of AML diagnoses (*Leukemia.* 2023;37:1413-1420).

WHO-HAEM5 includes eight differentiation-defined AML subtypes, classified by the degree of maturation and the predominant myeloid sublineage(s) as defined by cytochemistry, immunophenotype, and (to some extent) morphologic findings. The features are summarized in Table 12.7 and resemble the older French-American-British (FAB) system of AML subclassification by differentiation.

Clinical Characteristics and Prognosis

There are substantial older data characterizing the prognosis of AML by FAB subclass; however, genetic findings currently provide more precise risk stratification. Even in AML-NOS (by WHO-HAEM4R criteria), subclassification by differentiation provides relatively little additional prognostic information (*Blood.* 2013;121:2424-2431; *Am J Hematol.* 2017;92:344-350). The remaining clinical relevance for differentiation assessment in AML includes the association of monocytic differentiation with central nervous system (CNS) involvement and MS, and poor prognosis associated with AEL (described further) and adult acute megakaryoblastic leukemia (see e-Figures 12.3-1 to 12.3-3 for an example of monocytic AML).

TABLE 12.7 Characteristics of AML Defined by Differentiation (WHO-HAEM5)

AML Subtypes	Presentation	Morphology and Cytochemistry	Immunophenotype
AML with minimal differentiation *(FAB: M0)*	<5% of AML; adults > children. Associated with *BCL11B* translocation	Lacks morphologic/cytochemical evidence of myeloid differentiation or maturation. Blasts lack granules or Auer rods. Negative (<3% of blasts) for MPO, SBB, CAE, NSE	Positive for ≥2 myeloid markers (ie, CD13, CD33, CD117). Usually CD34+, CD38+, CD123+. MPO–. Markers are insufficient for Dx of other AML categories, ALL, or MPAL.
AML without maturation *(FAB: M1)*	Adults> children, cytopenias, sometimes marked leukocytosis	Granulocytic maturation is present but limited (<10% of cells). Blasts may or may not have granules. MPO+ and/or SBB+; mostly CAE–, NSE–	Positive for ≥2 myeloid markers (ie, CD13, CD33, CD117, MPO). Usually CD34+, CD15–, CD11c–, CD14–, CD36–, CD64–
AML with maturation *(FAB: M2)*	Variable age and presentation. Usually cytopenias, sometimes marked leukocytosis	≥10% maturing granulocytic cells, <20% monocytic lineage. Blasts often have granules or Auer rods, maturing neutrophils may be dysplastic. Blasts are MPO+ and/or SBB+; mostly CAE–, NSE–	Blasts + for ≥2 myeloid markers. Blasts and maturing neoplastic cells + for granulocytic markers (CD11b, CD15, CD65) but mostly negative for monocytic markers.
Acute basophilic leukemia *(FAB: rare/NA)*	Very rare; may have hyperhistaminemia or skin involvement.	Blasts are toluidine blue+ (DDx: mast cells). Negative for MPO, SBB, CAE, and NSE	Usually CD11b+, CD13+, CD33+, CD34+, CD123+, CD9+; lacks strong CD117 (found in mast cells)

(continued)

TABLE 12.7 Characteristics of AML Defined by Differentiation (WHO-HAEM5) *(continued)*

AML Subtypes	Presentation	Morphology and Cytochemistry	Immunophenotype
Acute myelomonocytic leukemia *(FAB: M4)*	Anemia, fever, fatigue; usually leukocytosis	≥20% blasts (including promonocytes); ≥20% monocyte lineage and ≥20% granulocyte lineage; ≥3% of blasts MPO+, usually also has NSE+ subset	Populations of myeloblasts (CD13+, CD33+, CD34+, etc), more mature granulocytes (CD15+, CD11b+, etc), and monocytic cells (CD4+, CD14+, CD64+, etc)
Acute monocytic leukemia *(FAB: M5)*	Most common in adults, often presents with extramedullary disease, bleeding disorders	≥20% blasts (including promonocytes); ≥80% overall monocytic cells; <20% granulocyte lineage; Usually mostly MPO– but NSE+	Blasts/promonocytes usually CD13+, CD33+, HLA-DR+. Promonocytes often CD34– and CD117–. Positive for ≥2 monocytic markers (CD14, CD4, CD11b, CD11c, CD64, CD68, CD36, lysozyme)
Acute erythroid leukemia *(FAB: M6)*	Mostly elderly; anemia; very poor prognosis; most have biallelic *TP53* inactivation	≥80% of entire nucleated population is erythroid and ≥30% are immature erythroblasts. Myeloblasts <20%. May show coarse cytoplasmic PAS staining.	Erythroblasts usually CD36+, CD71+, CD117+; negative for CD34 and MPO. Usually E-cadherin+ in early erythroids and CD235+ in more mature erythroids
Acute megakaryoblastic leukemia *(FAB: M7)*	Cytopenias, sometimes thrombocytosis. Exclude genetically defined AMLs, Down syndrome–associated myeloid neoplasms, and progression of MPN	≥20% blasts with megakaryocytic differentiation; often have cytoplasmic blebs. Marrow usually shows admixed dysplastic maturing megas and variable fibrosis. MPO–	Usually CD36+, CD41+, CD42b+, and/or CD61+. Variably CD33+/–, CD34+/–; CD45, HLA-DR, CD13, CD117 usually negative

ALL, acute lymphoblastic leukemia; AML, acute myeloid leukemia; CAE, chloroacetate esterase; FAB, French-American-British classification; MPAL, mixed-phenotype acute leukemia; MPN, myeloproliferative neoplasm; MPO, myeloperoxidase; NSE, nonspecific esterase; PAS, periodic acid–Schiff; SBB, Sudan Black B; WHO-HAEM5, 5th edition of the World Health Organization

AEL, or pure erythroid leukemia, is a rare subtype of differentiation-defined AML (<1% of all AML) with unique diagnostic and prognostic considerations. It shows erythroid predominance with decreased maturation, defined in WHO-HAEM4R and WHO-HAEM5 as more than 80% erythroid cells in the bone marrow with more than 30% proerythroblasts (and <20% conventional myeloblasts). Erythroid predominance can be highlighted by IHC, including CD71 (pan-erythroid), CD117, E-cadherin (early erythroblasts), and glycophorin-A/CD235 (more mature erythroids). AEL has a very high prevalence of biallelic *TP53* loss-of-function genetic lesions, and AEL diagnosis is supported by genetic, cytogenic, and/or IHC studies targeting *TP53* and the 17p locus.

AEL has a particularly poor prognosis, with a median survival of 2 to 4 months. Of note, AEL is unique among differentiation-defined AML in that it supersedes a diagnosis of AML-MR in WHO-HAEM5. The ICC criteria do not explicitly discuss cell count cutoffs for AEL-subtype AML, and so they maintain the same cutoffs carried over from WHO-HAEM4R; however, the predominance of AEL cases are categorized as AML with mutated *TP53* by ICC criteria.

VI. MYELOID SARCOMA

MS is defined as a "tumor mass involving any anatomic site other than bone marrow (ie, extramedullary) that effaces tissue architecture and is composed of myeloid blasts, with or without maturation" (WHO-HAEM5). Related and previously used terms include extramedullary AML, granulocytic sarcoma, myeloblastoma, and chloroma (chlor—referring to the green coloration sometimes present due to MPO). MS usually occurs alongside, precedes, or follows a diagnosis of "intramedullary" AML, and MS is usually considered diagnostically equivalent to AML for clinical management purposes. The diagnostic criteria for MS specified in WHO-HAEM4R are largely unchanged in the WHO-HAEM5 and ICC (Table 12.8).

TABLE 12.8 Diagnostic Characteristics of MS (WHO-HAEM5)

Essential Diagnostic Criteria (WHO-HAEM5)

- Effacement of tissue architecture (of an extramedullary site) by a mass composed of myeloid blasts, with or without maturing elements
- Positive immunophenotyping for granulocytic and/or monocytic markers

Diagnostic Caveats

- Per WHO-HAEM5, "A complete workup including flow cytometry immunophenotyping, conventional cytogenetics, and molecular analyses is suggested in patients with de novo myeloid sarcoma."
- Detection of MS is equivalent to a diagnosis of AML.
- Blasts in MS are less likely to express CD34 than in conventional AML.
- Involvement of extramedullary tissues by AML blasts without effacement/mass formation should not be diagnosed as MS, but may still be clinically relevant.

AML, acute myeloid leukemia; MS, myeloid sarcoma; WHO-HAEM5, 5th edition of the World Health Organization.

Clinical Features

MS is a rare disease that can occur at any age, with a slightly younger average population than AML (reported median age ranges from 46 to 59 years) and moderate male predominance (52%-59%; *Blood Rev.* 2021;47:100773). MS is reported in approximately 2% to 9% of patients with AML, and is a relatively common manifestation of AML relapse after allo-HSCT, occurring in 5% to 12% of posttransplant patients (*Blood.* 2011;118:3785-3793; *Ann Hematol.* 2023;102: 1973-1984). Occasionally, MS results from the transformation of other myeloid neoplasms (ie, MDS, MPN, MDS/MPN). Isolated de novo MS is uncommon, and usually progresses to overt/intramedullary AML within 4 to 6 months (*Blood Rev.* 2021;47:100773). MS frequently has localized symptoms dependent on the organ(s) involved.

Morphology, Immunophenotype, and Genetics

MS shows a similar range of morphology and immunophenotype to AML cells in the marrow, although with a greater frequency of monocytic or myelomonocytic differentiation. Cytologic preparations demonstrate blasts with or without maturation, while hematoxylin and eosin (H&E) tissue sections are useful for confirming architectural effacement. The morphologic differential can be broad, including lymphomas and various poorly differentiated and small blue cell tumors, but diagnosis can usually be clarified by IHC/FC. Markers expressed in the majority of MS include CD68, CD33, MPO, and CD117; CD34 is positive in only about 30% (*Ann Hematol.* 2023;102:1973-1984). See e-Figures 12.4-1 to 12.4-4 for examples.

Of note, tissue involvement by AML blasts without mass formation or architectural effacement should not be classified as MS, but may still be clinically relevant. Dermatologists sometimes use the nonspecific term "leukemia cutis" for clinically identifiable skin lesions caused by a leukemic infiltration of any type (*Am J Clin Pathol.* 2008;129:130-142), while the WHO Skin Tumours guidelines suggest a descriptive diagnosis for myeloid blast involvement of the skin if criteria for MS are not met (WHO Classification of Tumours online, Skin Tumours 5th Ed.).

MS shares cytogenetic and molecular abnormalities with intramedullary AML. A comprehensive evaluation that includes cytogenetic analysis and molecular assessment is needed for classification, prognostication, and planning therapy. Cytogenetic abnormalities with reported enrichment in MS include *RUNX1::RUNX1T1*/t(8;21), which is associated with orbital involvement in children, and *CBFB-MYH11*/inv(16), which is associated with abdominal MS (*Blood Rev.* 2021;47:100773).

Prognosis and Treatment

AML patients with MS at diagnosis have a worse prognosis compared to those without MS (*Cancer Sci.* 2012;103:1513-1517), while isolated MS at presentation has a higher survival rate than non-MS AML (*Leuk & lymphoma.* 2015;56:1698-1703). Localized radiation can be palliative but is not usually curative, even in isolated MS cases. Systemic chemotherapy mirroring AML regimens is the mainstay of treatment for MS whether isolated or concurrent with AML, although little data are available regarding efficacy of newer AML therapeutics in MS (*Ann Hematol.* 2023;102:1973-1984).

SUGGESTED READINGS

1. Arber DA, Erba HP. Diagnosis and treatment of patients with acute myeloid leukemia with myelodysplasia-related changes (AML-MRC). *Am J Clin Pathol.* 2020;154(6):731-741.
2. Arber DA, Orazi A, Hasserjian RP, et al. International Consensus Classification of myeloid neoplasms and acute leukemias: integrating morphologic, clinical, and genomic data. *Blood.* 2022;140(11):1200-1228.
3. Döhner H, Wei AH, Appelbaum FR, et al. Diagnosis and management of AML in adults: 2022 recommendations from an international expert panel on behalf of the ELN. *Blood.* 2022;140(12):1345-1377.
4. Huber S, Baer C, Hutter S, et al. AML classification in the year 2023: how to avoid a Babylonian confusion of languages. *Leukemia.* 2023;37(7):1413-1420. doi:10.1038/s41375-023-01909-w
5. Loscocco GG, Vannucchi AM. Myeloid sarcoma: more and less than a distinct entity. *Ann Hematol.* 2023;102(8):1973-1984. doi:10.1007/s00277-023-05288-1
6. Shimony S, Stahl M, Stone RM. Acute myeloid leukemia: 2023 update on diagnosis, risk-stratification, and management. *Am J Hematol.* 2023;98(3):502-526. doi:10.1002/ajh.26822
7. Short NJ, Rytting ME, Cortes JE. Acute myeloid leukaemia. *Lancet.* 2018;392(10147):593-606.
8. Solary E, Gujral S, et al. Acute myeloid leukaemia. In: *WHO Classification of Tumours Editorial Board. Haematolymphoid Tumours* [Internet; beta version ahead of print]. International Agency for Research on Cancer; 2022.
9. Swerdlow SH, Campo E, Harris NL, et al. WHO revised 4th edition (2017), acute myeloid leukaemia. In: *WHO Classification of Tumours of Haematopoietic and Lymphoid Tissues: WHO Classification of Tumours.* Revised 4th ed. Vol 2. International Agency for Research on Cancer; 2017.
10. Wilson CS, Medeiros LJ. Extramedullary manifestations of myeloid neoplasms. *Am J Clin Pathol.* 2015;144(2):219-239.

13 Secondary Myeloid Neoplasms

Michael C. Horwath and Alexandra E. Kovach

I. CLASSIFICATION OF SECONDARY MYELOID NEOPLASMS (WHO-HAEM5 AND ICC)

Secondary myeloid neoplasms are a diverse group of diseases defined not only by morphologic, genetic, and clinical characteristics of the neoplasm itself but also by the preceding context in which the neoplasm arises. Both the WHO-HAEM5 (*Leukemia*. 2022;36:1703-1719) and ICC-2022 (*Blood*. 2022;140:1200-1228) classification systems provide criteria and recommendations for the diagnosis of myeloid neoplasms post-cytotoxic therapy (MN-pCT) as well as those arising in individuals with specific germline predispositions (MN-GP [myeloid neoplasms associated with germline predisposition]). While these classification systems diverge somewhat in their approach and nomenclature, similar information should be captured in the final report regardless of classification system(s) used.

In WHO-HAEM5, as in the WHO-HAEM4R, prior cytotoxic therapy for an unrelated disorder can qualify a myeloid neoplasm otherwise meeting criteria for acute myeloid leukemia (AML), myelodysplastic syndrome (MDS), or MDS/myeloproliferative neoplasm (MPN) for a diagnosis of MN-pCT. This separation of MN-pCTs as a distinct category was based on studies showing that classic microscopic findings used in MDS and AML classification (morphology and blast count) have relatively little impact on the prognosis of MN-pCTs, which is generally poor (*Am J Clin Pathol*. 2007;127:197-205). However, in the last decade, there has been increasing evidence that subclassifying MN-pCTs utilizing genetic/cytogenetic information does provide meaningful prognostic and therapeutic information (*Leukemia*. 2021;35:835-849; *Br J Haematol*. 2022;197:736-744). Therefore, WHO-HAEM5 emphasized that MN-pCTs should be additionally subclassified according to the relevant criteria for specific *de novo* myeloid disease where possible. An example is "AML with *KMT2A* rearrangement post-cytotoxic therapy."

Similarly, in MN-GP diagnoses, both the underlying germline syndrome/disorder as well as the identity of the specific myeloid neoplasm carry prognostic and therapeutic significance. WHO-HAEM5 again recommends a composite diagnosis utilizing the predisposing factor as a descriptor, for example, "MDS with low blasts associated with germline *RUNX1* variant."

In the International Consensus Classification (ICC) system, "therapy-related" and "germline predisposition-related" neoplasms are not considered diagnoses in themselves but are instead conceptualized as diagnostic qualifiers that should be appended to the neoplastic diagnosis. In practice, this should result in similar information included in the diagnostic line as in WHO-HAEM5. Examples using ICC nomenclature include "AML with myelodysplasia-related cytogenetic abnormality, therapy-related" and "AML with myelodysplasia-related gene mutation, germline RUNX1 mutation." Of note, when appropriate, these ICC diagnostic qualifiers can also be applied to precursor myeloid lesions (such as CCUS [clonal cytopenia of uncertain significance]) and to nonmyeloid neoplasms (such as acute lymphoblastic leukemia [ALL]). This contrasts somewhat with WHO-HAEM5, in which the diagnosis of MN-pCT is reserved for myeloid neoplasms meeting criteria for AML, MDS, or MDS/MPN, and the diagnosis of MN-GP is generally applied only to non-precursor myeloid lesions (usually meeting criteria for AML, MDS, MDS/MPN, or MPN).

Whether using ICC or WHO criteria, in the case of germline predisposition, special care must be taken to distinguish true progression to malignancy from background or premalignant changes associated with the underlying genetic lesion and to apply any special diagnostic criteria specific to that syndrome. The most well-established special diagnostic criteria are those for myeloid proliferations associated with trisomy 21 (Down syndrome [DS]), which have unique clinicopathologic characteristics and are classified as transient abnormal myelopoiesis (TAM) or myeloid leukemia of Down syndrome (ML-DS).

In some instances, MN-pCT and MN-GP diagnoses can overlap. Some germline mutations carry increased risk for both myeloid and nonmyeloid neoplasms, and cytotoxic treatment for a nonmyeloid malignancy can multiply the risk for later developing myeloid malignancy. This pattern is seen in Li-Fraumeni syndrome (germline *TP53* mutation) and *BRCA1/BRCA2*-related syndromes. Even in patients without overt genetic syndromes, germline variants likely influence the risk for developing MN-pCT due to varying sensitivity to chemotherapy toxicity as well as varying incidence of underlying clonal hematopoiesis, which may progress to MN-pCT under selective pressure of cytotoxic therapy (*Nat Rev Cancer*. 2017;17:513-527; *Cancers (Basel)*. 2023;15:1483). The currently published versions of WHO-HAEM5 and ICC criteria do not provide specific guidance on diagnostic terminology when germline-related and therapy-related etiologies overlap. However, it seems reasonable to include both the prior therapy and the germline predisposition in the diagnostic line if criteria for both are met.

Finally, myeloid malignancies can also be considered "secondary" if they progress from an underlying lower-grade myeloid neoplasm, such as AML progressing from MPN (blast-phase MPN), from MDS, or from MDS/MPN. These forms of "secondary" myeloid neoplasms are described under Chapters 9 and 12.

II. MYELOID NEOPLASMS POST-CYTOTOXIC THERAPY

Introduction

MN-pCT encompass a continuum of malignancies including acute myeloid leukemias (AML-pCT), myelodysplastic neoplasms (MDS-pCT), and myelodysplastic/myeloproliferative neoplasms (MDS/MPN-pCT), occurring in patients with prior DNA-damaging therapy for an unrelated disorder. The WHO diagnostic criteria are summarized in Table 13.1.

The most common prior disorders requiring cytotoxic therapy are solid tumors (breast cancer the single most common), followed by prior hematolymphoid malignancies (such as Hodgkin lymphoma or multiple myeloma). A small proportion of cases involve cytotoxic therapy administered for autoimmune disease or as pre-hematopoietic stem cell transplantation (pre-HSCT) conditioning for nonmalignant indications, such as sickle cell disease. Cytotoxic therapy is thought to induce MN-pCT by causing new genetic lesions and by selective pressure resulting in expansion of preexisting clonal hematopoiesis, and these two mechanisms likely

TABLE 13.1 — WHO-HAEM5 Diagnostic Criteria for Myeloid Neoplasms Post-cytotoxic Therapy

Essential

- Myeloid neoplasm[a] meeting diagnostic criteria of any myelodysplastic neoplasm, myelodysplastic/myeloproliferative neoplasm, or acute myeloid leukemia
- History of prior exposure to cytotoxic therapy and/or large-field radiation therapy for an unrelated disorder (see below)
- Not meeting diagnostic criteria for a myeloproliferative neoplasm

Desirable

- Detection of clonal molecular and/or chromosomal alterations

Cytotoxic agents

- **Alkylating agents**
  - Melphalan, cyclophosphamide, nitrogen mustard, chlorambucil, busulfan, carboplatin, cisplatin, dacarbazine, procarbazine, carmustine, mitomycin C, thiotepa, lomustine
- **Ionizing radiation therapy**[b]
  - Large fields containing active bone marrow
- **Topoisomerase II inhibitors**[c]
  - Etoposide, teniposide, doxorubicin, daunorubicin, mitoxantrone, amsacrine, actinomycin
- **Others**
  - Antimetabolites: thiopurines, mycophenolate mofetil, fludarabine
  - Antitubulin agents (usually in combination with other agents): vincristine, vinblastine, vindesine, paclitaxel, docetaxel
  - poly(ADP-ribose) polymerase 1 (PARP1 inhibitors)

[a]Precursor myeloid neoplasms such as clonal cytopenia of uncertain significance (CCUS) are excluded from myeloid neoplasms post-cytotoxic therapy (MN-pCT) in WHO-HAEM5, although by ICC 2022 criteria they can receive the "post-cytotoxic therapy" qualifier.
[b]Per WHO-HAEM5, the incidence of MN-PCT due to the genetic effects of modern limited-field radiation therapy needs further study.
[c]May also be associated with therapy-related lymphoblastic leukemia (ALL).
Based on the WHO Classification of Tumours Editorial Board. Haematolymphoid tumours [Internet]. Lyon (France): International Agency for Research on Cancer; 2024 (WHO classification of tumours series, 5th ed.; vol. 11). Available from: https://tumourclassification.iarc.who.int/chapters/63.

have greater importance in the etiology of pediatric and adult MN-pCT, respectively (*Blood*. 2022;140:1345-1377).

An estimated 10% to 20% of all AML, MDS, and MDS/MPN are cytotoxic therapy-related (*Leukemia*. 2017;31:1391). Estimates of absolute and relative risk for MN-pCT following cytotoxic therapy vary based on the study, the specific neoplasms, and specific therapies involved; however, one seminal study of over 400,000 patients treated with chemotherapy found a 4.7-fold increased risk of developing AML (*Blood*.

2013;121:2996-3004). The cytotoxic therapies generally accepted to cause MN-pCT are broad-field radiation involving bone marrow, alkylating agents, topoisomerase II inhibitors, and other DNA-damaging agents including antitubulins and some antimetabolites. Therapies for which myeloid neoplasm risk is low or less well-established, including modern limited-field radiation and immune modulators such as methotrexate and thalidomide, do not generally qualify for a diagnosis of MN-pCT per WHO-HAEM5.

Excluded from diagnosis of MN-pCT per WHO-HAEM5 are precursor myeloid neoplasms (CHIP [clonal hematopoiesis of indeterminate potential], CCUS), MPN, and nonmyeloid neoplasms (such as ALL). In contrast, by ICC criteria all of these diagnoses may be given the "post-cytotoxic therapy" qualifier. Under either system, the final diagnosis should include the specific neoplastic subcategory and statement of the post-therapy etiology. Of note, cases of a myeloid neoplasm treated with cytotoxic therapy which then recur or progress to higher-grade malignancy are excluded from MN-pCT under both WHO and ICC.

Clinical Features

The presentation of MN-pCT varies, with clinical signs and symptoms similar to the corresponding de novo myeloid neoplasms. The most common initial presentation is an MDS-like picture including persistent cytopenias and symptoms such as fatigue, bleeding/bruising, and infection susceptibility. MDS-pCT and AML-pCT form a clinical and biologic continuum, with MDS-pCT frequently progressing to AML-pCT, and AML-pCT frequently showing MDS-related features. A smaller number of cases initially present as MDS/MPN or as AML. The clinical picture for MN-pCT patients can also be complicated by comorbidities associated with the prior diagnosis.

The latency period from prior therapy to diagnosis of MN-pCT varies but is often at least 5 to 7 years following alkylating agents (*Haematologica*. 2009;94:454-459; *J Clin Oncol*. 2015;33:3641-3649). For most therapy modalities, early occurrence of MN pCT with less than 1 year latency is very uncommon, and findings such as cytopenias or abnormal marrow morphology are more likely to be treatment-related. Myeloid neoplasms occurring very late (>10 years) after cytotoxic therapy are also uncommon and may have a sporadic rather than therapy-related etiology. However, no absolute cutoffs for latency period are included in the diagnostic criteria for MN-pCT.

Of note, the usual clinical picture varies somewhat by treatment modality. In particular, topoisomerase II inhibitors are associated with shorter latency to MN-pCT, higher likelihood of AML (or sometimes ALL) rather than MDS at presentation, and better prognosis of the MN-pCT compared to other cytotoxic therapies (*Int J Environ Res Public Health*. 2012;9:2075-2091).

Morphology and Immunophenotype

MN-pCTs usually exhibit multilineage dysplasia but lack specific morphologic or immunophenotypic features to distinguish them from their de novo AML, MDS, and MDS/MPN counterparts. Blasts frequently express aberrant lymphoid markers (*Ann Hematol*. 2018;97:2319-2324), and cases of acute leukemia with mixed or undifferentiated phenotype also occur. Per WHO-HAEM5, cases with ambiguous lineage can still be classified as MN-pCT, as the MN-pCT diagnosis "takes precedence" over the diagnosis of acute biphenotypic or acute undifferentiated leukemia *TP53* mutation is more common than in de novo disease and can be assessed by immunohistochemical staining (*Mod Pathol*. 2015;28:552-563). See e-Figures 13.1-1 to 13.1-4 for an example of AML-pCT.

Genetic Features

MN-pCT can show a broad range of genetic abnormalities, similar to those found in de novo MNs but with increased proportions of high-risk genetic lesions (*Nat Rev Cancer.* 2017;17:513-527). The majority of MN-pCT harbor chromosomal abnormalities, with increased frequency of complex karyotypes and unbalanced abnormalities including frequent deletions in chromosomes 5 and 7 (*Blood.* 2021;138:749-757; *Leukemia.* 2021;35:835-849). Mutation of *TP53* and/or deletion of 17p and mutations specific for myelodysplasia-related AML are also increased relative to de novo myeloid neoplasms (*Blood.* 2015;125:1367-1376; *Semin Diagn Pathol.* 2023;40:182-186). To some extent, the specific prior cytotoxic therapy influences the genetic profile. In particular, topoisomerase II inhibitors are associated with frequently balanced translocations, often involving *KMT2A* or *RUNX1*, but have lower incidence of unbalanced translocations or complex karyotypes (*Nat Rev Cancer.* 2017;17:513-527). Finally, some cases of MN-pCT arise in the context of germline genetic variants, which may predispose to nonmyeloid neoplasms requiring cytotoxic therapy and increase the risk for developing MN-pCT following treatment.

Prognosis and Treatment

MN-pCT is associated with poor prognosis compared to de novo disease, with most studies showing 5-year survival less than 10%. Prognosis varies somewhat by prior therapy modality (topo-II inhibitors are associated with a better prognosis). Blast count and morphologic classification into AML, MDS, or MDS/MPN have little impact on the prognosis of MN-pCTs (*Am J Clin Pathol.* 2007;127:197). However, cytogenetic and molecular findings as well as clinical characteristics of the patient do impact prognosis and treatment options (*Leukemia.* 2021;35:835-849; *Br J Haematol.* 2022;197:736). Many cases of MDS-pCT present in the high-risk category by risk stratification schemes such as IPSS-R (Revised International Prognostic Scoring System), but cases with lower IPSS-R stratification still carry worse prognosis than their de novo counterparts (*Leukemia.* 2017;31:1391).

Like other high-risk myeloid neoplasms, MN-pCT treatment is guided by specific biology of the disease, medical fitness for intensive chemotherapy, and goals of care, and may include allogeneic HSCT in select patients. Refractory or relapsed MN-pCT carries an especially poor prognosis.

Key Points

- Myeloid neoplasms post-cytotoxic therapy (MN-pCT) are myeloid neoplasms arising in patients with history of cytotoxic therapy for an unrelated disorder.
- Qualifying cytotoxic therapies include large-field ionizing radiation, alkylating agents, and other agents that induce DNA damage (topoisomerase II inhibitors, some antimetabolites, antitubulins, and PARP1 inhibitors).
- MN-pCT generally have poor prognosis, even in cases with low blast count, but the cytogenetic/genetic profile does carry prognostic and therapeutic significance.
- Topoisomerase II inhibitor-related MN-pCT is associated with shorter latency from treatment, higher incidence of acute myeloid leukemia (AML) rather than myelodysplastic syndrome (MDS), and better prognosis.
- Diagnostic description should combine the "post-cytotoxic therapy" descriptor with the specific myeloid malignancy present.

Diagnostic Caveats

- Under WHO-HAEM5 criteria, MN-pCT includes malignant diagnoses otherwise meeting criteria for AML, MDS, or MDS/myeloproliferative neoplasm (MPN) but **not** MPN, lymphoid malignancies, or precursor neoplasms such as CCUS (clonal cytopenia of uncertain significance).
- Under ICC 2022 criteria, the "post-cytotoxic therapy" qualifier can be applied more broadly, including acute lymphoblastic leukemia or precursors myeloid neoplasms when appropriate.
- Therapies for which myeloid neoplasm risk is lower or insufficiently studied, including limited-field radiation and immune modulators, do not generally qualify for a diagnosis of MN-pCT.

III. MYELOID NEOPLASMS ASSOCIATED WITH GERMLINE PREDISPOSITION

Introduction

An estimated 5% to 15% of myeloid malignancies occur in the context of an underlying germline genetic lesion associated with MN risk (*Hemasphere.* 2019;3:e321; *Br J Haematol.* 2022;196:1293-1310) and can be classified as myeloid neoplasms associated with germline predisposition (MN-GP). Many MN-GPs arise in syndromic disorders associated with underlying hematopoietic abnormalities, developmental abnormalities, and risk for nonmyeloid neoplasms, although some germline predispositions (such as *DDX41*-related) carry MN risk without other overt syndromic features. MN-GPs are heterogeneous, and some may present at any age (although unusually early presentation may prompt suspicion for germline workup). Many MN-GPs present as MDS or AML, but some of the most common syndromes are associated with other myeloid neoplasms (JMML [juvenile myelomonocytic leukemia] in RASopathies, TAM of DS, and ML-DS). Major groups of germline disorders associated with MN-GP are described later and in Table 13.2. As described in the introduction, both WHO-HAEM5 and ICC advocate combining the specific myeloid neoplasm and the germline predisposition in the diagnostic line. The WHO diagnostic criteria are summarized in Table 13.3.

Clinical Features

Germline predispositions to myeloid neoplasms without preexisting platelet disorder or organ dysfunction: Some germline disorders are associated with increased risk for myeloid malignancies (and potentially other neoplasms), without overt preneoplastic effects on hematopoiesis or other baseline constitutional manifestations. Germline *CEBPA* pathogenic variants are associated with high incidence of AML (nearly 100% penetrance in 5′ mutations), with risk for recurrence in the form of independent primary clones (*Blood.* 2015;126:1214-1223; *Semin Hematol.* 2017;54:87-93). Germline *DDX41* variants are associated with MDS and AML (and less frequently lymphoid neoplasms), generally presenting in adulthood with higher penetrance in male mutation carriers (*Cancers (Basel).* 2023;15:344; *Blood.* 2023;141:534-549). Li-Fraumeni syndrome, caused by *TP53* mutations, is associated with high incidence of solid tumors as well as increased risk for myeloid and lymphoid malignancies; there is also increased risk for secondary neoplasms after radio/cytotoxic therapy (*Cold Spring Harb Mol Case Stud.* 2019;5:a003210). Each of these disorders shows autosomal dominant

TABLE 13.2 Cancer Predisposing Syndromes Associated With Myeloid Neoplasms

Germline Predispositions to Myeloid Neoplasms	Genetic Disorder/Syndrome P/LP = Pathogenic/Likely Pathogenic	Gene(s) and Inheritance	Hematopoietic Neoplasms	Effects on Underlying Hematopoiesis and Other Systemic Manifestations
Without preexisting platelet disorder or organ dysfunction	*CEBPA* P/LP variant associated	*CEBPA* Inheritance: **AD**	AML with bi*CEBPA*, MDS, MDS/MPN. Wide age range	NA/unknown
	DDX41 P/LP variant associated	*DDX41* **AD**	AML, MDS, lymphoid Adult > childhood	Likely increased risk for nonheme malignancies
	Li-Fraumeni syndrome	*TP53* **AD**	ALL, AML, MDS, others. Wide age range	High risk for wide range of malignancies
With preexisting platelet disorders	*RUNX1* P/LP variant associated	*RUNX1* **AD**	AML, MDS, ALL. Wide age range	Thrombocytopenia and platelet dysfunction. May have eczema or psoriasis
	ANKRD26 P/LP variant associated	*ANKRD26* **AD**	MDS, AML, others. Adult > childhood	Variable thrombocytopenia and platelet dysfunction
	ETV6 P/LP variant associated	*ETV6* **AD**	ALL > AML, others. Wide age range	Thrombocytopenia

With potential organ dysfunction	**Bone marrow failure and related syndromes**	Severe congenital neutropenia	Multiple; most common *ELANE* **AD** or **AR**	AML, MDS. Often young adulthood (varies with genetics)	Neutropenia, severe opportunistic infections
		Fanconi anemia	*FANC (A-W)* genes Usually **AR**	MDS, AML. Childhood > adult	BMF/AA, congenital malformations, solid tumor risk
		Shwachman-Diamond syndrome	Multiple; most common *SBDS* Usually **AR**	MDS, AML, ALL. Childhood > adult	Neutropenia, other cytopenias, pancreatic insufficiency, skeletal dysplasia
		Telomere biology disorders	Multiple; variable inheritance	MDS, AML. Wide age range	BMF/AA, nail and skin abnormalities, hepatic and pulmonary fibrosis, SqCC
	RASopathies	Noonan syndrome	*PTPN11, NRAS, KRAS* **AD**	JMML, JMML-like MPN. Usually infancy	Developmental disorder with variable expression, including coag defects, solid tumor risk
		CBL syndrome	*CBL* **AD**	JMML, JMML-like MPN. Usually early childhood	Noonan-like development disorder with variable expression, often vasculopathy
		Neurofibromatosis 1	*NF1* **AD**	JMML, AML, ALL. Childhood > adult	Neurocutaneous manifestations including neurofibromas, nervous system tumors

(*continued*)

TABLE 13.2 Cancer Predisposing Syndromes Associated With Myeloid Neoplasms (continued)

Germline Predispositions to Myeloid Neoplasms	Genetic Disorder/Syndrome P/LP = Pathogenic/Likely Pathogenic	Gene(s) and Inheritance	Hematopoietic Neoplasms	Effects on Underlying Hematopoiesis and Other Systemic Manifestations
Others	GATA2 deficiency syndrome	*GATA2* **AD**	AML, MDS, CMML. Often adolescent/young adult	Variable manifestations including mono/B/T/NK deficiency, lymphedema, deafness, and others
	Down syndrome	Trisomy 21	TAM (infancy), ML-DS (early childhood), ALL (later)	Developmental disorder with variable intellectual disability and other manifestations
	Bloom syndrome	*BLM* **AR**	AML, MDS, ALL, lymphomas. Often young adulthood	Immunodeficiency, short stature, photosensitivity, T2DM, COPD, skin cancer risk
	SAMD9 P/LP variant associated	*SAMD9* **AD**	MDS/AML with monosomy 7/del(7q). Childhood > adult	Variable manifestations include: BMF, MIRAGE syndrome, adrenal insufficiency
	SAMD9L P/LP variant associated	*SAMD9L* **AD**		Variable manifestations include: BMF, ataxia-pancytopenia syndrome

AA, aplastic anemia; ALL, acute lymphoblastic leukemia; AML, acute myeloid leukemia; BMF, bone marrow failure; CMML, chronic myelomonocytic leukemia; COPD, chronic obstructive pulmonary disease; JMML, juvenile myelomonocytic leukemia; MDS, myelodysplastic syndrome; MIRAGE, myelodysplasia, infections, restriction of growth, adrenal hypoplasia, genital problems, and enteropathy; ML-DS, myeloid leukemia of Down syndrome; MPN, myeloproliferative neoplasm; NK, natural killer; SqCC, squamous cell carcinoma; TAM, transient abnormal myelopoiesis; T2DM, type 2 diabetes mellitus.

Based on the WHO Classification of Tumours Editorial Board. Haematolymphoid tumours [Internet]. Lyon (France): International Agency for Research on Cancer; 2024 (WHO classification of tumours series, 5th ed.; vol. 11). Available from: https://tumourclassification.iarc.who.int/chapters/63. and *Blood*. 2022;140:1345.

TABLE 13.3 WHO-HAEM5 Diagnostic Criteria for Myeloid Neoplasms With Germline Predisposition

Note: Per WHO-HAEM5, "The diagnostic criteria for the various specific myeloid neoplasms that are diagnosed in the setting of a germline predisposition take precedence over the broad essential and desirable criteria listed below."

Essential
- Detection of germline mutation with increased risk of myeloid malignancies
- Myeloid neoplasm meeting the diagnostic criteria of a specific disease type

Desirable
- Clonal molecular and cytogenetic abnormalities in addition to the germline mutation
- Positive family history as determined by formal genetic counseling

Based on the WHO Classification of Tumours Editorial Board. Haematolymphoid tumours [Internet]. Lyon (France): International Agency for Research on Cancer; 2024 (WHO classification of tumours series, 5th ed.; vol. 11). Available from: https://tumourclassification.iarc.who.int/chapters/63.

inheritance, with development of malignancy frequently associated with additional somatic mutation or loss-of-heterozygosity affecting the second allele.

Germline predispositions to myeloid neoplasms with preexisting platelet disorders: This group comprises several autosomal dominant disorders characterized by lifelong thrombocytopenia along with variable degrees of platelet dysfunction, dysmegakaryopoiesis, and myeloid malignancy risk. Three genes associated with these syndromes are noted in WHO-HAEM5 and ICC-2022: *ANKRD24*, which is associated with myeloid malignancies (MDS, AML); *RUNX1*, which is associated with myeloid and less commonly lymphoid malignancies as well as eczema/psoriasis; and *ETV6*, which is associated with B-ALL and less commonly myeloid malignancies (*Int J Lab Hematol.* 2019;41(suppl 1):131-141; *Blood.* 2023;141:1533-1543). In general, underlying thrombocytopenia and bleeding tendency are mild to moderate; solid tumor risk can also be increased.

Inherited bone marrow failure syndromes (IBMFS): WHO-HAEM5 makes note of three disorders under the general category of IBMFS: severe congenital neutropenia (SCN), Shwachman-Diamond syndrome (SDS), and Fanconi anemia (FA). Other hereditary syndromes associated with bone marrow failure (BMF) and myeloid malignancies include Diamond-Blackfan anemia (rare, primarily affects erythroid lineage) and telomere maintenance disorders (described later). Each of these syndromes can be caused by mutations in multiple different genes, with varying inheritance patterns, penetrance, and clinical features.

SCN is defined by neutropenia, usually without other cytopenias or congenital abnormalities, and is associated with recurrent/severe bacterial infections and risk of progression to MN-GP (MDS or AML) (*Nat Rev Dis Primers.* 2017;3:17032). Most cases of SCN respond to granulocyte colony-stimulating factor (G-CSF) therapy; however, long-term, high-dose G-CSF administration is associated with increased risk of MN-GP (*Br J Haematol.* 2010;150:196-199). The most commonly mutated gene in SCN is *ELANE* (neutrophil elastase, autosomal dominant inheritance). Cyclic neutropenia is a related but less severe congenital disorder with lower risk of MN-GP.

SDS is a rare disorder caused by mutations in genes affecting ribosomal function, most commonly *SBDS* (autosomal recessive inheritance). Patients have neutropenia with variable degrees of other cytopenias, exocrine pancreatic insufficiency, and skeletal abnormalities. SDS carries increased risk for myeloid malignancies (MDS more than for AML), often presenting in childhood or adolescence, with relatively poor prognosis (*Lancet Haematol.* 2020;7:e238).

FA is caused by mutations in a number of genes belonging to the FA/BRCA DNA-repair pathway, with mostly autosomal recessive inheritance (including the most commonly affected gene, *FANCA*) (*Nat Rev Cancer.* 2018;18:168-185). FA is characterized by progressive BMF and cytopenia, with 90% developing aplastic anemia by age 40. Congenital abnormalities are present in most patients and can include short stature, absent radii, abnormal thumbs, and endocrine dysfunction. FA carries increased risk for MDS, AML, and solid tumors; a study of 421 children with FA showed 11% developed cancer by age 18 (*J Clin Oncol.* 2022;40:32). Chromosome breakage analysis as well as mutational testing are frequently indicated in the diagnostic workup.

Of note, diagnosis of MDS in the context of IBMFS requires stricter criteria than in the de novo setting, due to frequent cytopenias, dysplasia, and even clonal hematopoiesis without malignant transformation. Detection of increased blasts or somatic genetic lesions that are unambiguously associated with malignant transformation is helpful to diagnosis of MDS in this setting. A recently proposed classification scheme for myeloid disorders in FA is included in WHO-HAEM5 and may serve as a template for other IBMFS-related neoplasms (*Haematologica.* 2021;106:3000).

Telomere maintenance disorders: Dyskeratosis congenita (DC) and related short telomere syndromes are caused by germline mutations in multiple genes resulting in defective maintenance of telomere length (*Genet Med.* 2010;12:753-764; *Best Pract Res Clin Haematol.* 2021;34:101282). Many patients eventually develop BMF, and there is increased risk for myeloid neoplasms (especially MDS). Other manifestations vary and can include the DC "mucocutaneous triad" of reticular skin hyperpigmentation, nail dystrophy, and oral leukoplakia; pulmonary and liver fibrosis; or squamous cell carcinomas of the head and neck. The inheritance pattern depends on the specific gene involved, and telomere length analysis as well as molecular testing is frequently utilized in the diagnostic workup.

RASopathies: Germline mutations causing overactivation of the *RAS* signaling pathway are associated with several syndromes that carry myeloid neoplasm risk; these include Noonan syndrome (associated with mutations in *PTPN11, NRAS, KRAS,* and other genes), CBL syndrome (*CBL*), neurofibromatosis-1 (*NF1*), and other Noonan-like and related syndromes (*Pract Res Clin Haematol.* 2020;33:101171; *Biomed J.* 2021;44:422-432). All are characterized by childhood risk for JMML, with varying risks for other hematolymphoid neoplasms, solid tumors, and developmental abnormalities. RASopathies generally have autosomal dominant inheritance with varying expressivity. The propensity for de novo germline mutations results in a high proportion of sporadic RASopathy cases without prior family history.

GATA2 deficiency: *GATA2* encodes a transcription factor involved in hematopoietic stem cell development and maintenance, and loss-of-function mutations result in an autosomal dominant syndrome with variable phenotype (*Hum Mutat.* 2021;42:1399). Effects on the hematolymphoid system generally develop over time and include leukocyte deficiencies (especially of monocytes, dendritic cells, and lymphocyte subsets), recurrent infections (commonly mycobacterial, viral, or fungal), autoimmune disease, and (less commonly) aplastic anemia. Effects on other body systems can include lymphedema, pulmonary alveolar proteinosis, and sensorineural hearing loss. The majority of people with *GATA2* insufficiency will eventually develop MDS; there is also increased risk for AML, chronic myelomonocytic leukemia (CMML), and rarely B-ALL (*Blood*. 2023;141:1524-1532).

Down syndrome: Trisomy 21, the usual cause of DS, is the most common congenital chromosomal abnormality. There are two DS-specific myeloid disorders: transient abnormal myelopoiesis (TAM) of DS and myeloid leukemia of Down Syndrome (ML-DS), both of which are characterized by somatic *GATA1* mutation and usually have a megakaryoblastic phenotype. DS also carries an increased risk of ALL (usually later in life). TAM and ML-DS have unique clinical and diagnostic considerations and are described in a separate section.

Bloom syndrome: Bloom syndrome, also called congenital telangiectatic erythema, is a very rare disorder caused by germline mutation in *BLM* (autosomal recessive). *BLM* encodes a DNA-helicase-family protein, and deficiency results in a high rate of somatic homologous recombination between sister chromatids and resulting cytogenetic abnormalities (*Mol Genet Metab*. 2021;133:35-48). Bloom syndrome shows variable effects across multiple body systems, including photosensitivity (associated with telangiectatic facial rash), immune deficiency, short stature, characteristic facies, and increased risk for type 2 diabetes and chronic obstructive pulmonary disease (*Mol Syndromol*. 2017;8:4-23). There is increased risk for myeloid malignancies, lymphoid malignancies, and solid tumors.

SAMD9 and SAMD9L related syndromes: SAMD9 and SAMD9L are two related genes on chromosome 7q, in which specific heterozygous germline mutations result in increased risk for BMF, childhood MDS and AML, and varying systemic manifestations (*Leukemia*. 2018;32:1106). *SAMD9* mutation causes MIRAGE syndrome (myelodysplasia, infection, restriction of growth, adrenal hypoplasia, genital phenotypes, and enteropathy), while *SAMD9L* causes ataxia-pancytopenia syndrome (with variable cerebellar atrophy). Somewhat paradoxically, *SAMD9/SAMD9L* functions as tumor suppressors, but germline mutations resulting in increased myeloid neoplasm risk are gain of function. Leukemogenic potential seems to be the result of selective pressure in hematopoietic cells to delete the mutated allele, resulting in somatic monosomy 7/del(7q) with characteristic retention of the wild-type allele (see e-Figures 13.2-1 to 13.2-5). Interestingly, monosomy 7 in this context is not MDS defining, as it can be seen in isolation in *SAMD9/SAMD9L*-associated disease in the absence of (prior too) the acquisition of additional secondary somatic mutations. In addition, monosomy 7 has been reported to revert in some cases to date (*Best Pract Res Clin Haematol*. 2020;33:101197).

Additional and emerging cancer predisposition syndromes: Multiple genetic syndromes classically associated with solid tumors also confer risk for MN-GP. Many of these syndromes involve disruption of DNA repair, including hereditary breast and ovarian cancer syndrome (*BRCA1/BRCA2*-related), Lynch syndrome (*MLH1/MSH2/MSH6/PMS2*-related), *CHEK2*-related syndrome, and some forms of xeroderma pigmentosum (*XPC*-related) (Leuk Res. 2018;70:74-78; *Cancer*. 2016;122(2):304-311; *Front Pediatr*. 2020;8:570084; *Haematologica*. 2020;105:e144-e146). In addition, several syndromes classically associated with nonneoplastic effects on the hematolymphoid system also carry some increased risk for myeloid malignancies; these include *MPL*-related thrombocytopenia/thrombocytosis syndromes, and Wiskott-Aldrich syndrome.

The WHO and ICC diagnostic frameworks for MN-GP are designed to be expandable, and descriptions of additional germline variants associated with myeloid malignancies continue to emerge. WHO-HAEM5 notes reports of myeloid neoplasm association with pathogenic/likely pathogenic variants in *CSF3R, ERCC6L2, JAK2, MBD4, MECOM/EVI1, NPM1, RBBP6, SRP72, TET2,* and *GATA1*.

Morphology and Immunophenotype

Morphology and immunophenotype of MN-GP are heterogeneous and reflect the specific myeloid malignancy present. Some germline predisposition syndromes are associated with cytomorphologic abnormalities in the blood or marrow at baseline or before true malignant transformation, potentially complicating diagnosis of MN. Syndromes associated with thrombocytopenia frequently exhibit dysmegakaryopoiesis, and IBMFS frequently exhibit dysplastic changes in one or more lineages and may show hypocellular marrow (aplastic anemia picture). Cases of hypoplastic MDS have increased likelihood of underlying germline predisposition and should raise the differential of MN-GP (*Blood*. 2023;142:643-657).

Genetic Features

Germline mutations associated with specific syndromes are discussed earlier. When a germline predisposition is suspected, genetic testing as well as formal genetic counseling is often indicated. Testing for genetic syndromes may involve targeted molecular panels, next-generation sequencing, or testing modalities specific to a particular syndrome (ie, chromosomal breakage test for FA). Testing for germline mutations on blood, marrow, or other tissue containing hematolymphoid cells carries risk of either a false-positive result (due to somatic mutation) or a false-negative result (due to somatic reversion of a germline mutation). Therefore, testing on a source such as cultured skin fibroblasts may be indicated. In general, the germline variant must be classified as pathogenic or likely pathogenic ("P/LP") to diagnose MN-GP; criteria for P/LP are provided by the American College of Medical Genetics (*Genet Med*. 2015;17:405). Cases with germline mosaicism or variants of uncertain significance can be especially challenging to diagnose accurately.

Development of MN-GP is associated with the accumulation of additional (somatic) pathogenic mutations and cytogenetic abnormalities. These have a broad range and include both genetic lesions common in non-germline-related myeloid neoplasms and some which are enriched in specific germline disorders. In many GPs with autosomal dominant inheritance (such as *CEBPA*, *DDX41*, *TP53*, *RUNX1*, and *NF1*-associated syndromes), neoplastic progression involves inactivation or loss of the wild-type allele. As discussed earlier, clonal hematopoiesis is common in some syndromes, and the finding of a somatic genetic lesion does not always represent transformation to malignancy.

Prognosis and Treatment

Reflecting the heterogeneity of MN-GP diagnoses, there is a wide range of prognoses and appropriate treatments. Both the specific germline disorder and the specific myeloid neoplasm subtype influence the clinical features and prognosis. However, several special considerations are common across multiple germline disorders. Treatment options may be complicated by increased chemotherapy toxicity/low tolerance (eg, in the setting of FA) and require syndrome-specific protocols. Long-term prognosis and all-cause mortality are often affected by comorbidities associated with the underlying disorder, and by increased risk for new primary neoplasms. Therefore, allogeneic bone marrow transplants can carry additional long-term survival benefits. Evaluation of potential related bone marrow donors should include investigation for the presence of the germline variant in the donor (*Blood*. 2022;140:1345-1377).

> **Key Points**
>
> - Myeloid neoplasms associated with germline predisposition (MN-GP) are a heterogeneous group of neoplasms arising in individuals with a genetic condition predisposing to myeloid malignancy.
> - Clues prompting germline workup can include prior personal or family malignant history, presence of syndromic signs/symptoms, myeloid malignancy (MDS [myelodysplastic syndrome]) at unusually early age, or presence of potential germline allele on molecular profiling.
> - Diagnostic description should combine the specific myeloid malignancy present and the specific germline disorder.
>
> **Diagnostic Caveats**
>
> - It is necessary to distinguish features of the underlying germline disorder (sometimes including cytopenias, morphologic abnormalities, or clonal hematopoiesis) from true malignant clonal evolution.
> - Germline predisposition disorders often have associated family history but can also be sporadic resulting from de novo germline mutations.
> - A variant allele frequency of ~50% may suggest workup for germline variant but does not exclude somatic mutation.
> - To confirm MN-GP, the variant must be pathogenic/likely pathogenic and confirmed as germline (ie, by testing on skin fibroblasts or detection in relatives).

IV. MYELOID PROLIFERATIONS ASSOCIATED WITH DOWN SYNDROME

Introduction

Trisomy 21/DS is the most common congenital chromosomal condition, with an incidence of approximately 1 in 700 live births in the United States (*Birth Defects Res.* 2019;111:1420-1435). About 10% of neonates with DS have clinical or hematologic manifestations of TAM, a clonal myeloproliferative/leukemic process that generally resolves spontaneously; another 15% have "silent TAM" diagnosable only by molecular studies (*Blood.* 2013;122:3908-3917). Approximately 20% of children with a history of clinical TAM, as well as some children with DS but no prior TAM diagnosis, develop ML-DS (*Pediatr Int.* 2019;61:222-229; Leukemia. 2021;35:1480-1484). ML-DS presents in early childhood as an acute leukemia, often with an MDS-like prodromal phase. Both TAM and ML-DS have characteristic somatic *GATA1* mutations and usually show a megakaryoblastic phenotype. The diagnostic criteria for TAM and ML-DS are summarized in Table 13.4. Of note, children and adults with trisomy 21 can also develop other hematolymphoid neoplasms that must be distinguished from TAM/ML-DS; this includes an increased risk for B-ALL (*J Clin Oncol.* 2024;42:218-227).

Clinical Features

Clinical TAM usually presents in the first week of life with increased blasts in the peripheral blood and ranges from asymptomatic to severe and life threatening. Some cases display extreme leukocytosis more than $100 \text{ k} \times 10^9/\text{L}$ (*Blood.* 2011;118:6752-6996). TAM is thought to originate from fetal hematopoiesis in the liver, and reflecting this, involvement of liver and peripheral blood is frequently greater than bone marrow involvement. Hepatomegaly is common, and severe cases show progressive fibrosis,

TABLE 13.4 WHO-HAEM5 Diagnostic Criteria for Myeloid Proliferations Associated With Down Syndrome

Transient abnormal myelopoiesis associated with Down syndrome

Essential

- Confirmation of constitutional trisomy 21
- Peripheral blood leukocytosis with increased blasts
- Detection of exon 2/3 *GATA1* mutation (*GATA1* exon 2/3 sequencing should be performed in all cases with peripheral blood blasts >10%.)

Myeloid leukemia associated with Down syndrome

Essential	Desirable
• Confirmation of constitutional trisomy 21 • Myeloid neoplasm with persistent increased peripheral blood and bone marrow blasts (may be <20%) • Detection of exon 2/3 *GATA1* mutation	• Mutation profiling and detection of mutations in other genes, for example, cohesin complex, *EZH2*, *KANSL1*, and *JAK3*

EZH2, enhancer of zeste homolog 2; JAK3, Janus kinase 3; KANSL1, KAT8 regulatory NSL complex subunit 1.
Based on the WHO Classification of Tumours Editorial Board. Haematolymphoid tumours [Internet]. Lyon (France): International Agency for Research on Cancer; 2024 (WHO classification of tumours series, 5th ed.; vol. 11). Available from: https://tumourclassification.iarc.who.int/chapters/63.

---

ascites, and liver failure. Other common manifestations include splenomegaly, skin rash, and pleural or pericardial effusions. Most cases spontaneously resolve within the first few months of life; however, children with a history of TAM have increased risk for later developing ML-DS.

ML-DS usually presents outside the neonatal period in the first 4 years of life, with a median age of 1.7 years (*Blood*. 1998;91:608-615). In many cases, ML-DS is preceded by a pancytopenic MDS-like phase without overtly increased blasts, which can last for several months before progressing to an AML-like phase. A minority have elevated blast count at presentation similar to do novo acute leukemia. Some cases display extramedullary involvement including the liver and spleen, but the central nervous system (CNS) is usually spared. Unlike TAM, ML-DS does not resolve spontaneously and usually requires treatment with chemotherapy.

Morphology and Immunophenotype

Both TAM and ML-DS frequently show blasts with megakaryoblastic morphology, including granular basophilic cytoplasm and cytoplasmic blebs, but in some cases, blasts have nonspecific/undifferentiated morphology. While not required for diagnosis, blasts usually have a characteristic immunophenotype with expression of CD117, CD13, CD33, and CD36; frequent expression of CD7, CD56, CD71, and the megakaryocyte-lineage markers CD41, CD42b, and CD61; variable expression of CD34 (often negative in ML-DS); and negative MPO (myeloperoxidase) (*Klin Padiatr.* 2005;217:126-134). The morphologic differential of pediatric megakaryoblastic leukemias includes AML with *RBM15::MRTFA*, AML with other specific translocations (ie, subsets of *CBFA2T3::GLIS2*, *NUP98* rearranged, or *KMTA* rearranged AML), and acute megakaryoblastic leukemia NOS (*Front Cell Dev Biol.* 2023;11:1170622).

TAM often shows greater blast counts in peripheral blood than in marrow. Blood may show circulating atypical erythroid precursors and circulating mature atypical megakaryocytes, and marrow biopsy often shows dysplastic erythropoiesis and megakaryopoiesis. ML-DS in the MDS-like phase typically shows multilineage dysplastic features without overtly increased blasts, while the AML-like phase is characterized by increased blasts in the marrow and sometimes peripheral blood. Proliferation of atypical mature megakaryocytes is variably present. Like other myeloid malignancies with megakaryocytic differentiation, ML-DS often shows marrow fibrosis, which may result in a "dry tap." Of note, there is no absolute cutoff for blast percentile for diagnosis of either TAM or ML-DS. See e-Figures 13.3-1 to 13.3-5 for an example of ML-DS morphology and immunophenotype.

Genetic Features

By definition, TAM and ML-DS occur in patients with constitutional trisomy 21, although occasional cases occur in the setting of trisomy 21 mosaicism without the usual manifestations of DS. Somatic *GATA1* exon 2/3 mutation (usually resulting in a truncated protein) underlies both TAM and ML-DS. This mutation is thought to occur prenatally in a fetal hematopoietic stem cell. Clonality studies support etiology for ML-DS as arising from a persistent/recurrent TAM subclone (*Nat Genet.* 2013;45:1293-1299). ML-DS typically shows additional cytogenetic abnormalities and somatic mutations, with common targets including cohesin complex genes (*STAG2*, *RAD21*), epigenetic regulator genes (*EZH2*, *KANSL1*), and activation/proliferation signaling pathway genes (*JAK3*, *NRAS*) (*Cancer Cell.* 2019;36:123-138).

Prognosis and Treatment

TAM has a generally good prognosis and resolves spontaneously within 3 months of birth in the majority of patients. However, early deaths occur in approximately 10% of cases, often associated with progressive liver failure (*Pediatr Int.* 2019;61:222-229). Chemotherapy is indicated for cases with high-risk features including severe hepatic dysfunction, hyperleukocytosis, or coagulopathy. Blast counts usually respond well to low-dose cytarabine, although there is increased risk for treatment-related myelosuppression in these patients (*Blood.* 2011;118:6752-6996; *Blood Adv.* 2018;2:1532-1540). Approximately 20% of children with a history of clinical TAM later develop ML-DS regardless of treatment.

ML-DS does not resolve spontaneously; however, it carries a better prognosis than most other forms of childhood AML. When treated with ML-DS-specific chemotherapy regimens, 5-year event-free survival (EFS) is approximately 90% (*Blood.* 2017;129:3304-3313). ML-DS blasts are highly sensitive to chemotherapy, but there is risk for significant treatment toxicity including severe cytopenia, viral infections, and cardiotoxicity. Recent clinical trials have focused on optimizing regimens to maintain high EFS while reducing toxicity (*Blood.* 2021;138:2337-2346). Refractory or relapsed cases of ML-DS are rare but have a poor prognosis.

Key Points

- Both transient abnormal myelopoiesis (TAM) and myeloid leukemia of Down syndrome (ML-DS) are associated with constitutional trisomy 21 and *GATA1* mutation.
- Both TAM and ML-DS usually have a megakaryoblastic phenotype.
- TAM occurs in early infancy and usually resolves spontaneously, but patients carry risk of later developing ML-DS.
- ML-DS generally occurs in the first 4 y of life and usually responds well to chemotherapy.

Diagnostic Caveats

- Peripheral blood blasts in TAM can decrease rapidly after birth, and *GATA1* mutation analysis after the first week of life may result in a false negative.
- Children and adults with Down syndrome can also develop other hematolymphoid neoplasms that must be distinguished from TAM/ML-DS.
- Morphologic differential of megakaryoblastic leukemias includes acute myeloid leukemia (AML) with *RBM15::MRTFA*, subsets of AML with *CBFA2T3::GLIS2*, *NUP98*-r, or *KMTA*-r, and acute megakaryoblastic leukemia NOS.

ACKNOWLEDGMENTS

The case of *SAMD9L*-associated monosomy 7 myelodysplasia and leukemia syndrome-1 (M7MLS1) (e-Figures 13.2-1 to 13.2-5) was presented by Dr Kovach in "Germline predisposition variants in pediatric and adult myelodysplasic syndromes (MDS)" at the 2023 American Society of Clinical Pathology meeting on October 20, 2023 in Long Beach, CA.

SUGGESTED READINGS

Behrens YL, Göhring G, Bawadi R, et al. A novel classification of hematologic conditions in patients with Fanconi anemia. *Haematologica*. 2021;106(11):3000-3003. doi:10.3324/haematol.2021.279332

Döhner H, Wei AH, Appelbaum FR, et al. Diagnosis and management of AML in adults: 2022 recommendations from an international expert panel on behalf of the ELN. *Blood*. 2022;140(12):1345-1377. doi:10.1182/blood.2022016867

Kennedy AL, Shimamura A. Genetic predisposition to MDS: clinical features and clonal evolution. *Blood*. 2019;133(10):1071-1085. doi:10.1182/blood-2018-10-844662

Kuendgen A, Nomdedeu M, Tuechler H, et al. Therapy-related myelodysplastic syndromes deserve specific diagnostic sub-classification and risk-stratification: an approach to classification of patients with t-MDS. *Leukemia*. 2021;35(3):835-849.

McNerney ME, Godley LA, Le Beau MM. Therapy-related myeloid neoplasms: when genetics and environment collide. *Nat Rev Cancer*. 2017;17(9):513-527. doi:10.1038/nrc.2017.60

1. Patel N, Calvo KR. How I diagnose myeloid neoplasms with germline predisposition. *Am J Clin Pathol*. 2023;160(4):352-364. doi:10.1093/ajcp/aqad075

14. Myeloid/Lymphoid Neoplasms With Eosinophilia and Tyrosine Kinase Gene Fusions

Rohan Kodgule, Ranjit Chauhan, and Anjum Hassan

Eosinophilia is generally defined as a peripheral blood absolute eosinophilic count (AEC) of $\geq 0.5 \times 10^9$/L. The term "hypereosinophilia" is used when the AEC is $\geq 1.5 \times 10^9$/L (*Am J Hematol.* 2023;98:1286-1306). Clinical evaluation of eosinophilia is necessary to differentiate reactive conditions from clonal (neoplastic) disorders. The exclusion of reactive (non-clonal) causes of eosinophilia relies on various tests based on the clinical context, including morphologic review of blood and bone marrow, cytogenetics, fluorescence in situ hybridization (FISH), and immunophenotypic and clonality studies, to establish histopathologic evidence of acute or chronic clonal hematologic malignancy. A diagnostic algorithm for differential diagnosis of hypereosinophilia is illustrated in Figure 14.1.

One of the categories of hematologic malignancies associated with eosinophilia includes myeloid/lymphoid neoplasms with gene fusions causing constitutive tyrosine kinase signaling (M/LN-eo-TK) (Table 14.1). Both the International Consensus Classification (ICC) and WHO-HAEM5 recognize rearrangements of *PGFRA, PDGFRB, FGFR1, JAK2, FLT3*, and/or *ETV6::ABL1* as genetic abnormalities with relatively distinct clinicopathologic and therapeutic implications.

I. GENERAL FEATURES OF M/LN-eo-TK

With the growing list of recurrent molecularly defined primary eosinophilias, the basic difference between the ICC and WHO-HAEM5, to date, is the number of listed gene rearrangements (*Am J Hematol.* 2022;97:129-148; *Leukemia.* 2022;36:1703-1719). The ICC system categorizes M/LN-eo-TK into six groups of gene rearrangements, while WHO-HAEM5 identifies seven groups of M/LN-eo-TK gene abnormalities (with "other TK gene fusions" as the novel addition to the WHO diagnostic criteria), as summarized in Figure 14.2.

Clinical Features

M/LN-eo-TK encompasses a spectrum of presentations depending on the subgroup. Age at onset varies, yet the late fifth decade is a common presenting age across subtypes. Gender is skewed toward male predominance, especially evident in cases with *PDGFRA* rearrangement (7:1 male-to-female), *PDGFRB* rearrangement (2:1 male-to-female), *FGFR1* rearrangement (1.5:1 male-to-female), and *JAK2* rearrangement (27:5 male-to-female). Cases with *PDGFRA* rearrangement show systemic

SECTION III: NEOPLASTIC

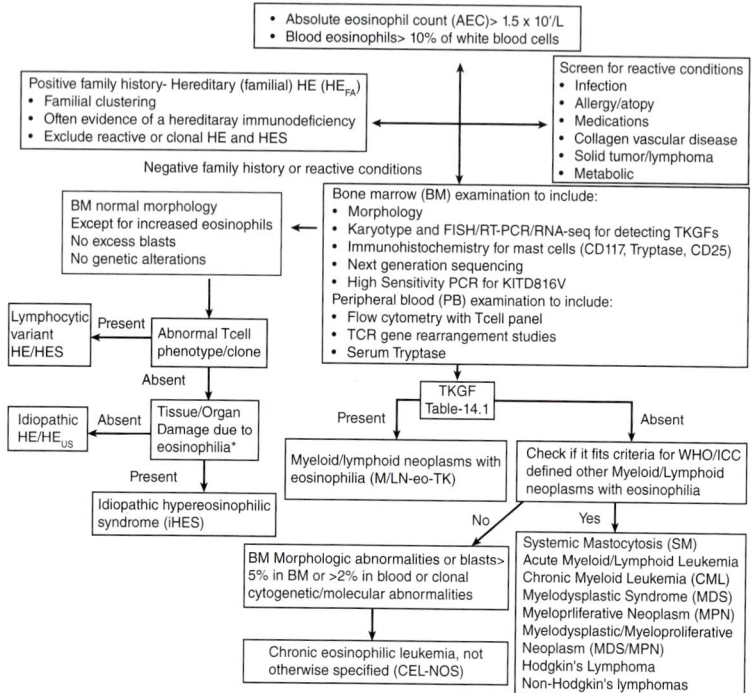

Figure 14.1. Diagnostic algorithm for hypereosinophilia. Eosinophilia-induced organ damage can be seen in familial, reactive, and clonal conditions. FISH, fluorescent in situ hybridization; HE, hypereosinophilia; HES, hypereosinophilic syndrome; HE$_{US}$, hypereosinophilia of unknown significance; PCR, polymerase chain reaction; RNA-seq, RNA sequencing; RT-PCR, real-time reverse transcription polymerase chain reaction; TCR, T-cell receptor; wgss, tyrosine kinase gene fusions. (Modified from *Am J Hematol.* 2023;98:1286-1306; *Am J Hematol.* 2022;97:129-148; *Allergy.* 2023;78:47-59.)

mastocytosis, elevated serum tryptase (>12 ng/mL), or elevated serum vitamin B$_{12}$ levels (*Head Neck Pathol.* 2021;15:1399-1403); splenomegaly is also observed in the majority of cases. Cases with *PDGFRB* rearrangement are characterized by splenomegaly, hepatomegaly, and varying degrees of B-symptoms.

Morphology

Peripheral blood and bone marrow eosinophilia remains a predominant finding in most cases (e-Figures 14.1-1, 14.1-2, 14.2-1, 14.2-2, and 14.3-3). Since M/LN-eo-TK neoplasms can differentiate into myeloid and/or lymphoid lineages, heterogeneous disease morphology resembling myeloproliferative neoplasm (MPN), myelodysplastic syndrome (MDS), systemic mastocytosis, MDS/MPN, acute myeloid leukemia (AML), T-cell acute lymphoblastic leukemia (T-ALL), B-cell acute lymphoblastic leukemia (B-ALL), mixed-phenotype acute leukemia (MPAL), chronic eosinophilic leukemia (CEL)–like features with extramedullary involvement, and nodal T-ALL/LBL can be expected. Additionally, M/LN-eo-TK with *PDGFRA* rearrangement frequently show increased loose aggregates of mast cells (e-Figure 14.1-3). Bone marrow fibrosis is commonly seen in cases with *PDGFRA* or *PDGFRB* rearrangement. In cases with *PDGFRB* rearrangement, abnormal megakaryocytes resembling MDS and

TABLE 14.1 Features of Myeloid/Lymphoid Neoplasms With Eosinophilia and TK Gene Fusions

TK Gene	Most Common Genetic Alteration	Other Partner Genes	Clinical Features	Other Features	Associated Mutations	Primary Diagnostic Techniques	Treatments
PDGFRA	FIP1L1::PDGFRA (cytogenetically cryptic deletion of chromosome 4q12 resulting in FIP1L1::PDGFRA)	KIF5B, CDK5RAP2, STRN, ETV6, BCR, and TNKS2	Show common features of chronic eosinophilic leukemia. Pulmonary, cardiac, or respiratory symptoms, fatigue, and pruritus. Results of hypereosinophilia	Male:female ratio ~7:1	ASXL1, BCOR, DNMT3A, RUNX1, SRSF2, TET2	RT-PCR for FIP1L1::PDGFRA fusion; FISH for PDGFRA rearrangement; RNA-seq for more cryptic rearrangements	Excellent treatment response to a multikinase inhibitor and a TKI, imatinib. In vitro and in vivo efficacy to midostaurin and sorafenib TKIs
PDGFRB	ETV6::PDGFRB fusion gene or other rearrangement of PDGFRB due to chromosome 5q32 rearrangements t(5;12)(q32;p13.2)	>30 other partner genes (eg, SART3)	Often resemble CML with prominent eosinophilia; extramedullary involvement of skin and heart; splenomegaly, hepatomegaly, and B-symptoms to varying degrees	Male:female ratio ~2:1. Initial diagnosis in the fifth decade of life	ASXL1, BCOR, DNMT3A, NRAS, STAG2, STAT5B, TET2, ZSRS2	Break-apart FISH for PDGFRB; RT-PCR for PDGFRB fusion gene; RNA-seq	Excellent response to TKI imatinib

(continued)

TABLE 14.1 Features of Myeloid/Lymphoid Neoplasms With Eosinophilia and TK Gene Fusions (*continued*)

TK Gene	Most Common Genetic Alteration	Other Partner Genes	Clinical Features	Other Features	Associated Mutations	Primary Diagnostic Techniques	Treatments
FGFR1	ZMYM2::FGFR1 (T-lymphoblastic leukemia)	BCR::FGFR1 (MPN), TPR::FGFR1 (MPN), CEP43::FGFR1 (CML), CNTRL::FGFR1 (CML), and CEP43G::FGFR1 (polycythemia vera)	Heterogeneous group of neoplasms; manifests as CMN or blast-phase disease associated with eosinophilia; B cell, T cell, myeloid or mixed-phenotype leukemia or MPN or myelodysplastic/ myeloproliferative neoplasms	Male:female ratio ~1.5:1 Initial detection in the fourth decade of life	RUNX1, ASXL1, CSFR3, STAG2	Conventional karyotyping of alternations of FGFR1 at 8p11; break-apart FISH for FGFR1; RNA-seq	Responds effectively to FGFR inhibitor such as pemigatinib
JAK2	PCM1::JAK2 (due to chromosome 9p24.1 alterations)	ASXL1, BCOR, ETV6, RUNX1, SRSF2, TET2, and TP53	Commonly presented with eosinophilia; associated with neutrophilia, eosinophilia, and/or monocytosis; present features of CMN or myelodysplastic/myeloproliferative neoplasms; hepatosplenomegaly and lymphadenopathy are seen	Male:female ratio 27:5 Diagnosed first in the fifth decade of life	ASXL1, BCOR, BCORL1, CD36, EP300, ETV6, RUNX1, SRSF2, TET2, TP53	Routine karyotyping of alterations of 9p24.1; break-apart FISH for JAK2 rearrangement; RT-PCR for specific gene fusions	Limited responses to the JAK2 inhibitor, ruxolitinib. Allogeneic hematopoietic stem cell transplantation as alternate treatment

FLT3	ETV6::FLT3 due to chromosome t(12;13)(p13.2;q12.2)	BCR/22q11, ZMYM2/13q12, TRIP11/14q32, SPTBN1/2p16, GOLGB1/3q13, CCDC88C/14q32, ZBTB44/11q24, and MYO18A/17q12	Hematopoietic stem cell neoplasms associated with eosinophilia; Peripheral blood abnormalities (ie, leukocytosis, anemia, and thrombocytopenia)	Male:female ratio 1.4:1 Diagnosed first in the 5th decade	ASXL1, RUNX1, STAT5B, SRSF2, TET2, TP53, U2AF1	Routine karyotyping of 13q12 rearrangements; break-apart FISH of FLT3; RT-PCR; RNA-seq	Various responses to specific FLT3 inhibitors (eg, sorafenib, sunitinib, or midostaurin)
ETV6::ABL1	ETV6::ABL1 fusion due to t(9;12)(q34;p13)	Not reported	Hematopoietic stem cell neoplasms; splenomegaly, leukocytosis, anemia, thrombocytopenia, and basophilia are common; most cases are present with eosinophilia	Male:female ratio 1.9:1 Diagnosed first in the fifth decade of life	ARID2, CDKN1B, TP53, SMC1A	Chromosome banding analysis; FISH with a combination of ETV6 and ABL1 probes; RT-PCR; RNA-seq	Effective response to ABL1-inhibitors (eg, dasatinib, nilotinib, imatinib, bosutinib, and ponatinib)
Other TK gene fusions	ETV6::FGFR2; ETV6::LYN; ETV6::NTRK3; RANBP2::ALK; BCR::RET; FGFR1OP::RET	Unknown	Still under investigation	Not known		RNA-seq; karyotyping; break-apart FISH	Not known

B-ALL, B-cell acute lymphoblastic leukemia; BM, bone marrow; CML, chronic myeloid leukemia; CMN, chronic myelomonocytic leukemia; FISH, fluorescent in situ hybridization; MPN, myeloproliferative neoplasms; Ph chromosome, Philadelphia chromosome; RNA-seq, RNA sequencing; RT-PCR, real-time reverse transcription polymerase chain reaction; TK, tyrosine kinase; TKI, tyrosine kinase inhibitor; WHO, World Health Organization.
Modified from the WHO-HAEM5 and *Virchows Arch.* 2023;482:85-89.

WHO 2022

- PDGFRA rearrangement
- PDGFRB rearrangement
- FGFR1 rearrangement
- JAK2 rearrangement
- FLT3 rearrangement
- ETV6::ABL1 fusion
- Other tyrosine kinase gene fusions
  ETV6::FGFR2, ETV6::LYN; ETV6::NTRK3, RANBP2::ALK, BCR::RET and FGFR1OP::RET

ICC 2022

- PDGFRA rearrangement
- PDGFRB rearrangement
- FGFR1 rearrangement
- JAK2 rearrangement
- FLT3 rearrangement
- ETV6::ABL1 fusion

Figure 14.2. Genetic alterations that define myeloid/lymphoid neoplasms with eosinophilia and tyrosine kinase gene fusions (M/LN-eo-TK) based on the WHO-HAEM5 (myeloid and histiocytic/dendritic neoplasms) (WHO 2022) and the International Consensus Classification system of myeloid neoplasms and acute leukemias (ICC 2022).

elevated mast cells may be seen. Cases with *FGFR1* rearrangement have cytologic features that are diverse with a mix of immature myeloid cells, small lymphoblasts, mature eosinophils, and sometimes mast cells (e-Figures 14.3-1 and 14.3-2). *JAK2*-rearranged neoplasms show hypercellular bone marrow in association with eosinophilia with abnormal morphology, increased pronormoblasts in clusters (erythroid microtumors), and myelofibrosis.

Genetic Features

Although M/LN-eo-TK gene fusions involving *PDGFRA, PDGFRB, FGFR1, JAK2, ETV6::ABL1, FLT3,* and others all originate in pluripotent stem cells and result in constitutive tyrosine kinase signaling, the mechanisms for tyrosine kinase activation differ. Truncation of PDGFRA between two conserved tryptophan residues in the juxtamembrane (JM) domain is required for kinase activation and the transforming potential of *FIP1L1::PDGFRA* (*PNAS.* 2006;103:8078-8083). *PDGFRB* and *FGFR1* translocation activation of tyrosine kinase signaling is dependent on the homodimerization of fusion partners like *ETV6* or *ZNF198* (*IJLH.* 2013;35:491-500). Interphase/metaphase FISH using break-apart or fusion probes, nested real-time reverse transcription polymerase chain reaction (RT-PCR), and targeted anchored multiplex assays using next-generation sequencing (NGS), RNA sequencing (RNA-seq), or whole genome sequencing (WGS) can be used to detect the translocations that are used to subcategorize cases of M/LN-eo-TK. Diagnostic criteria, as per updated WHO guidelines, are listed in Table 14.2.

Differential Diagnosis

M/LN-eo-TK should be differentiated from Ph-like B-ALL and de-novo T-ALL, which sometimes can show similar translocations without features of myeloid involvement. It is important to identify any prior history of MPN, relevant translocations, and persistent gene fusions in remission before categorizing a case as belonging to the

TABLE 14.2   WHO-HAEM5 Diagnostic Criteria

TK Gene	Criteria
PDGFRA	**Essential:** A myeloid (more frequent) or lymphoid neoplasm, usually with prominent peripheral and/or tissue eosinophilia AND Presence of a *PDGFRA* fusion gene, usually with *FIP1L1* **Desirable:** In the absence of molecular demonstration of the fusion gene, the diagnosis should be suspected if there is a *BCR::ABL1*–negative myeloproliferative neoplasm with prominent eosinophilia associated with splenomegaly Marked elevation of serum vitamin B_{12}, increased serum tryptase, and increased bone marrow mast cells
PDGFRB	**Essential:** A myeloid or lymphoid neoplasm, often with prominent eosinophilia with varying degrees of neutrophilia or monocytosis associated with the formation of a *PDGFRB* fusion gene. Cases of *BCR::ABL1*–like B-ALL without evidence of an associated myeloid neoplasm are excluded from this category. **Desirable:** Cytogenetic and molecular identification of the partner gene, for example, t(5;12)(q32;p13.2) with *ETV6::PDGFRB* or other partner genes
FGFR1	**Essential:** Demonstration of t(8;13)(p11.2;q12.1) or a different translocation leading to formation of an *FGFR1* fusion gene is required. Phenotypically the disease may present as a myeloproliferative or myelodysplastic/myeloproliferative neoplasm with prominent eosinophilia, with or without neutrophilia or monocytosis or with increased blasts of myeloid, T-cell or B-cell lineage, or mixed phenotype, usually with eosinophilia. **Desirable:** Molecular identification of the partner gene of *FGFR1*
JAK2	**Essential:** A myeloid or lymphoid neoplasm, often with prominent eosinophilia and the presence of a *JAK2* fusion gene Cases of *BCR::ABL1*–like B-ALL without evidence of an associated myeloid neoplasm are excluded from this category. **Desirable:** Cytogenetic identification of the translocation and molecular identification of the fusion gene, for example, *PCM1::JAK2*

| TABLE 14.2 | WHO-HAEM5 Diagnostic Criteria (*continued*) |

TK Gene	Criteria
FLT3	**Essential/Desirable:**
	A myeloid or lymphoid neoplasm, with or without associated eosinophilia with chromosomal rearrangements leading to the formation of a *FLT3* fusion gene
ETV6::ABL1	**Essential:**
	A hematopoietic (myeloid or lymphoid) neoplasm in chronic phase associated with *ETV6::ABL1*
	Desirable:
	Cytogenetic confirmation of t(9;12)(q34;p13) or complex aberrations involving other chromosomes
Other TK gene fusions	**Essential:**
	A myeloid and/or lymphoid neoplasm
	Detection of a *TK* fusion gene, other than those specifically defined as distinct entities (ie, *PDGFRA*, *PDGFRB*, *FGFR1*, *JAK2*, *FLT3*, and *ETV6::ABL1*)
	Desirable:
	Eosinophilia; cytogenetic identification of a translocation, suggesting the involvement of a *TK* gene and prompting the selection of appropriate break-apart FISH probes and/or other molecular investigation

FISH, fluorescence in situ hybridization; TK, tyrosine kinase.
Based on the WHO Classification of Tumours Editorial Board. Haematolymphoid tumours [Internet]. Lyon (France): International Agency for Research on Cancer; 2024 (WHO classification of tumours series, 5th ed.; vol. 11). Available from: https://tumourclassification.iarc.who.int/chapters/63.

M/LN-eo-TK subset. *PDFGRA* fusion cases sometimes resemble systemic mastocytosis but lack *KIT* D816V mutation.

II. M/LN-eo-TK WITH *PDGFRA* REARRANGEMENT

This entity is the most common among M/LN-eo-TK and shows cryptic deletion of 4q12, resulting in the fusion of the *PDGFRA* gene with a partner gene, most frequently *FIP1L1*; other partner genes such as *KIF5B*, *CDK5RAP2*, *STRN*, *FOXP1*, *ETV6*, *BCR*, and *TNKS2* have also been identified (*Am J Hematol.* 2023;98:1286-1306). Laboratory evaluation of primary causes of eosinophilia should ideally begin with screening of the peripheral blood for *FIPL1L1-PDGFRA* gene fusion (usually by RT-PCR or interphase/metaphase FISH). As noted earlier, there is a striking male predominance (*Blood.* 2017;129:704-714). While this disorder shows common features of chronic eosinophilic leukemia, rare manifestations of AML or lymphoblastic leukemia have also been reported (*Head Neck Pathol.* 2021;15:1399-1403).

The eosinophil population primarily consists of mature cells that exhibit cytologic abnormalities (ie, large size, abnormal cytoplasmic granule distribution, cytoplasmic vacuolation, changes in granule size or color, or abnormal nuclear lobation). Atypical and spindle-shaped forms of mast cells may be present. Serum tryptase levels are usually elevated.

Genetic Features

FISH probes that hybridize between the *FIPL1L1* and *PDGFRA* genes can also detect the presence of the cytogenetically occult 800-kb deletion on 4q12 that results in the diagnostic *FIP1L1::PDGFRA* gene fusion. The *CHIC2* gene is located in this segment, and separate FISH testing can be performed to detect *CHIC2* gene deletion.

Prognosis and Treatment

First-line therapy for patients with M/LN-eo-TK with a *PDGFRA* fusion gene employs a multikinase inhibitor and a tyrosine kinase inhibitor (TKI) such as imatinib (*N Engl J Med.* 2003;348:1201-1214). An excellent treatment response to imatinib has been reported in both the chronic phase and blast phase of the disease. Additionally, midostaurin and sorafenib TKIs have also shown potential for use in cases of acquired imatinib resistance (*Blood.* 2005;106:3206-3213).

III. M/LN-eo-TK WITH *PDGFRB* REARRANGEMENT

The disease entity M/LN-eo-TK is characterized by chromosome 5q32 rearrangements that lead to the formation of a *PDGFRB* fusion. This disorder has a 2:1 male-to-female predominance, and patients usually have their initial diagnosis in the fifth decade of life.

Extramedullary involvement of skin and heart (often associated with cardiac failure) is present. Ph-like B-ALL with *PDGFRB* rearrangements should be excluded before a diagnosis of this type of M/LN-eo-TK is made.

Genetic Features

The most common genetic feature of M/LN-eo-TK with *PDGFRB* rearrangement is t(5;12)(q32;p13.2), which results in the *ETV6::PDGFRB* fusion gene. The second most common rearrangement is *CCDC88C::PDGFRB*. Additional fusions with more than 30 gene partners have also been identified. While most of the *PDGFRB* translocations are detected in conventional karyotypes, some cryptic rearrangements require DNA sequence analysis (*Histopathology.* 2020;76:1042-1054). Of note, some cases with translocations involving 5q32 may not have *PDGFRB* fusion genes and do not respond to imatinib, and are excluded from this category (*Leukemia.* 2007;21:1839-1841). Therefore, break-apart FISH for *PDGFRB*, RT-PCR, or RNA-sequencing tests are strongly recommended to confirm the presence of a *PDGFRB* fusion gene.

Prognosis and Treatment

The first line of therapy for patients with M/LN-eo-TK with *PDGFRB* rearrangement is the TKI imatinib. Cases with a complex karyotype are associated with a poor prognosis (*Acta Haematol.* 2002;107:113-122).

IV. M/LN-eo-TK WITH *FGFR1* REARRANGEMENT

This is a rare subset that arises from pluripotent hematopoietic stem cells and manifests with variable phenotypes such as chronic myeloid neoplasms or blast phase of myeloid, T cell, B cell, or mixed phenotype associated with eosinophilia. Genetically, it is characterized by *FGFR1* fusion genes. Patients are most often initially diagnosed in the fourth decade of life.

Genetic Features

FISH with break-apart probes for *FGFR1* can be used to diagnose this entity by demonstrating the characteristic *FGFR1* fusion genes. The most commonly seen fusions and their associations are: t(8;13)(p11;q12)/*ZMYM2::FGFR1* (T-lymphoblastic leukemia), *BCR::FGFR1* (MPN), *TPR::FGFR1* (MPN), *CEP43::FGFR1* (chronic myelomonocytic leukemia), *CNTRL::FGFR1* (chronic myelomonocytic leukemia), and *CEP43G::FGFR1* (polycythemia-vera). *RUNX1* is often mutated in this subset of cases (*Leuk Lymphoma*. 2018;59:1672-1676).

Prognosis and Treatment

This disease has an aggressive course and a poor prognosis. Treatment with third-generation TKIs such as ponatinib and fibroblast growth factor receptors (FGFR) inhibitors such as pemigatinib has shown promising results, especially in chronic phase disease (*Blood*. 2022;140:1200-1228).

V. M/LN-eo-TK WITH *JAK2* REARRANGEMENT

These are M/LN-eo-TKs associated with genetic rearrangements involving chromosome 9p24.1 resulting in a *JAK2* fusion gene. This type of M/LN-eo-TK is usually first diagnosed in the fifth decade of life. The disease is often associated with neutrophilia, eosinophilia, and/or monocytosis (*Mod Pathol*. 2019;32:490-498), and hepatosplenomegaly and lymphadenopathy are also commonly seen. Some specific fusions are associated with unique histopathologic features, such as with *PCM1::JAK2*, which presents with a typical triad of bone marrow hypercellularity with eosinophilia, large aggregates of immature erythroid precursors (frequently seen in extramedullary lesions), and myelofibrosis.

Genetic Features

Alterations of 9p24.1 that lead to *JAK2* fusion products are unique to this type of M/LN-eo-TK. The most common fusion product is *PCM1::JAK2*, but a number of other fusion partners with *JAK2* have been demonstrated, including *ETV6* and *BCR*. Phenotypic and clinical heterogeneity of the resulting neoplasms may be the results of additional somatic gene mutations in *ASXL1, BCOR, ETV6, RUNX1, SRSF2, TET2*, and *TP53* genes (*Mod Pathol*. 2019;32:490-498). *PCM1::JAK2* can sometimes be observed in AML at relapse as an acquired event, which should be excluded from this subset of LN/M-eo-TK.

Prognosis and Treatment

Limited short-term responses (1-2 years in duration) to the JAK2 inhibitor ruxolitinib have been reported among patients with *JAK2* fusions. Alternative treatments include allogeneic hematopoietic stem cell transplantation.

VI. M/LN-eo-TK WITH *FLT3* REARRANGEMENT

These are hematopoietic stem cell neoplasms associated with eosinophilia caused by gene rearrangements involving 13q12 leading to *FLT3* gene fusions. Patients are often first diagnosed in the fifth decade of life. Some patients present with relative and/or absolute monocytosis, and imaging studies may show lytic bone lesions.

Genetic Features

The most common *FLT3* gene fusion partner is *ETV6*, and other partner genes include *BCR, ZMYM2, TRIP11, SPTBN1, GOLGB1, CCDC88C, ZBTB44,* and *MYO18A*. Somatic mutations have also been reported in *ASXL1, SETBP1, U2AF1, STAT5B, TP53, SRSF2, TET2, RUNX1,* and *PTPN11* (*Mod Pathol.* 2021;34:1673-1685). In this type of M/LN-eo-TK, constitutive phosphorylation of the chimeric protein encoded by the *FLT3* fusion gene results in growth factor/ligand-independent proliferation (*Exp Hematol.* 2007;35:1723-1727).

Prognosis and Treatment

Because the disease typically progresses aggressively, responses to specific FLT3 inhibitors (eg, sorafenib, sunitinib, or midostaurin) have been reported (*Blood.* 2011;118:2239-2242). An alternative treatment is allogeneic hematopoietic stem cell transplantation (*Leukemia.* 2014;28:2090-2092).

VII. M/LN-eo-TK WITH *ETV6::ABL1* FUSION

This M/LN-eo-TK entity is often diagnosed first in the fifth decade of life and resembles chronic myelomonocytic leukemia (CML) with eosinophilia (*Haematologica.* 2016;101:1082-1093).

Genetic Features

The translocation t(9;12)(q34;p13) leads to the *ETV6::ABL1* gene fusion (*Mol Cytogenet.* 2013;6:39), which is ultimately responsible for the activation of the nonreceptor tyrosine kinase ABL1 via downstream pathways similar to those in *BCR::ABL1* translocated hematopoietic malignancies.

Prognosis and Treatment

The disease has an aggressive course and a poor prognosis. ABL1 inhibitors (eg, dasatinib, nilotinib, imatinib, bosutinib, and ponatinib) have shown some efficacy in achieving remission (*Haematologica.* 2021;106:614-618).

VIII. M/LN-eo-TK WITH OTHER TK GENE FUSIONS

The other TK fusions categorized under M/LN-eo-TK to date include *ETV6::FGFR2, ETV6::LYN, ETV6::NTRK3, RANBP2::ALK, BCR::RET,* and *FGFR1OP::RET* (*Leukemia.* 2022;36:1703-1719). Due to the limited number of cases reported to date, the epidemiology, clinical features, and pathogenesis of these rare variants are still under investigation.

SUGGESTED READINGS

Arber DA, Orazi A, Hasserjian RP, et al. International Consensus Classification of myeloid neoplasms and acute leukemias: integrating morphologic, clinical, and genomic data. *Blood.* 2022;140(11):1200-1228. doi:10.1182/blood.2022015850

Khoury JD, Solary E, Abla O, et al. The 5th edition of the World Health Organization classification of haematolymphoid tumours: myeloid and histiocytic/dendritic neoplasms. *Leukemia.* 2022;36(7):1703-1719. doi:10.1038/s41375-022-01613-1

Thiele J, Kvasnicka HM, Orazi A, et al. The International Consensus Classification of myeloid neoplasms and acute leukemias: myeloproliferative neoplasms. *Am J Hematol.* 2023;98(1):166-179. doi:10.1002/ajh.26751

Tzankov A, Reichard KK, Hasserjian RP, et al. Updates on eosinophilic disorders. *Virchows Arch.* 2023;482(1):85-97.

World Health Organization. 5th Edition of the WHO classification of hematolymphoid tumours (myeloid and histiocytic/dendritic neoplasms). World Health Organization. Accessed July 23, 2023. https://tumourclassification.iarc.who.int/welcome/#

15. Mastocytosis
Omar M. Al-Rusan and Brooj Abro

Mastocytosis encompasses a group of rare diseases that involve the accumulation of abnormal and clonal mast cells (MCs) in one or more organ systems. Based on the disease distribution, mastocytosis is classified into three main types by the WHO-HAEM5: cutaneous mastocytosis (CM), systemic mastocytosis (SM), and mast cell sarcoma (MCS). CM and SM are further divided into subtypes, determined by the extent and behavior of the disease (Table 15.1). Mastocytosis shows variable clinical behavior ranging from indolent to aggressive disease with most cases falling under the indolent category, including CM, bone marrow mastocytosis (BMM), indolent SM (ISM), and smoldering SM (SSM). The aggressive variants, which are collectively known as advanced SM (AdvSM), include aggressive SM (ASM), SM with an associated hematologic neoplasm (SM-AHN), and mast cell leukemia (MCL). The development of mastocytosis is linked to somatic activating mutations in the *KIT* gene, responsible for encoding a receptor tyrosine kinase essential in the growth and differentiation of MCs. Mutations in the *KIT* gene (most commonly *KIT* p.D816V) lead to proliferation and abnormal accumulation of MCs. MCs are involved in immune responses and allergic reactions. The accumulation of MCs in various tissues leads to diverse clinical symptoms. MCs in mastocytosis usually show atypical morphology and aberrant immunophenotype by immunohistochemistry (IHC) and/or flow cytometry (FC) (see Table 15.2).

TABLE 15.1 WHO-HAEM5 Classification of Mastocytosis

Cutaneous mastocytosis (CM)
- Maculopapular CM (MPCM): monomorphic and polymorphic forms
- Diffuse CM (DCM)
- Mastocytoma: isolated and multifocal forms

Systemic mastocytosis (SM)
- Bone marrow mastocytosis (BMM) ⎱
- Indolent SM (ISM) ⎬ Indolent forms
- Smoldering SM (SSM) ⎰
- Aggressive SM (ASM) ⎱
- SM with an associated hematologic neoplasm (SM-AHN) ⎬ Aggressive forms/AdvSM
- Mast cell leukemia (MCL) ⎰

Mast cell sarcoma (MCS)

Extracutaneous mastocytoma

Based on the WHO Classification of Tumours Editorial Board. Haematolymphoid tumours [Internet]. Lyon (France): International Agency for Research on Cancer; 2024 (WHO classification of tumours series, 5th ed.; vol. 11). Available from: https://tumourclassification.iarc.who.int/chapters/63.

TABLE 15.2 Features of Normal/Reactive and Atypical Mast Cells

Normal/Reactive/Typical MC

Morphology:
- BM aspirate smears (Wright Giemsa): mature MCs (usually within the spicules) with round shape, abundant cytoplasmic metachromatic dark-purple granules often obscuring the nucleus
- BM core and tissue sections (H&E-stained): round to ovoid cells with bland nuclei, pale pink granular cytoplasm (individual cells may be difficult to identify on H&E)

Immunophenotype:
- Positive for CD117/c-kit (bright) and tryptase
- Negative for CD25, CD2, and CD30

Atypical/Neoplastic MC

Morphology:
- Type 1: spindle-shaped cells with round-ovoid nucleus and decreased granulation
- Type 2: MCs with pleomorphic multilobated nuclei
- Immature: blastoid cell resembling basophil precursor (may be seen in acute MCL)

Immunophenotype:
- Positive for CD117/c-kit and tryptase
- Aberrant expression of one or more of the following: CD25, CD2, and CD30

MCs are normally present in epithelial tissues, most vascularized tissues, and BM. They are usually a few scattered cells (<1% in the BM). Reactive mast cell hyperplasia (MCH) may be seen in chronic inflammatory conditions and other malignancies (eg, BM involved by lymphoplasmacytic lymphoma typically shows increased reactive MCs). MCs in MCH show typical MC morphology. In mastocytosis, MCs usually show atypical morphology and form compact aggregates. A small subset of SM cases may show typical MC morphology (well-differentiated SM).
BM, bone marrow; MC, mast cell; MCL, mast cell leukemia.

I. CUTANEOUS MASTOCYTOSIS

CM primarily affects the skin, with a predilection for the trunk, proximal extremities, and scalp and usually sparing the palms, soles, and face. It is the most common form of mastocytosis and usually occurs in children. The diagnostic criteria are summarized in Table 15.3.

Clinical Features

CM presents as solitary or multiple reddish-brown macules or papules, often with pruritus. When lesions are stroked or rubbed, they may become urticarial (Darier sign). Based on the number and type of lesions, CM is subclassified into the following three subtypes: maculopapular cutaneous mastocytosis (MPCM) also known as urticaria pigmentosa, diffuse cutaneous mastocytosis (DCM), and mastocytoma. MPCM typically shows varying numbers of maculopapular lesions usually involving the extremities and trunk. Polymorphic lesions (heterogeneous lesions with varying sizes and shapes) are common in children and monomorphic lesions (homogenous

TABLE 15.3 WHO-HAEM5 Diagnostic Criteria for Cutaneous Mastocytosis

Essential	Desirable
• Classic mastocytosis skin lesions • Increased number of MCs in lesions • MCs expressing CKIT/CD117 and tryptase. SM was ruled out clinically or with bone marrow evaluation when indicated	• Lesional MCs aberrantly expressing one or more of the following: CD2, CD25, and CD30 • Detection of *KIT* mutations

MC, mast cell.
Based on the WHO Classification of Tumours Editorial Board. Haematolymphoid tumours [Internet]. Lyon (France): International Agency for Research on Cancer; 2024 (WHO classification of tumours series, 5th ed.; vol. 11). Available from: https://tumourclassification.iarc.who.int/chapters/63.

---

small lesions) are more common in adults. DCM is characterized by generalized skin involvement with diffuse erythema and thickening and is usually accompanied by severe systemic symptoms. Mastocytoma(s) is defined as solitary skin lesions (≤3 lesions). Systemic symptoms in CM arise from the activation of MCs and release of mediators such as tryptase, histamine, interleukins, etc. Systemic symptoms include flushing, hypotension, abdominal pain, diarrhea, respiratory symptoms, and rarely anaphylaxis. Serum tryptase levels are usually not elevated.

Morphology

CM is characterized by an increased number of atypical MCs in the dermis. On hematoxylin and eosin (H&E) stained sections, atypical MCs usually show histiocytoid morphology and appear as round-oval or spindle in shape with moderate to abundant pale variably hypogranular cytoplasm (type I). In some cases, MCs may show pleomorphic, multilobated nuclei (type II) (*J Allergy Clin Immunol.* 2016;137:168-178. e1). In MPCM, MCs form loose aggregates with perivascular and periadnexal distribution. Polymorphic lesions show predominance of round to oval MCs and monomorphic lesions more often show spindled MC infiltrates. In DCM, diffuse sheets of MCs are present within the dermis. Mastocytoma(s) show diffuse sheets or nodular aggregates of MCs with abundant cytoplasm and may extend to the subcutis.

Immunophenotype

Both normal and neoplastic MCs show co-expression of CD117 (c-KIT) and tryptase, and these stains are very sensitive in detecting MC infiltrates. In mastocytosis, MCs can show aberrant expression of one or more of the following markers: CD25, CD2, and CD30.

Genetic Features

Somatic mutations involving the *KIT* gene are detected in most cases. Germline *KIT* mutations have been reported in some cases. Adult CM cases most frequently harbor the *KIT* p.D816V mutation in exon 17 (~80%), which is also present in children albeit at a lower frequency (~25%) (*Oncotarget.* 2015;6:18250-18264). A significant proportion of pediatric cases (~45%) show other activating *KIT* mutations (most commonly in exons 8, 9, and 11) and a small subset show wild-type *KIT* (*J Invest Dermatol.* 2010;130:804-815).

Prognosis and Treatment

CM in children is usually a self-limited disease with excellent prognosis, and lesions may completely resolve by adolescence. Adult-onset disease is persistent; however, it shows an indolent clinical course and overall survival is similar to the general population. Most adult patients may also have bone marrow involvement (such cases would be classified as SM). Treatment options include corticosteroids and other immunomodulating agents such as pimecrolimus.

II. SYSTEMIC MASTOCYTOSIS

SM is defined by the clonal expansion of MCs in organs outside the skin, although skin lesions can also occur. Bone marrow involvement occurs in nearly all cases, and less frequently, other organs like lymph nodes, spleen, liver, and gastrointestinal (GI) tract may also be affected. In contrast to CM which mostly affects children, SM is most often diagnosed in adults. The diagnostic criteria of SM and various subtypes (indolent and aggressive forms) are summarized in Tables 15.4 and 15.5, respectively. Identifying the presence or lack of "B" and "C" findings is important for subclassification (listed in Table 15.6).

TABLE 15.4 WHO-HAEM5 Diagnostic Criteria for Systemic Mastocytosis

The diagnosis of SM requires fulfillment of the major and one minor criterion or three minor criteria.

Major criterion
- Multifocal dense MC infiltrates (≥15 mast cells in aggregates) in bone marrow and/or extracutaneous organ(s).

Minor criteria
- >25% of all MCs show atypical morphology (type I or II) in bone marrow smears or show spindled morphology within dense MC infiltrates in sections of bone marrow core or other extracutaneous organs(s).
- *KIT* p.D816V mutation or other activating *KIT* mutation in bone marrow or extracutaneous organ(s)
- MCs aberrantly expressing one or more of the following: CD2, CD25, and CD30
- Serum tryptase level >20 ng/mL in the absence of an associated myeloid neoplasm[a]

MC, mast cell; SM, systemic mastocytosis.
[a]Elevated levels of serum tryptase can be seen in other myeloid neoplasms. The tryptase levels should be adjusted in hereditary α-tryptasemia.
Based on the WHO Classification of Tumours Editorial Board. Haematolymphoid tumours [Internet]. Lyon (France): International Agency for Research on Cancer; 2024 (WHO classification of tumours series, 5th ed.; vol. 11). Available from: https://tumourclassification.iarc.who.int/chapters/63.

TABLE 15.5 WHO-HAEM5 Diagnostic Criteria for SM Subtypes

SM Subtype	Diagnostic Criteria[a]
BMM	• No B-finding • No skin lesions • Serum tryptase <125 ng/mL • No dense MC infiltrates in an extramedullary organ
ISM	• ≤1 B-finding and typical skin lesions • ISM *without* skin lesions: ≤1 B-finding and/or serum tryptase ≥125 ng/mL and/or dense MC infiltrates in an extramedullary organ
SSM	• ≥2 B-findings • No C-finding
ASM	• ≥1 C-finding
SM-AHN	• Criteria met for SM and a WHO-defined hematologic neoplasm (HN). • Both diseases (SM and associated HN) are classified according to WHO diagnostic criteria.
MCL	• ≥20% MCs in BM smears • C-Findings present in cute MCL • C-Findings are not present in chronic MCL (better prognosis than acute MCL).

ASM, aggressive systemic mastocytosis; BMM, bone marrow mastocytosis; ISM, indolent systemic mastocytosis; MCL, mast cell leukemia; SSM, smoldering systemic mastocytosis; SM, systemic mastocytosis; SM-AHN, systemic mastocytosis with an associated hematologic neoplasm; WHO, World Health Organization.
[a]Fulfillment of SM criteria (see Table 15.4) is required in all subtypes. Identifying the presence or lack of B- and C-findings is important for subclassification (listed in Table 15.6).
Based on the WHO Classification of Tumours Editorial Board. Haematolymphoid tumours [Internet]. Lyon (France): International Agency for Research on Cancer; 2024 (WHO classification of tumours series, 5th ed.; vol. 11). Available from: https://tumourclassification.iarc.who.int/chapters/63.

Clinical Features

SM manifests a wide range of clinical behavior, and symptoms range from mild to severe. Common signs and symptoms include constitutional symptoms (fever, weight loss, fatigue, etc), MC mediator release–associated symptoms (flushing, hypotension, abdominal pain, diarrhea, respiratory symptoms anaphylaxis, etc), musculoskeletal manifestations (arthralgias, osteopenia, fractures), cytopenia(s), eosinophilia, hepatosplenomegaly, and lymphadenopathy. Skin manifestations including urticaria, pruritus, and dermographism may be present. Serum tryptase levels are persistently high (>20 ng/mL). Indolent forms of SM show milder symptoms and limited disease with a prolonged clinical course. Aggressive forms present with severe systemic

TABLE 15.6 B- and C-Findings

B-Findings	C-Findings
1. High MC burden • MC infiltration in the BM ≥30% and/or • Serum total tryptase level ≥200 ng/mL and/or • *KIT* p.D816V VAF ≥10% (BM or PB) **2. Myeloproliferative and/or myelodysplastic features** • Myeloproliferative features: leukocytosis, eosinophilia, increased BM cellularity • Myelodysplasia involving neutrophils, erythrocytes, or megakaryocytes (<10%) **3. Organomegaly** • Hepatomegaly without ascites • Splenomegaly without hypersplenism or weight loss • Lymphadenopathy (palpable or on imaging: >20 mm)	**1. Cytopenia(s) ≥1 of the following:** • ANC $<1 \times 10^9$/L • Hb < 10 g/dL • PLT $< 1.0 \times 10^9$/L **2. Hepatopathy** • Ascites and elevated liver enzymes ± hepatomegaly or cirrhotic liver ± portal hypertension **3. Splenomegaly** • Palpable splenomegaly with hypersplenism ± weight loss ± hypoalbuminemia **4. GI symptoms** • Malabsorption with hypoalbuminemia ± weight loss **5. Bone abnormalities** • Large-sized osteolysis (≥2 cm) with pathologic fracture ± bone pain

B-findings indicate a significant MC burden, involvement of various organ systems, and abnormalities of multiple myeloid lineages, but without any organ damage. In contrast, C-findings are indicative of organ damage caused by SM.
ANC, absolute neutrophil count; BM, bone marrow; GI, gastrointestinal; Hb, hemoglobin; MC, mast cell; PB, peripheral blood; PLT, platelet.
Modified from Valent P, Akin C, Hartmann K, et al. Updated diagnostic criteria and classification of mast cell disorders: a consensus proposal. *Hemasphere*. 2021;5(11):e646.

manifestations and progressive disease leading to multiorgan dysfunction and decreased life expectancy.

Morphology

Since bone marrow is almost always involved, the diagnosis of SM usually requires a bone marrow biopsy. Bone marrow core biopsy sections typically show a variable number of compact MC aggregates (≥15 MCs within an aggregate) predominantly in paratrabecular or perivascular distribution (e-Figure 15.1). A significant proportion of MCs show atypical morphology (usually type I) (see Table 15.2). Intermixed histiocytes, lymphocytes, eosinophils, and reticulin fibrosis may be present within the MC aggregates. The adjacent bone may show sclerotic changes. Atypical MCs can be seen on aspirate smears within and outside the spicules (e-Figure 15.1). The MC burden is low in the indolent forms, BMM and ISM (usually <10%) and higher in

SSM, ASM, and MCL. Diffuse sheets of MCs in bone marrow core biopsy sections and ≥20% MCs in aspirate smears is a feature of MCL (e-Figure 15.2). SM can be associated with other hematologic neoplasms and in some cases, the associated non-mast cell hematologic neoplasm may obscure SM. Careful bone marrow evaluation should be performed in all SM cases to exclude the presence of another hematologic neoplasm.

A subset of SM cases (<5%) show well-differentiated morphology, known as well-differentiated SM (WDSM). The MC aggregates in these cases show round MCs with prominent cytoplasmic granules (resembling normal/reactive MCs). WDSM also frequently lacks *KIT* p.D816V (*Cancers (Basel)*. 2022;14:3474).

Immunophenotype

MCs (both reactive and neoplastic) show co-expression of CD117 and tryptase. Neoplastic MCs typically show aberrant expression of one or more of the following: CD25, CD2, and CD30. The most common aberrant marker in SM is CD25 (*Am J Surg Pathol*. 2004;28:1319-1325). WDSM usually lacks expression of CD25 and CD2 but often shows CD30 co-expression, which is a helpful feature in differentiating from MC hyperplasia (*J Allergy Clin Immunol*. 2016;137:168-178.e1).

Genetic Features

KIT p.D816V (exon 17) is the most common mutation in SM. A small subset of cases (particularly WDSM) harbor other *KIT* mutations. Patients with SM-AHN may show additional mutations involving other genes. Mutations in *SRSF2*, *ASXL1*, *DNMT3A*, and *RUNX1* have been associated with worse outcomes (*Lancet Haematol*. 2021;8:e194-e204).

Prognosis and Treatment

Indolent SM has an excellent prognosis, and patients usually have a normal life expectancy. A small subset of cases may progress to AdvSM. Detection of *KIT* mutation with high variant allele frequency (VAF) at diagnosis increases the risk of progression. AdvSM (ASM, SM-AHN, and MCL) usually have poor prognosis. Treatment options include interferon-α and corticosteroids for symptomatic relief and cytoreductive therapies to decrease MC burden. Some patients with aggressive disease may benefit from hematopoietic stem cell transplant. Patients with SM-AHN also require therapy directed to the AHN.

III. MAST CELL SARCOMA

MCS is a very rare aggressive variant of mastocytosis, which can manifest as a *de novo* solid tumor or develop from preexisting SM. It occurs more frequently in adults. Unlike most other types of mastocytosis, *KIT* p.D816V mutations are rarely reported in MCS (*Oncotarget*. 2016;7:66299-66309). MCS usually presents as a localized destructive tumor and can occur at many sites, most commonly reported in the bones and GI tract, and less frequently in the lymph nodes, skin, spleen, and liver (*Oncotarget*. 2016;7:66299-66309).

Neoplastic MCs in MCS usually show markedly atypical morphology with immature appearing or highly pleomorphic cells. Intermixed eosinophils are frequently present. The differential diagnosis is broad on H&E sections including other

TABLE 15.7 WHO-HAEM5 Diagnostic Criteria for Mast Cell Sarcoma

Essential
- Localized tumor with infiltrative/destructive growth
- Tumor composed of MCs with marked atypia (MC lineage demonstrated by expression of CD117 and tryptase)
- Criteria for SM is not met in classic MCS cases.

Desirable

Aberrant expression of one or more of the following: CD2, CD25, and CD30

MC, mast cell; MCS, mast cell sarcoma.
Based on the WHO Classification of Tumours Editorial Board. Haematolymphoid tumours [Internet]. Lyon (France): International Agency for Research on Cancer; 2024 (WHO classification of tumours series, 5th ed.; vol. 11). Available from: https://tumourclassification.iarc.who.int/chapters/63.

sarcomas and poorly differentiated carcinoma. MC lineage of the tumor cells can be demonstrated by positive staining with CD117 and tryptase IHC. Similar to other types of mastocytosis, MCs in MCS may show aberrant expression of CD25, CD2, and CD30. Other nonspecific markers that can be positive include CD45, CD43, and CD68.

MCS is an aggressive disease with a poor prognosis. The disease shows rapid progression, may transform to AdSM, and resembles MCL in the terminal phase (*Br J Haematol.* 2020;189:e160-e164). The diagnostic criteria are summarized in Table 15.7.

Key Points

- Mastocytosis is a group of rare diseases characterized by clonal proliferation of MCs.
- *KIT* p.D816V is overall the most common mutation in mastocytosis.
- Neoplastic MCs often show atypical morphology: usually spindled cells with pale hypogranular cytoplasm.
- Both reactive and neoplastic MCs show expression of CD117 and tryptase. Neoplastic MCs usually show aberrant expression of one or more of the following markers: CD25, CD2, and CD30.
- CM is mostly diagnosed in children whereas SM is more common in adults.
- CM and indolent forms of SM usually have excellent prognosis in contrast to AdvSM, which shows poor prognosis.

Diagnostic caveats

- Neoplastic MCs show atypical morphology that overlaps with other neoplasms (eg, histiocytic and soft tissue tumors). Expression of CD117 and tryptase is required to demonstrate MC lineage.
- SM may be associated with another hematologic neoplasm (SM-AHN). It is critical to examine bone marrow samples to evaluate for concurrent AHN.
- A small subset of cases show typical MC morphology (WDSM) and also lack aberrant expression of CD2 and CD25. Aberrant expression of CD30 can be helpful in such cases.

SUGGESTED READINGS

Matito A, Azaña JM, Torrelo A, Alvarez-Twose I. Cutaneous mastocytosis in adults and children: new classification and prognostic factors. *Immunol Allergy Clin North Am*. 2018; 38(3):351-363.

Monnier J, Georgin-Lavialle S, Canioni D, et al. Mast cell sarcoma: new cases and literature review. *Oncotarget*. 2016;7(40):66299-66309.

Pardanani A. Systemic mastocytosis in adults: 2021 update on diagnosis, risk stratification and management. *Am J Hematol*. 2021;96(4):508-525.

Valent P, Akin C, Hartmann K, et al. Updated diagnostic criteria and classification of mast cell disorders: a consensus proposal. *Hemasphere*. 2021;5(11):e646.

16 Plasmacytoid Dendritic Cell Neoplasms
Xi Zhang, Alnoor, and Brooj Abro

Plasmacytoid dendritic cell (pDC) neoplasms include two distinct entities that are discussed in this chapter: blastic plasmacytoid dendritic cell neoplasm (BPDCN), an aggressive disease showing overlapping features with other blastoid neoplasms particularly acute myeloid leukemia (AML), and mature plasmacytoid dendritic cell proliferation associated with myeloid neoplasm (MPDCP), a clonal process arising in association with an underlying myeloid neoplasm.

I. BLASTIC PLASMACYTOID DENDRITIC CELL NEOPLASM

BPDCN, a rare and aggressive type of hematologic malignancy, is derived from pDC precursors and shows frequent skin and systemic involvement. BPDCN has a bimodal age distribution and most commonly affects men over the age of 60; however, cases have been reported in all age groups. The diagnostic criteria are summarized in Table 16.1.

Clinical Features

- **Clinical presentation:** Skin lesions are the most common initial manifestation; however, leukemic presentation without extramedullary disease has also been reported. Skin lesions are heterogeneous and can appear as bruise-like or erythematous papules, plaques, or tumor-like growths, commonly on the face, trunk, and extremities. Bone marrow involvement can lead to cytopenia(s). Some patients may also have lymphadenopathy.
- **Sites of involvement:** Skin (most common site), bone marrow, peripheral blood, lymph nodes, and central nervous system (CNS) may be involved at initial disease presentation or relapse.

Morphology

- **Bone marrow aspirate and blood smear:** On smear preparations, BPDCN tumor cells may resemble lymphoblasts or myeloblasts. The cells are typically small to medium sized, with scant agranular cytoplasm, round, irregular or elongated nuclei, fine chromatin, and variable nucleoli. The tumor cells may show eccentric nuclei and unipolar pseudopod-like cytoplasmic projections or blebs and cytoplasmic vacuoles (e-Figure 16.1).
- **Tissue sections:** On tissue sections, BPDCN is characterized by a monomorphic infiltrate with blastoid morphology. Frequent mitosis and apoptosis and intermixed tingible body macrophages imparting a "starry-sky appearance" may be present. Occasionally, the tumor cells may show immunoblastic morphology. Bone marrow involvement on core biopsy sections shows variable interstitial or diffuse infiltrate replacing hematopoietic cells (e-Figure 16.2). Background marrow elements may show dysplastic changes. In skin lesions, a diffuse dermal infiltrate with epidermal

TABLE 16.1 WHO-HAEM5 Diagnostic Criteria for Blastic Plasmacytoid Dendritic Cell Neoplasm (BPDCN)

Essential
- Morphology: immature, blastoid cells
- Immunophenotype: consistent with pDC differentiation (see criteria below)

Desirable
- Absence of lymphoid or myeloid lineage–specific markers
- Absence of CD34 expression
- High Ki-67 proliferation index

Immunophenotypic criteria for BPDCN
- Expression of CD123 and one other pDC marker (listed below) in addition to CD4 and/or CD56
- Expression of any three pDC markers and absence of all expected negative markers (listed below)

pDC markers	Expected negative
1. CD123	1. CD3
2. TCF4	2. CD14
3. TCL1	3. CD19
4. CD303	4. CD34
5. CD304	5. Lysozyme
	6. Myeloperoxidase

pDC, plasmacytoid dendritic cell.
Based on the *WHO Classification of Tumours Editorial Board. Haematolymphoid tumours* [Internet]. Lyon (France): International Agency for Research on Cancer; 2024 (WHO classification of tumours series, 5th edition; vol. 11). Available from: https://tumourclassification.iarc.who.int/chapters/63.

sparing is the typical histologic finding (e-Figure 16.3). The infiltrate may extend to the subcutaneous tissue. Lymph nodes involved by BPDCN show partial or complete effacement. In cases with partial nodal involvement, paracortical and medullary regions are typically involved, and the B cell follicles may be spared.

Immunophenotype

The tumor cells are positive for pDC markers (CD123, TCL-1, TCF4, and CD303/BDCA-2), CD4, CD56, and HLA-DR. Loss of one or more pDC markers may be observed. Except CD303, all these markers can be positive in AML. Other nonspecific markers that may be positive in BPDCN include the following: CD43, CD45, CD79a, TdT, S100, CD2, CD7, PD-1, and certain myelomonocytic markers including CD33, CD36, CD68, and CD117 (*Am J Surg Pathol.* 2014;38:673-680). It is important to evaluate for the expression of myeloid and lymphoid lineage–specific markers to exclude acute lymphoblastic leukemia (ALL) and AML. Comprehensive immunophenotyping using flow cytometry and immunohistochemistry is helpful in establishing the diagnosis of BPDCN. BPDCN is negative for CD3, CD19, CD20, myeloperoxidase, lysozyme, CD14, and CD34. See Table 16.1 for the immunophenotypic criteria required for the diagnosis of BPDCN.

Genetic Features

BPDCN does not have specific disease-defining molecular abnormalities. Most BPDCN cases (~75%) demonstrate a complex karyotype. *MYC* and *MYB* rearrangements have been reported (*Hematol Oncol Clin North Am.* 2020;34:523-538). Next generation sequencing (NGS) studies have shown recurrent mutations in genes associated with myeloid neoplasms including *ASXL1, TET2, DNMT3A, ZRSR2, NRAS, SRSF2, IDH2, JAK2, KRAS,* and *TP53* (*Cancers (Basel).* 2021;13:5888).

Prognosis and Treatment

BPDCN is an aggressive disease with poor outcomes. A recent multicenter study reported a median overall survival of 24 months in 59 patients (*Blood.* 2019;134:678-687). Similar outcomes were reported in patients with primary skin or systemic disease at presentation. Treatment options include Hyper-CVAD (cyclophosphamide, vincristine, doxorubicin/adriamycin, dexamethasone)-based therapy, CD123 and BCL-2 targeted therapy, and allogeneic hematopoietic stem cell transplantation in eligible patients (*Blood Adv.* 2022;6:3027-3035). BPDCN in pediatric patients is less aggressive with better outcomes compared to adults and responds to high-risk ALL chemotherapy regimens (*Haematologica.* 2010;95:1873-1879).

Differential Diagnosis

The major differential diagnosis is AML. AML with monocytic differentiation is particularly challenging to exclude. Strong expression of pDC markers and negative expression of myeloid lineage–specific markers helps in establishing the diagnosis of BPDCN. BPDCN does not harbor AML-defining genetic abnormalities. MPDCP should also be excluded (discussed below). The morphology of MPDCP is usually similar to mature pDCs in contrast to blastoid morphology of BPDCN, and CD56 is generally negative.

Key Points

- BPDCN is a rare aggressive neoplasm derived from pDC precursors.
- Patients with BPDCN present with skin lesions (most common site of involvement) and/or leukemic disease.
- The tumor cells typically show blastoid morphology and the following immunophenotypic findings: CD4 (+), CD56 (+), CD123 (+), TCL-1 (+), HLA-DR (+), CD34 (−), CD117 (−/+), myeloperoxidase (−), lysozyme (−), CD14 (−), CD3 (−), CD19 (−).
- Complex karyotype is frequent, and recurrent mutations in genes associated with myeloid neoplasms have been reported (*ASXL1, TET2,* and others). BPDCN does not have a specific disease-defining genetic abnormality.

Diagnostic Caveats

- The clinical presentation, morphology, and immunophenotype overlap with other myeloid and lymphoid leukemias.
- A comprehensive immunophenotypic profile is necessary to exclude ALL and AML.
- BPDCN should also be distinguished from MPDCP.

II. MATURE PLASMACYTOID DENDRITIC CELL PROLIFERATION ASSOCIATED WITH MYELOID NEOPLASM

MPDCP represents a clonal expansion of pDCs in association with a myeloid neoplasm, most commonly found in the bone marrow and skin and occasionally in lymph nodes. The diagnostic criteria are summarized in Table 16.2.

MPDCP predominantly affects men and is most frequently reported in association with chronic myelomonocytic leukemia (CMML). Other associated myeloid neoplasms include myelodysplastic syndrome/neoplasms (MDS) and AML. Studies have shown that MPDCP in association with AML (pDC-AML) demonstrates a similar genetic profile as the AML blasts, indicating that pDCs originate from blasts in pDC-AML, and *RUNX-1* was found to be the most frequently mutated gene in these cases (*Haematologica*. 2021;106(12):3056-3066).

Morphologically, MPDCP typically shows nodular aggregates or clusters of cells with plasmacytoid morphology without significant atypia or pleomorphism. The immunophenotype is similar to that of mature pDCs; positive expression of CD123, CD4, TCL1, TCF4, CD303, and CD304. According to the WHO-HAEM5, MPDCP may show loss of normal pDC antigen expression, and aberrant expression of CD34, CD56, and TdT may also be observed. The clinical picture is generally reflective of the underlying myeloid neoplasm, which also determines the treatment. MPDCP has been shown to be a poor prognostic factor, and its recognition may be important for prognostication and therapeutic decision making (*Blood Adv*. 2020;4:5425-5430; *Blood*. 2021;137:1377-1391).

TABLE 16.2 WHO-HAEM5 Diagnostic Criteria for Mature Plasmacytoid Dendritic Cell Proliferation Associated With Myeloid Neoplasm (MPDCP)

Essential	Desirable
- Morphology: mature plasmacytoid cells - Immunophenotype: expression of CD123 and/or other pDC antigens - Presence of a defined myeloid neoplasm	- Aberrant pDC immunophenotype - Absence or low expression of CD56

pDC, plasmacytoid dendritic cell.
Based on the *WHO Classification of Tumours Editorial Board. Haematolymphoid tumours* [Internet]. Lyon (France): International Agency for Research on Cancer; 2024 (WHO classification of tumours series, 5th edition; vol. 11). Available from https://tumourclassification.iarc.who.int/chapters/63.

SUGGESTED READINGS

Julia F, Dalle S, Duru G, et al. Blastic plasmacytoid dendritic cell neoplasms: clinico-immunohistochemical correlations in a series of 91 patients. *Am J Surg Pathol*. 2014;38(5):673-680.

Lucas N, Duchmann M, Rameau P, et al. Biology and prognostic impact of clonal plasmacytoid dendritic cells in chronic myelomonocytic leukemia. *Leukemia*. 2019;33(10):2466-2480.

Yin CC, Pemmaraju N, You MJ, et al. Integrated clinical genotype-phenotype characteristics of blastic plasmacytoid dendritic cell neoplasm. *Cancers (Basel)*. 2021;13(23):5888.

Zalmaï L, Viailly PJ, Biichle S, et al. Plasmacytoid dendritic cells proliferation associated with acute myeloid leukemia: phenotype profile and mutation landscape. *Haematologica*. 2021;106(12):3056-3066.

PART 2: Lymphoid Neoplasms

Overview and Classification of Lymphoid Neoplasms

Amna Qureshi and Cecilia C. S. Yeung

In the fast-paced world of genomic sequencing, evidence-based classification, and targeted therapies, an updated classification system became imperative to guide personalized patient care. Advancements in sequencing techniques empowered pathologists not only to diagnose neoplastic lymphoid proliferations but also provide valuable insights for prognosis and treatment. Molecular data enabled identification of therapy targets and facilitated the detection of minimal residual disease.

In 2022, two similar classifications emerged: one proposed by International Consensus Classification (ICC) and the other by WHO 5th Edition (WHO-HAEM5). These classifications were built upon the foundation laid by the revised European American classification of lymphoid neoplasms (REAL) in 1994, which provided the basis of WHO classification published in 2001 followed by updates in 2008 and 2017 (*Leukemia*. 2022;36(7):1720-1748). Although most of the entities' diagnostic criteria remained unchanged, there were refinements in nomenclature based on clinical information, immunophenotype, and molecular data. New entities were introduced, provisional entities were upgraded to definite entities, and old entities were deleted. A distinctive feature of the WHO-HAEM5 is the inclusion of essential and desirable diagnostic criteria for each entity. Unlike the ICC, WHO-HAEM5 did not incorporate provisional entities. Notably, the WHO-HAEM5 introduced the category of tumor-like lesions with B-cell or T-cell predominance, aiming to prevent overdiagnosis of lymphomas. The classification of lymphoid neoplasms and updates (WHO-HAEM5 and ICC) are summarized in Table 17.1.

TABLE 17.1 Classification of Lymphoid Neoplasms (WHO-HAEM5 and ICC)

Tumor-Like Lesions With B-Cell Proliferation

ICC

Multicentric Castleman disease

WHO-HAEM5

- Reactive B-cell-rich lymphoid proliferations that can mimic lymphoma
- Unicentric Castleman disease
- Idiopathic multicentric Castleman disease
- KSHV-/HHV-8-associated multicentric Castleman disease
- IgG4-related disease

Preneoplastic Small Lymphocytic Proliferations

ICC

Monoclonal B-cell lymphocytosis
- CLL type (low and high count)
- Non-CLL type
- Atypical CLL type

WHO-HAEM5

Monoclonal B-cell lymphocytosis
- Low-count or clonal B-cell expansion
- CLL/SLL type
- Non-CLL/SLL type

B-Cell Lymphomas

ICC

Chronic lymphocytic leukemia/small lymphocytic lymphoma (CLL/SLL)

B prolymphocytic leukemia (B PLL)

Splenic B-cell lymphomas
- Splenic marginal zone lymphoma
- Hairy cell leukemia (HCL)
- Hairy cell leukemia variant (provisional)
- Splenic diffuse red pulp small B-cell lymphoma (provisional)

Marginal zone lymphoma
- Nodal marginal zone lymphoma
- Pediatric nodal marginal zone lymphoma
- Primary cutaneous marginal zone lymphoproliferative disorder
- Extranodal marginal zone lymphoma of mucosa-associated lymphoid tissue (MALT)

WHO-HAEM5

Chronic lymphocytic leukemia/small lymphocytic lymphoma (CLL/SLL)

Removed

Splenic B-cell lymphomas
- Splenic marginal zone lymphoma
- Hairy cell leukemia
- Splenic B-cell lymphoma/leukemia with prominent nucleoli (distinct from HCL and includes all previous CD5-negative B PLL)
- Splenic diffuse red pulp small B-cell lymphoma

Marginal zone lymphoma
- Nodal marginal zone lymphoma
- Pediatric nodal marginal zone lymphoma
- Primary cutaneous marginal zone lymphoma
- Extranodal marginal zone lymphoma of mucosa-associated lymphoid tissue (MALT)

(continued)

TABLE 17.1 Classification of Lymphoid Neoplasms (WHO-HAEM5 and ICC) (*continued*)

Follicular lymphoma
- In situ follicular neoplasia
- Follicular lymphoma
- Duodenal type follicular lymphoma
- Primary cutaneous follicle center lymphoma
- Bcl-2 rearrangement negative, CD23 positive follicle center lymphoma
- Pediatric-type follicular lymphoma
- Testicular follicular lymphoma

Mantle cell lymphoma
- In situ mantle cell neoplasia
- Mantle cell lymphoma
- Leukemic nonnodal mantle cell lymphoma

Not included as a separate entity

Large B-cell lymphoma
- Diffuse large B-cell lymphoma, NOS
- T-cell/histiocyte-rich B-cell lymphoma
- Plasmablastic lymphoma
- EBV-positive diffuse large B-cell lymphoma
- Primary diffuse large B-cell lymphoma of central nervous system
- Primary diffuse large B-cell lymphoma of testes
- Diffuse large B-cell lymphoma associated with chronic inflammation
- Intravascular large B-cell lymphoma
- ALK-positive large B-cell lymphoma

Follicular lymphoma
- In situ follicular neoplasm
- Follicular lymphoma
- Duodenal type follicular lymphoma
- Primary cutaneous follicle center lymphoma
- Follicular lymphoma with a predominantly diffuse pattern
- Pediatric-type follicular lymphoma

Mantle cell lymphoma
- In situ mantle cell neoplasm
- Mantle cell lymphoma
- Leukemic nonnodal mantle cell lymphoma

Transformations of indolent B-cell lymphomas

Large B-cell lymphoma
- Diffuse large B-cell lymphoma, NOS
- T-cell/histiocyte-rich B-cell lymphoma
- Plasmablastic lymphoma
- EBV-positive diffuse large B-cell lymphoma
- Primary large B-cell lymphoma of immune-privileged sites
- Diffuse large B-cell lymphoma associated with chronic inflammation
- Intravascular large B-cell lymphoma
- ALK-positive large B-cell lymphoma
- Large B-cell lymphoma with *IRF4* rearrangement
- Fibrin-associated large B-cell lymphoma

TABLE 17.1 Classification of Lymphoid Neoplasms (WHO-HAEM5 and ICC) (*continued*)

- Large B-cell lymphoma with *IRF4* rearrangement
- Fibrin-associated large B-cell lymphoma
- Mediastinal gray zone lymphoma
- High-grade B-cell lymphoma with *MYC* and *BCL2* rearrangements (provisional entity)
- High-grade B-cell lymphoma with *MYC* and *BCL6* rearrangement
- High-grade B-cell lymphoma, NOS
- Large B-cell lymphoma with 11 q aberration
- Lymphomatoid granulomatosis
- HHV-8 and EBV8-negative primary effusion-based lymphoma
- Primary cutaneous diffuse large B-cell lymphoma, leg type
- Burkitt lymphoma

- Mediastinal gray zone lymphoma
- Diffuse large B-cell lymphoma/high-grade B-cell lymphoma with *MYC* and *BCL2* rearrangements (previous high-grade B-cell lymphoma with *MYC* and *BCL6* rearrangements is designated as DLBCL, NOS)
- High-grade B-cell lymphoma, NOS
- High-grade B-cell lymphoma with 11 q aberration
- Lymphomatoid granulomatosis
- Fluid overload–associated large B-cell lymphoma
- Primary cutaneous diffuse large B-cell lymphoma, leg type
- Burkitt lymphoma

Hodgkin Lymphomas

ICC

- Nodular lymphocyte predominant B-cell lymphoma
- Classic Hodgkin lymphoma

WHO-HAEM5

- Nodular lymphocyte predominant Hodgkin lymphoma
- Classic Hodgkin lymphoma

Plasma Cell Neoplasms

ICC

- Multiple myeloma (MM), NOS
- MM with recurrent genetic abnormality
  - MM with *MAF* family translocation
  - MM with hyperdiploidy
  - MM with *CCND* family translocation
  - MM with *NSD2* family translocation
- Extraosseous plasmacytoma
- Solitary plasmacytoma of bone

WHO-HAEM5

- Plasma cell myeloma

- Extraosseous plasmacytoma
- Solitary plasmacytoma of bone

(*continued*)

TABLE 17.1	Classification of Lymphoid Neoplasms (WHO-HAEM5 and ICC) (*continued*)
• Plasma cell neoplasm with associated paraneoplastic syndrome 　• TEMPI 　• POEMS • IgM monoclonal gammopathy of undetermined significance (IgM MGUS) 　• IgM MGUS, NOS 　• IgM MGUS, plasma cell type • Non-IgM monoclonal gammopathy of undetermined significance • Primary cold agglutinin disease	• Plasma cell neoplasm with associated paraneoplastic syndrome 　• AESOP 　• TEMPI 　• POEMS • IgM monoclonal gammopathy of undetermined significance • Non-IgM monoclonal gammopathy of undetermined significance • Monoclonal gammopathy of renal significance • Cold agglutinin disease

AESOP, adenopathy and extensive skin patch overlying a plasmacytoma; ALK, anaplastic lymphoma kinase; EBV, Epstein-Barr virus; HHV8, human herpesvirus-8; ICC, International Consensus Classification; KSHV, Kaposi sarcoma–associated herpesvirus; NOS, not otherwise specified.

I. OVERVIEW OF B-CELL LYMPHOID PROLIFERATIONS AND LYMPHOMAS

WHO-HAEM5 broadens the classification of B-cell lymphoid proliferations and lymphomas, which now includes five subcategories: tumor-like lesions with B-cell predominance, precursor B-cell neoplasms, mature B-cell lymphomas, Hodgkin lymphomas, and plasma cell neoplasms and related diseases with paraproteins.

II. OVERVIEW OF TUMOR-LIKE LESIONS WITH B-CELL PREDOMINANCE

These lesions can disrupt the normal nodal architecture and often contain atypical cells raising important differential diagnostic concerns. The entities in this group include Castleman disease, IgG4-related disease, progressive transformation of germinal centers, infectious mononucleosis, florid reactive lymphoid hyperplasia/lymphoma-like lesion of the female genital tract, and systemic lupus erythematosus. It is, however, crucial to make a precise diagnosis by integrating the patient's clinical history, histologic findings, and serologic results to prevent overdiagnosis of lymphoma.

III. OVERVIEW OF ACUTE LEUKEMIA/LYMPHOMAS

Acute lymphoblastic leukemias are hematopoietic neoplasms characterized by clonal proliferation of immature B cells or T cells. In the updated WHO-HAEM5 classification, precursor B-cell neoplasms are categorized into 12 entities of B lymphoblastic leukemia/lymphoma (B-LBL) with defined genetic alterations and B lymphoblastic lymphoma/leukemia, not otherwise specified (NOS). Diagnosis of B acute lymphoblastic leukemia (B-ALL) involves morphology and immunophenotyping, with further subclassification based on specific cytogenetic and/or molecular abnormalities. Most of the B-ALL cases can therefore be diagnosed as such, with hyperdiploidy and hypodiploidy, chromosomal rearrangements such as iAMP21, BCR: ABL1 fusion, KMT2A rearrangement, ETV 6: RUNX1 fusion. B-ALL with TCF3: HLF fusion has been added to the WHO-HAEM5 and is characterized by aggressive behavior (*Eur J Biochem*. 1990;188(1):147-153). The NOS category is used for cases that lack specific genetic abnormalities following comprehensive testing.

The T-ALL/LBL arise from mutations in tumor suppressive pathways, ribosomal dysfunction, and formation of long noncoding RNA strands, disrupting T-cell development. These mutations affect crucial cell pathways like JAK/STAT, NOTCH 1, RAS-MAPK, CDKN2A, and PI3K/AKT, involved in signal transduction, cell cycle progression, and thymocyte specification. However, genetically defined T-ALL subtypes are quite heterogeneous, the most common being the mutations in NOTCH1 and CDKN2A noted in up to 50% of cases (*Genes (Basel)*. 2021;12(8):1118).

NK lymphoblastic leukemia/lymphoma, previously a provisional entity in the 4th edition of WHO, is not listed in WHO-HAEM5 due to insufficient diagnostic criteria and overlap with other conditions like blastic plasmacytoid dendritic cell neoplasm, acute myeloid leukemia, and CD56-positive acute undifferentiated leukemia (AUL). Acute leukemias of ambiguous lineage (ALAL) encompass AUL and mixed phenotype acute leukemia (MPAL) (*Br J Haematol*. 1993;84(1):49-60). Immunophenotyping by flow cytometry is the best way for lineage assignment. In AUL, the blasts lack clear-cut criteria for any specific lineage and in MPAL blasts show expression of multiple lineage-specific antigens. A wide variety of molecular and genetic abnormalities are also associated with ALAL such as KMT2A rearrangement. These leukemias are usually B/myeloid immunophenotype but can be B/T lineage, indicating lineage plasticity in progenitor cells (*Blood*. 2011;117(11):3163-3171).

IV. OVERVIEW OF MATURE B-CELL LYMPHOMAS

In the realm of B cell lymphoproliferative disorders, a distinction exists between clonal and nonclonal manifestations. Nonclonal B-cell lymphoproliferative disorders can emerge in the context of infections and autoimmune disorders, whereas B-cell lymphomas signify a clonal expansion of mature B cells. The WHO-HAEM5 classification adheres to the traditional approach of characterizing lymphoid neoplasms based on their cell lineage. While some neoplasms may resemble normal B cells at various stages of maturation, others deviate, necessitating classification based on characteristic genetic/genomic changes, specific clinical features, and association with infectious agents such as Epstein-Barr virus (EBV) and human herpesvirus-8 (HHV-8). The WHO-HAEM5 recognizes 17 specific entities, classifying them according to their site of origin, genetic features, and clinical context. In some entities, the term "large B-cell lymphoma" is used when the diffuse growth pattern cannot be entirely assessed, as seen in fibrin-associated large B-cell lymphoma and fluid overload large B-cell lymphoma. The WHO-HAEM5 introduces the concept of low-count monoclonal B-cell lymphocytosis or clonal B-cell expansion, denoting clonal B-cell counts below 0.5×10^9/L. It also addresses the prolymphocytic progression of chronic lymphocytic leukemia (CLL) and Richter's transformation, characterized by transformation into large cells only after ruling out the treatment effect of ibrutinib (*Br J Haematol*. 2020;191(1):e22-e25).

A new entity, splenic B-cell lymphoma/leukemia with prominent nucleoli is included, encompassing hairy cell leukemia variant and CD5-negative B prolymphocytic leukemia. B prolymphocytic leukemia is no longer recognized as a distinct category and can be categorized under mantle cell lymphoma with IGH:CCND1, prolymphocytic progression of CLL/small lymphocytic lymphoma (SLL), and splenic B-cell lymphoma/leukemia with prominent nucleoli. ICC still recognizes B prolymphocytic leukemia, but the diagnosis should only be made in cases without prior history of B-cell lymphomas.

In the WHO-HAEM5 classification, three morphologic subtypes of follicular lymphoma are recognized based on BCL-2 rearrangement. These include classic follicular lymphoma with t(14;18)(q32;q21)/IGH::BCL2 fusion, follicular large B-cell lymphoma which corresponds to previous grade 3B but lacks BCL-2 translocation (IRF4 rearrangement analysis should be performed by fluorescence in situ hybridization [FISH] studies) and follicular lymphoma with uncommon features. Because follicular lymphoma grades 1, 2, and 3A have shown similar clinical outcomes as well as immunohistochemistry and genetic profiles (*J Clin Oncol*. 2019;37(31):2815-2824; *Ann Oncol*. 2016;27(7):1323-1329) and reproducibility of grading has been challenging, this grading is no longer mandated. Furthermore, FL grade 3B is now termed follicular large B-cell lymphomas based on clinical behavior, which is more closely aligned with DLBCL. In contrast, the consensus in ICC is to retain morphologic grading of follicular lymphoma as it is important to distinguish between FL 3A which is treated as grade 1 or grade 2 and grade 3B is usually treated as DLBCL. ICC also includes provisional entity: BCl-2 rearrangement negative, CD23 positive follicular center lymphoma. Additionally, testicular follicular lymphoma is another new entity recognized by ICC.

Pediatric marginal zone lymphoma is now a distinct category in WHO-HAEM5 but in ICC this is a provisional entity.

Notably, both the WHO HAEM5 and ICC recognize fibrin-associated large B-cell lymphoma as a novel entity. Furthermore, primary large B-cell lymphoma of immune-privileged sites includes diffuse large B-cell lymphoma of extranodal sites including central nervous system (CNS), vitreoretinal compartment, and testes in WHO-HAEM5. This conclusion is based on several common morphologic, immunophenotypic, and genetic findings including but not limited to concordant *MYD88* and *CD79a* mutations.

High-Grade B-Cell Lymphomas

High-grade B-cell lymphoma with 11 q aberration, previously termed Burkitt-like lymphoma with 11 q aberration (a provisional entity), is now officially recognized as a distinct new entity in WHO-HAEM5. However, it remains a provisional entity in ICC. For Burkitt lymphoma, WHO-HAEM5 recommends using EBV status for its subtyping rather than considering epidemiologic factors.

Large B-cell lymphoma with IRF4 rearrangement, previously a provisional entity, is now a distinct entity in both WHO and ICC. Additionally, high-grade B-cell lymphoma with MYC and BCL-2 and/or BCL6 rearrangements previously classified as a single entity are now two separate entities due to differences in genetic profiles and mutational landscape. B-cell lymphoma with MYC and BCL-2 rearrangement is now renamed as diffuse large B-cell lymphoma/high-grade B-cell lymphoma with MYC and BCL-2 rearrangements in WHO-HAEM5. High-grade B-cell lymphoma with MYC and BCL6 rearrangement is a provisional entity in ICC whereas WHO-HAEM5 recognizes this entity as diffuse large B-cell lymphoma, NOS or high-grade lymphoma, NOS based on its cytomorphologic features.

The term "mediastinal gray zone lymphoma" has replaced B-cell lymphoma, unclassifiable with features intermediate between diffuse large B-cell lymphoma and classical Hodgkin lymphoma. This category now encompasses B-cell lymphomas with overlapping features between primary mediastinal B-cell lymphoma and classic Hodgkin lymphoma especially nodular sclerosis type.

WHO has introduced the concept of "transformation of indolent B-cell lymphomas," recognizing the genetic alterations leading to the transformation of indolent lymphomas like CLL, follicular or marginal zone lymphoma into large B-cell lymphomas. These transformed lymphomas maintain the immunophenotype of their low-grade counterparts.

Lymphoid Proliferations and Lymphomas Associated With Immune Deficiency and Dysregulation

This is the new terminology used in WHO-HAEM5, which is based on histologic features, viral association (notably EBV and Kaposi sarcoma–associated herpesvirus [KSHV]/HHV-8), and type of immunodeficiency/dysregulation. The subcategories include hyperplasia, polymorphic lymphoproliferative disorder, mucocutaneous ulcer, and lymphomas with diagnostic criteria similar to immunocompetent patients. Immune deficiency/dysregulation settings include inborn errors of immunity, HIV infection, posttransplant (solid organ or bone marrow), autoimmune disease, iatrogenic/therapy-related conditions, and immune senescence (*Leukemia*. 2022;36(7): 1720-1748). Additional details are discussed in Chapter 22.

V. OVERVIEW OF HODGKIN LYMPHOMA

In classic Hodgkin lymphoma, Reed-Sternberg cells originate from germinal center B cells due to malfunctioning B-cell pathways like JAK-STAT pathway, leading to alterations in STAT3, STAT5B, JAK1, JAK2, and PTPN1 (*Blood*. 2018;131(22): 2454-2465). The diagnostic criteria for classical Hodgkin lymphoma remain consistent in both WHO-HAEM5 and ICC classifications. However, in the ICC, nodular lymphocyte-predominant Hodgkin lymphoma (NLPHL) has been renamed as nodular lymphocyte-predominant B-cell lymphoma. Although NLPHL is recognized as a distinct neoplasm from classic Hodgkin lymphoma, the WHO-HAEM5 continues to use the NLPHL terminology to avoid confusion in clinical trials and practice.

VI. OVERVIEW OF PLASMA CELL NEOPLASMS AND OTHER DISEASES WITH PARAPROTEINS

Monoclonal gammopathy of renal significance (MGRS), cold agglutinin disease (CAD), and AESOP syndrome (adenopathy and extensive skin patch overlying a plasmacytoma) are new conditions added to the category of "plasma cell neoplasms (PCNs) and other diseases with paraproteins" in WHO-HAEM5.

VII. OVERVIEW OF T CELL LYMPHOMAS

In WHO-HAEM5, the T-cell and NK-cell neoplasms are grouped under a comprehensive category of T-cell and NK-cell lymphoid proliferations and lymphomas.

This category also includes tumor-like lesions with T-cell predominance and precursor T-cell neoplasms, allowing classification based on presentation, cell of origin, morphology, and shared immunophenotypic features.

WHO-HAEM5 introduces non-neoplastic entities including Kikuchi-Fujimoto disease, indolent T-lymphoblastic proliferation, and autoimmune lymphoproliferative syndrome. Additionally, new entities like primary cutaneous peripheral T-cell lymphoma NOS, indolent NK-cell lymphoproliferative disorder of the gastrointestinal tract, and EBV-positive nodal T- and NK-cell lymphoma are included.

Advances in molecular testing, particularly next-generation sequencing, have enhanced our biologic understanding of T- and NK-cell lymphomas. These techniques provide crucial insights into the mechanisms underlying the malignant behavior of these neoplasms, offering valuable data for prognosis, and identifying therapeutic targets. For instance, anaplastic lymphoma kinase (ALK)-positive anaplastic large-cell lymphoma demonstrates NPM: ALK fusion, while ALK-negative anaplastic large T-cell lymphoma shows gene fusions like DUSP22, TP63, ROS1, and TYK2, serving as important genetic events and prognostic indicators. Point mutations and copy number changes are also identified in several T-cell lymphomas that lead to the activation of targetable pathways such as JAK/STAT and PI3K/AKT (*Cancers (Basel)*. 2022;14(15):3716).

Mature T-cell and NK-cell neoplasms consist of nine subcategories based on the cell of origin, clinical scenario, location of the disease, and cytomorphology. While most of the T-cell and NK-cell lymphomas can be classified according to cell lineage, certain lymphomas exhibit overlapping features or an indeterminant phenotype, as seen in EBV-positive nodal T- and NK-cell lymphomas and extranodal NK-/T-cell lymphomas. These overlapping cases are classified accordingly.

Furthermore, primary cutaneous T-cell lymphoid proliferations and lymphomas, newly recognized entities in the mature T-cell and NK-cell neoplasms category, are distinct due to their specific clinical features and genetic landscape.

SUGGESTED READINGS

Alaggio R, Amador C, Anagnostopoulos I, et al. The 5th edition of the World Health Organization Classification of haematolymphoid tumours: lymphoid neoplasms. *Leukemia*. 2022;36:1720-1748. doi:10.1038/s41375-022-01620-2

Campo E, Jaffe ES, Cook JR, et al. The International Consensus Classification of mature lymphoid neoplasms: a report from the Clinical Advisory Committee. *Blood*. 2022;140(11):1229-1253.

Falini B, Martino G, Lazzi S. A comparison of the International Consensus and 5th World Health Organization classifications of mature B-cell lymphomas. *Leukemia*. 2023;37(1):18-34. doi:10.1038/s41375-022-01764-1

Fend F, van den Brand M, Groenen PJ, et al. Diagnostic and prognostic molecular pathology of lymphoid malignancies. *Virchows Arch*. 2023. doi:10.1007/s00428-023-03644-0

Li W. The 5th edition of the World Health Organization classification of hematolymphoid tumors. In: Li W, ed. *Leukemia* [Internet]. Exon Publications; 2022.

WHO Classification of Tumors Editorial Board. Hematolymphoid tumors [Internet; beta version ahead of print (in progress)]. In: *WHO Classification of Tumors Series*. 5th ed. International Agency for Research on Cancer; 2022 [cited 2022 Aug 29]. https://tumourclassification.iarc.who.int

18 Precursor Lymphoid Neoplasms and Leukemias of Ambiguous Lineage

18.1 B-Lymphoblastic Leukemia/Lymphoma

Ishaq A. Asghar and Alexandra E. Kovach

B-lymphoblastic leukemia/lymphoma (B-ALL/LBL) is a neoplasm of precursor B lymphocytes. ALL represents 12% of all leukemia cases, with a worldwide incidence projected to be 1 to 4.75 per 100,000 people. The highest incidences of ALL occur in Italy, the United States, Switzerland, and Costa Rica (*Eur J Cancer Care (Engl).* 2005;14(1):53-62). B-ALL is the most common malignancy of childhood, with 80% of all cases presenting in patients aged less than 6. B-LBL is 10% of all LBL cases and is more common in patients aged less than 18 years (*Am J Clin Pathol.* 2001;115(6):868-875; *Mayo Clin Proc.* 2016;91(11):1645-1666). Down syndrome (DS) children have a 10-fold higher risk of developing B-ALL. Patients with DS-associated B-ALL have different associated somatic mutations; 50% of cases harboring *CRLF2* rearrangements (CRLF2-R), compared with only 5% to 10% of non-DS cases, experience increased rates of relapse and have increased mortality (*J Clin Oncol.* 2024;42(2):218-227). The diagnosis of B-ALL/LBL requires a combination of morphologic and immunophenotypic findings, along with further classification based on cytogenetic and/or molecular abnormalities. Both the WHO-HAEM5 and International Consensus Classification (ICC) offer similar classifications of B-ALL/LBL with some differences and a few provisional subtypes in each, based on whole transcriptome analysis and gene expression studies (*Leukemia.* 2022;36(7):1720-1748; *Blood.* 2022;140(11):1200-1228). See Table 18.1-1.

Clinical Features

- **B-ALL:** B-ALL involves bone marrow, with or without peripheral blood or other extramedullary sites, including the central nervous system (CNS), testis, lymph nodes, spleen, and liver.
- **B-LBL:** B-LBL (extramedullary B-ALL) forms tissue masses involving lymph nodes, skin, soft tissue, and bone.

This distinction between B-ALL and B-LBL is not exclusive and they can overlap. There is no strict quantity required to diagnose B-ALL/LBL, unlike myeloid neoplasms; nevertheless, the presence of at least 20% to 25% blasts is used by most treatment protocols. The diagnostic criteria for B-ALL/LBL are summarized in Table 18.1-2.

TABLE 18.1-1 Classification of B-Lymphoblastic Leukemia/Lymphoma (B-ALL)

WHO-HAEM5	ICC
B-ALL, NOS	B-ALL, NOS
B-ALL with recurrent genetic abnormalities	
B-ALL with *BCR::ABL1* fusion	B-ALL with t(9;22)(q34.1;q11.2)/*BCR::ABL1*
	• With lymphoid-only involvement
	• With multilineage involvement
B-ALL with *BCR::ABL1*–like features	B-ALL *BCR::ABL1*–like, *ABL-1* class rearranged
	B-ALL *BCR::ABL1*–like, *JAK-STAT* activated
	B-ALL *BCR::ABL1*–like, NOS
B-ALL with high hyperdiploidy	B-ALL hyperdiploid
B-ALL with hypodiploidy (low-hypodiploid/near-hypodiploid)	B-ALL low-hypodiploid
	B-ALL near-haploid
B-ALL with *KMT2A* rearrangement	B-ALL with t(v;11q23.3)/*KMT2A* rearranged
B-ALL with *iAMP21*	B-ALL with *iAMP21*
B-ALL with *ETV6::RUNX1* fusion	B-ALL with t(12;21)(p13.2;q22.1)/*ETV6::RUNX1*
B-ALL with *TCF3::PBX1* fusion	B-ALL with t(1;19)(q23.3;p13.3)/*TCF3::PBX1*
B-ALL with *IGH::IL3* fusion	B-ALL with t(5;14)(q31.1;q32.3)/*IL3::IGH*
B-ALL with *TCF3::HLF* fusion	B-ALL with *HLF* rearrangement
B-ALL with other defined genetic alterations	
B-ALL with *DUX4* rearrangement	B-ALL with *DUX4* rearrangement
B-ALL with *MEF2D* rearrangement	B-ALL with *MEF2D* rearrangement
B-ALL with *ZNF384* rearrangement	B-ALL with *ZNF384* rearrangement
B-ALL with *PAX5*alt	Not included
B-ALL with *PAX5* p.P80R	B-ALL with *PAX5* P80R
B-ALL with *NUTM1* rearrangement	B-ALL with *NUTM1* rearrangement
B-ALL with *MYC* rearrangement	B-ALL with *MYC* rearrangement
Not included	B-ALL with *IKZF1* N159Y
Not included	B-ALL with UBTF::ATXN7L3/*PAN3*, CDX2 ("CDX2/UBTF")

TABLE 18.1-1 Classification of B-Lymphoblastic Leukemia/Lymphoma (B-ALL) (*continued*)

Provisional entities

B-ALL with *ZNF384*-like rearrangement	B-ALL *ZNF384* rearranged–like
B-ALL with *IKZF1 N1597* mutation	B-ALL with *PAX5* alteration
B-ALL with *KMT2A*-like features	B-ALL *KMT2A*–like
B-ALL with *ZEB2* exon mutation	B-ALL *ETV6::RUNX1*–like
B-ALL with *CRLF2* (non–Ph-like) rearrangement	B-ALL with mutated *ZEB2* (p. H1038R)/*IGH::CEBPE*
B-ALL with *CBEPE* rearrangement	

ICC, International Consensus Classification.

Morphology

Lymphoblasts vary in cytology from small cells with scant cytoplasm, round nuclei, relatively condensed chromatin, and indistinct nucleoli, to large cells with convoluted nuclei, pale blue-gray cytoplasm, vacuolization, dispersed chromatin, and multiple variably prominent nucleoli (e-Figure 18.1-1). Cytoplasmic granules are rare, but may be numerous, occasionally mimicking Auer rods, and cytoplasmic pseudopods may be present (hand-mirror cells). In bone marrow core biopsies, blasts form sheets and pseudoclusters that displace normal marrow elements (e-Figures 18.1-2 and 18.1-3). Lymph nodes may show a diffuse, paracortical, or sinusoidal (leukemia) infiltration pattern (e-Figure 18.1-4). There are no reliable morphologic features to distinguish B- and T-lineage lymphoblasts. Benign B-cell precursors (hematogones) have a similar cytomorphologic appearance, and morphologic discrimination between B-ALL and normal B-cell precursors is challenging.

TABLE 18.1-2 WHO-HAEM5 Diagnostic Criteria for B-Lymphoblastic Leukemia/Lymphoma (B-ALL/LBL))

Essential

- B-ALL: peripheral blood or bone marrow B lymphoblasts (≥20%) by flow cytometry with B-cell lineage markers (CD19, CD22, cCD79a, and/or PAX5)
- B-LBL: a histologically effaced lymph node architecture or diffuse infiltration of an organ by a monomorphic population of blasts with immunophenotype (CD19, CD22, cCD79a, and/or PAX5) and markers of immaturity (TdT, CD34, and/or CD10), surface immunoglobulin negative. CD34 and TdT expression may be absent in rare cases.

Desirable

- Immunophenotypic profiles associated with specific recurrent genetic abnormalities
- Identification of specific recurrent genetic abnormalities

Based on the WHO Classification of Tumours Editorial Board. Haematolymphoid tumours [Internet]. Lyon (France): International Agency for Research on Cancer; 2024 (WHO classification of tumours series, 5th ed.; vol. 11). Available from: https://tumourclassification.iarc.who.int/chapters/63.

Cytochemical Stains

Although rarely used today, cytochemical staining of lymphoblasts shows the absence of myeloperoxidase (MPO) and may show light gray weak staining with Sudan Black B. Nonspecific esterase (NSE) shows a Golgi staining pattern. Periodic acid-Schiff (PAS) staining may show coarse, chunky cytoplasmic staining.

Immunophenotype

Lineage-defining B-cell markers are expressed by lymphoblasts. These include CD19, CD79a, and CD22 (cytoplasmic and surface), typically demonstrated by flow cytometry (FC). Immunohistochemical stains including the B-cell transcription factor PAX5, as well as CD19 and cCD79a, can be used in combination to increase sensitivity and specificity, as these can be expressed in some forms of acute myeloid leukemia (AML) and T-ALL/LBL. CD10 is expressed with moderate to high intensity in a majority of B-ALL, but specific genetic subtypes are characterized by variable to absent CD10 expression (eg, B-ALL with *KMT2A* rearrangement). CD20, CD34, and TdT are variably expressed. Surface light chain expression is typically absent.

The myeloid-associated antigens CD13 and CD33 can be present at low intensity on subsets of B-ALL/LBL, particularly B-ALL with *BCR::ABL1* rearrangement (Ph+ ALL). MPO can also be expressed rarely in so-called cases of B-ALL with isolated MPO expression (*Am J Clin Pathol.* 2017;147(4):374-381; *Cytometry B Clin Cytom.* 2021;100(4):446-453; *Blood.* 2018;131(5):573-577). In the absence of other myeloid lineage-defining antigens (CD14, CD64), a diagnosis of B-ALL (and not mixed phenotype acute leukemia [MPAL], B/myeloid) should be rendered.

Molecular Classification of B-Lymphoblastic Leukemia/Lymphoma

a. **B-lymphoblastic leukemia/lymphoma with recurrent genetic abnormalities**
   - **B-lymphoblastic leukemia/lymphoma with *BCR::ABL1* fusion:** This subtype of B-ALL/LBL is characterized by the rearrangement between the *BCR* gene on chromosome 22q.11.2 and the *ABL1* oncogene on chromosome 9q34.1 with most frequently observed 190-kDa fusion protein in 80% to 90% cases. Various methods, including karyotyping, fluorescence in situ hybridization (FISH), polymerase chain reaction (PCR), and DNA or RNA sequencing, can be used to identify this fusion for diagnosis, quantifying disease burden and monitoring therapeutic response. Ph+ ALL is more common in adults than children (*Blood.* 2008;112(3):918-919). *BCR::ABL1* B-ALL/LBL is associated with poor prognosis, and measurable residual disease (MRD) is a strong predictor of relapse and overall survival (*Blood.* 2016;128(4):504-507).
   - **B-lymphoblastic leukemia/lymphoma with *BCR::ABL1*–like features:** This subtype of B-ALL/LBL is characterized by DNA alterations that share similar gene expression profile to that of *BCR::ABL1*+, but in the absence of the *BCR::ABL1* rearrangement (*Nat Genet.* 2022;54(9):1376-1389). These include *JAK/STAT*, *ABL*-class, or other kinase signaling pathway activation through alternative pathways, including *CRLF2* rearrangements with *IGH* or *P2RY8* deletion leading to aberrant expression of *CRLF2*. A subset of the kinase-driven fusions in this category may be sensitive to targeted pharmacologic inhibition (*N Engl J Med.* 2014;371(11):1005-1015; *Blood.* 2017;129(25):3352-3361). Several molecular methods, including whole transcriptome sequencing and quantitative real-time polymerase chain reaction (qRT-PCR), can be used to identify

the specific genetic alteration due to its therapeutic and prognostic implications (*Blood.* 2012;119(8):1872-1881).

- **B-lymphoblastic leukemia/lymphoma with high hyperdiploidy:** This subtype is defined as a karyotype comprising between 51 and 65 chromosomes, including nonrandom gains of one or more copies of entire chromosomes, in the absence of type-defining translocations. The most common gains are of chromosomes X, 4, 6, 10, 14, 17, 18, and 21. FC of DNA, cytogenetics, and several molecular techniques can be used to detect hyperdiploidy (*Blood.* 2003;102(8):2756-2762). Chromosomal microarray can be used to detect "pseudo-hyperdiploidy." Due to consistent presence of extra copies of chromosome 21, FISH studies for *RUNX1* gene can be used as surrogate marker for hyperdiploidy (*Br J Haematol.* 2010;151(2):132-142). B-ALL with high hyperdiploidy is among the most common subtypes in the pediatric population and is associated with a favorable prognosis, particularly when chromosomes 4 and 10 gains are present (so-called "double trisomy") (*J Clin Oncol.* 2023;41(35):5422-5432).

- **B-lymphoblastic leukemia/lymphoma with hypodiploidy:** Hypodiploidy in B-ALL is characterized by a karyotype comprising less than or equal to 43 chromosomes. There are three subtypes: near-haploid (24-31 chromosomes), low-hypodiploid (32-39 chromosomes), and high-hypodiploid (40-43 chromosomes). FC of DNA, cytogenetics, and several molecular techniques can be used to detect hypodiploidy. More than 90% of cases with low haploid chromosomes are associated with somatic *TP53* alterations or Li-Fraumeni syndrome (germline *TP53* mutation). Near-haploid is associated with tyrosine kinase or *RAS* pathway alterations. SNP (single-nucleotide polymorphism) array analysis is important for detection of "pseudohyperdiploidy" and correct assessment of prognosis (*J Clin Oncol.* 2019;37(10):770-779).

- **B-lymphoblastic leukemia/lymphoma with *KMT2A* rearrangement:** This disease typically affects infants (<1 year of age, occasionally congenital) and is characterized by the presence of a rearrangement between the *KMT2A* gene (11q23) with breakpoints at an 8.3-kb region with various fusion partners, most commonly with *AFF1* (*DNA Repair (Amst).* 2006;5(9-10):1265-1272). Other fusion partners include *MLLT1, MLLT3, MLLT10, AFDN, EPS15,* and *AFF3.* Rearrangements of the *KMT2A* gene are also present in myeloid leukemia, where they alter methylation properties and upregulate *HOXA* genes, resulting in leukemogenesis. Immunophenotypically, B-ALL with *KMT2A* rearrangement is negative for CD10 and TdT and may express variable CD15. PCR and FISH can be used to detect *KMT2A* rearrangements, but next-generation sequencing (NGS) is the best method as it can detect cryptic breakpoints (*Hematol Oncol.* 2017;35(4):760-768).

- **B-lymphoblastic leukemia/lymphoma with iAMP21:** It is defined by the presence of gains and gross rearrangements of the long arm of chromosome 21. Karyotyping, SNP array, and FISH for *RUNX1* gene on chromosome 21 can be used as a surrogate marker for structural abnormality. FISH results involving five or more copies of *RUNX1* per cell with three or more copies on a single abnormal chromosome 21 are considered diagnostic (*Blood.* 2015;125(9):1383-1386). iAMP21 is associated with adverse prognosis and high risk of relapse (*J Clin Oncol.* 2013;31(27):3389-3396).

- **B-lymphoblastic leukemia/lymphoma with *ETV6::RUNX1* fusion:** It is defined by the presence of rearrangement between the *ETV6* gene on chromosome

12p13.2 and the *RUNX1* gene on chromosome 21q22.1. FISH, RT-PCR, and RNA sequencing methods can be used to evaluate this fusion (*Blood Adv.* 2020;4(5):930-942). It is generally not identified by conventional karyotype. B-ALL with *ETV6::RUNX1* fusion is the most common subtype of pediatric B-ALL and is associated with a favorable prognosis (*Blood.* 2004;104(8):2452-2457).

- **B-lymphoblastic leukemia/lymphoma with *ETV6::RUNX1*–like features:** It is defined by a gene expression profile similar to B-ALL with *ETV6::RUNX1* in the absence of the *ETV6::RUNX1* translocation. Combined *ETV6* and *IKZF1* rearrangements or deletions appear commonly in this entity, suggesting alternate pathways of *RUNX1* disruption. Many partners of *ETV* have been identified so far, including *BCL2L14, CREBBP,* and *BRCOS5* (*Nat Commun.* 2016;7:11790). Although *IKZF1* alterations are associated with poor prognosis in ALL (specifically Ph+), they do not appear to be associated with poor outcome in this subtype (*N Engl J Med.* 2009;360(5):470-480). This subtype lacks specific laboratory findings; a combination of CD27-positive/CD44 low-to-negative expression along with a high *RAG1* signature may be seen (*Cancer Med.* 2021;10(12):3997-4003).

- **B-lymphoblastic leukemia/lymphoma with *TCF3::PBX1* fusion:** It is defined by the presence of a rearrangement between the *TCF3* gene on chromosome 19 and the *PBX1* gene on chromosome 1. This fusion leads to production of oncogenic transcriptional activator on chromosome 19 (*Front Biosci.* 2003;8:s206-s222). Karyotype, FISH, and other molecular studies can be used to diagnose this fusion gene as well as cryptic translocations (*Genes Chromosomes Cancer.* 2022;61(1):22-26). NGS can help detect other fusion partners of *TCF3,* as they are not included in this category and can be misdiagnosed by break-apart FISH (*Blood Cancer J.* 2019;9(10):81). This fusion is associated with an intermediate to favorable prognosis and increased risk of CNS relapse (*Leukemia.* 2009;23(8):1406-1409).

- **B-lymphoblastic leukemia/lymphoma with *IGH::IL3* fusion:** A rare subtype (<1%) defined by the presence of fusion of *IGH* enhancer and the *IL3* promoter. IL3 activation leads to peripheral eosinophilia with infiltration of solid organs (*Pediatr Blood Cancer.* 2015;62(6):1055-1057). Karyotype and FISH can detect this fusion but may be challenging due to commonly low blast counts at diagnosis. NGS can be used to increase the sensitivity (*Ann Diagn Pathol.* 2021;53:151761). This subtype has a poor prognosis, and reemergence of eosinophilia may be a harbinger of relapse (*Front Oncol.* 2019;9:1374).

- **B-lymphoblastic leukemia/lymphoma with *TCF3::HLF* fusion:** This is a rare subtype isolated to the pediatric population and defined by the presence of a rearrangement between *TCF3* at 19p13.3 and *HLF* at 17q22. FISH and molecular methods can be used to detect this fusion (*Nat Genet.* 2019;51(2):296-307). NGS can detect all partners of the *TCF3* gene, as FISH cannot distinguish all partners of *TCF3* (*Blood.* 1994;83(10):2970-2977). It is associated with poor outcome despite CD19 directed treatment. Importantly, *TCF3* break-apart FISH probes are not recommended to identify the presence of the *TCF3::PBX1* fusion because of their differing prognoses.

- **B-lymphoblastic leukemia/lymphoma with other defined genetic alterations:** A number of other subtypes of B-ALL have recently been described through large-scale genomic studies. Details of these subtypes are beyond the scope of this chapter, but they are included in the WHO-HAEM5 and ICC and listed in Table 18.1-3. The recognition of these subtypes, each with diagnostic, prognostic, and therapeutic implications, underscores the increasing need for comprehensive genomic characterization of B-ALL at diagnosis.

TABLE 18.1-3 Key Features of B-Lymphoblastic Leukemia/Lymphoma (B-ALL/LBL) Subtypes

Subtype	Clinical Features	Morphology	Immunophenotype	Prognosis
BCR::ABL1 fusion	Incidence increases with age	Like other subtypes with high peripheral blood WBC count	In addition to B-ALL/LBL markers, myeloid markers may be expressed (CD13, CD33, CD25).	Historically poor Improving with the use of TKIs Worse if associated with IKZF1 mutation, it causes TKI resistance
BCR::ABL1-like fusion	Male:female ratio ~2:1 Incidence increases with age and 50%-60% in Down syndrome	Like other subtypes with high peripheral blood WBC count	Classic B-ALL/LBL profile	Historically poor Improving with the use of TKIs Worse if associated with IKZF1 mutation
High hyperdiploidy	More common in children Rare in infants and less common in adults	Like other subtypes with low peripheral blood WBC count	Classic B-ALL/LBL profile	Very favorable (>90% in children)
Hypodiploidy	Rare in children (<1%), increased incidence with age	Like other subtypes	Classic B-ALL/LBL profile	Poor Worse prognosis with increased loss of chromosomes
KMT2A rearrangement	Infants <1 y (80% cases) CNS involvement	Like other subtypes with high peripheral blood WBC count	CD19$^+$, with CD10$^-$, CD24$^-$, and TdT$^-$ Positive for myeloid markers, CD15, and CD65	Poor

(continued)

TABLE 18.1-3 Key Features of B-Lymphoblastic Leukemia/Lymphoma (B-ALL/LBL) Subtypes (*continued*)

Subtype	Clinical Features	Morphology	Immunophenotype	Prognosis
iAMP21	Older children Rare in adults	Like other subtypes with low peripheral blood count	Classic B-ALL/LBL profile	Poor
ETV6::RUNX1 fusion	Most common in children (2-10 y) Rare in infants and adults	Like other subtypes	CD9−, CD20−, and CD66c− CD27+ and CD44+/− Myeloid markers may be expressed (CD13, CD33)	Favorable
ETV6::RUNX1–like fusion	Common in children Rare in infants and adults	Like other subtypes	CD9−, CD20−, CD66c−, CD27+, and CD44+/−	Undetermined with common relapse
TCF3::PBX1 fusion	Common in children (5%) Rare in infants	Like other subtypes	CD9+, CD10+, CD19+, CD34−, and at least partial absence of CD20	Favorable with increased risk of CNS relapse
IGH::IL3 fusion	Children and young	Blood and bone marrow eosinophilia	Classic B-ALL/LBL profile with CD13+ and CD33+	Poor
TCH3::HLF fusion	Hypercalcemia and coagulopathy	Like other subtypes	Classic B-ALL/LBL profile	Poor

CNS, central nervous system; TKI, tyrosine kinase inhibitor; WBC, white blood cell.

b. **B-lymphoblastic leukemia/lymphoma, not otherwise specified (NOS)**
The genetic drivers of some B-ALL/LBL cases remain unknown even after comprehensive genomic testing. In most laboratories, approximately 5% to 10% are left as "NOS," but its frequency is decreasing with the newly identified genetic alterations and comprehensive testing method adoption. As such, B-ALL NOS is a diagnosis of exclusion. It has intermediate prognosis in children, with about 86% 5-year survival, likely reflecting the heterogeneous nature of these cases (*Blood Cancer Discov.* 2021;2(4):326-337).

Prognosis and Treatment

Several risk factors, including age, ethnicity, presenting white blood cell (WBC) count, leukemic versus lymphomatous presentation, syndromic associations (eg, constitutional trisomy 21 or DS), CNS or testicular involvement, genetics, and molecular subtype, can predict the prognosis and treatment outcome. See Table 18.1-4. Minimal/MRD is also a key indicator of response (*Haematologica.* 2020;105(11):2524-2539; *Semin Diagn Pathol.* 2023;40(6):457-471).

Differential Diagnosis

Burkitt lymphoma: The neoplastic cells of Burkitt lymphoma can show blastoid cytomorphology similar to that of B-ALL/LBL, but they tend to be larger and have multiple peripheral nucleoli. They express clonal surface immunoglobulin light chain and lack of CD34 and TdT expression.

Hematogones: Hematogones are difficult to distinguish from lymphoblasts by morphology in the assessment of residual disease. Hematogones are typically smaller than lymphoblasts and have simplified round nuclei. Their highly stereotyped immunophenotype is the basis of MRD testing by FC for B-ALL.

TABLE 18.1-4 Prognostic Factors of B-Lymphoblastic Leukemia/Lymphoma Subtypes

Favorable Prognosis	Unfavorable Prognosis
1-10 y	<1 or >10 y
Caucasian and Asian	Hispanic and African American
WBC <50,000/μL	WBC ≥50,000/μL
Fast blast clearance with therapy	Slow blast clearance with therapy
MRD+	MRD−
High hyperdiploidy (>50 chromosomes)	Near (24-31) and low hypodiploidy (32-39)
CNS+/−	CNS+
Testicular involvement−	Testicular involvement+
ETV6::RUNX1 fusion	Ph-positive or Ph-like ALL, *KMT2A*, *MEF2D* or *BCL2/MYC* rearrangements or *TCF3::HLF* fusion

CNS, central nervous system; MRD, measurable residual disease; WBC, white blood cell.

SUGGESTED READINGS

Alaggio R, Amador C, Anagnostopoulos I, et al. The 5th edition of the World Health Organization classification of haematolymphoid tumours: lymphoid neoplasms [published correction appears in *Leukemia*. 2023;37(9):1944-1951]. *Leukemia*. 2022;36(7):1720-1748.

Arber DA, Orazi A, Hasserjian RP, et al. International Consensus Classification of myeloid neoplasms and acute leukemias: integrating morphologic, clinical, and genomic data. *Blood*. 2022;140(11):1200-1228.

Duffield AS, Mullighan CG, Borowitz MJ. International Consensus Classification of acute lymphoblastic leukemia/lymphoma. *Virchows Arch*. 2023;482(1):11-26.

Kovach AE, Raca G. Modern classification and management of pediatric B-cell leukemia and lymphoma. *Surg Pathol Clin*. 2023;16(2):249-266.

18.2 T-Lymphoblastic Leukemia/Lymphoma

Barina Aqil and Anjum Hassan

I. T-LYMPHOBLASTIC LEUKEMIA/LYMPHOMA, NOS

T-cell acute lymphoblastic leukemia/lymphoma (T-ALL/LBL) accounts for 85% to 90% of all LBL cases (*Leuk Lymphoma*. 2019;60:1171-1178). It can present with peripheral blood (PB) and bone marrow (BM) involvement (leukemia) or in lymph nodes, extranodal sites, or thymus (lymphoma) or both. It accounts for 15% of childhood ALL cases and is more common in adolescents. Adult T-ALL comprises 25% of ALL cases. **The diagnostic criteria are summarized in Table 18.2-1.**

Clinical Features
- **Clinical presentation:** T-ALL presents classically as a mediastinal mass with or without pleural or pericardial effusion, but leukemic presentation with high white blood cell count, and lymphadenopathy and hepatosplenomegaly are also reported.

TABLE 18.2-1 WHO-HAEM5 Diagnostic Criteria for T-ALL

Essential	Desirable
• Immature/progenitors of T-cell lineage, defined by expression of sCD3 and cCD3 with abnormal phenotype	• Blasts/progenitors >20% in PB/BM/extramedullary site • Unlike AML, a defined cutoff for blasts is not required for the diagnosis of T-ALL/LBL.

Based on the WHO Classification of Tumours Editorial Board. Haematolymphoid tumours [Internet]. Lyon (France): International Agency for Research on Cancer; 2024 (WHO classification of tumours series, 5th ed.; vol. 11). Available from: https://tumourclassification.iarc.who.int/chapters/63.

AML, acute myeloid leukemia; cCD3, cytoplasmic CD3; PB/BM, peripheral blood/bone marrow; sCD3, surface CD3; T-ALL/LBL, T-cell acute lymphoblastic leukemia/lymphoma.

Morphology

The lymphoblasts are small to medium in size with high nuclear to cytoplasmic ratio, round to irregular nuclear contour, fine to condensed chromatin, variably conspicuous nucleoli, and scant or vacuolated cytoplasm (e.Figure 18.2.1A-D). The lymph nodes may show variable architectural effacement with paracortical involvement and residual germinal centers. Thymic involvement is usually noted as disruption/replacement of thymic epithelial cell networks and adipose tissue infiltration.

Immunophenotype

Lymphoblasts in T-ALL/LBL are positive for lineage-specific markers, cytoplasmic CD3 (cCD3), and/or surface CD3 (sCD3); cCD3 is more commonly expressed. Other T-cell antigens include CD7, CD5, and CD2. Precursor T- and B-cell markers, such as CD34, terminal deoxynucleotidyl transferase (TdT), CD1a, and CD99, are also positive, but they are not lineage specific (*Mod Pathol*. 1997;10:277-282) (e.Figure 18.2.1E-G).

T-ALL/LBL recapitulates stages of normal counterparts of T-cell maturation/differentiation (*Am J Clin Pathol*. 2015;144:411-422) (Table 18.2-2). However, some B-cell antigens, such as CD79a and CD19 (heterogeneous), can be present (*J Pathol*. 1998;186:140-143; *Br J Haematol*. 2012;159:454-461). Myeloid lineage antigens, such as CD13, CD33, and CD117, are also reportedly expressed. CD117 expression is associated with activating mutations of *FLT3*.

Genetic Features

Clonal rearrangements of the *TCRB* and *TCRG* genes in more than 90% of cases are noted. In addition, 20% cases demonstrate *IGH* gene rearrangement. Immunophenotypically immature T-ALL/LBL (early T-precursor lymphoblastic leukemia/lymphoma; ETP-ALL) may lack T-cell receptor (*TCR*) gene rearrangement. The common recurrent genetic abnormalities in T-ALL/LBL are presented in Table 18.2-3.

WHO-HAEM5 has proposed to divide T-ALL into five distinct genetic subgroups based on specific translocations leading to aberrant expression of specific genes

TABLE 18.2-2 Stages of T-Cell Differentiation and Maturation

Postulated Stages of T-Cell Maturation	Immunophenotype
Early/Pro-T cell	CD1a−, CD8−, CD5+/weak and positivity for one or more stem cell (CD34, HLA-DR) and myeloid (CD117, CD13, CD33, CD11b, CD65) antigens
Pre-T cell	CD1a−, CD7+, CD8−, TdT+
Cortical T cell	CD1a+, CD4+, CD8+
Medullary T cell	CD1a−, CD4+ or CD8+, sCD3+

Based on the WHO Classification of Tumours Editorial Board. Haematolymphoid tumours [Internet]. Lyon (France): International Agency for Research on Cancer; 2024 (WHO classification of tumours series, 5th ed.; vol. 11). Available from: https://tumourclassification.iarc.who.int/chapters/63.
CD, cluster of differentiation; HLA-DR, human leukocyte antigen-DR; sCD3+, surface CD3+; TdT+, terminal deoxynucleotidyl transferase.

TABLE 18.2-3 Common Genetic Abnormalities in T-ALL/LBL

Antigen receptor genes

- *TCRB* and *TCRG* genes rearrangement (>90%)
- Negative *TCR* gene rearrangement seen mostly in ETP-ALL
- *IGH* gene rearrangement (~20%)

Cytogenetic abnormalities

- Rearrangements of α and δ *TCR* loci at 14q11.2
- Rearrangements of β locus at 7q34
- Rearrangements of γ locus at 7p14.1
- del(9p)

Transcriptional gene dysregulation

- *TLX1, TLX3, TAL1, TAL2, LMO1, LMO2, LYL1, NKX2-1,2,5, OLIG2, HOXA*
- *MYC, MYB, LCK*
- *MLLT10, KMT2A, ABL1, NUP98*

Inactivated/deleted tumor suppressor genes

- *BCL11B, LEF1, WT1, NF1 ETV6, RUNX1, GATA3*

Signaling pathway mutations

- *NOTCH1, FBXW7*

Epigenetic mutations

- *PHF6, SUZ12, EZH2, TET2, H3F3A, KDM6A, EED, SETD2, DNMT3A*

Based on the WHO Classification of Tumours Editorial Board. Haematolymphoid tumours [Internet]. Lyon (France): International Agency for Research on Cancer; 2024 (WHO classification of tumours series, 5th ed.; vol. 11). Available from: https://tumourclassification.iarc.who.int/chapters/63.
ETP-ALL, early T-precursor lymphoblastic leukemia/lymphoma; T-acute lymphoblastic leukemia/lymphoma, T-cell acute lymphoblastic leukemia/lymphoma.

TABLE 18.2-4 Genetic Subgroups of T-ALL

Groups	Affected Genes	Notable Findings
1	*TAL* or *LMO*	
2	*TLX1*	Favorable prognosis
3	*TLX3*	
4	*HOXA*	
5	*LYL1*	Resemble ETP-ALL

Based on the WHO Classification of Tumours Editorial Board. Haematolymphoid tumours [Internet]. Lyon (France): International Agency for Research on Cancer; 2024 (WHO classification of tumours series, 5th ed.; vol. 11). Available from: https://tumourclassification.iarc.who.int/chapters/63.
ETP-ALL, early T-precursor lymphoblastic leukemia/lymphoma; T-acute lymphoblastic leukemia/lymphoma, T-cell acute lymphoblastic leukemia.

(Table 18.2-4) (*Best Pract Res Clin Haematol.* 2010;23:307-318). On the other hand, the International Consensus Classification (ICC) of acute lymphoblastic leukemia/lymphoma has incorporated *BCL11B*-activating rearrangements into ETP-ALL. In addition, eight new provisional entities are added to the T-ALL subclassification (Table 18.2-5) (*Virchows Archiv.* 2023;482:11-26).

Prognosis and Treatment

Long-term response rates are approximately 85% in children and adolescents, and approximately 60% in adults (*J Clin Oncol.* 2020;38:3282-3293; *Pediatr Blood Cancer.* 2021;68:e28719). Minimal residual disease (MRD) at the end of consolidation is the most significant predictor of clinical outcome. The prognosis of T-LBL relies on the patient's age, disease stage, and lactate dehydrogenase levels. Chemotherapy, in combination with dexamethasone and nelarabine in children and young adults, is known to be associated with better outcomes (*J Clin Oncol.* 2020;38:3282-3293).

Differential Diagnosis

- **Thymoma:** Pancytokeratin (AE1/AE3) highlights an extensive epithelial cell network which is not seen in T-LBL. In addition, lymphoid cells demonstrate a normal thymocyte maturational spectrum by flow cytometry (FC), leaning toward more cortical thymocyte maturation. *TCR* gene rearrangement is polyclonal.
- **MPAL (mixed-phenotype acute leukemia), T/myeloid:** These cases show expression of cytoplasmic myeloperoxidase (MPO) or markers of monocytic differentiation. *NOTCH1* mutations and *CDKN2A/CDKN2B* deletions are less commonly seen in MPAL-T/M in comparison to T-ALL and ETP-ALL (*Haematologica.* 2020;105:e294-e297).
- **Acute undifferentiated leukemia (AUL):** This is a rare entity that expresses no lineage-specific markers. It may express one of the myeloid markers (CD13, CD33, and CD117) and CD7 or CD56.
- **Mature T-cell leukemia/lymphoma:** The cases of T-ALL/LBL with expression of sCD3 may overlap with mature T-cell leukemia/lymphoma, especially with dual expression of CD4+/CD8+ in T-cell prolymphocytic leukemia (T-PLL), and CD10 expression with nodal T follicular helper (TFH) lymphoma-angioimmunoblastic type (nTFHL-AI). It is important to remember that mature T-cell leukemia/lymphoma is negative for CD34, TdT, and CD1a, and shows negative to dim CD7 expression, unlike T-ALL/LBL that demonstrates all these and a brighter CD7 expression. Detection of *NOTCH1* mutation favors T-ALL/LBL whereas TCL1 expression or rearrangement supports T-PLL.

Key Points

- Lymphoblasts in ETP-ALL have a unique immunophenotype with cytoplasmic CD3+ (cCD3+), CD1a−, CD8−, MPO−, negative to dim CD5 (<75% blasts), and positivity for ≥1 myeloid and/or stem cell markers.
- The majority of ETP-ALL cases are negative for *TRG* gene rearrangement.

Diagnostic Caveats

- Lack of standardization of CD5 leads to underdiagnosis of ETP-ALL. Some studies have reported negative CD4 expression, or gene expression profiling for detection of ETP-ALL.

TABLE 18.2-5 New Provisional Entities Under T-ALL Subclassification

Subtype	Frequency	Immunophenotype	Partner Genes/Other Rearrangements	Prognosis
BCL11B-activated	30% ETP-ALL, MPAL, T/myeloid, <5% AML and AUL[a]	Variable immunophenotype	BETA (BCL11B enhancer tandem amplification at 14q32, ~700 kb distal of BCL11B); *ARID1B, CCDC26/MYC; CDK6; TAB1; ETV6; ZEB2; RUNX1*	
TAL1/2-R	30%–40%	CD4+, CD8+	*TCRA/D; TCRB (TAL2);* 1p32 deletion (*STIL*); intergenic SNV generating a *TAL1*-dergulating superenhancer	Intermediate
TLX1-R	Adults	CD4+, CD8+, CD1a+	*TCR*	Good
TLX3-R	Children		*TCR; BCL11B; CDK6*	
HOXA	15%–25%	Immature immunophenotype, some meeting criteria of ETP-ALL	*HOXA::TCRB/TCRG; KMT2A-R; PICALM::MLLT10; SET::NUP214*	
LMO1/2-R	15%	Immature immunophenotype	*TCR*; cryptic deletion; enhancer/promoter mutations *LMO* complex with bHLH factors; extremely high LMO1/2 expression	
NKX2-R	<5%, children		*NKX2.1/NKX2.2/NKX2.5::TCR; BCL11B; CDK6*	
SPI1-R	<5%, children	HLA-DR+	*STMN1; TCF7; BCL11B*	Very poor prognosis
BHLH, other	<2%		*TCRB::LYL1* *TCR::BHLHB1*; high LMO expression	

Modified from Duffield AS, Mulligan CG, Borowitz MJ. International Consensus Classification of acute lymphoblastic leukemia/lymphoma. *Virchows Archiv.* 2023;482:11-26.

AML, acute myeloid leukemia; AUL, acute undifferentiated leukemia; bHLH, basic helix-loop-helix; CD, cluster of differentiation; ETP-ALL, early T-precursor lymphoblastic leukemia/lymphoma; HLA-DR, human leukocyte antigen-DR; LMO, LIM domain-only; MPAL, mixed-phenotype acute leukemia; SNV, single nucleotide variant; T-acute lymphoblastic leukemia/lymphoma, T-cell acute lymphoblastic leukemia.

TABLE 18.2-6 WHO-HAEM5 Diagnostic Criteria for ETP-ALL

Essential

- Presence of blasts
- Expression of specific immunophenotypic markers:
  - Positive for cytoplasmic CD3
  - Lack of (<5% positive blasts) CD1a and CD8 expression
  - Negative or dim (<75% positive blasts) CD5 expression
  - Positive (≥25% positive blasts) for ≥1 myeloid (CD11b, CD13, CD33, CD65, CD117) and stem cell (CD34, HLA-DR) markers
  - Negative myeloperoxidase (<3% by cytochemistry and <10% by flow cytometry)

Based on the WHO Classification of Tumours Editorial Board. Haematolymphoid tumours [Internet]. Lyon (France): International Agency for Research on Cancer; 2024 (WHO classification of tumours series, 5th ed.; vol. 11). Available from: https://tumourclassification.iarc.who.int/chapters/63.
CD, cluster of differentiation; ETP-ALL, early T-precursor lymphoblastic leukemia/lymphoma; HLA-DR, human leukocyte antigen-DR.

- **Indolent T-lymphoblastic proliferation (IT-LBP):** Implies indolent extra-thymic expansion of T-lymphoblasts with preservation of the overall architecture. These proliferations are commonly seen in the lymph nodes and are positive for CD3 and TdT but negative for CD34. LMO2 is negative in IT-LBP but positive in T-ALL. *TCR* gene rearrangement is negative.

II. EARLY T-PRECURSOR LYMPHOBLASTIC LEUKEMIA/LYMPHOMA

ETP-ALL is an immature neoplasm with T-cell lineage-specific blasts with a unique immunophenotype, accounting for 12%-17% of pediatric T-ALL cases and 20%-40% of adult cases. **The diagnostic criteria are summarized in Table 18.2-6.**

Clinical Features
- **Clinical presentation:** The white blood cell count is usually not elevated, rather these patients may present with cytopenias. Symptoms pertaining to extramedullary site involvement may be seen.

Morphology
ETP-ALL has similar morphology to T-ALL, NOS; blasts may show cytoplasmic blebs (e.Figure 18.2.2A-E).

Immunophenotype
ETP-ALL has unique immunophenotypic selection criteria (e.Figure 18.2.3A-O):

1. cCD3 expression, which may be heterogeneous (negative to positive)
2. Negative MPO (<10% by FC and <3% by cytochemistry)
3. Lack of CD8 and CD1a (<5% positive blasts)
4. Negative to dim CD5 expression (<75% positive blasts)

5. Expression (≥25% blasts) of one or more myeloid (CD13, CD33, CD117, CD11b, CD65) and stem cell (CD34, HLA-DR) antigens
6. **Near ETP-ALL**: cCD3+, CD8−, CD1a−, MPO−, positive for one or more myeloid and stem cell markers but 75% or more blasts are CD5+.

These proposed immunophenotypic criteria may not identify all ETP-ALL cases that can potentially be detected by gene expression profiling, due to lack of standardization for CD5 expression by FC. Therefore, it has been proposed that CD4 negativity instead of dim CD5 expression be used as an alternative, which has allowed identification of most of the ETP-ALL cases (*Haematologica.* 2014;99:94-102; *Haematologica.* 2020;105:e294-e297). Other authors have devised immunophenotype scoring systems based on antigen expression to differentiate ETP-ALL from T-ALL (*Br J Haematol.* 2012;156:358-365; *Br J Haematol.* 2019;186:538-548) (Tables 18.2-7 and 18.2-8).

Genetic Features

The majority of ETP-ALL cases are negative for *TRG* gene rearrangement and show the absence of biallelic *TRG* deletions (*Blood Adv.* 2021;5:2890-2900). ETP-ALL

TABLE 18.2-7	Comparison of Immunophenotypic Expression Between ETP-ALL and Other T-ALL Subgroups, Including Near ETP-ALL		
Markers	**ETP-ALL**	**Near ETP-ALL**	**Other T-ALL**
cCD3	+++	+++	+++
CD7	+++	+++	+++
CD2	+++	+++	+++
CD38	+++	+++	+++
CD34	+++	+++	++
TdT	++	+++	+++
HLA-DR	++	++	+
CD4	+/−	++	+++
CD10	+/−	+++	+++
CD117	+++	+	+/−
CD13	+++	++	+/−
CD33	+++	++	+/−

Modified from Khogeer H, Rahman H, Jain N, et al. Early T precursor acute lymphoblastic leukaemia/lymphoma shows differential immunophenotypic characteristics including frequent CD33 expression and in vitro response to targeted CD33 therapy. *Br J Haematol.* 2019;186(4):538-548.
CD, cluster of differentiation; ETP-ALL, early T-precursor lymphoblastic leukemia/lymphoma; HLA-DR, human leukocyte antigen-DR; near ETP-ALL, near early T-precursor lymphoblastic leukemia/lymphoma; T-ALL, T-lymphoblastic leukemia/lymphoma, TdT, terminal deoxynucleotidyl transferase.

| TABLE 18.2-8 | Scoring System Based on 11 Cell Surface Antigens for ETP-ALL as Described in TCCSG L99-15 Study With Specificity (100%) and Sensitivity (94%) |

Antigens	Score			
	+2	+1	−1	−2
CD34	≥75%	≥25%		
HLA-DR	≥75%	≥25%		
CD3		<20%	≥75%	
CD2		<20%	≥75%	
CD5	<75%			≥75%
CD4		<20%	≥75%	
CD8	<5%			≥5%
CD10		<20%	≥75%	
CD13	≥75%	≥25%		
CD33	≥75%	≥25%		
CD56		≥20%		

Total score of T-ALL cases was ≤6 while ETP-ALL cases had a score of ≥7.

Modified from Inukai T, Kiyokawa N, Campana D, et al. Clinical significance of early T-cell precursor acute lymphoblastic leukaemia: results of the Tokyo Children's Cancer Study Group Study L99-15. Br J Haematol. 2012;156(3):358-365.
CD, cluster of differentiation; FTP-ALL, early T-precursor lymphoblastic leukemia/lymphoma; HLA-DR, human leukocyte antigen-DR; T-ALL, T-lymphoblastic leukemia/lymphoma; TCCSG, T-Cell Consortium Study Group.

has a distinct gene expression pattern with dysregulation of *MEF2C*, *IGFBP7*, *WT1*, and *GATA3*. ETP-ALL frequently demonstrates myeloid-associated gene alterations such as *FLT3*, *NRAS/KRAS*, *DNMT3A*, *IDH1*, and *IDH2* mutations with more frequent deletions of *ETV6* and *RPL22* and lower frequencies of other T-ALL-associated mutations such as *NOTCH1* and *CDKN2A/B* gene mutations (*Am J Hematol.* 2021;96:312-319; *Blood Adv.* 2021;5:2890-2900).

ETP-ALL with *BCL11B* alterations is reported to have interchromosomal rearrangements in 80% of cases, while the remaining cases have focal amplifications that generate a neo-enhancer distal to *BCL11B* (*Blood.* 2021;138:773-784; *Cancer Discov.* 2021;11:2846-2867). Both mechanisms produce leukemias with similar genetic profiles, so this group has been termed "*BCL11B* activated" (*BCL11B*a), excluding *BCL11B*-r cases such as *BCL11B::TLX3*, which do not lead to activation of *BCL11B*. MPAL-T/M (mixed-phenotype acute leukemia with T/myeloid) (T-lymphoid and myeloid phenotype) and less than 5% of acute myeloid leukemia (AML) cases also show similar *BCL11B* alterations and gene expression profile to ETP-ALL, thereby leading to the hypothesis that it represents a distinct molecular group of acute leukemia.

> **Key Points**
> - cCD3 is the most lineage specific and defines T-lineage differentiation, as does surface CD3 (sCD3), but the latter is present less frequently and usually at a decreased level compared to mature T cells.
> - Lack of or weak expression of CD5 points toward ETP-ALL diagnosis.
>
> **Diagnostic Caveats**
> - CD56 is expressed in a subset of cases that overlap with ETP-ALL but does not suggest NK-cell differentiation.
> - Cases with mediastinal presentation may be difficult to distinguish from thymoma. PanCK, LMO2 (positive in T-LBL but not in thymocytes), and *TCR* gene rearrangement studies are helpful in this setting.

Prognosis and Treatment

ETP-ALL confers a poor prognosis with the use of conventional induction treatment and significantly poorer overall event-free survival than the T-ALL subgroup. Despite a higher rate of MRD positive disease post-induction, several recent studies have reported better outcomes in ETP-ALL cases with intensive chemotherapy, use of nelarabine, and stem cell transplantation.

Differential Diagnosis

- **MPAL, T/myeloid:** See Chapter 18.3.
- **AML cases that also exhibit T-cell lymphoid features:** A subset of AMLs harbor clonal *TCR* or immunoglobulin (*IG*) gene rearrangements. These AML cases can also express CD7, CD2, and CD4 (*Mod Pathol.* 2013;26:195-203). *STIL::TAL1*, *FBXW7* mutation, and *CDKN2A/B* deletions have been found only in ETP-ALL, while *NOTCH1*, *FLT3*, *N/KRAS* mutations, *TLX3*, and *KMT2A* rearrangements have been reported in both T/M-MPAL and ETP-ALL cases (*Cancer Manag Res.* 2019;11:3933-3943).

III. NK-LYMPHOBLASTIC LEUKEMIA/LYMPHOMA

NK-lymphoblastic leukemia/lymphoma (NK-ALL/LBL) was considered a provisional entity in WHO-HAEM4R due to CD56 expression by the blasts and difficulty in distinguishing it from T-ALL (CD2+, CD7+, CD5+, cCD3+, and sCD3−). CD56 expression can, however, be seen in other neoplasms such as blastic plasmacytoid dendritic cell neoplasm, T-ALL, AML, and AUL. Although expression of some immature NK-cell markers, such as CD94 and CD161, can help in this distinction, there is a lack of reliable published data in this regard. This entity is no longer included in WHO-HAEM5, although ICC still considers it a provisional entity.

SUGGESTED READINGS

1. Liu Y, Easton J, Shao Y, et al. The genomic landscape of pediatric and young adult T-lineage acute lymphoblastic leukemia. *Nat Genet.* 2017;49:1211-1218.
2. Duffield AS, Mullighan CG, Borowitz MJ. International Consensus Classification of acute lymphoblastic leukemia/lymphoma. *Virchows Archiv.* 2023;482:11-26.
3. Swerdlow SH, Campo E, Harris NL, et al. *WHO Classification of Tumors of Haematopoietic and Lymphoid Tissues.* IARC; 2017.

4. Girardi T, Vicente C, Cools J, De Keersmaecker K. The genetics and molecular biology of T-ALL. *Blood.* 2017;129:1113–1123.
5. Falini B, Lazzi S, Pileri S. A comparison of the International Consensus and 5th WHO classifications of T-cell lymphomas and histiocytic/dendritic cell tumours. *Br J Haematol.* 2023;203:369-383.

18.3 Acute Leukemias of Mixed or Ambiguous Lineage

Barina Aqil, Cara Lunn Shirai, and Anjum Hassan

Acute leukemias of ambiguous lineage (ALAL) are a diverse group that includes acute undifferentiated leukemia (AUL), when the blasts fail to show commitment to either myeloid or lymphoid lineage, and mixed-phenotype acute leukemia (MPAL) when there is evidence of commitment to more than one lineage in the blast population. MPALs can have distinct blast populations each of a different lineage, one blast population with multiple antigens of different lineages, or a combination. AUL and MPAL both require 20% or more blasts/progenitor cells for diagnosis. Other WHO-defined leukemias, such as acute myeloid leukemia (AML) with myelodysplasia-related changes (now called as AML, myelodysplasia-related), therapy-related AML (now called AML post cytotoxic changes), blast-phase chronic myeloid leukemia, or AML with balanced translocations, such as core-binding leukemia [t(8;21), inv(16)] and *PML::RARA*/t(15;17)], are excluded from MPAL.

Lineage assignment is most commonly performed by flow cytometry (FC) and less frequently by cytochemistry and immunohistochemistry. The lineage specificity depends on the strength of each antigen in question; the closer the antigen expression profile matches the intensity or expression pattern of a normal population, the more likely the commitment to that particular lineage.

The lineage characterization in MPAL can be based on EGIL (European Group of Immunological Characterization of Leukemia) and WHO classification systems. In the EGIL scoring system, cases are defined based on the number of points by a lymphoid or myeloid marker. When the scores are over two points for myeloid lineage and one of the two lymphoid lineages, the lineage is characterized as biphenotypic. Acute leukemias demonstrating an otherwise consistent antigenic profile associated with a particular type of acute leukemia with isolated aberrancies should not be classified as MPAL (see Table 18.3-1).

The WHO classification likewise recommends focusing on the strength of association between various markers expressed on the blasts and the lineage being assigned. Also, variation in the intensity of expression and its correlation with normal patterns of expression weighs in heavily in assigning lineage (see Table 18.3-2 and e-Figure 18.3.1).

TABLE 18.3-1 European Group of Immunological Classification of Leukemia Scoring System

Lineage	2 Points	1 Point	0.5 Points
Myeloid lineage	Myeloperoxidase (MPO)	CD117	CD14
	Lysozyme	CD13	CD64
		CD33	CD15
		CD65a	
B-lymphoid lineage	CD79a	CD19	CD24
	Cytoplasmic CD22 (CytoCD22)	CD20	TdT
	CytoIgM	CD10	
T-lymphoid lineage	CD3 (surface/cytoplasmic)	CD2	TdT
	TCR α/α	CD5	CD7
	TCR α/α	CD8	CD1a
		CD10	

Modified from Bene MC, Castoldi G, Knapp W, et al. Proposals for the immunological classification of acute leukemias. European Group for the Immunological Characterization of Leukemias (EGIL). *Leukemia.* 1995;9:1783-1786.
CD, cluster of differentiation; IgM, immunoglobulin M; TCR, T-cell receptor; TdT, terminal deoxynucleotidyl transferase.

TABLE 18.3-2 Lineage Assignment Criteria for MPAL by WHO-HAEM5

Lineage	Criteria
B-lineage	
Strong CD19 (exceeds 50% of expression intensity of normal B cell progenitor by flow cytometry)	One or more also strongly expressed: CD10, CD22, or CD79a
OR	Two or more also strongly expressed: CD10, CD22, or CD79a
Weak CD19 (does not exceed 50% of normal B cell progenitor by flow cytometry)	
T-lineage	
CD3 (surface or cytoplasmic)	Intensity, in part, exceeds 50% of expression intensity of mature T cells by flow cytometry
	OR
	Immunocytochemistry positive with non-ζ chain reagent
Myeloid lineage	
MPO	Intensity, in part, exceeds 50% of expression intensity of granulocytes in two or more expressed: Nonspecific esterase, CD11c, CD14, CD64, or lysozyme
OR	
Monocytic differentiation	

CD, cluster of differentiation; MPO, myeloperoxidase.
Based on the WHO Classification of Tumours Editorial Board. Haematolymphoid tumours [Internet]. Lyon (France): International Agency for Research on Cancer; 2024 (WHO classification of tumours series, 5th ed.; vol. 11). Available from: https://tumourclassification.iarc.who.int/chapters/63.

In general, the prognosis of MPAL is considered poor. Older age, higher white blood cell (WBC) count, increased creatinine or uric acid at presentation, extramedullary involvement, and *KMT2A/MLL* rearrangement are additional poor risk factors (*Leuk Res.* 2015;39:606-616; *Ann Hematol.* 2014;93:595-601). Wide accessibility of molecular studies is helpful in identifying targetable mutations in genes such as *IDH1/2, BRAF, NOTCH1,* and *FLT3*.

I. ACUTE LEUKEMIA OF AMBIGUOUS LINEAGE WITH DEFINING GENETIC ABNORMALITIES

A number of molecular and genetic abnormalities have been associated with MPAL, but only a subset of them have been classified as "defining" based on specific genetic associations (see Table 18.3-3). A brief account of each of these entities follows:

A. Mixed-Phenotype Acute Leukemia With *BCR::ABL1* Fusion (MPAL With *BCR::ABL1*)

By definition, this should be a new acute leukemia with *BCR::ABL1* fusion that fulfills diagnostic criteria for MPAL. Prior myeloproliferative or myelodysplastic neoplasms, MPAL post cytotoxic therapy, and secondary *BCR::ABL1* acquisition during disease course have to be excluded. About 15%-20% of MPAL cases fall in this category (<1%), usually presenting in adults with male predominance.

TABLE 18.3-3 Key Features of MPAL/ALAL With Defining Genetic Abnormalities

Entity	Immunophenotype	Defining Genetic Features	Diagnostic Criteria[a]
MPAL *BCR::ABL1* fusion	• B/M: most frequent • T/M, B/T, B/T/M: rare	• *BCR::ABL1* or t(9;22)(q34;q11.2)	• ≥20% blasts in bone marrow and/or blood with MPAL immunophenotype • Defining genetic features • No previous cytotoxic therapy
MPAL with *KMT2A* rearrangement	• B/M: most frequent • B/T: rare	• *KMT2A* rearrangement	
ALAL with other defined genetic alterations • MPAL with *ZNF386* • ALAL with *BCL11B*	• HSCAs + B/M (*ZNF386* subtype) • HSCAs + T/M and rarely any lineage differentiation (*BCL11B* subtype)	• *ZNF386* or *BCL11B* rearrangement	• ≥20% blasts in bone marrow and/or blood with mixed or ambiguous immunophenotype • Defining genetic features

ALAL, acute leukemia of ambiguous lineage; B, B-cell lineage; HSCAs, hematopoietic stem cell antigens (CD34, HLA-DR, and/or CD117); M, myeloid lineage; MPAL, mixed-phenotype acute leukemia; T, T-cell lineage.
[a]Diagnostic criteria per the WHO-HAEM5.
Note: Diagnosis of MPAL with *BCR::ABL1* also requires the absence of a history of CML and the differential diagnosis includes AML and B-ALL with *BCR::ABL1*.

Genetic Features

Chromosome analysis or fluorescence in situ hybridization studies (FISH) identify either a sole t(9;22)(q34;q11.2) abnormalities or additional chromosomal aberrations such as trisomy or hyperdiploidy. Alternatively, a complex karyotype (three or more clonal structural chromosomal abnormalities) can be seen with relatively frequent involvement of chromosome 6q and abnormalities of chromosomes 5 and 7. Expression of p190 (*BCR::ABL1*) is more common than that of p210 (*BCR::ABL1*). *NOTCH1*, *FLT3*, and *RUNX1* are detected frequently in MPAL (*Nature*. 2018;562:373-379).

Prognosis and Treatment

Females and patients with high WBC ($>100 \times 10^9$/L) at baseline have a lower clinical remission (CR) rate. Current treatment utilizes acute lymphoblastic leukemia (ALL)-directed therapy. The addition of tyrosine kinase inhibitors (TKIs), such as imatinib, nilotinib, or ponatinib, to standard chemotherapy has been beneficial (*Lancet Haematol*. 2018;5:e618-e627). Some patients have also benefited from an allogeneic hematopoietic stem cell transplantation (HSCT).

Differential Diagnosis

- **B-ALL with *BCR::ABL1*:** In addition to B-lineage markers, blasts frequently express the myeloid-associated antigens CD13 and CD33 which could be misdiagnosed as MPAL, so careful evaluation of myeloperoxidase (MPO) expression on the blasts is required. These cases have deletion or splicing abnormalities of *IKZF1*, deletions, mutations, or rearrangements of *PAX5*, and deletion of *CDKN2A* and/or *CDKN2B* (*Leukemia*. 2009;23:1989-1998).
- **AML with *BCR::ABL1*:** Additional cytogenetic abnormalities are observed in MPAL with *BCR::ABL1* (13%-30%), as compared to 50%-60% in AML with *BCR::ABL1*, and 70%-80% in chronic myeloid leukemia blast phase (CML-BP). Mutations in *TP53*, *NRAS*, *IDH2*, *FLT3*, *PHF6*, *ASXL1*, *ETV6*, and *DNMT3A* occur in higher frequency in MPAL.
- **Mixed-phenotype (MP) blast phase of CML:** These cases have higher peripheral blood basophil count with increased frequency of splenomegaly. The bone marrow in CML with MP blasts has an elevated myeloid/erythroid ratio at diagnosis. Abnormalities commonly seen in myeloid blast phase of CML, such as 3q26.2

Key Points

- MPAL with *BCR::ABL1* is a de novo acute leukemia that meets the criteria for MPAL and demonstrates *BCR::ABL1* at initial diagnosis, without evidence of CML.
- Presents with leukocytosis with or without hepatosplenomegaly.

Diagnostic Caveats

- CML with MP blasts is in the differential, but no basophilia or increased M:E ratio is noted in MPAL with *BCR::ABL1*, and cryptic deletions within immunoglobulin and T-cell receptor genes accompanied by losses of the *IKZF1* and/or *CDKN2A/B* genes help in the differential diagnosis.
- Mutations in *TP53*, *NRAS*, *IDH2*, *FLT3*, *PHF6*, *ASXL1*, *ETV6*, and *DNMT3A* occur in higher frequency in MPAL, but no *NPM1* mutation has been described.

rearrangement, monosomy 7, trisomy 8, isochromosome 17q, trisomy 19, trisomy 21, and additional Ph chromosome and complex karyotype, are typically present (*Leukemia.* 2017;31:585-559).

B. Mixed-Phenotype Acute Leukemia With *KMT2A/MLL* Rearrangement

These cases are commonly present in children, especially in infants. Mixed-phenotype acute leukemia with *KMT2A/MLL* rearrangement (MPAL-*KMT2A*r) meets the criteria set for MPAL (B, T, or myeloid lineages) and has *KMT2A* (also known as *MLL*, located at 11q23.3) rearrangement with multiple known partner genes. It is noteworthy that *KMT2A*-rearrangement is seen in only 8% of MPAL cases, which usually are B/myeloid, with very few T/myeloid MPAL cases reported (*Leuk Res Rep.* 2022;17:100306). Blasts may be myeloblasts, monoblasts, lymphoblasts and display a dimorphic or undifferentiated population.

Genetic Features

Common translocations involving the *KMT2A* gene include t(4;11)(q21;q23), t(11;19)(q23;p13), and t(9;11)(p22;q23). In addition, *KMT2A* fusion partner genes such as *SNX9* (6q25.3), *USP8* (15q21.2), *SEPT3* (22q13.2), and *USP2* (1 Mbp telomer to *KMT2A* at 11q23.3) have been described (*Leukemia.* 2019;33:2306–2340).

The mutational profile of MPAL-B/M is quite different from that of MPAL-T/M. The T/M type has more frequent somatic mutations and a less complex karyotype than B/myeloid MPAL (*Oncotarget.* 2018;9:8441-8449). Mutations in MPAL-T/M involve the *IDH2*, *WT1*, *CEBPA*, *DNMT3A*, *EZH2*, *PHF6*, *FLT3*, *KRAS*, *NRAS*, *CDKN2A/B*, *ETV6*, *NOTCH1*, *IL7R*, *FBXW7*, and *JAK/STAT* signaling proteins while MPAL-B/M has mutations in *RUNX1*, *ASXL1*, *EZH2*, and *TET2*, and deletions in *IKZF1* (*Exp Hematol.* 2016;44:740-744; *Nature.* 2018;562:373-379). *PICALM* mutation has been reported in AML and T-ALL, including MPAL, and is seen in younger men with extramedullary disease (*Ann Lab Med.* 2010;30:117-121).

Prognosis and Treatment

This entity is considered high risk with poor survival. Most published treatment strategies are in childhood leukemias with beneficial results on ALL-type protocols. HSCT is considered an option only in patients with a poor response to treatment (*Blood.* 2018;132:264-276).

Differential Diagnosis

- **Early T precursor lymphoblastic leukemia/lymphoma (ETP-ALL):** ETP-ALL has poor outcomes and is considered an ALL intermediate between MPAL-T/M and T-ALL. It is characterized by a lack of CD1a and CD8, with weak (<75% positive blasts) CD5 expression and the presence of one or more markers of myeloid or hematopoietic progenitors (CD117, CD34, HLA-DR, CD13, CD33, CD11b, or CD65). *NOTCH1* mutations and *CDKN2A/CDKN2B* deletion are less commonly seen in MPAL-T/M (*Haematologica.* 2020;105:e294-e297).

> **Key Points**
>
> - MPAL with *KMT2A* rearrangement is usually B/myeloid with rare T/myeloid MPAL cases. The latter can be confused with ETP-ALL.
> - Common translocations involving the *KMT2A* gene include t(4;11)(q21;q23), t(11;19)(q23;p13), and t(9;11)(p22;q23).
>
> **Diagnostic Caveats**
>
> - Additional *KMT2A* fusion partner genes such as *SNX9* (6q25.3), *USP8* (15q21.2), *SEPT3* (22q13.2), and *USP2* (1Mbp telomer to *KMT2A* at 11q23.3) have been described.
> - Conventional karyotyping may detect only a subset of cases. Some cryptic rearrangements may require alternate techniques (FISH [fluorescence in situ hybridization] or NGS [next-generation sequencing]).
> - *KMT2A::USP2* may be undetectable by FISH.

C. Acute Leukemia of Ambiguous Lineage With Other Defined Genetic Alterations

ALAL are acute leukemias with newly described genetic alterations. The two entities recognized in this group include the following:

1. MPAL with *ZNF384* rearrangement (MAPL-*ZNF384r*): Seen predominantly in children and comprises 20% of MPAL cases and 48% of MPAL-B/M cases.
2. ALAL with *BCL11B* rearrangement (ALAL-*BCL11Br*): Comprises 10%-15% of MPAL and 30%-40% of MPAL-T/M cases. Some AUL cases have shown this rearrangement.

Genetic Features

1. MPAL-*ZNF384r* has a distinct pattern of genomic alterations. *ZNF384r* is most commonly rearranged with *TCF3*, but *KDM6A* alterations, higher *FLT3* expression, focal heterozygous *IKZF1* deletion, and a focal homozygous deletion of *CDKN2A* and *CDKN2B* also occur (*Nature*. 2018;562:373-379).
2. ALAL-*BCL11Br* shows *WT1* mutations and activating *FLT3* alterations as previously reported in T/myeloid MPAL (*Nature*. 2018;562:373-379) and ETP-ALL (*Nat Genet*. 2017;49:1211-1218). However, these leukemias pose significant diagnostic and therapeutic challenges due to the poorly understood role of *BCL11B*, in as much as oncogenic dysregulation of the gene is driven by a variety of structural alterations that result in this distinct type of ALAL. Furthermore, this subtype-defining event indicates that some T/myeloid MPAL and ETP-ALL originate in a hematopoietic progenitor cell before the initiation of T-lineage differentiation.

> **Key Points**
>
> - Two new subtypes have been recently described: MAPL-*ZNF384r* and ALAL-*BCL11Br*.
>
> **Diagnostic Caveats**
>
> - These acute leukemias must be differentiated from ETP-ALL and AUL.

Prognosis and Treatment

ALAL shows overexpression of *FLT3* and has shown remarkable responsiveness in limited studies to nonselective *FLT3* inhibitors (midostaurin and sorafenib) (*Leuk Lymphoma*. 2020;61:3275-3277).

II. ACUTE LEUKEMIA OF AMBIGUOUS LINEAGE, IMMUNOPHENOTYPICALLY DEFINED

The diagnostic criteria and common features of this category of MPAL are summarized in Table 18.3-4. Examples of biphenotypic leukemic blasts in patients with MPAL as assessed by FC are shown in e-Figures 18.3.2 and 18.3.3.

TABLE 18.3-4 Key Features of MPAL, Immunophenotypically Defined and ALAL

Entity	Immunophenotype	Diagnostic Criteria[a]	Genetic Findings[b]
MPAL-B/M ~6% of MPAL	HSCAs + B/M	• ≥20% blasts in bone marrow and blood • No MPAL defining genetic features • No previous cytotoxic therapy	Trisomy 4, del(6q), 12p11.2, monosomy 7, *ZNF384* rearrangement among others
MPAL-T/M	HSCAs + B/T/M		• t(12;21) with *ETV6::RUNX1* fusion • t(10;11) with *PICALM::MLLT10* • Mutations reported include *DNMT3A, WT1, TP53, IDH1/2, BCOR NOTCH1, NRAS, PHF6, ETV6, RUNX1, FLT3, TET2,* and *ASXL1*
MPAL Rare	HSCAs + various combinations of B/T/M and Mk	All of the above and exclusion of a previous h/o AML	• Complex karyotype, monosomy 7, and t(10;11)(p15;q21) • NGS heterogeneous genetic alterations, with *PHF6* most common
ALAL—NOS	HSCAs/no lineage-defining markers	Exclude all other AML/MPAL	

ALAL, acute leukemia of ambiguous lineage; AML, acute myeloid leukemia; B, B-cell lineage; h/o, history of; HSCAs, hematopoietic stem cell antigens (CD34, HLA-DR, and CD117); M, myeloid lineage; Mk, megakaryocytic lineage; MPAL, mixed-phenotype acute leukemia; NGS, next-generation sequencing; T, T-cell lineage.
[a]Diagnostic criteria per the WHO Classification of Hematolymphoid Tumors (5th Edition).
[b]Some commonly noted genetic findings associated with the entity.

III. MIXED-PHENOTYPE ACUTE LEUKEMIA, RARE TYPES

Mixed-phenotype acute leukemia, rare types (MPAL-rt) are defined by expression of rare T, B, myeloid, and megakaryocytic lineage-specific markers that do not meet the criteria for MPAL with defined genetic alterations (Table 18.3-4). These leukemias are commonly seen in children and young adults. There are three subtypes:

1. MPAL, B/T (MPAL-B/T): Constitutes approximately 6% of MPAL-rt cases.
2. MPAL, B/T/myeloid (MPAL-B/T/M): Constitutes approximately 3% of MPAL-rt cases.
3. MPAL, T/megakaryocytic (MPAL-T/Mk): The incidence is unknown due to its rarity. This type has been reported in infants.

IV. ACUTE UNDIFFERENTIATED LEUKEMIA

AUL is a rare entity that expresses no markers considered to be specific for lymphoid or myeloid lineages (e-Figure 18.3-4) and hence the term "undifferentiated." The incidence is higher in older populations, with a median age of 74 years (*Leukemia Res.* 2020;89:106301).

Genetic Features

AUL has been reported to have del(5q), trisomy of chromosome 13, and a complex karyotype (*Cancer Genet Cytogenet.* 1996;92:31-36). Somatic mutations seen in AUL include the genes *PHF6*, *SRSF2*, *RUNX1*, *ASXL1,* and *BCOR* (*Mod Pathol.* 2019;32:1373-1385). Gene fusions such as *SET::NUP214* are also detected in a subset of cases (*Nature.* 2018;562:373-379).

> **Key Points**
>
> - There is no expression of lineage-specific markers, but the cells are positive for CD34, HLA-DR, and TdT (terminal deoxynucleotidyl transferase).
> - Recurrent mutations *PHF6*, *RUNX1*, *SRSF2*, *ASXL1,* and *BCOR* have been identified.
>
> **Diagnostic Caveats**
>
> - M0 acute leukemia is in the differential and expresses at least two of the myeloid-associated markers (CD13, CD33, or CD117).

SUGGESTED READINGS

1. Lin N, Yan X, Cai D. et al. Leukemia with *TCF3-ZNF384* rearrangement as a distinct subtype of disease with distinct treatments: perspectives from a case report and literature review. *Front Oncol.* 2021;11:709036.
2. Montefiori L, Mullighan CG. Redefining the biological basis of lineage-ambiguous leukemia through genomics: BCL11B deregulation in acute leukemias of ambiguous lineage. *Best Pract Res Clin Haematol.* 2021;34:101329.
3. Alexander TB, Gui Z, Iacobucci I. et al. The genetic basis and cell of origin of mixed phenotype acute leukaemia. *Nature.* 2018;562:373-379.
4. Kurosawa S, Toya T, Kishida Y. et al. Outcome of patients with acute undifferentiated leukemia after allogeneic hematopoietic stem cell transplantation. *Leuk Lymphoma.* 2018;59:3006-3009.
5. Padella A, Simonetti G, Paciello G et al. Novel and rare fusion transcripts involving transcription factors and tumor suppressor genes in acute myeloid leukemia. *Cancers (Basel).* 2019;11:1951.

19 Mature B-cell and Plasma Cell Neoplasms

19.1 Chronic Lymphocytic Leukemia/Small Lymphocytic Lymphoma, Monoclonal B-Cell Lymphocytosis, and B-Cell Prolymphocytic Leukemia

Brooj Abro and Anjum Hassan

I. CHRONIC LYMPHOCYTIC LEUKEMIA/SMALL LYMPHOCYTIC LYMPHOMA

Chronic lymphocytic leukemia/small lymphocytic lymphoma (CLL/SLL) is the most common leukemia in adults, accounting for 25% to 30% of adult leukemias in Western countries (*CA Cancer J Clin.* 2015;65:5-29). It is a low-grade neoplasm of monomorphic small, mature B cells infiltrating the peripheral blood and bone marrow (CLL) and/or involving lymph nodes and extranodal sites (SLL). The characteristic CLL/SLL phenotype consists of mature B cells with weak expression of CD20, dim monotypic surface immunoglobulin (sIg) expression, and co-expression of CD5 and CD23. The distinction between CLL and SLL is based on the disease distribution, and they can overlap. The incidence increases with age, and the median age at diagnosis is approximately 70 years. It is more common in men (male-to-female ratio approximately 2:1). There is a strong genetic predisposition, with an approximately 7- to 8-fold increased risk in first-degree relatives of patients with CLL (*Blood.* 2015;126:2265-2273). The diagnostic criteria for CLL/SLL are summarized in Table 19.1-1.

Clinical Features

- **Clinical presentation:** Most patients are asymptomatic, with lymphocytosis identified incidentally during routine complete blood count (CBC). Clinical findings include lymphocytosis, lymphadenopathy, and splenomegaly, with some patients presenting with autoimmune cytopenias. Serum monoclonal paraprotein (usually IgM) is detected in some patients.
- **Sites of involvement:** CLL/SLL primarily affects the peripheral blood, bone marrow, lymph nodes, and spleen. However, it may also involve other sites such as central nervous system (CNS), skin, kidneys, gastrointestinal tract, and liver in a subset of patients.

TABLE 19.1-1 WHO-HAEM5 Diagnostic Criteria for CLL/SLL

Essential

- Absolute B-cell count $>5 \times 10^9$/L (peripheral blood)
- Effacement of architecture (lymph node/tissues)
- Classic CLL/SLL morphology
- Characteristic immunophenotype by FC/IHC (positive: B-cell markers (CD20 positive/weak), CD5, CD23 [variable], weak monotypic light chain expression; negative: cyclin D1)

Desirable

FC:
- Positive: CD200, ROR1, CD43
- Negative: FMC7, CD10, CD81, CD79b$^{weak/-}$

IHC:
- Positive: LEF1, CD43, MUM1
- Negative: SOX11, CD10

FC, flow cytometry, IHC, immunohistochemistry.
Based on the WHO Classification of Tumours Editorial Board. Haematolymphoid tumours [Internet]. Lyon (France): International Agency for Research on Cancer; 2024 (WHO classification of tumours series, 5th ed.; vol. 11). Available from: https://tumourclassification.iarc.who.int/chapters/63.

Morphology

- **Lymph nodes and spleen:** Lymph nodes typically show diffuse effacement of architecture by small, mature lymphocytes with clumped chromatin and round nuclei (e-Figure 19.1-1). Proliferation centers (also known as pseudofollicles) is a characteristic low-power feature of SLL appreciated as ill-defined pale areas of larger prolymphocytes and paraimmunoblasts compared to the surrounding darker, more closely packed small lymphocytes (e-Figure 19.1-2). Mitotic activity is typically very low, and an interfollicular pattern of involvement with preservation of follicles has also been described (*Mod Pathol.* 2000;13:1161-1166). In the spleen, the white pulp is primarily involved, although red pulp infiltration is also frequently present.
- **Peripheral blood:** On blood smears, the neoplastic cells typically appear as small, mature lymphocytes with scant cytoplasm, condensed chromatin (soccer ball pattern), and inconspicuous nucleoli (e-Figure 19.1-3). Smudge cells may also be observed (ethylenediaminetetraacetic acid [EDTA] artifact). Prolymphocytes (medium-sized lymphocytes with a moderate amount of basophilic cytoplasm and prominent nucleoli) may be present, usually comprising less than 15% of the lymphocytes (e-Figure 19.1-4). Greater than 15% prolymphocytes are seen in prolymphocytic progression of CLL.
- **Bone marrow:** Typically, infiltrates in the bone marrow exhibit a non-paratrabecular pattern, with interstitial, nodular, or diffuse involvement (e-Figure 19.1-5). Proliferation centers are not as frequently observed as in lymph nodes and are usually present when there is diffuse marrow involvement.

Immunophenotype

By immunohistochemistry (IHC), neoplastic cells express B-cell markers and are typically positive for CD5, CD23, CD43, and LEF-1, while being negative for CD10, BCL6, cyclin D1, and SOX-11. Patchy cyclin D1 positivity may be observed in cells within proliferation centers. Flow cytometry (FC) analysis usually shows positive expression of CD19, CD20 (weak), CD5, CD23, CD200, CD11c (variable), ROR1, and monotypic light chain (dim to negative) expression. Markers that are typically negative include CD10, FMC7, CD81, CD25, and CD103. Expression of CD38 and CD49d is associated with a worse prognosis. CLL/SLL cases with atypical immunophenotypes have been reported, and careful evaluation for exclusion of other B-cell lymphomas is warranted in such cases.

Genetic Features

Common cytogenetic abnormalities in CLL/SLL include trisomy 12, deletions in 13q14, 11q22, and 17p13. Genes recurrently mutated include *TP53, SF3B1, ATM, NOTCH1,* and *BIRC3* (*Nature.* 2015;526:525-530). More than 50% of CLL/SLL cases are *IGHV* mutated and have a better prognosis than those that are *IGHV* unmutated (*J Mol Diagn.* 2020;22:1114-1125). Mutations involving *BTK* and *PLCG2* are associated with treatment resistance to Bruton tyrosine kinase (BTK) inhibitors (*J Clin Oncol.* 2017;35:1437-1443), while *BCL2* mutations are associated with treatment resistance to venetoclax (*Cancer Discov.* 2019;9:342-353).

Disease Progression and Transformation

- **Aggressive histologic features and prolymphocytic progression:** Confluent proliferation centers ($>20\times$ field) and high Ki-67 proliferation index ($>40\%$) are features of aggressive disease (*Haematologica.* 2010;95:1526-1533). Prolymphocytic progression of CLL is characterized by more than 15% prolymphocytes and often associated with *TP53* mutations.
- **Richter transformation:** CLL/SLL most commonly transforms into diffuse large B-cell lymphoma (DLBCL) and rarely into classic Hodgkin lymphoma (cHL) (*Am J Surg Pathol.* 2007;31:1605-1614). The diagnosis of cHL requires an appropriate cellular background; isolated Reed-Sternberg–like cells may be seen in cases without transformation. CLL/SLL transformation into DLBCL is characterized by diffuse proliferation of large B cells (e-Figure 19.1-6), usually with a nongerminal center B-cell phenotype, and the classic CLL/SLL markers CD5 and CD23 tend to be negative (*Blood.* 2018;131:2761-2772).

Prognosis and Treatment

CLL/SLL typically has an indolent clinical course. Clinical staging systems (Rai/Binet) and genetic features help assess prognosis and the need for therapy (Table 19.1-2). A comprehensive international prognostic score (International Prognostic Index for patients with chronic lymphocytic leukemia [CLL-IPI]) integrates various clinical and genetic features to stratify risk groups in CLL (*Lancet Oncol.* 2016;17:779-790).

Observation alone in early-stage disease is sufficient unless there are indications for therapy, such as worsening clinical symptoms, advancing lymphadenopathy, high-stage disease, eligibility for a clinical trial, or certain medical complications of CLL/SLL, such as immune hemolysis, thrombocytopenia, and recurrent infections (*Blood.* 2018;131:2745-2760).

Differential Diagnosis

- **Monoclonal B-cell lymphocytosis (MBL):** Asymptomatic clonal B-lymphocytosis with a count of less than 5×10^9/L, without evidence of lymphoma at other sites
- **Mantle cell lymphoma (MCL):** While both CLL/SLL and MCL are typically CD5 positive, other immunophenotypic differences help distinguish between the two. Fluorescence in situ hybridization (FISH) for t(11;14) can be performed in

TABLE 19.1-2 Prognostic Markers in CLL/SLL

Category	Clinical/Laboratory	Histology/FC	Genetic
Favorable	• Female • Age <60 y • Low Rai/Binet stage	• CD38⁻ • ZAP70⁻ • CD49d⁻	• *IGHV* hypermutated • Del(13q14)
Unfavorable	• Male • Age >60 y • High Rai/Binet stage • Elevated β_2-microglobulin • Elevated serum thymidine kinase	• Confluent proliferation centers • Diffuse marrow involvement • CD38⁺ • ZAP70⁺ • CD49d⁺	• *IGHV* unmutated • Complex karyotype • Trisomy 12 • Del(11q23) • Del(17p13) • *TP53* mutations

CLL, chronic lymphocytic leukemia; FC, flow cytometry; SLL, small lymphocytic lymphoma.
(Modified from *Blood*. 2013;121:1403-1412; *N Engl J Med*. 2005;352:804-815; Nat Rev Cancer. 2010;10:37-50; Nature. 2015;526:525-530; *J Mol Diagn*. 2020;22:1114-1125).

difficult cases. MCL usually has the following features: CD20^{bright}, sIg^{bright}, CD5$^+$, CD23$^-$, cyclin D1$^+$, LEF1$^-$, SOX11$^+$, CD200$^-$, t(11;14)$^+$.
- **Other small B-cell lymphomas:** A subset of CLL cases may show atypical (nonclassic) morphology and/or immunophenotype, overlapping with other small B-cell lymphomas. A complete workup should be performed to exclude other B-cell lymphomas.

Key Points

- The diagnosis of CLL/SLL requires circulating clonal B cells ≥5 × 10^9/L or nodal/extranodal involvement.
- The characteristic CLL/SLL phenotype is small, mature CD20^{dim}, sIg^{dim}, CD5$^+$, and CD23$^+$ monoclonal B cells.
- Proliferation centers or "pseudofollicles" are a classic feature of SLL best appreciated at low power.
- Favorable prognostic markers include CD38/ZAP70 negativity, mutated *IGHV*, and isolated del(13q).
- Unfavorable prognostic markers include CD38/ZAP70 positivity, unmutated *IGHV*, del(17p), *TP53* mutation, del(11q), and complex karyotype.

Diagnostic Caveats

- Cyclin D1$^+$ cells can be seen in proliferation centers of SLL, causing potential concern for MCL. SOX11 expression and t(11;14) should test negative.
- Isolated Epstein-Barr virus (EBV)/CD30 + Reed-Sternberg cells may be seen occasionally. This should be distinguished from cHL transformation, which can be challenging on small biopsies.
- A small subset of CLL/SLL cases have an atypical phenotype: CD20^{bright}, CD23$^{dim/-}$, or CD5$^-$.

TABLE 19.1-3 MBL Subtypes

Subtype	Features
CLL/SLL type	• Most common type • Classic CLL/SLL phenotype • **Low-count MBL:** <0.5 × 10^9/L clonal B cells, usually does not progress to CLL • **High-count MBL:** ≥0.5 × 10^9/L and <5 × 10^9/L, may progress to CLL
Non-CLL/SLL type	• Non-CLL/SLL phenotype and no other features of lymphoma • Most commonly shows marginal zone lymphoma phenotype

CLL, chronic lymphocytic leukemia; MBL, monoclonal B-cell lymphocytosis; SLL, small lymphocytic lymphoma.

II. MONOCLONAL B-CELL LYMPHOCYTOSIS

MBL is defined by the presence of asymptomatic clonal B-lymphocytosis with a count of less than 5 × 10^9/L. Similar cytogenetic and molecular features to CLL can be present (*Br J Haematol.* 2012;157;86-96). MBL can be detected in bone marrow and lymphoid tissues, with lymph nodes involved by MBL measuring less than 15 mm and showing preserved architecture. Bone marrow usually shows less than 30% involvement (*Blood.* 2018;131:2745-2760). MBL is classified into three subtypes: low count, CLL type, and non-CLL type (Table 19.1-3). It is crucial to exclude low-level peripheral blood involvement by other B-cell lymphoproliferative disorders.

III. B-CELL PROLYMPHOCYTIC LEUKEMIA

The WHO-HAEM5 has removed B-cell prolymphocytic leukemia (B-PLL) from its classification system (*Leukemia.* 2022;36:1720-1748). Based on the new diagnostic criteria, B-PLL cases may now be classified as prolymphocytic progression of CLL/SLL or under a new category called "splenic B-cell lymphoma/leukemia with prominent nucleoli (SBLPN)," as discussed in Chapter 19.4. However, the International Consensus Classification (ICC) still retains B-PLL as a diagnosis of exclusion.

SUGGESTED READINGS

Hallek M, Cheson BD, Catovsky D, et al. iwCLL guidelines for diagnosis, indications for treatment, response assessment, and supportive management of CLL. *Blood.* 2018;131(25):2745-2760.

Lee J, Wang YL. Prognostic and predictive molecular biomarkers in chronic lymphocytic leukemia. *J Mol Diagn.* 2020;22(9):1114-1125.

19.2 Extranodal, Nodal, and Pediatric Nodal Marginal Zone Lymphoma

Brooj Abro

Marginal zone lymphomas (MZLs) are indolent small B-cell lymphomas characterized by the proliferation of marginal zone B cells, usually negative for CD5 and germinal center markers (CD10, BCL6), with or without plasmacytic differentiation. In the WHO-HAEM4R, three distinct entities with overlapping morphologic and immunophenotypic features were included: extranodal marginal zone lymphoma (EMZL) of mucosa-associated lymphoid tissue (MALT) lymphoma, splenic marginal zone lymphoma (SMZL), and nodal marginal zone lymphoma (NMZL). The recent WHO-HAEM5 recognizes two additional distinct categories: primary cutaneous marginal zone lymphoma (PCMZL, previously part of EMZL) and pediatric nodal marginal zone lymphoma (PNMZL). While the histologic features may be similar, these entities have distinct biologic and clinical features. This chapter will focus on EMZL, NMZL, and PNMZL. SMZL and PCMZL are discussed in Chapters 19.4 and 19.10, respectively.

I. MARGINAL ZONE LYMPHOMA GENERAL FEATURES

Morphology

The infiltrate in MZL is typically composed of a heterogeneous population of mature B cells, predominantly consisting of small centrocyte-like and monocytoid cells. In addition, admixed centroblasts and immunoblasts are usually present. MZL can show various growth patterns (namely, follicular, interfollicular, parafollicular, diffuse), and plasmacytic differentiation may be present, which is also commonly seen in lymphoplasmacytic lymphoma (e-Figure 19.2-1). The infiltrate typically causes the expansion of marginal zones around reactive-appearing follicles, with areas of confluent growth replacing follicles (e-Figure 19.2-2). Colonization of follicles can mimic follicular lymphoma. MZL can closely resemble reactive lymphoid tissue; however, demonstration of light chain restriction (B cells and/or plasma cells [PCs]) helps in distinguishing MZL from reactive lesions. When bone marrow is involved by MZL, it usually shows nodular, interstitial, or intrasinusoidal pattern.

Site-specific morphologic features are mentioned later under various categories of MZL.

Immunophenotype

MZL does not have defining immunophenotypic or molecular features, which can make the diagnosis difficult. Therefore, the workup for MZL should include a comprehensive evaluation to exclude other B-cell lymphomas.

MZL shows expression of pan B-cell antigens (CD19, CD20, PAX5, etc) and is usually negative for CD5, CD10, and BCL6. Co-expression of CD43 is present in a subset of cases (e-Figure 19.2-2). Cyclin D1 and SOX11 are negative (rules out mantle cell lymphoma). CD138 shows increased PCs in cases with plasmacytic differentiation (e-Figure 19.2-1). CD21 and CD23 typically show expanded follicular dendritic meshworks. Monotypic light chain restriction in B cells and/ or PCs can be demonstrated by flow cytometry (FC), while kappa and lambda immunohistochemistry/in situ hybridization studies can be helpful to demonstrate PC clonality. PCs in MZL are usually $CD19^+$, $CD20^-$, and $CD56^-$, in contrast to PCs in PC neoplasm (more likely to be negative for CD19 and positive for CD56 and/or CD20).

Transformation

MZL can transform to diffuse large B-cell lymphoma (DLBCL). While a few scattered larger centroblast-like and immunoblast-like cells can be present, areas with confluent sheets of large cells with increased proliferation index are features of transformation to DLBCL.

Differential Diagnosis

- **Reactive lymphoid hyperplasia:** Polyclonal κ and λ light chain expression
- **Lymphoplasmacytic lymphoma (LPL):** LPL and MZL have overlapping morphology and immunophenotype. Features that favor LPL include an increased IgM paraprotein (Waldenström macroglobulinemia) and the detection of the *MYD88* L265P mutation (rare in MZL).
- **Other small B-cell lymphomas (see Figure 19.2-1):** Other lymphomas such as follicular lymphoma, mantle cell lymphoma, and chronic lymphocytic leukemia/lymphoma should be excluded. A panel of immunohistochemical stains should be performed to exclude other B-cell lymphomas, and in challenging cases, fluorescence in situ hybridization (FISH) studies can be helpful (eg, evaluation of *BCL2* and *BCL6* rearrangements in cases with features of follicular lymphoma).

II. EXTRANODAL MARGINAL ZONE LYMPHOMA OF MUCOSA-ASSOCIATED LYMPHOID TISSUE

As the name implies, EMZL occurs at extranodal sites and is characterized by a heterogeneous B-cell infiltrate typically involving acquired MALT at sites that are normally devoid of organized lymphoid tissue (also known as MALT lymphoma). EMZL accounts for 7% to 8% of B-cell lymphomas, and the median age at presentation is 60 to 70 years (*Ann Lymphoma.* 2021;5:1). EMZL is associated with chronic antigenic stimulation. Several microorganisms and autoimmune conditions have been implicated in the pathogenesis of EMZL at various sites (Table 19.2-1). The diagnostic criteria for EMZL are summarized in Table 19.2-2.

Clinical Features

- **Clinical presentation:** Symptoms vary depending on the site of involvement. Serum monoclonal paraprotein is present in a subset of patients and is associated with plasmacytic differentiation (*Clin Cancer Res.* 2004;10:7179).
- **Sites of involvement:** The most common site is the stomach, followed by the eye/ocular adnexa, lung, skin, salivary glands, breast, thyroid, etc (*Br J Haematol.* 2014;165:67). Approximately 25% to 50% of patients present with disease at multiple sites, and 2% to 20% have bone marrow involvement (*Ann Oncol.* 2020;31:17). Disseminated disease is more common in nongastric MALT lymphomas (*Blood.* 2003;101:2489).

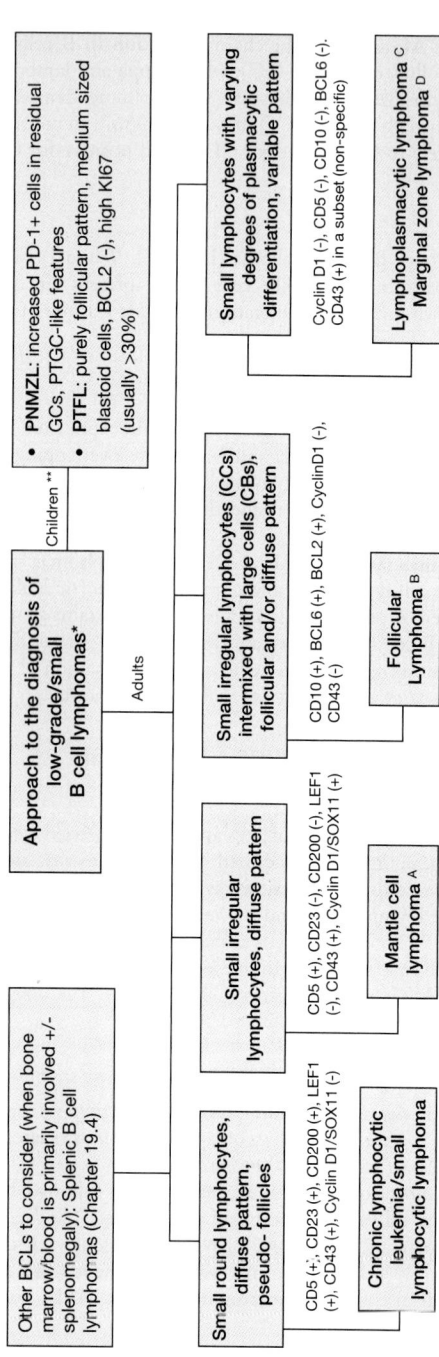

Figure 19.2-1. Diagnosis and workup of small B cell lymphomas.

Abbreviations: CCs = centrocytes, CBs = centroblasts, PNMZL = pediatric nodal marginal zone lymphoma, PTFL = pediatric-type follicular lymphoma, BCL = B cell lymphoma, GCs = germinal centers, PTGC = progressive transformation of GCs.

*Features listed here are characteristic of the respective BCLs, but there are exceptions. For more details see the respective chapters. The morphologic patterns refer to the typical patterns in involved nodal/extra-nodal tissue (not bone marrow/blood). IHC panel for workup of low-grade BCLs: CD20, PAX5, CD3, CD10, BCL6, BCL2, CD21, CD23, Ki67, CD5 and Cyclin D1 (CD138, Kappa and lambda IHC/ISH can be added when plasmacytic differentiation is noted or MZL/LPL is suspected). Additional stains e.g., SOX11, CD43, LEF1 can be added when needed. **Low-grade BCLs are rare in children, and the diagnosis should made with caution. Some features are distinct, and some features overlap with adult counterparts.

A. Cyclin D1 is rarely negative, SOX11 is (+); leukemic non-nodal MCL is usually SOX11 (-). **B.** Certain FL variants are negative for CD10 and/or BCL2. **C.** *MYD88* mutation (>90%). **D.** *MYD88* mutation is uncommon. Note: other BCLs may also show plasmacytic differentiation.

TABLE 19.2-1 Etiologies Implicated in EMZL

Etiology	Site
Infectious	
Helicobacter pylori	Stomach
Chlamydia psittaci	Ocular adnexa
Achromobacter xylosoxidans	Lungs
Borrelia burgdorferi	Skin
Campylobacter jejuni	Small intestine
Autoimmune	
Hashimoto thyroiditis	Thyroid
Sjogren syndrome	Salivary glands

EMZL, extranodal marginal zone lymphoma.
From *Blood.* 2016;127:2082; *CA Cancer J Clin.* 2016;66:153.

Morphology and Immunophenotype

In addition to the features previously described, lymphoepithelial lesions (LELs) are commonly seen in glandular tissues (e-Figure 19.2-2C). LELs are defined as distortion or destruction of epithelial structures caused by aggregates of three or more lymphoma cells.

See "Immunophenotype" section previously marginal zone lymphoma general features.

TABLE 19.2-2 WHO-HAEM5 Diagnostic Criteria for EMZL

Essential	Desirable
• Extranodal site • Atypical B-cell lymphoid infiltrate of small-medium sized cells resembling reactive MALT with architectural distortion • Exclusion of other small B-cell lymphomas	• Demonstration of clonality: light chain restriction or immunoglobulin gene rearrangement • Lymphoepithelial lesions • Reactive inflammatory background

EMZL, extranodal marginal zone lymphoma; MALT, mucosa-associated lymphoid tissue.
Based on the WHO Classification of Tumours Editorial Board. Haematolymphoid tumours [Internet]. Lyon (France): International Agency for Research on Cancer; 2024 (WHO classification of tumours series, 5th ed.; vol. 11). Available from: https://tumourclassification.iarc.who.int/chapters/63.

TABLE 19.2-3 Common Rearrangements in EMZL

Translocation	Genes Involved	Comments
t(11;18)(q21;q21)	*BIRC3* and *MALT1*	Most commonly in lungs, stomach, and ocular adnexa (20%-30%)
t(14;18)(q32;q21)	*IGH* and *MALT1*	Most commonly in liver, skin, and ocular adnexa (10%-15%)
t(3;14)(p14.1;q32)	*FOXP1* and *IGH*	Approximately 10% of cases, commonly seen in thyroid, skin, and ocular adnexa
t(1;14)(p22;q32)	*BCL10* and *IGH*	Approximately 5% of cases, commonly seen in lungs, small intestine, and stomach

EMZL, extranodal marginal zone lymphoma.
Modified from Medeiros LJ. *Ioachim's Lymph Node Pathology*. 5th ed. Wolters Kluwer; 2021.

Genetic Features

Common chromosomal abnormalities in EMZL include trisomy of chromosomes 3, 8, and 12. Various translocations are associated with EMZL and the frequency varies by location (Table 19.2-3).

Prognosis and Treatment

The prognosis is good, with a 10-year survival rate of approximately 80% (*CA Cancer J Clin*. 2016;66:153). Recurrences involving the same location or other extranodal sites can occur after several years. Gastric EMZL usually responds well to *Helicobacter pylori* treatment. Localized disease at other sites can be treated with radiation therapy. Systemic therapy is indicated for disseminated or transformed disease.

See "Differential Diagnosis" section previously marginal zone lymphoma general features.

III. NODAL MARGINAL ZONE LYMPHOMA

NMZL primarily involves the lymph nodes without significant involvement of extranodal sites at initial diagnosis. It is uncommon and accounts for less than 2% of all non-Hodgkin lymphomas (*Pathology*. 2020;52:15). The diagnostic criteria for NMZL are summarized in Table 19.2-4.

Clinical Features

- **Clinical presentation**: Patients may present with localized or widespread lymphadenopathy. Some individuals are asymptomatic. B symptoms are uncommon.
  Sites of involvement: Peripheral lymph nodes most commonly in the head and neck region are involved. Bone marrow involvement is often present. While peripheral blood involvement can occur, lymphocytosis is rare.

TABLE 19.2-4 WHO-HAEM5 Diagnostic Criteria for NMZL

Essential

- Proliferation of small mature B cells with a variable amount of pale cytoplasm, with or without plasmacytic differentiation causing architectural distortion
- Growth patterns: follicular, parafollicular, interfollicular, diffuse
- Exclusion of other small B-cell lymphomas

Desirable

- Residual follicles with follicular colonization
- Demonstration of clonality: light chain restriction or immunoglobulin gene rearrangement

NMZL, nodal marginal zone lymphoma.
Based on the WHO Classification of Tumours Editorial Board. Haematolymphoid tumours [Internet]. Lyon (France): International Agency for Research on Cancer; 2024 (WHO classification of tumours series, 5th ed.; vol. 11). Available from: https://tumourclassification.iarc.who.int/chapters/63.

Morphology and Immunophenotype

In NMZL, affected lymph nodes usually show some degree of nodal architectural distortion or effacement (usually partial) caused by a proliferation of small mature B cells with various growth patterns (e-Figure 19.2-3).

See "Morphology and Immunophenotype" section previously marginal zone lymphoma general features.

Genetic Features

Clonal *IGH/IGK* gene rearrangements are present, and this finding can be helpful to distinguish NMZL from reactive changes, especially when FC is not available. NMZL does not show specific recurrent translocations. The presence of recurrent translocations associated with other lymphomas (eg, *BCL2* and *BCL6* translocation in follicular lymphoma) excludes diagnosis of NMZL. Recurrently mutated genes include *MLL2/KMT2D*, *PTPRD*, *NOTCH2*, and *KLF2*, with *PTPRD* mutations being the most common in NMZL (*Blood.* 2016;128:1362). *BRAF* V600E mutation has also been reported (*Leukemia.* 2018;32:2412).

Prognosis and Treatment

NMZL is an indolent lymphoma with favorable outcomes. However, progression of disease after treatment and transformation to large cell lymphoma indicates a worse prognosis. Treatment options include radiation for localized disease and immunochemotherapy regimens, for disseminated disease (*Blood.* 2016;127:2064).

See "Differential Diagnosis" section previously marginal zone lymphoma general features.

IV. PEDIATRIC NODAL MARGINAL ZONE LYMPHOMA

PNMZL is a rare childhood lymphoma, accounting for less than 2% of all childhood non-Hodgkin lymphomas. It primarily affects male adolescents and shares many features with the adult counterpart (NMZL); however, there are clinical and morphologic differences between the two. The diagnostic criteria for PNMZL are summarized in Table 19.2-5.

TABLE 19.2-5 Diagnostic Criteria for PNMZL

Essential

- Partial effacement of nodal architecture
- Interfollicular infiltrate of cells with monocytoid and centrocytic-like morphology and immunophenotype of marginal zone B cells
- Clonal *IGH/IGK* gene rearrangements

Desirable

- Follicular colonization
- Monotypic light chain restriction
- Reactive follicles with increased PD1$^+$ cells and PTGC-like features

PNMZL, pediatric nodal marginal zone lymphoma; PTGC, progressive transformation of germinal centers.
Based on the WHO Classification of Tumours Editorial Board. Haematolymphoid tumours [Internet]. Lyon (France): International Agency for Research on Cancer; 2024 (WHO classification of tumours series, 5th ed.; vol. 11). Available from: https://tumourclassification.iarc.who.int/chapters/63.

Clinical Features

- **Clinical presentation:** PNMZL most commonly presents with localized lymphadenopathy, with systemic symptoms being rarely reported.
- **Sites of involvement:** Lymph nodes in the head and neck regions are most often involved.

Morphology and Immunophenotype

Like other types of MZLs, PNMZL lacks specific biomarkers. Morphologic and immunophenotypic features overlap with NMZL. PNMZL typically shows expansion of interfollicular spaces by mature polymorphic B cells with varying amounts of pale cytoplasm and a marginal zone phenotype. The nodal architecture is usually partially effaced, with residual follicles showing increased PD-1$^+$ cells and progressive transformation of germinal centers (PTGC)–like features (highlighted by IgD). Neoplastic B cells show expression of pan B-cell antigens, are usually negative for germinal center markers (rarely CD10$^+$), and often show co-expression of CD43 (*Virchows Arch.* 2016;468:141). Plasmacytic differentiation may also be present.

Genetic Features

Clonal *IGH/IGK* gene rearrangements are present and can be helpful in supporting the diagnosis of PNMZL. Trisomy 8 is the most common cytogenetic abnormality (*Mod Pathol.* 2010;23:866).

Prognosis and Treatment

For limited localized disease, which is usually the case, conservation management including excision and watchful waiting is sufficient (*Pediatr Blood Cancer.* 2018;65:10). The prognosis is excellent, with disease relapse and progression being rare.

Differential Diagnosis

- **Atypical marginal zone hyperplasia (AMZH):** AMZH can show overlapping features with PNMZL, including the detection of light chain restriction by FC.

IGH/IGK gene rearrangement studies are recommended for the diagnosis of PNMZL.
- Other small B-cell lymphomas should be excluded.

> **Key Points**
>
> - MZLs are indolent small B-cell lymphomas without specific biomarkers.
> - According to the recent WHO-HAEM5, the following types are recognized as distinct entities: EMZL/MALT lymphoma, SMZL, PCMZL, NMZL, and PNMZL.
> - MZLs have overlapping morphologic and immunophenotypic features. Typically, a polymorphic B-cell infiltrate composed of centrocyte-like or monocytoid B cells without expression of CD5, CD10, and BCL6 is observed. Expanded follicular dendritic cell meshworks, aberrant co-expression of CD43, and the presence of clonal PCs can give clues to the diagnosis.
>
> **Diagnostic Caveats**
>
> - MZLs show various growth patterns that can mimic other small B-cell lymphomas (eg, follicular colonization pattern mimics follicular lymphoma). A comprehensive workup should be performed to rule out other B-cell lymphomas.
> - LPL is an important differential diagnosis, especially when there is bone marrow involvement. Features that favor LPL include increased IgM paraprotein (Waldenström macroglobulinemia) and the detection of the *MYD88* L265P mutation (rare in MZL).
> - PNMZL typically shows residual germinal centers with PTGC-like features. Both AMZH and PNMZL can show light chain restriction by FC. *IGH/IGK* gene rearrangement studies are recommended to establish a definitive diagnosis.

SUGGESTED READINGS

Attarbaschi A, Abla O, Arias Padilla L, et al. Rare non-Hodgkin lymphoma of childhood and adolescence: a consensus diagnostic and therapeutic approach to pediatric-type follicular lymphoma, marginal zone lymphoma, and nonanaplastic peripheral T-cell lymphoma. *Pediatr Blood Cancer*. 2020;67(8):e28416.

Di Rocco A, Petrucci L, Assanto GM, Martelli M, Pulsoni A. Extranodal marginal zone lymphoma: pathogenesis, diagnosis and treatment. *Cancers (Basel)*. 2022;14(7):1742.

Nakamura S, Ponzoni M. Marginal zone B-cell lymphoma: lessons from Western and Eastern diagnostic approaches. *Pathology*. 2020;52(1):15-29.

19.3 Lymphoplasmacytic Lymphoma

Tanya Sajan Ponnatt, Omar Al-Rusan, and Brooj Abro

Lymphoplasmacytic lymphoma (LPL) is a rare, indolent B-cell lymphoma composed of small mature B cells and a variable spectrum of plasmacytic differentiation. LPL commonly involves the bone marrow and is often accompanied by serum IgM paraprotein; the combination of these features is known as Waldenström macroglobulinemia (WM). The presence of serum IgM paraprotein is not specific to LPL and can be detected in other B-cell lymphomas. LPL is mostly diagnosed in older adults

TABLE 19.3-1 WHO HAEM5 Diagnostic Criteria for LPL

Essential

- **Morphology:** Bone marrow involved by >10% lymphoplasmacytic infiltrate (mixture of small lymphocytes and plasmacytoid lymphocytes/plasma cells)
- **Immunophenotype:** Positive for B-cell antigens, IgM (IgA or IgG rare), CD25 and negative for CD10[a], CD23, and CD103. CD138[+/−]

Desirable

- *MYD88* (p.L265P) and *CXCR4* somatic mutation
- Presence of monoclonal IgM

Based on the WHO Classification of Tumours Editorial Board. Haematolymphoid tumours [Internet]. Lyon (France): International Agency for Research on Cancer; 2024 (WHO classification of tumours series, 5th edition; vol. 11). Available from: https://tumourclassification.iarc.who.int/chapters/63.
[a]A subset of cases are CD10+

(>60 years) and is more common in males (*Leuk Lymphoma.* 2012;53:1625). The diagnostic criteria for LPL are summarized in Table 19.3-1.

The WHO-HAEM5 recognizes two subtypes of LPL: IgM LPL/WM type and non-IgM LPL/WM type. The non-IgM LPL/WM type is quite rare (<5% of LPL cases) and includes LPL with IgG or IgA paraprotein, nonsecretory LPL, and IgM LPL without marrow involvement (*Leukemia.* 2022;36:1720).

Clinical Features

- **Clinical presentation:** Patients may be asymptomatic. Common signs and symptoms are associated with bone marrow and/or tissue infiltration and the presence of IgM paraprotein. Bone marrow involvement can result in cytopenias. Various clinical manifestations associated with IgM paraprotein include hyperviscosity syndrome, an increased bleeding tendency, neuropathy, and symptoms of autoimmunity such as hemolytic anemia. Patients may present with constitutional symptoms such as fever and fatigue. Lymphadenopathy and hepatosplenomegaly may be present. Non-IgM LPL/WM type is less frequently associated with serum paraprotein and bone marrow infiltration. These patients are less likely to present with hyperviscosity syndrome and neuropathy. Extramedullary disease is more common in the non-IgM LPL/WM type (*Leuk Lymphoma.* 2020;61:1388).
- **Sites of involvement:** The bone marrow is the most frequent site involved at presentation. Lymph nodes and other extranodal sites such as the liver, spleen, skin, and central nervous system (CNS) can be involved.

Morphology

- **Blood and bone marrow:** Rouleaux formation in the blood is common in cases with high IgM levels. Few circulating plasmacytoid lymphocytes may be present; however, lymphocytosis is uncommon. The bone marrow typically shows a lymphoplasmacytic infiltrate composed of varying proportions of small B cells, plasmacytoid lymphocytes, and plasma cells (PCs) (e-Figure 19.3-1). The infiltration patterns include paratrabecular, interstitial, diffuse, and nodular. Plasmacytic differentiation with Dutcher bodies, an increase in reactive mast cells, and

hemosiderin-laden histiocytes serve as helpful clues in the diagnosis of LPL (*Am J Clin Pathol.* 2015;143:797). Light chain amyloid deposition can be present. In some cases, the PC component is predominant and the lymphoid component may be absent, particularly after treatment. Increased large cells and mitosis may be present, described as the "polymorphous variant" in some studies, and these features may represent evolution to large cell transformation.
- **Lymph node and spleen:** Lymph nodes involved by LPL may show partial or complete effacement of architecture. Residual follicles, intact sinuses, hemosiderin-laden macrophages, and increased mast cells may be present. The cytologic features are similar to those seen in bone marrow. Splenic involvement is usually characterized by infiltration of both red and white pulp by a lymphoplasmacytic infiltrate.

Transformation

LPL can transform to diffuse large B-cell lymphoma (DLBCL). Increased large cells can be seen in the polymorphous variant; however, confluent sheets of large cells with an increased proliferation index are features of transformation to DLBCL.

Immunophenotype

Like marginal zone lymphoma (MZL), LPL does not have specific immunophenotypic markers. The neoplastic B cells in LPL express pan B-cell antigens (CD20, PAX5, CD79a, etc), IgM (majority of cases), and are usually negative for CD10, BCL6, CD5, cyclin D1, CD23, and CD103. A subset of cases may show an atypical phenotype, including variable expression of CD5, CD23, or CD10. CD10-positive cases are usually negative for BCL6. Neoplastic B cells may show aberrant co-expression of CD43. CD138 highlights the PC component. PCs in LPL are usually positive for CD19 and negative for CD20 and CD56. Light chain restriction can be demonstrated in both the B-cell and PC components using flow cytometry. Kappa and lambda immunohistochemistry/in situ hybridization studies can be helpful in demonstrating PC clonality.

Genetic Features

Molecular testing for *MYD88* and *CXCR4* mutations is helpful in the workup of LPL. *MYD88* (p.L265P) mutations are identified in the majority of cases (>90%), while *CXCR4* mutations are detected in approximately 30% to 40% of cases, and both mutations can co-occur (*Blood.* 2016;128:827). It should be noted that *MYD88* mutations can be detected in other lymphomas; however, the detection of the *MYD88* (p.L265P) mutation can be used to support the diagnosis of LPL in the appropriate clinicopathologic context. Deletions involving chromosome 6q are the most frequent chromosomal abnormality reported (*Am J Clin Pathol.* 2001;116:543).

Prognosis and Treatment

According to the WM International Prognostic Scoring System (IPSSWM), the following five adverse factors can be used to stratify patients into low-risk, intermediate-risk, and high-risk disease: advanced age (>65 years), hemoglobin 11.5 g/dL and less, platelets 100×10^9/L and less, β_2-microglobulin more than 3 mg/L, and serum monoclonal protein concentration more than 7.0 g/dL. Patients with two or more adverse features are considered high-risk and showed decreased 5-year survival (36% vs 68% in intermediate-risk and 87% in low-risk categories) in a multicenter study (*Blood.* 2009;113:4163). LPL without *MYD88* mutation (wild type) is associated with shorter overall survival and an increased risk of transformation to DLBCL (*Br J Haematol.* 2018;180:374; *Blood.* 2014;123:2791). Not all patients require treatment at the initial diagnosis, and therapy is usually reserved for patients with symptomatic disease. Common regimens include rituximab in combination with other agents, including alkylating agents and proteasome inhibitors (*Hematol Oncol Clin North Am.* 2019;33:639).

Differential Diagnosis

- **Marginal zone lymphoma (MZL):** Both LPL and MZL can show plasmacytic differentiation and have a nonspecific immunophenotype (CD5 and CD10 negative). Differentiating LPL from MZL by histology alone can be challenging. Extensive bone marrow involvement, high IgM paraprotein, and detection of *MYD88* mutation favors the diagnosis of LPL.
- **IgM MGUS (monoclonal gammopathy of unknown significance):** IgM MGUS shows less than 10% bone marrow involvement by a lymphoplasmacytic infiltrate, less than 3 g/dL serum IgM monoclonal protein, and no evidence of clinical signs or symptoms associated with lymphoma. *MYD88* mutation can be present.
- **Other small B-cell lymphomas** can show plasmacytic differentiation. Conversely, some LPL cases do not show prominent plasmacytic differentiation, and morphologic features may overlap with other small B-cell lymphomas such as chronic lymphocytic leukemia/small lymphocytic lymphoma (CLL/SLL) and mantle cell lymphoma. A panel of immunohistochemical stains should be performed to exclude other B-cell lymphomas.

Key Points

- LPL is an indolent lymphoma composed of small B lymphocytes, plasmacytoid lymphocytes, and PCs.
- The combination of LPL in the bone marrow and presence of IgM paraprotein in the blood is known as Waldenström macroglobulinemia (WM).
- Like MZL, LPL does not have specific immunophenotypic markers, but it is usually negative for CD5, CD23, CD10, and BCL6.
- *MYD88* (p.L265P) mutation is present in >90% of cases, and *CXCR4* mutations are seen in 30%-40% of cases.

Diagnostic Caveats

- The diagnosis of LPL requires clinicopathologic correlation, and a diagnosis of "B-cell lymphoma with plasmacytic differentiation" is often rendered by histologic evaluation alone.
- LPL and MZL show overlapping morphologic and immunophenotypic features. Extensive bone marrow involvement, high IgM paraprotein, and detection of *MYD88* mutation favor the diagnosis of LPL.
- Rarely, LPL can show atypical immunophenotype (positivity for CD5, CD23, or CD10). A complete workup should be performed to exclude other B-cell lymphomas.

SUGGESTED READINGS

Gertz MA. Waldenström macroglobulinemia: 2021 update on diagnosis, risk stratification, and management. *Am J Hematol.* 2021;96(2):258-269.

Wang W, Lin P. Lymphoplasmacytic lymphoma and Waldenström macroglobulinaemia: clinicopathological features and differential diagnosis. *Pathology.* 2020;52(1):6-14.

19.4 Splenic B-Cell Leukemias/Lymphomas

Brooj Abro

Splenic B-cell leukemias/lymphomas are rare mature B-cell neoplasms primarily involving the spleen, bone marrow, and blood. The diagnosis often relies on examining blood and bone marrow samples as spleen biopsies/splenectomies are uncommonly performed. The following entities were included in the WHO-HAEM4R: hairy cell leukemia (HCL), splenic marginal zone lymphoma (SMZL), and two provisional entities, hairy cell leukemia variant (HCL-v) and splenic diffuse red pulp small B-cell lymphoma (SDRPL). While the International Consensus Classification (ICC) retains the same categories, the WHO-HAEM5 has made a few notable changes. The term "HCL-v" is removed in recognition that these cases have significant biologic and clinical differences from HCL, and a new category, "splenic B-cell lymphoma/leukemia with prominent nucleoli (SBLPN)," has been introduced. This new diagnostic category encompasses cases of HCL-v and some cases of B-cell prolymphocytic leukemia (B-PLL). Notably, the latter category has also been removed from the WHO-HAEM5 while retained in the ICC.

I. HAIRY CELL LEUKEMIA

HCL is a rare distinct entity characterized by "hairy" cytoplasmic projections and a unique immunophenotype. It accounts for approximately 2% of all leukemias. HCL is more common in Caucasians and predominantly affects adult men (male-to-female ratio ~4:1) with a median age of presentation in the sixth decade. *BRAF* V600E mutation–mediated constitutive activation of the RAF-MEK-ERK protein kinase pathway is the key pathogenic event, and this mutation is identified in almost all cases (*N Engl J Med*. 2011;364:2305). While the *BRAF* V600E mutation is also detected in other malignancies, this mutation is rare in other mature B cell neoplasms. The diagnostic criteria for HCL are summarized in Table 19.4-1.

Clinical Features

- **Clinical presentation:** Common signs and symptoms include fatigue, infections, pancytopenia, and splenomegaly. Monocytopenia is a characteristic finding in HCL.
- **Sites of involvement:** The spleen and bone marrow are primarily involved. Circulating hairy cells (usually few) can be seen in the peripheral blood. Involvement of lymph nodes and other extranodal sites is uncommon.

Morphology

- **Peripheral blood:** Small- to medium-sized lymphocytes with oval or bean-shaped nuclei, inconspicuous nucleoli, moderate to abundant cytoplasm, and circumferential cytoplasmic projections (e-Figure 19.4-1)
- **Bone marrow:** Interstitial and diffuse patterns of involvement with increased reticulin fibrosis are common, resulting in a "dry tap." The neoplastic cells have moderate to abundant cytoplasm and widely spaced nuclei, giving a "fried egg"

TABLE 19.4-1	WHO-HAEM5 Diagnostic Criteria for Hairy Cell Leukemia (HCL)
Essential	**Desirable**
• **Morphology:** Small- to medium-sized lymphocytes with oval-indented nucleus, inconspicuous nucleoli, and cytoplasmic projections in blood/bone marrow smear or a "fried egg" appearance in bone marrow biopsy • **Immunophenotype:** Strong CD20 and annexin A1 expression, or co-expression of CD20, CD11c, CD103, and CD25	• *BRAF* p.V600E mutation • Expression of CD123, bright CD22, bright CD200, bright surface light chain, cyclin-D1, and TBX21/T-Bet

Based on the WHO Classification of Tumours Editorial Board. Haematolymphoid tumours [Internet]. Lyon (France): International Agency for Research on Cancer; 2024 (WHO classification of tumours series, 5th ed.; vol. 11). Available from: https://tumourclassification.iarc.who.int/chapters/63.

appearance in core biopsy sections (e-Figure 19.4-2). Some cases show subtle, patchy low-level involvement.
- **Spleen, liver, and lymph nodes:** The spleen shows diffuse splenic red pulp infiltration with expansion of the red pulp and atrophic or absent white pulp. "Pseudosinuses" (blood lakes lined by hairy cells) are a characteristic feature. In the liver, the sinuses are commonly involved. Lymph node involvement is uncommon and typically shows infiltration of paracortex and sinuses.

Immunophenotype

HCL shows expression of pan B-cell antigens (CD20 is usually bright on flow cytometry [FC]), annexin A1, classic HCL markers by FC (bright CD11c, CD25, CD103, and CD123), CD200, FMC7, bright monotypic surface light chain, DBA-44/CD76, BCL-2, TRAP, and BRAF V600E (e-Figure 19.4-2). HCL is usually negative for CD23, CD5, and CD10. Cyclin D1 is variably positive. Rare cases with variant immunophenotypic features have been described, including expression of CD23/CD5/CD10 and lack of CD103 (*Am J Clin Pathol.* 2006;125:251; *Cytometry B Clin Cytom.* 2016;90:467).

Genetic Features

Loss of 7q is the most common cytogenetic abnormality in HCL (*Blood.* 2017; 130:1644). Although cyclin D1 immunohistochemistry (IHC) positivity can be present, t(11;14) is negative. Most cases show *IGHV* gene hypermutations (*Am J Hematol.* 2017;92:1382). The *BRAF* V600E mutation is present in virtually all cases and is considered a disease-defining event.

Prognosis and Treatment

HCL generally has a good prognosis (~90% 10-year survival), with high response rates to purine analogs (*Blood.* 2017;129:553). Unfavorable prognostic factors include unmutated *IGHV*, *IGHV4-34* immunoglobulin variable heavy chain rearrangement, massive splenomegaly, high white blood cell (WBC) count ($>10^9$/L), increased circulating hairy cells (>5 G/L), high β_2-microglobulin levels, and CD38 expression (*Am J Hematol.* 2019;94:1413).

Differential Diagnosis

Due to its clinical presentation of pancytopenia, splenomegaly, and "dry tap" (marrow fibrosis), the differential diagnosis includes myeloid disorders. Dysplastic features may be present in hematopoietic cells. Cases with adequate biopsy material and diffuse infiltrate with classic HCL morphology are easily identified; however, in some cases, HCL may show atypical morphology or subtle infiltrate on hematoxylin and eosin (H&E) sections. Detection of a clonal B-cell population by FC with positive expression of classic HCL antigens (CD11c, CD123, CD25, and CD103) is helpful, and in difficult cases, *BRAF* V600E mutation testing can be performed to confirm the diagnosis. HCL has some overlapping features with other splenic B-cell neoplasms. See the discussion at the end of the chapter and Table 19.4-5.

Key Points

- Key points are summarized in Table 19.4-5.

Diagnostic Caveats

- HCL is not common, and the clinical findings at presentation (pancytopenia, splenomegaly, dry tap due to marrow fibrosis) overlap with myeloid disorders.
- In some cases, HCL may show atypical morphology or a subtle infiltrate on bone marrow core biopsy H&E sections. Detection of clonal B-cell population by FC with positive expression of classic HCL antigens is a clue to the diagnosis.
- In difficult cases, *BRAF* V600E mutation testing can be helpful.

II. SPLENIC MARGINAL ZONE LYMPHOMA

SMZL is a mature B-cell lymphoma characterized by prominent involvement of the splenic white pulp, circulating villous lymphocytes, and a nonspecific immunophenotype. SMZL is uncommon and accounts for less than 2% of all lymphoid neoplasms. Most patients are over 50 years old at diagnosis, and the incidence is similar in men and women. The diagnostic criteria for SMZL are summarized in Table 19.4-2.

Clinical Features

- **Clinical presentation:** Some patients are asymptomatic. Common signs and symptoms include splenomegaly, cytopenias, lymphocytosis, and clinical manifestations associated with autoimmunity. A small monoclonal paraprotein is present in one-third of patients. Association with hepatitis C virus infection has been reported (*N Engl J Med.* 2002;347:89).
- **Sites of involvement:** The spleen and splenic hilar lymph nodes are primarily involved, with frequent involvement of the bone marrow and peripheral blood. Peripheral lymphadenopathy and involvement of other extranodal sites are uncommon.

TABLE 19.4-2 WHO-HAEM5 Diagnostic Criteria for Splenic Marginal Zone Lymphoma (SMZL)

Essential

- **Morphology:** Small lymphocytes with villous processes
- **Immunophenotype:** Positive for pan B-cell antigens, IgM, and IgD, and negative for BCL6, annexin A1, CD103, cyclin D1, SOX11, and LEF1
- Exclusion of other B-cell lymphomas
- Splenomegaly

Desirable

- Negative for CD5 and CD10

Based on the WHO Classification of Tumours Editorial Board. Haematolymphoid tumours [Internet]. Lyon (France): International Agency for Research on Cancer; 2024 (WHO classification of tumours series, 5th ed.; vol. 11). Available from: https://tumourclassification.iarc.who.int/chapters/63.

Morphology

- **Spleen and splenic hilar lymph nodes:** On gross examination, the spleen is enlarged with multiple nodules representing expansion of the white pulp. On microscopic examination, the white pulp is predominantly involved with variable infiltration of the red pulp. Neoplastic small mature lymphocytes surround follicles or infiltrate and replace germinal centers (e-Figure 19.4-3). A biphasic or target-like pattern can be appreciated in some cases (central residual germinal center surrounded by a dark zone of small lymphocytes and a pale outer zone of monocytoid cells). In the red pulp, the neoplastic cells invade the sinuses. Scattered larger B cells resembling immunoblasts and centroblasts, as well as epithelioid histiocytes, can be seen. Plasmacytic differentiation is present in a subset of cases. The involved splenic hilar lymph nodes typically show dilated sinuses and partial to complete effacement by the neoplastic cells.
- **Peripheral blood and bone marrow:** Circulating mature lymphocytes with unipolar or bipolar cytoplasmic projections (villous lymphocytes) may be present (e-Figure 19.4-4). Bone marrow involvement is variable, with a combination of various patterns of infiltration including paratrabecular, intrasinusoidal, interstitial nodular, or diffuse.

Immunophenotype

Neoplastic cells show expression of pan B-cell antigens, FMC7, $CD25^{+/-}$, and $DBA-44^{+/-}$ and are mostly negative for CD5, CD10, BCL6, cyclin D1, LEF1, CD123, CD103, and annexin A1. CD21 highlights associated follicular dendritic cell meshworks (e-Figure 19.4-3). In contrast to other marginal zone lymphomas (MZLs), SMZL can show expression of both IgM and IgD, while CD43 is usually negative. CD5-positive SMZL cases have been reported and are associated with a higher disease burden (higher lymphocyte count and diffuse marrow involvement) compared to classic CD5-negative SMZL (*Haematologica.* 2010;95:604).

Genetic Features

The most common cytogenetic abnormality is hemizygous deletion of 7q, identified in 30% to 40% of cases (*Blood.* 2011;117:1595). Other less frequent chromosomal abnormalities include gain of 3q and 18q, 14q aberrations, and del(17p13) resulting in loss of *TP53* (*Best Pract Res Clin Haematol.* 2017;30:56). SMZL is not associated with recurrent translocations seen in other lymphomas. Approximately 50% of cases are *IGHV* mutated, and IGHV1-2 usage is most frequent (~30%) (*Leukemia.* 2012;26:1638). *NOTCH2* and *KLF2* (involved in marginal zone differentiation) are the most frequently mutated genes. The combination of deletion 7q31-32 and *NOTCH2* mutations is most specific to SMZL among other B-cell neoplasms (*Blood.* 2016;127:2072).

Prognosis and Treatment

SMZL has an indolent clinical course with a good prognosis and a 10-year survival of up to 95% (*Leuk Res.* 2016;44:53). Transformation to DLBCL has been reported in approximately 10% to 15% of cases, which portends a worse prognosis (*Best Pract Res Clin Haematol.* 2017;30:56). Other unfavorable prognostic markers include anemia, thrombocytopenia, high lactate dehydrogenase (LDH) level, extra-hilar lymphadenopathy, unmutated *IGHV*, and mutations involving *NOTCH2, KLF2,* and *TP53* (*Clin Cancer Res.* 2015;21:4174; *Blood.* 2016;127:2072). A prognostic index has been developed to stratify patients into low-, intermediate-, and high-risk groups using the following parameters: hemoglobin level, platelet count, LDH level, and extra-hilar lymphadenopathy (*Br J Haematol.* 2012;159:164). A watchful waiting approach is recommended for asymptomatic patients. Treatment options for symptomatic patients include rituximab (as monotherapy or in combination with other agents) and splenectomy (*Blood.* 2018;132:666).

Differential Diagnosis

The differential diagnosis includes other splenic B-cell neoplasms and other small B-cell lymphomas such as CLL/SLL, mantle cell lymphoma, follicular lymphoma, MZLs, and lymphoplasmacytic lymphoma (LPL). A panel of immunohistochemical studies and fluorescence in situ hybridization (FISH) studies (as needed) can help exclude other B-cell lymphomas. However, differentiating other MZLs involving blood and marrow and LPL from SMZL can be difficult since all have nonspecific immunophenotypic features and can show plasmacytic differentiation. The identification of the *MYD88* mutation favors LPL. The diagnosis of SMZL requires the integration of clinical, morphologic, immunophenotypic, and genetic features. See the discussion at the end of the chapter and Table 19.4-5.

Key Points

- Key points are summarized in Table 19.4-5.

Diagnostic Caveats

- SMZL does not have a distinct immunophenotype or defining genetic features. Other B-cell lymphomas should be excluded.
- Other MZLs can also involve blood and bone marrow. The diagnosis of SMZL often requires the integration of clinical, radiologic, morphologic, immunophenotypic, and genetic features.

III. SPLENIC DIFFUSE RED PULP SMALL B-CELL LYMPHOMA/LEUKEMIA

SDRPL is a rare entity characterized by circulating villous lymphocytes, intrasinusoidal bone marrow infiltration, and diffuse red pulp involvement in the spleen (key features summarized in Table 19.4-5). Recently, a study identified increased expression of cyclin D3 and recurrent *CCND3* mutations in a series of 23 SDRPL cases (*Blood.* 2017;129:1042). The diagnosis of this entity can be difficult and requires the exclusion of other small B-cell lymphomas. The diagnostic criteria for SDRPL are summarized in Table 19.4-3.

IV. SPLENIC B-CELL LYMPHOMA/LEUKEMIA WITH PROMINENT NUCLEOLI

This newly introduced category (encompassing cases of HCL-v and some cases of B-PLL) is characterized by neoplastic medium- to large-sized mature B cells with moderate to abundant cytoplasm and usually a prominent nucleolus (e-Figure 19.4-5). SBLPN involves the spleen, bone marrow, and blood and has some features resembling HCL, such as circulating lymphocytes with cytoplasmic projections and splenic red pulp involvement. However, it does not have all the classic features of HCL (key features summarized in Table 19.4-5). Notably, the *BRAF* V600E mutation is absent. It is important to differentiate these cases from HCL as they do not respond to conventional HCL therapy. The diagnostic criteria for SBLPN are summarized in Table 19.4-4.

TABLE 19.4-3 WHO-HAEM5 Diagnostic Criteria for Splenic Diffuse Red Pulp Small B-Cell Lymphoma/Leukemia (SDRPL)

Essential	Desirable
• **Spleen**[a]: Diffuse infiltration of red pulp by neoplastic small B cells and atrophic white pulp • **Blood:** Small lymphocytes with abundant cytoplasm, cytoplasmic projections, inconspicuous nucleoli • **Immunophenotype:** Compatible with SDRPL	• Absence of *BRAF* p.V600E mutation • Absence of lymphadenopathy (exception: splenic hilar lymph nodes)

Based on the WHO Classification of Tumours Editorial Board. Haematolymphoid tumours [Internet]. Lyon (France): International Agency for Research on Cancer; 2024 (WHO classification of tumours series, 5th ed.; vol. 11). Available from: https://tumour-classification.iarc.who.int/chapters/63.
[a]Splenectomy is uncommon, hence the classification of SDRPL may not be definitive; however, the diagnosis can be speculated from other findings.

TABLE 19.4-4   WHO-HAEM5 Diagnostic Criteria for Splenic B-Cell Lymphoma/Leukemia With Prominent Nucleoli (SBLPN)

Essential	Desirable
• **Morphology:** Circulating medium-sized lymphocytes with prominent nucleoli/convoluted nuclei • **Immunophenotype:** Positive for pan B-cell antigens and negative for characteristic HCL markers: annexin A1, CD25, TRAP, cyclin D1	• Spleen (if available): Diffuse involvement of red pulp and atrophic white pulp • Absence of *BRAF* p.V600E mutation

Based on the WHO Classification of Tumours Editorial Board. Haematolymphoid tumours [Internet]. Lyon (France): International Agency for Research on Cancer; 2024 (WHO classification of tumours series, 5th ed.; vol. 11). Available from: https://tumourclassification.iarc.who.int/chapters/63.

V. DIFFERENTIAL DIAGNOSIS OF SPLENIC B-CELL LEUKEMIAS/LYMPHOMAS

Splenic B-cell leukemias/lymphomas (SBCLs) have overlapping morphologic features in the blood and bone marrow, and usually, spleen biopsy/splenectomy is not performed, precluding histologic evaluation of the spleen. Among the subtypes discussed, HCL is the easiest to distinguish due to its distinctive immunophenotype and the presence of the *BRAF* V600E mutation. Annexin A1 is a specific IHC marker for HCL (negative in other SBCLs). SBLPN cases usually present with higher WBC counts and circulating atypical cells with a prominent nucleolus, features not common in other SBCLs. While SMZL and SDRPL have distinctive features in the spleen, the morphology in blood/bone marrow and immunophenotype overlap. Other B-cell lymphomas such as CLL/SLL, follicular lymphoma, and mantle cell lymphoma should be excluded. Integration of cytogenetic and molecular findings may be helpful. According to the WHO-HAEM5, when a definitive diagnosis cannot be established, the term, "splenic B-cell leukemia/lymphoma NOS" is appropriate. Key features of SBCLs are summarized in Table 19.4-5.

TABLE 19.4-5 Key Features of HCL, SMZL, SDRPL, and SBLPN

		HCL	SMZL	SDRPL	SBLPN
CBC		Pancytopenia including monocytopenia	Lymphocytosis	Lymphocytosis	High lymphocytosis and cytopenia(s) without monocytopenia
Morphology	Blood	Small- to medium-sized lymphocytes with circumferential villi, inconspicuous nucleoli	Small- to medium-sized lymphocytes with polar villi, inconspicuous nucleoli	Small- to medium-sized lymphocytes with polar villi, inconspicuous nucleoli	Medium- to large-sized lymphocytes with variable poorly defined cytoplasmic projections and usually a single prominent nucleolus
	Bone marrow	Usually diffuse interstitial infiltrate with "fried egg" appearance, fibrosis	Variable pattern: Nodular/intrasinusoidal	Variable pattern: Intrasinusoidal/interstitial/nodular	Variable pattern: Usually interstitial and intrasinusoidal
	Spleen	Diffuse red pulp involvement, pseudosinuses, atrophic white pulp	Predominant white pulp involvement	Diffuse red pulp involvement and atrophic white pulp	Diffuse red pulp involvement and atrophic white pulp

(continued)

TABLE 19.4-5 Key Features of HCL, SMZL, SDRPL, and SBLPN (continued)

	HCL	SMZL	SDRPL	SBLPN
Immunophenotype[a]	• Annexin A1+ • BRAF V600E+ • Cyclin D1+/− • DBA.44+ • CD25+ • CD123+ • CD103+ • CD11c+	• Annexin A1− • BRAF V600E− • Cyclin D1− • DBA.44+/− • CD25+/− • CD123−/+ • CD103− • CD11c −/+	• Annexin A1− • BRAF V600E− • Cyclin D1− • DBA.44+ • CD25− • CD123−/+ • CD103−/+ • CD11c −/+	• Annexin A1− • BRAF V600E− • Cyclin D1− • DBA.44+ • CD25− • CD123− • CD103+/− • CD11c+/−
Common genetic features	• *BRAF* V600E (~100%)	• Del(7q) ~40% • Mutations in *NOTCH2* (~25%) and *KLF2* (30%–40%)	• Del(7q) in a few cases • *NOTCH2* and *KLF2* mutations are rare. • Commonly mutated genes: *CCND3* (~20%), *MAP2K1*, *BCOR*, etc	• Del(17p) leading to loss of *TP53* (~30%) • Commonly mutated genes: *MAP2K1* (~50%), *TP53*, *KMT2C*, *CCND3*, etc

CBC, complete blood count; HCL, hairy cell leukemia; SBLPN, splenic B-cell lymphoma/leukemia with prominent nucleoli; SDRPL, splenic diffuse red pulp small B-cell lymphoma; SMZL, splenic marginal zone lymphoma.

[a]All entities have a mature B-cell phenotype and usually negative for CD10 and CD5.

Expert Rev Hematol. 2021;14:355; *Blood.* 2017;130:1644; *Blood.* 2016;127:2072; *Blood.* 2017;129:1042; *Am J Surg Pathol.* 2016;40:192; Based on the WHO Classification of Tumours Editorial Board. Haematolymphoid tumours [Internet]. Lyon (France): International Agency for Research on Cancer; 2024 (WHO classification of tumours series, 5th ed.; vol. 11). Available from: https://tumourclassification.iarc.who.int/chapters/63.

SUGGESTED READINGS

Maitre E, Cornet E, Troussard X. Hairy cell leukemia: 2020 update on diagnosis, risk stratification, and treatment. *Am J Hematol.* 2019;94(12):1413-1422.

Arcaini L, Rossi D, Paulli M. Splenic marginal zone lymphoma: from genetics to management. *Blood.* 2016;127(17):2072-2081.

Nakamura S, Ponzoni M. Marginal zone B-cell lymphoma: lessons from Western and Eastern diagnostic approaches. *Pathology.* 2020;52(1):15-29.

Yilmaz E, Chhina A, Nava VE, Aggarwal A. A review on splenic diffuse red pulp small B-cell lymphoma. *Curr Oncol.* 2021;28(6):5148-5154.

19.5 Follicular Lymphoma

Anurag Khanna and Brooj Abro

Follicular lymphoma (FL) is a germinal center (GC) B-cell neoplasm, with most cases showing varying degrees of follicular growth pattern. The subtyping of FL has been updated in the new classifications, WHO-HAEM5 and International Consensus Classification (ICC) (Table 19.5-1). The majority of FL cases (>80%) are characterized by *BCL2 rearrangement* (*BCL2*-R)/t(14;18)(q32;q21), which juxtaposes the immunoglobulin heavy chain (IGH) locus at 14q32 with the B-cell lymphoma 2 (BCL2) oncogene at 18q21. Certain distinct types of FL typically lack the *BCL2*-R (see Table 19.5-3 for key features of FL types). The grading of adult nodal/systemic FL is retained in the ICC but optional in the WHO-HAEM5. According to the WHO-HAEM5, this recommendation is supported by studies that have shown poor

TABLE 19.5-1 Classification of Follicular Lymphomas

WHO-HAEM5	ICC
• In situ follicular B-cell neoplasm	• In situ follicular neoplasia
• Follicular lymphoma[a]	• Follicular lymphoma[a]
• Classic follicular lymphoma	• *BCL2*-R-negative, CD23-positive follicle center lymphoma[b]
• Follicular lymphoma with unusual cytologic features	• Pediatric-type follicular lymphoma
• Follicular lymphoma with a predominantly diffuse growth pattern[b]	• Duodenal-type follicular lymphoma
• Follicular large B-cell lymphoma	• Testicular follicular lymphoma
• Pediatric-type follicular lymphoma	
• Duodenal-type follicular lymphoma	

BCL2-R, *BCL2* rearrangement.
[a]Grading of nodal/systemic FL is retained in the ICC but not required per the WHO-HAEM5. [b]dFL and *BCL2*-R-negative, CD23-positive follicle center lymphoma are similar entities.

TABLE 19.5-2 WHO-HAEM5 Diagnostic Criteria for Follicular Lymphoma

Essential
- **Morphology:** intermixed CCs and CBs, with predominance of CCs in majority of cases
- **Immunophenotype:** consistent with GC B-cell origin (positive for B-cell markers and GC markers such as CD10, BCL6, HGAL, LMO$_2$, etc)

Desirable
- Follicular growth pattern (may be partial or focal)
- Presence of *BCL2*-R or *BCL6*-R and/or lack of *IRF4*-R (in equivocal cases)

CB, centroblast; CC, centrocyte; GC, germinal center; R, rearrangement.
Based on the WHO Classification of Tumours Editorial Board. Haematolymphoid tumours [Internet]. Lyon (France): International Agency for Research on Cancer; 2024 (WHO classification of tumours series, 5th ed.; vol. 11). Available from: https://tumourclassification.iarc.who.int/chapters/63.

reproducibility in morphologic grading of FL and a lack of significant clinical differences between FL grades 1, 2, and 3A (*Leukemia.* 2022;36:1720-1748).

I. FOLLICULAR LYMPHOMA

FL is a common type of non-Hodgkin lymphoma (NHL), accounting for approximately 20% to 25% of NHLs in Western countries (*Nat Rev Dis Primers.* 2019;5:83). The disease mainly affects older adults, and the median age at diagnosis is approximately 60 years. The neoplastic cells of FL are primarily composed of varying proportions of centrocytes (CCs) and centroblasts (CBs). FL is divided into four subtypes (discussed later) based on morphology and immunophenotype. The diagnostic challenge lies in differentiating higher-grade FLs or FLs with large or unusual cells from large B-cell lymphomas. The diagnostic criteria are summarized in Table 19.5-2.

Clinical Features
- **Clinical presentation:** Widespread disease (stages III-IV) at diagnosis is common. Patients may be asymptomatic or present with lymphadenopathy and other signs/symptoms associated with the site(s) involved. B symptoms are uncommon and usually associated with disease progression/transformation. FL generally shows a chronic relapsing clinical course.
- **Sites of involvement:** Lymph nodes are the most common site. Many extranodal sites can be involved, including the spleen, bone marrow, gastrointestinal (GI) tract, and soft tissue. Peripheral blood and Waldeyer's ring are rarely involved. Primary testicular involvement is also reported, and testicular FL is recognized as a distinct entity in the ICC.

Morphology, Immunophenotype, and Genetic Features
The WHO-HAEM5 categorizes nodal/systemic FL into four subtypes: (1) classic follicular lymphoma (cFL), (2) FL with unusual cytologic features (ucFL), (3) FL with

predominantly diffuse growth pattern (dFL), and (4) follicular large B-cell lymphoma (FLBCL). The morphologic, immunophenotypic, and genetic features of these subtypes are discussed below.

i. Classic Follicular Lymphoma

- **Cytomorphology:** The neoplastic cells primarily consist of CCs and CBs. CCs are typically small, with cleaved/angulated/twisted nuclei, inconspicuous nucleoli, dense chromatin, and scant cytoplasm. CBs are large cells with non-cleaved round-oval nuclei, vesicular chromatin, single or multiple prominent nucleoli, and moderate cytoplasm (e-Figure 19.5-1). Monocytoid B cells are present in cases with marginal zone differentiation. Plasmacytic differentiation is uncommon, and these cases show the presence of monotypic plasma cells, usually in interfollicular areas. Occasionally, immunoblast-like and Hodgkin-Reed-Sternberg (HRS)-like cells may be present (*Virchows Arch.* 2016;468(2):127-139). Signet-ring cell morphology has been reported in rare cases (*Ann Diagn Pathol.* 2017;26:38-42).
- **Grading:** Histologic grading of FL is optional in the WHO-HAEM5 and retained in the ICC. The grading is based on the average number of CBs in 10 consecutive 400× high-power microscopic fields (HPF) and consists of grades 1, 2, 3A, and 3B. The number of CBs in each grade is the following: grade 1: 5 or less CBs/HPF, grade 2: more than 5 but less than or equal to 15 CBs/HPF, and grade 3: more than 15 CBs/HPF. Grade 3 is subdivided into 3A and 3B, which may be challenging to distinguish, especially in small biopsies. In grade 3A, CBs are abundant, but intermixed CCs are present, whereas in grade 3B, the neoplastic cells are primarily composed of sheets of CBs. The significance of grades 1 to 3A is debatable, and these may be lumped together for treatment purposes. Clinically, grade 3B is usually considered equivalent to diffuse large B-cell lymphoma (DLBCL). As mentioned above, the WHO-HAEM5 considers grading optional, which applies to grades 1 to 3A. Grade 3B is recognized as a morphologic subtype (FLBCL), discussed in a later section.
- **Morphology in lymph nodes and extranodal sites:** Varying proportions of CCs and CBs are arranged in a follicular/nodular pattern (e-Figure 19.5-2). In some cases, this pattern may not be prominent in H&E (hematoxylin and eosin) sections, and diffuse areas may be present. Immunohistochemical (IHC) studies are helpful in highlighting nodularity and demonstrating intact follicular dendritic cell (FDC) meshworks. The neoplastic follicles efface the nodal architecture and are usually densely packed (back-to-back) with attenuated mantle zones and lack features of normal GCs (polarization and tingible body macrophages). Scattered neoplastic cells may be seen in the interfollicular regions. Background hyalinization or sclerosis may be present, and, in some cases, prominent fibrotic bands, mimicking the pattern of nodular sclerosis classic Hodgkin lymphoma (CHL), can be seen at low power. Some cases display a "floral" pattern. This pattern is characterized by neoplastic follicles with prominent mantle zones, mimicking progressive transformation of germinal centers (PTGC). Pale areas outside the follicles can be seen in cases with marginal zone differentiation, consisting of neoplastic cells with monocytoid appearance.
- **Morphology in the bone marrow and peripheral blood:** FL frequently involves bone marrow and typically shows a paratrabecular pattern (e-Figure 19.5-3). The aggregates are usually composed of CCs and, less frequently, CBs. The

typical follicular/nodular pattern seen in the lymph nodes and other extranodal sites is rarely observed in the bone marrow. The peripheral blood may be involved in a small subset of cases. The neoplastic cells in the peripheral blood are also described as "buttock cells" due to their distinctly indented nuclei (e-Figure 19.5-4).
- **Immunophenotype:** FL cells express pan B-cell markers (CD19, CD20, PAX-5, etc), monotypic surface immunoglobulin light chain, and usually co-express CD10 and BCL6, among other GC markers (HGAL, LMO_2, etc). CD10 may be negative in some cases, particularly in those with higher histologic grade. BCL2 is expressed in most cases, which also helps establish the neoplastic phenotype of FL (nonneoplastic secondary follicles are negative for BCL2). BCL2 may be negative in some cases due to mutation in the *BCL2* gene or lack of *BCL2*-R. Grade 3 FL is more likely to be negative for CD10 and BCL2. Ki-67 proliferation indices are highly variable but tend to be lower than those of reactive follicles (*J Clin Oncol.* 2007;25:3330-3336). FDC meshworks within the neoplastic follicles show variable expression of FDC markers (CD21, CD23, CD35). FL cells may express CD23 and are typically negative for CD43. Expression of CD5, MUM1, and EBV (Epstein-Barr virus) is rare. CD30 is also usually negative but may be expressed in a subset of cases in grade 3 FL.
- **Genetic features:** Most cases of cFL show *BCL2*-R, and some may also harbor *BCL6*-R. A small subset of cases (<20%) are negative for *BCL2*-R and *BCL6*-R. Other abnormalities including chromosomal gains (1q, 2p, 17q, 2q, etc) and deletions (1p, 6q, 9p etc) can be present. Recurrent somatic mutations involving the following genes have been identified: *KMT2D, CREBBP, EZH2, ARID1A, TNFRSF14, BCL2, STAT6, BTK, NOTCH1/2,* among others (*Blood.* 2019;133:81-93).

ii. Follicular lymphoma with Unusual Cytological Features

According to the WHO-HAEM5, this morphologic category includes rare cases of FL primarily composed of cells with unusual cytologic features: medium-sized immature/blastoid cells or large cells with cleaved/irregular nuclei ("large CCs"), and these cases also have a higher frequency of atypical immunophenotypic and genetic features (*Leukemia.* 2022;36:1720-1748). The Ki-67 proliferation index and proportion of cells with MUM1 expression may be higher, while *BCL2*-R is found at a lower frequency than cFL. In cases with strong diffuse MUM1 expression, fluorescence in situ hybridization (FISH) testing for *IRF4*-R may be needed to rule out large B-cell lymphoma with *IRF4*-R. Additional studies may be needed to determine the clinical significance of this morphologic subtype.

iii. Follicular Lymphoma with Predominantly Diffuse Growth Pattern

This variant is characterized by a diffuse growth pattern with minimal to absent FDC meshworks, and the neoplastic cells are predominantly CCs. The inguinal lymph nodes are typically involved, and the disease is often localized. Other features associated with this variant include expression of CD23 and lack of *BCL2*-R (*Mod Pathol.* 2016;29:570-581). CD10 expression may be negative, and *STAT6* mutations are more frequent in this subtype (*Blood Adv.* 2020;4:5652-5665). Some cases of cFL may show partial diffuse morphology; hence, the diagnosis of dFL should not be rendered on limited material. The ICC describes a similar entity, "*BCL2*-R-negative, $CD23^+$ follicle center lymphoma." According to the ICC, this subtype frequently, but not always, shows a diffuse pattern, involves the pelvic/inguinal region, and is frequently associated with *STAT6* mutations (*Blood.* 2022;140:1229-1253).

iv. Follicular Large B-Cell Lymphoma

FLBCL is the new terminology used by the WHO-HAEM5 for FL grade 3B. This variant shows a follicular pattern with sheets of large cells or CBs and a lack of CCs. In contrast to cFL, CD10 and BCL2 expression is frequently negative. In some cases, areas with lower-grade morphology (cFL) may be present. FLBCL is often associated with DLBCL. Careful inspection and adequate sampling are required to rule out DLBCL. *BCL2*-R is often negative, and the frequency of *BCL6*-R is higher in this subtype (*Am J Pathol.* 2004;165:481-490).

Transformation

FL can transform to DLBCL, which is the most common histologic type of FL transformation. Rarely, transformation to other types, including B-cell acute lymphoblastic leukemia (B-ALL), CHL, and histiocytic sarcoma, has been reported (*J Clin Exp Hematop.* 2023;63:12-18).

Prognosis and Treatment

FL is an indolent disease with an overall 10-year survival of approximately 80% (*Nat Rev Dis Primers.* 2019;5:83). Relapses are common. Treatment options include rituximab as a single agent for low-stage disease and as combination therapy (eg, Rituximab, cyclophosphamide, hydroxydaunorubicin (doxorubicin), oncovin® (vincristine), prednisone [RCHOP]) for advanced disease. To assess the prognosis of patients with FL, the FL-International Prognostic Index (FLIPI) was developed (*Blood.* 2004;104:1258-1265). The FLIPI comprises the following adverse factors: age above 60 years, hemoglobin levels below 12 g/dL, elevated serum lactate dehydrogenase, Ann Arbor stage III/IV, and more than four involved nodal areas. Based on the number of these factors present, the disease is categorized as low risk (0-1 factors), intermediate risk (2 factors), or high risk (3-5 factors). Other adverse prognostic factors include histologic transformation, *TP53* mutations, and 17p deletion. Differential diagnosis, key points, and diagnostic caveats are discussed in Table 19.5-3.

II. DUODENAL-TYPE FOLLICULAR LYMPHOMA

Duodenal-type follicular lymphoma (DFL) is an indolent GC B-cell neoplasm with a follicular architecture, and the disease is limited to the intestine. The most common location is the second portion of the duodenum. Lesions may be present throughout the GI tract. The disease is often asymptomatic and discovered incidentally. The histologic and immunophenotypic features of DFL are similar to cFL.

On histologic examination, DFL shows a follicular pattern, a mixture of CCs and CBs, often with grades 1-2 morphology (e-Figure 19.5-5). The neoplastic cells are often limited to the mucosa, but the submucosa may be involved to a limited extent. A characteristic feature of DFL is the "glove-balloon sign," which is the expansion/ballooning of villi by infiltrating neoplastic cells. This is a helpful morphologic feature, particularly in limited biopsies (*Pathol Int.* 2019;69:48-50). The immunophenotype is consistent with GC B-cell origin (positive for B-cell markers, CD10, BCL6), and the neoplastic cells co-express BCL2 (e-Figure 19.5-5). The FDC meshworks,

TABLE 19.5-3 Key Features of Follicular Lymphoma Subtypes

FL Subtype	Key Points	Diagnostic Caveats and Differential Diagnosis
cFL[a]	- **Morphology:** follicular pattern, intermixed CCs and CBs - **IHC**[b]**:** CD10 (+) and BCL2 (+) in majority - **Genetics:** *BCL2*-R is common (>80%), *BCL6*-R in a subset	- FFH may mimic FL. GCs in FFH usually show polarization, tingible body macrophages, and high Ki-67. - Some FL patterns overlap with other lymphomas, for example, MZ and plasmacytic differentiation mimic MZL. - FL with floral pattern mimics PTGC.
ucFL[a]	- **Morphology:** medium-sized blastoid cells or large centrocytic cells - **IHC:** MUM1 (+/−), CD10 (+/−) BCL2 (+/−) - **Genetics:** lower frequency of *BCL2*-R	- Morphology may overlap with immature lymphoid neoplasms (excluded by IHC and FC). - Cases with high MUM1 expression may require *IRF4* FISH testing to exclude LBCL with *IRF4* rearrangement.
dFL[a]	- **Morphology:** diffuse pattern, cells are predominantly CCs. - **IHC:** CD10 (+/−), CD23 (+), and BCL2 (−), FDC markers show minimal or lack of FDC meshworks. - **Genetics:** lack *BCL2*-R, *STAT6* mutations are common. - **Other:** inguinal/pelvic region is typically involved.	- cFL may show partial diffuse pattern. The diagnosis of dFL should not be rendered on limited material. - Unlike cFL, dFL typically presents as low-stage localized disease in the inguinal region and outcomes are more favorable.
FLBCL[a]	- **Morphology:** follicular pattern, sheets of CBs without CCs - **IHC:** CD10 (+/−), BCL2 (+/−) - **Genetics:** *BCL2*-R may be negative. Higher frequency of *BCL6*-R	- Adequate sampling is required to exclude DLBCL. FISH for *BCL2*, *BCL6*, and *MYC* rearrangements is helpful. - Cases with high MUM1 expression may require *IRF4* FISH to exclude LBCL with *IRF4* rearrangement.
PTFL	- **Morphology:** purely follicular pattern, medium-sized blastoid cells - **IHC:** CD10 (+), BCL2 (−), MUM1 (−), Ki-67 (high proliferation, usually >30%) - **Genetics:** lack of *BCL2*, *BCL6*, *IRF4*, and *MYC* rearrangements - **Other:** localized nodal disease in children and young adults	- PNMZL has some overlapping features with PTFL such as large GCs. - Features that favor PNMZL: PTGC-like features, expansion of MZ B cells, increased PD-1 (+) T cells in GCs - FFH can mimic PTFL. Evidence of B-cell clonality distinguishes PTFL from FFH.

TABLE 19.5-3 Key Features of Follicular Lymphoma Subtypes (*continued*)

FL Subtype	Key Points	Diagnostic Caveats and Differential Diagnosis
DFL	• **Morphology:** follicular pattern similar to cFL, infiltrate usually limited to the mucosa and may cause villous expansion "glove-balloon sign" • **IHC and genetics:** similar to cFL	• Involvement by systemic FL should be excluded.
TFL	• **Morphology:** follicular pattern. Many cases are grade 3A. • **Immunophenotype:** CD10 (+), BCL2 (−) • **Genetics:** *BCL2*-R is usually absent. • **Other:** affects young boys and is localized to the testis. A distinct entity in the ICC	• Involvement by systemic FL should be excluded.
ISFN	• **Morphology:** reactive appearing GCs, nodal architecture is preserved. • **IHC:** neoplastic cells in GC show strong expression of BCL2. • **Genetics:** *BCL2*-R is present. • **Other:** usually an incidental finding	• ISFN may coexist with FL and the latter should be excluded.

BCL2, B-cell lymphoma 2; *BCL2*-R, *BCL2* rearrangement; *BCL6*-R, *BCL6* rearrangement; CB, centroblasts; CC, centrocytes; CD10, cluster of differentiation 10; cFL, classic follicular lymphoma; DFL, duodenal-type follicular lymphoma; dFL, follicular lymphoma with predominantly diffuse pattern; DLBCL, diffuse large B-cell lymphoma; FC, flow cytometry; FFH, florid follicular hyperplasia; FISH, fluorescence in situ hybridization; FL, follicular lymphoma; FLBCL, follicular large B-cell lymphoma; GC, germinal center; IHC, immunohistochemistry; ISFN, in situ follicular B-cell neoplasm; LBCL, large B-cell lymphoma; MUM1, multiple myeloma 1; MZ, marginal zone; MZL, marginal zone lymphoma; PD-1, programmed cell death protein 1; PNMZL, pediatric nodal marginal zone lymphoma; PTFL, pediatric-type follicular lymphoma; PTGC, progressive transformation of germinal centers; TFL, testicular follicular lymphoma; ucFL, follicular lymphoma with unusual cytologic features.

[a]Subtypes of nodal/systemic FL in the WHO-HAEM5. A new provisional entity in the ICC "*BCL2*-R-negative, CD23+ follicle center lymphoma," has similar features as dFL.
[b]All subtypes of FL show expression of B-cell markers and variable expression of GC markers. CD10 and BCL6 are the most common markers used to determine GC phenotype. FL subtypes are mostly positive for BCL6, but CD10 may be negative particularly in the non-classic subtypes.

demonstrated by FDC markers (CD21, CD23, CD35), are typically located at the periphery of neoplastic follicles. Almost all the cases show *BCL2*-R and recurrent somatic mutations similar to cFL have been identified, including *KMT2D, CREBBP, EZH2,* and *TNFRSF14* (*Blood.* 2018;132(16):1695-1702).

DFL has an excellent prognosis with a 10-year overall survival of approximately 100%. The clinical course is highly indolent, and patients usually remain asymptomatic even without treatment. In most cases, it appears that adopting a "watch and wait" approach is the best course of action (*J Clin Oncol.* 2011;29:1445-1451). The diagnostic criteria are summarized in Table 19.5-4.

III. PEDIATRIC-TYPE FOLLICULAR LYMPHOMA

Pediatric-type follicular lymphoma (PTFL) is an indolent nodal B-cell lymphoma of GC origin with a pure follicular pattern and high-grade cytologic features, occurring predominantly in the pediatric and adolescent age group. The disease most commonly occurs in males with a male-to-female ratio of greater than 10:1. Most patients present with isolated lymphadenopathy (stage I disease). The most common sites are the head and neck lymph nodes, and extranodal involvement is absent.

Histologic examination shows partial or complete effacement of the nodal architecture by large expansile or serpiginous follicles. The neoplastic follicles predominantly comprise intermediate-sized blastoid cells (usually smaller than typical CBs), lack polarity, and contain tingible body macrophages, imparting a starry sky appearance (e-Figure 19.5-6). Some cases may have typical CB morphology. Mantle zones are attenuated or absent. A "node-in-node" appearance has been described, which can be appreciated at low power. This appearance results from a rim of residual reactive nodal tissue at the periphery. Diffuse large cell areas or features diagnostic of DLBCL should not be present.

The immunophenotype is consistent with GC B-cell origin (positive for B-cell markers, CD10, and BCL6). The expression of CD10 is usually strong, and BCL2 is typically negative (weak/partial expression may be present). FDC markers (CD21, CD23, CD35) highlight FDC meshworks demonstrating the pure follicular architecture. Ki-67 is usually high (>30% and often up to 90%). The neoplastic cells show

TABLE 19.5-4 WHO-HAEM5 Diagnostic Criteria for Duodenal-Type Follicular Lymphoma

Essential	Desirable
- **Morphology:** follicular pattern, neoplastic cells are predominantly CCs, and mostly confined to the mucosa of intestine. - **Immunophenotype:** B cell and GC markers (+), BCL2 (+)	- Exclusion of secondary involvement from nodal/systemic FL

BCL2, B-cell lymphoma 2; CC, centrocyte; FL, follicular lymphoma; GC, germinal center
Based on the WHO Classification of Tumours Editorial Board. Haematolymphoid tumours [Internet]. Lyon (France): International Agency for Research on Cancer; 2024 (WHO classification of tumours series, 5th ed.; vol. 11). Available from: https://tumourclassification.iarc.who.int/chapters/63.

monotypic surface immunoglobulin light chain expression by flow cytometry. A novel IHC marker, FOXP-1, was found to be positive in the neoplastic cells of PTFL and negative in reactive GCs. This marker can help distinguish PTFL from florid follicular hyperplasia (*Virchows Arch*. 2019;475:771-779). MUM1 is usually negative. In cases with positive MUM1 expression, FISH for *IRF4*-R may be considered to rule out large B-cell lymphoma with *IRF4*-R.

PTFL is negative for *BCL2, BCL6, MYC,* and *IRF4* rearrangements. *IGH/IGK* gene rearrangement studies show evidence of clonality. PTFL is a neoplasm with low genomic complexity. Chromosome analysis shows a simple karyotype. Copy number neutral loss of heterozygosity of 1p36 locus is a common finding (*Int J Hematol Oncol*. 2022;11:IJH41). Unlike nodal/systemic FL in adults, PTFL usually lacks mutations involving histone-modifying genes, and there is a high frequency of *TNFRSF14* mutations (*Blood*. 2016;128:1101-1111). Recurrent mutations in mitogen-activated protein kinase (MAPK) pathway genes have also been identified (*Blood*. 2016;128:1093-1100). PTFL is a highly indolent disease and has an excellent prognosis. A watchful waiting approach after surgical excision is recommended (*Pediatr Blood Cancer*. 2020;67:e28416). The diagnostic criteria of PTFL are summarized in Table 19.5-5.

IV. IN SITU FOLLICULAR B-CELL NEOPLASM

In situ follicular B-cell neoplasm (ISFN) is characterized by GC B cells with strong BCL2 co-expression, colonizing GCs in an otherwise reactive lymph node/extranodal lymphoid tissue. The involved follicles are not expanded, and the lymph node

TABLE 19.5-5 WHO-HAEM5 Diagnostic Criteria for Pediatric-Type Follicular Lymphoma

Essential

- **Clinical features:** localized nodal disease in pediatric/young adult patients
- **Morphology:** Purely follicular growth with marked architectural distortion. Neoplastic cells are predominantly large/blastoid cells with high proliferation. Diffuse proliferation of large cells and features of DLBCL are not present.
- **Immunophenotype:** expression of B cell and GC markers
- **Genetics:** absence of *BCL2, BCL6,* and *MYC* rearrangements. If increased MUM1 expression: absence of *IRF4* rearrangement
- B-cell monoclonality demonstrated by immunophenotyping or genetic studies

Desirable

- Markedly expansile follicles
  Mutations in *MAP2K1* and *TNFRSF14*

DLBCL, diffuse large B-cell lymphoma; GC, germinal center.
Based on the WHO Classification of Tumours Editorial Board. Haematolymphoid tumours [Internet]. Lyon (France): International Agency for Research on Cancer; 2024 (WHO classification of tumours series, 5th ed.; vol. 11). Available from: https://tumourclassification.iarc.who.int/chapters/63.

TABLE 19.5-6	WHO-HAEM5 Diagnostic Criteria for In Situ Follicular B-Cell Neoplasm

Essential

- **Morphology:** preserved lymphoid architecture, lack of FL features
- **Immunophenotype:** variable proportion of GC B cells showing strong BCL2 expression

Desirable

- Strong CD10 expression in the BCL2 positive B cells within the GCs

FL, follicular lymphoma; GC, germinal center.
Based on the WHO Classification of Tumours Editorial Board. Haematolymphoid tumours [Internet]. Lyon (France): International Agency for Research on Cancer; 2024 (WHO classification of tumours series, 5th ed.; vol. 11). Available from: https://tumourclassification.iarc.who.int/chapters/63.

architecture is preserved. ISFN is typically an incidental finding. ISFN can also co-occur with overt FL and other lymphomas. The cells in ISFN are positive for *BCL2*-R and clonal *IGH* gene rearrangements. Some patients with ISFN may develop overt FL or other lymphomas (*Hum Pathol.* 2013;44:1328-1340). The diagnostic criteria are summarized in Table 19.5-6.

SUGGESTED READINGS

Attarbaschi A, Abla O, Arias Padilla L, et al. Rare non-Hodgkin lymphoma of childhood and adolescence: a consensus diagnostic and therapeutic approach to pediatric-type follicular lymphoma, marginal zone lymphoma, and nonanaplastic peripheral T-cell lymphoma. *Pediatr Blood Cancer.* 2020;67(8):e28416.

Freedman A, Jacobsen E. Follicular lymphoma: 2020 update on diagnosis and management. *Am J Hematol.* 2020;95(3):316-327.

Khanlari M, Chapman JR. Follicular lymphoma: updates for pathologists. *J Pathol Transl Med.* 2022;56(1):1-15.

19.6 Mantle Cell Lymphoma

Julia An and Brooj Abro

This chapter includes a discussion on three distinct categories of mantle cell lymphoma (MCL) and related neoplasms that are recognized by both the International Consensus Classification (ICC) and the WHO-HAEM5: MCL, non-nodal mantle cell lymphoma (nnMCL), and in situ mantle cell neoplasm (ISMCN).

I. MANTLE CELL LYMPHOMA

MCL is an aggressive B-cell lymphoma typically composed of monomorphic small mature B lymphocytes co-expressing CD5, cyclin D1, and SOX11. It accounts for 3% to 10% of non-Hodgkin lymphomas (*CA Cancer J Clin.* 2016;66:443). The median age of presentation is approximately 70 years, with a male predominance.

Two molecular subtypes are recognized by the WHO: cyclin D1–positive MCL and cyclin D1–negative MCL. Translocation (11;14)(q13;q32)/*CCND1* rearrangement is the hallmark genetic feature of cyclin D1–positive MCL. Cyclin D1–negative MCL constitutes a small subset of MCL cases (<5%) that are negative for cyclin D1 expression and *CCND1* rearrangement but show typical MCL morphology and SOX11 expression. Studies have shown that cyclin D1–negative MCL demonstrates *CCND2/CCND3* rearrangements (*Blood.* 2019;133:940). The diagnostic criteria for MCL are summarized in Table 19.6-1.

Clinical Features

- **Clinical presentation:** Most patients present at an advanced stage (Ann Arbor stages III and IV) with diffuse lymphadenopathy. B symptoms are commonly observed at initial presentation.
- **Sites of involvement:** Lymph nodes are the most common sites. Extranodal sites can also be involved and include the spleen, peripheral blood, bone marrow, Waldeyer ring, and the gastrointestinal (GI) tract. MCL in the GI tract can present with multiple polyps, known as lymphomatous polyposis. Dissemination to other sites such as the skin, central nervous system (CNS), etc, is more common in progressive or relapsed disease.

TABLE 19.6-1 WHO-HAEM5 Diagnostic Criteria for MCL

Essential	Desirable
Cyclin D1+ MCL	
- Neoplastic cells of B-lineage (CD20+ and usually CD5+)	- SOX11+
- Classic morphology (monomorphic and centrocyte-like) or variant morphology	
- Cyclin D1+/*CCND1* rearrangement+	
Cyclin D1− MCL	
- Neoplastic B cells (CD20+ and usually CD5+)	- *CCND2* rearrangement
- Classic morphology (monomorphic and centrocyte-like) or variant morphology	
- Immunophenotype consistent with MCL and SOX11+	
- Absence of cyclin D1 and *CCND1* rearrangement	

MCL, mantle cell lymphoma.
Based on the WHO Classification of Tumours Editorial Board. Haematolymphoid tumours [Internet]. Lyon (France): International Agency for Research on Cancer; 2024 (WHO classification of tumours series, 5th ed.; vol. 11). Available from: https://tumourclassification.iarc.who.int/chapters/63.

Morphology

MCL typically demonstrates a monomorphic lymphoid proliferation composed of small- to medium-sized lymphoid cells with dispersed nuclear chromatin, inconspicuous nucleoli, and irregular nuclear contours (e-Figures 19.6-1 to 19.6-3). Various growth patterns may include diffuse (most common), nodular, and, rarely, mantle zone or follicular patterns.

Variant morphologic subtypes such as blastoid, pleomorphic, small cell, and marginal zone-like are encountered infrequently (*Br J Haematol.* 2005;131:29). The blastoid and pleomorphic variants have been associated with aggressive features such as increased proliferation index, a high frequency of *TP53* alterations, and worse clinical outcomes (*Genes Chromosomes Cancer.* 2020;59:484). The blastoid variant is characterized by cells resembling lymphoblasts, while the pleomorphic variant shows variable morphology, including large cells with prominent nucleoli, which may resemble diffuse large B-cell lymphoma (DLBCL). Other morphologic features associated with MCL include hyalinized small blood vessels (e-Figure 19.6-1A) and scattered epithelioid histiocytes.

MCL in the bone marrow can show variable patterns of infiltration, including nodular, diffuse, and paratrabecular (e-Figure 19.6-3C).

Immunophenotype

MCL expresses pan B-cell markers (CD20, PAX5, CD79a, etc) and typically demonstrates moderate to strong expression of surface IgM/IgD, more often with λ than κ immunoglobulin light chain restriction by flow cytometric analysis. In addition, MCL usually tests positive for CD5, BCL2, FMC7, and CD43 and negative for CD10, BCL6, and CD200. A small subset of cases show variant immunophenotypic features such as expression of CD23, CD10, CD200, and lack of CD5 (*Am J Clin Pathol.* 2009;132:699). Expression of CD10 and BCL6 is reported more often in aggressive morphologic variants. Cyclin D1 expression is detected in the vast majority (>95%) of cases due to *CCND1* rearrangements. In addition, SOX11 is expressed, which aids in identifying cyclin D1–negative cases; however, it is important to note that SOX11 expression may also be seen in other hematologic malignancies such as Burkitt lymphoma (*Haematologica.* 2009;94:1555).

In rare cases, MCL with typical morphologic and immunophenotypic characteristics lack cyclin D1 expression and *CCND1* rearrangements (termed as cyclin D1–negative MCL).

Genetic Features

The t(11;14)(q13;q32) translocation, which involves the juxtaposition of *CCND1* to *IGH* on chromosome 14q32, is present in over 95% of cases and is considered the genetic hallmark of MCL. This translocation results in the overexpression of cyclin D1, which is involved in cell cycle regulation. Variant *CCND1* translocations with IG light chain genes (IGK or IGL) have been reported. Rare cases of MCL lack *CCND1* translocations (termed as cyclin D1–negative MCL). These cases are usually associated with other genetic alterations such as *CCND2/CCND3* translocations (*Blood.* 2019;133:940). Of note, there are very rare cases of MCL in which cyclin D1 expression cannot be demonstrated by immunohistochemistry despite the presence of the *CCND1* rearrangement due to mutations in *CCND1* (*Haematologica.* 2018;103:e432).

Secondary genomic alterations, such as copy-number changes with chromosomal gains or amplifications, as well as loss of chromosomes, are present in a large proportion of cases and may contribute to disease development. Abnormal expression of SOX11 is also thought to play a role in pathogenesis. The most commonly mutated genes include *ATM*, *TP53*, *CCND1*, and *KMT2D* (*J Intern Med.* 2017;282:371).

Prognosis and Treatment

The prognosis of MCL has greatly improved with novel and improved therapeutic approaches. Poor prognostic factors include an increased Ki-67 proliferation index (>30%), high TP53 expression (>50%), complex karyotype, and aggressive morphologic variants (blastoid and pleomorphic) (Blood. 2018;131:417; *J Clin Oncol.* 2016;34:1386).

Differential Diagnoses

The differential diagnosis includes other cyclin D1 or CD5-positive lymphoid neoplasms such as hairy cell leukemia (HCL) and chronic lymphocytic leukemia/small lymphocytic lymphoma (CLL/SLL). HCL has a distinct immunophenotype (see Chapter 19.4), and cyclin D1 expression is usually variable (MCL shows diffuse strong expression). CLL/SLL can show focal cyclin D1 expression in proliferation centers. The pleomorphic variant of MCL mimics DLBCL, and the blastoid variant mimics Burkitt lymphoma and B-cell acute lymphoblastic leukemia (B-ALL). Cyclin D1 and SOX11 expression are helpful in establishing the diagnosis of MCL. At least one of these markers (usually Cyclin D1) should be included in the initial panel for the work-up of both small and large B-cell lymphomas.

> **Key Points**
>
> - MCL typically consists of monomorphic small mature B lymphocytes with irregular nuclear contours, which are positive for CD5, BCL2, SOX11, cyclin D1, and *CCND1* translocation.
> - Cases of cyclin D1–negative MCL lack *CCND1* translocation and often possess genetic alterations that lead to increased expression of cyclin D2 or cyclin D3.
>
> **Diagnostic Caveats**
>
> - Cyclin D1 may be expressed in other lymphomas (often weakly/focally) such as CLL/SLL, DLBCL, and HCL.
> - Variant morphologic subtypes such as pleomorphic and blastoid MCL can mimic DLBCL, Burkitt lymphoma, and B-ALL.
> - MCL with a mantle-like growth pattern should be distinguished from mantle cell neoplasia in situ.

II. LEUKEMIC NON-NODAL MANTLE CELL LYMPHOMA

Leukemic non-nodal mantle cell lymphoma (nnMCL) is characterized by MCL with a leukemic presentation, minimal lymph node involvement, and usually a lack of symptoms. While nnMCL shares many similar features with nodal MCL, such as cyclin D1 expression and *CCND1* rearrangement, there are distinct clinical and biologic differences between the two entities. The diagnostic criteria for nnMCL are summarized in Table 19.6-2.

Features That Distinguish Non-nodal Mantle Cell Lymphoma From Nodal Mantle Cell Lymphoma

The following features favor diagnosis of nnMCL:

- **Clinical presentation:** Usually asymptomatic, and lymphocytosis is discovered incidentally. Peripheral blood, bone marrow, and spleen are commonly involved, with minimal to absent lymph node involvement.

TABLE 19.6-2   WHO-HAEM5 Diagnostic Criteria for nnMCL

Essential
- Typical asymptomatic clinical presentation with lymphocytosis without significant nodal involvement
- Monomorphic small- to medium-sized cells of B-lineage (CD20$^+$)
- Cyclin D1$^+$/*CCND1* rearrangement

Desirable
- SOX11 (commonly negative)

nnMCL, non-nodal mantle cell lymphoma.
Based on the WHO Classification of Tumours Editorial Board. Haematolymphoid tumours [Internet]. Lyon (France): International Agency for Research on Cancer; 2024 (WHO classification of tumours series, 5th ed.; vol. 11). Available from: https://tumourclassification.iarc.who.int/chapters/63.

- **Immunophenotype:** SOX11 expression is usually negative, and the KI-67 proliferation index is low.
- **Genetic features:** Mutated *IGHV* and fewer genetic abnormalities

Prognosis and Treatment

The clinical course and outcomes of nn MCL are more favorable than nodal MCL. Patients often remain asymptomatic for long periods without requiring treatment. However, aggressive disease may develop in some cases (*Curr Treat Options Oncol.* 2019;20:85).

Differential Diagnosis

Other small B-cell lymphomas such as CLL/SLL and marginal zone lymphoma can show similar disease presentation and should be excluded.

III. IN SITU MANTLE CELL NEOPLASM

ISMCN is characterized by cyclin D1–positive B cells, usually with *CCND1* rearrangement, confined to the mantle zones of lymphoid follicles. It shows an indolent clinical behavior and a very low risk of transformation to MCL (*Am J Surg Pathol.* 2016;40:943; *Haematologica.* 2012;97:270). ISMCN is very rare, with an estimated prevalence of less than 0.5% in reactive lymph nodes (*Semin Diagn Pathol.* 2018;35:76).

ISMCN is usually an incidental finding, often discovered in lymph nodes being evaluated for other reasons. It typically involves multiple follicles with preserved architecture and reactive hyperplasia. Cyclin D1–positive cells are mostly confined to the inner mantle zone, although a few cells may be present in other areas. The mantle zones of involved follicles may show minimal expansion without significant atypia.

ISMCN cells express pan B-cell antigens, cyclin D1, BCL2, and IgD. SOX11 expression is variable, and the cells are often negative for CD5 and CD43 (*Semin Diagn Pathol.* 2018;35:76). A diagnosis of ISMCN requires careful evaluation and staging to exclude overt MCL. The diagnostic criteria for ISMCN are summarized in Table 19.6-3.

| TABLE 19.6-3 | WHO-HAEM5 Diagnostic Criteria for ISMCN |

Essential	Desirable
- Preservation of lymphoid architecture - Cyclin D1–positive B cells predominantly restricted to the inner mantle zones of follicles - Exclusion of MCL	- Detection of *CCND1* rearrangement (may be performed in unclear cases)

ISMCN, in situ mantle cell neoplasm.
Based on the WHO Classification of Tumours Editorial Board. Haematolymphoid tumours [Internet]. Lyon (France): International Agency for Research on Cancer; 2024 (WHO classification of tumours series, 5th ed.; vol. 11). Available from: https://tumourclassification.iarc.who.int/chapters/63.

SUGGESTED READINGS

Armitage JO, Longo DL. Mantle-cell lymphoma. *N Engl J Med*. 2022;386(26):2495-2506.
Jain P, Wang M. Mantle cell lymphoma: 2019 update on the diagnosis, pathogenesis, prognostication, and management. *Am J Hematol*. 2019;94(6):710-725.

19.7 Large B-Cell Lymphomas

Anurag Khanna and Brooj Abro

Large B-cell lymphomas (LBCLs) encompass diverse tumors with large-cell or high-grade cytomorphology and mature B-cell or plasmablastic immunophenotype. The WHO-HAEM5 recognizes 18 entities in this category, including diffuse large B-cell lymphoma, not otherwise specified (DLBCL-NOS), a heterogeneous disease and the most prevalent type, and 17 others. The classification of LBCLs is mostly similar in the WHO-HAEM5 and International Consensus Classification (ICC), with a few exceptions (*Blood*. 2023;142(suppl 1):3708) (see Table 19.7-1). The most comprehensive discussion in this chapter is centered on the most prevalent entity, DLBCL-NOS. Other LBCLs, particularly the rare types, are discussed more briefly, focusing primarily on their key characteristics. To facilitate discussion, several LBCL types are grouped into categories based on shared features such as morphologic patterns, immunophenotype, and association with specific anatomic sites. Key features of LBCLs are summarized in Table 19.7-15.

Diagnosis and workup of LBCLs: On routine histologic evaluation, the diagnosis of LBCL is usually considered when a proliferation of diffuse noncohesive medium-to-large neoplastic cells is encountered. The diagnosis of LBCL requires a comprehensive panel of immunohistochemical (IHC) stains and other studies (see Chapter 31, Table 31.4). Morphologic patterns and clinical features may guide in formulating a differential diagnosis and further workup of LBCLs. Although the morphology usually provides clues to the diagnosis of a hematologic malignancy, it may be deceiving in some cases. Before a lineage is established, the differential diagnosis of large-cell proliferation is broad and should include poorly differentiated carcinomas, sarcomas, and other hematopoietic neoplasms, including T-cell lymphomas and immature/

TABLE 19.7-1 Classification of Large B-Cell Lymphomas

WHO-HAEM5 classification of large B-cell lymphomas

1. Diffuse large B-cell lymphoma, not otherwise specified
2. T-cell/histiocyte-rich large B-cell lymphoma
3. Diffuse large B-cell lymphoma/high-grade B-cell lymphoma with *MYC* and *BCL2* rearrangements
4. ALK-positive large B-cell lymphoma
5. Large B-cell lymphoma with *IRF4* rearrangement
6. High-grade B-cell lymphoma with 11q aberrations
7. Lymphomatoid granulomatosis
8. EBV-positive diffuse large B-cell lymphoma
9. Diffuse large B-cell lymphoma associated with chronic inflammation
10. Fibrin-associated large B-cell lymphoma
11. Fluid overload–associated large B-cell lymphoma
12. Plasmablastic lymphoma
13. Primary large B-cell lymphoma of immune-privileged sites
14. Primary cutaneous diffuse large B-cell lymphoma, leg type[a]
15. Intravascular large B-cell lymphoma
16. Primary mediastinal large B-cell lymphoma
17. Mediastinal gray zone lymphoma
18. High-grade B-cell lymphoma, not otherwise specified

Key differences in the ICC

The ICC and WHO-HAEM5 classification of large B-cell lymphomas is mostly similar. There are minor differences in the nomenclature of some entities. Key differences in diagnostic categories are as follows:

- **High-grade B-cell lymphoma with *MYC* and *BCL6* rearrangements** is a provisional entity in the ICC.
- **Fluid overload–associated large B-cell lymphoma** is a new entity introduced in the WHO-HAEM5. The ICC also includes a new entity that overlaps with this entity, "**HHV8 and EBV-negative primary effusion-based lymphoma**." There is a slight difference in the diagnostic criteria. The ICC requires that EBV should be negative, whereas the WHO-HAEM5 mentions that EBV may be positive.
- **Primary large B-cell lymphoma of immune-privileged sites** is an umbrella term used by the WHO-HAEM5 that encompasses primary large B-cell lymphoma of the CNS, testis, and vitreoretina. The ICC includes the first two as distinct entities and does not specifically mention large B-cell lymphoma of the vitreoretina.

CNS, central nervous system; EBV, Epstein-Barr virus; HHV8, human herpesvirus-8; ICC, International Consensus Classification.
[a]Discussed in Chapter 19.10.

precursor neoplasms. The workup may be straightforward in patients with a previous diagnosis; however, in new cases, other possible diagnoses should also be considered before ordering an extensive LBCL IHC panel, particularly when the tissue is limited. A limited panel may be helpful initially (eg, CD45, CD3, CD20, PAX5, CD30, MUM1), and depending on the degree of suspicion of a nonhematologic neoplasm, other stains may be added. Ideally, more than one B-cell marker should be included in the initial workup, as some LBCLs may lose one or more B-cell markers, and T-cell lymphomas may aberrantly express CD20 (*Am J Surg Pathol.* 2008;32:1593-1607). Most cases of suspected hematolymphoid malignancies also have concurrent flow cytometry (FC), which is very helpful in the diagnosis of a B-cell lymphoma when a clonal B-cell population is detected; the FC findings can guide further workup. However, in some cases, FC does not capture large-cell populations.

I. DIFFUSE LARGE B-CELL LYMPHOMA, NOT OTHERWISE SPECIFIED

Diffuse large B-cell lymphoma, not otherwise specified (DLBCL-NOS) is the most common type of non–Hodgkin lymphoma (NHL) worldwide and accounts for more than 80% of all LBCL cases (*N Engl J Med.* 2021;384:842-858). The disease typically affects adults over the age of 60 and is rare in children. The diagnostic criteria for DLBCL-NOS are summarized in Table 19.7-2.

Clinical Features

- **Clinical presentation:** Patients typically present with enlarging mass lesion(s) in nodal/extranodal sites. Symptoms vary depending on the sites involved, and systemic B symptoms are common. Patients frequently present with advanced-stage disease (stage III-IV).
- **Sites of involvement:** In most cases, lymph nodes are involved. Primary involvement of extranodal sites is also common. DLBCL-NOS can involve almost any extranodal site, with the gastrointestinal (GI) tract and head and neck region being the most common. The bone marrow is involved in 15% to 20% of the cases at initial staging (*N Engl J Med.* 2021;384:842-858).

Morphology

Typically, a diffuse infiltrate of large monomorphic or pleomorphic lymphoid cells effacing the nodal architecture or infiltrating extranodal tissue is present. Increased

TABLE 19.7-2 WHO-HAEM5 Diagnostic Criteria for DLBCL-NOS

Essential	Desirable
- **Morphology:** large cells with a diffuse or vaguely nodular growth pattern - **Immunophenotype:** mature B cell - Exclusion of other LBCL types	- Cell of origin subtyping - Reporting of isolated *MYC* or dual *MYC* and *BCL6* rearrangements - Genetic testing, if clinically relevant

DLBCL-NOS, diffuse large B-cell lymphoma, not otherwise specified; LBCL, large B-cell lymphoma.
Based on the WHO Classification of Tumours Editorial Board. Haematolymphoid tumours [Internet]. Lyon (France): International Agency for Research on Cancer; 2024 (WHO classification of tumours series, 5th ed.; vol. 11). Available from: https://tumourclassification.iarc.who.int/chapters/63.

mitosis, apoptosis, and necrosis may be present. A subset of cases show increased tingible-body macrophages, imparting a "starry sky" appearance, mimicking Burkitt lymphoma (BL) and other high-grade lymphomas. Cytomorphologic features of large cells can vary (e-Figures 19.7-1 and 19.7-2), and the most common morphologic subtype is centroblastic (see Table 19.7-3).

Immunophenotype

The lymphoma cells demonstrate a mature B-cell phenotype and usually express CD45 and pan B-cell markers (CD19, CD20, PAX5, etc). CD45 expression may be decreased, and one or more B-cell markers may be lost in some cases. It is generally

TABLE 19.7-3 Morphologic Subtypes of DLBCL-NOS

Subtype	Features
Centroblastic	• Most common (~80% of cases)
• Cytomorphology: large lymphocytes with round-oval nuclei, vesicular chromatin, and multiple small peripheral nucleoli (e-Figure 19.7-1)
• DLBCL with centroblastic morphology may be monomorphic (>90% centroblastic cells) or pleomorphic (contain a mixture of centroblastic cells and other types of LBCs: large centrocytic cells, immunoblastic cells, etc).
Immunoblastic	• Second most common (~10% of cases). Immunoblastic cells comprise ~90% of tumor cells. Centroblastic cells may be present but should comprise <10% of the tumor cells.
• Cytomorphology: large lymphocytes with a single prominent central nucleolus (e-Figure 19.7-2). May have plasmacytoid differentiation
• Frequently associated with the presence of *MYC* translocations
Anaplastic	• Rare, accounting for ~3% of cases
• Cytomorphology: large pleomorphic cells with moderate-to-abundant cytoplasm (may resemble HRS cells)
• CD30 is often positive, mimicking CHL with syncytial growth pattern and ALCL.
• Frequently associated with *TP53* mutations
Other	• Other rare morphologic subtypes include signet-ring and spindle cell type, mimicking nonhematologic malignancies such as gastric carcinoma and sarcoma.

ALCL, anaplastic large-cell lymphoma; CHL, classic Hodgkin lymphoma; HRS, Hodgkin Reed-Sternberg; LBC, large B cell.
Based on the WHO Classification of Tumours Editorial Board. Haematolymphoid tumours [Internet]. Lyon (France): International Agency for Research on Cancer; 2024 (WHO classification of tumours series, 5th ed.; vol. 11). Available from: https://tumourclassification.iarc.who.int/chapters/63.

recommended to use more than one B-cell marker to confirm B-cell lineage, and in cases where one or more markers are lost, an expanded panel of multiple B-cell markers should be used. Most cases express BCL2. Expression of MYC and CD30 is variable. A small subset of cases co-express CD5 (*Oncotarget*. 2015;6:5615-56330). Cyclin D1 can rarely be positive; however, unlike mantle cell lymphoma, SOX11 expression and *CCND1* rearrangement are negative in DLBCL (*Histopathology*. 2012;61:685-693). In most cases, Ki-67 shows a high proliferation index (>50%). CD10, BCL6, and MUM1 markers are commonly used to subtype DLBCL-NOS into germinal center B-cell (GCB) and non–GCB types (see Figure 19.7-1, and discussion later).

Subtyping Diffuse Large B-Cell Lymphoma, Not Otherwise Specified, by Cell of Origin

- **Gene expression profiling (GEP) studies:** The term DLBCL-NOS encompasses a clinically and biologically heterogeneous disease. DLBCL can develop *de novo* or evolve from an existing low-grade B-cell lymphoma. GEP studies have demonstrated that DLBCL cases show a GEP profile similar to distinct B-cell differentiation stages. A subset of DLBCL cases show a GEP similar to GCBs and another subset shows a GEP similar to activated B cells (ABCs) or post-GCBs, thus classifying DLBCL into two subtypes: GCB and ABC/non–GCB types. However, a subset of cases show a GEP that does not fit into either of these categories, and these cases have been designated as unclassified DLBCL. Common genetic changes predominantly observed in GCB-type DLBCL include *BCL2* translocation, mutations in the *EZH2* gene, amplification of the *REL* locus, and mutations or deletions in the *PTEN* gene (*Curr Oncol Rep*. 2022;24:13-21). Genetic alterations typically seen in the ABC subtype include mutations involving B-cell receptor and nuclear factor kappa B (NF-κB) pathway (*CD79A, CD79B, MYD88*) (*Curr Oncol Rep*. 2022;24:13-21). While the ABC subtype typically does not show *BCL2* translocations, amplification of the *BCL2* locus is common. Deletions or lack of expression of the *CDKN2A/2B* tumor suppressor genes is also seen (*Semin Hematol*. 2015;52:67-76).
- **Immunohistochemical (IHC) studies:** Since genetic studies are not always available or cost-effective, alternative techniques using IHC markers have been devised to identify subtypes of DLBCL-NOS. The most widely used method is the Hans algorithm, which uses CD10, BCL6, and MUM1 IHC (Figure 19.7-1). The concordance between this IHC algorithm and GEP is 70% to 80% (*Am J Hematol*. 2020;95:57-67).

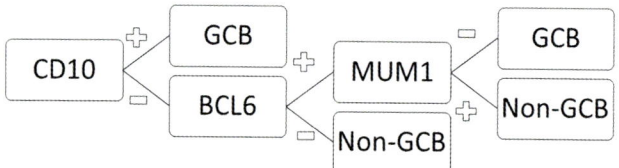

Figure 19.7-1. The Hans algorithm using immunohistochemistry to predict GCB and non–GCB subtypes of DLBCL-NOS. CD10, BCL6, and MUM1 are each considered positive if there is positive staining in 30% or more of the neoplastic cells (*Blood*. 2004;103(1):275-282).

GCB = Germinal center B-cell type, Non-GCB = Non-germinal center or activated B-cell type

- **Clinical significance of subtyping DLBCL-NOS by cell of origin**
  After the initial cell of origin (COO) classification of DLBCL by GEP, studies showed that the ABC subtype has worse outcomes than the GCB subtype, adding prognostic significance to this classification (*Nature*. 2000;403:503-511). Subsequent studies using IHC algorithms have shown varying results (*Lancet*. 2013;381:1817-1826). Currently, although GEP is considered the gold standard for subtyping DLBCL and is superior in predicting differences in overall survival, due to lack of availability in routine clinical practice, the Hans algorithm is still widely used.

Genetic Features

In addition to the common genetic alterations in GCB and ABC subtypes of DLBCL-NOS as discussed, several studies have proposed additional genetic subtyping of DLBCL-NOS based on clustering algorithms and shared genomic abnormalities different from the COO classification (*Cancer Cell*. 2020;37:551-568.e14; *N Engl J Med*. 2018;378:1396-1407). However, currently, no standard molecular classification system is used in routine clinical practice.

Nonetheless, the routine workup of a case showing DLBCL features should include fluorescence in situ hybridization (FISH) studies for *MYC, BCL2*, and *BCL6* rearrangements. DLBCL-NOS can show isolated *MYC, BCL2*, and *BCL6* rearrangements or simultaneous *MYC* and *BCL-6* rearrangements, which should be reported. The presence of dual *MYC* and *BCL2* rearrangements excludes DLBCL-NOS, and such cases should be diagnosed as DLBCL/high-grade B-cell lymphoma (HGBL) with *MYC* and *BCL2* rearrangements. FISH for *IRF4* rearrangement can be performed in young patients with disease limited to the head and neck region and strong MUM1/IRF4 expression. Detection of *IRF4* rearrangement also excludes DLBCL-NOS; such cases are diagnosed as LBCL with *IRF4* rearrangement.

Prognosis and Treatment

The International Prognostic Index (IPI) uses clinical parameters (age, lactate dehydrogenase [LDH] levels, Ann Arbor stage, Eastern Cooperative Oncology Group [ECOG] performance status, and number of extranodal sites involved) to stratify risk groups and is a commonly used prognostic tool for DLBCL-NOS in clinical practice (*N Engl J Med*. 1993;329:987-994). The National Comprehensive Cancer Network IPI (NCCN-IPI) enhances the IPI by providing a more detailed stratification of high-risk groups (*N Engl J Med*. 2021;384:842-858). Other factors associated with adverse prognosis that are not part of a validated prognostic index include ABC phenotype, CD5 expression, co-expression of MYC and BCL2 proteins (double-expresser), *MYC* rearrangement, and *TP53* mutations.

Treatment of DLBCL-NOS requires systemic chemotherapy. R-CHOP is the standard first-line therapy. Treatment options for relapsed and/or refractory disease include autologous stem cell transplantation and chimeric antigen receptor (CAR) T-cell therapy, and other novel drugs are being studied (*N Engl J Med*. 2021;384:842-858).

II. LARGE B-CELL LYMPHOMA WITH *IRF4* REARRANGEMENT

Introduction: Large B-cell lymphoma with *IRF4* rearrangement (LBCL-IRF4r) is a rare mature B-cell lymphoma defined by a structural chromosomal abnormality juxtaposing the *IRF4/MUM1* gene (6p25) next to an *IG* locus (most commonly *IGH*), leading to overexpression of IRF4/MUM1. Most cases are diagnosed in children and young adults, and the disease is usually localized to the head and neck region; the Waldeyer ring is the most common site (*Blood.* 2011;118:139-147). Involvement of other sites has been reported (*Pediatr Blood Cancer.* 2019;66:e27770). The diagnostic criteria for LBCL-IRF4r are summarized in Table 19.7-4.

Morphology, immunophenotype, and genetic features: The morphology overlaps with follicular LBCL (FLBCL) (FL grade 3B) and DLBCL; a case may show features of either, or both morphologies may coexist. IHC studies show strong expression of BCL6 and MUM1. Most cases are also positive for CD10 and BCL2. When the immunophenotypic pattern raises suspicion for LBCL-IRF4r, FISH testing for *IRF4* rearrangement can be performed. Rearrangements involving *MYC* and *BCL2* are absent.

Differential diagnosis: The differential diagnosis includes pediatric-type follicular lymphoma and FLBCL; however, strong expression of MUM1 is rare in these entities. FISH testing to confirm *IRF4* rearrangement may not be available, and in such cases, the diagnosis may be proposed based on clinical, morphologic, and immunophenotypic features.

Prognosis and treatment: The treatment protocols are similar to DLBCL-NOS, and outcomes are usually favorable (*Br J Haematol.* 2020;190:753-763).

III. HIGH-GRADE B-CELL LYMPHOMAS

The WHO-HAEM5 recognizes three entities in this category: DLBCL/HGBL with *MYC* and *BCL2* rearrangements, HGBL with 11q aberrations, and HGBL-NOS. These entities cannot be distinguished by morphology and immunophenotype; genetic studies are required to establish the diagnosis. The diagnostic criteria for HGBLs are summarized in Table 19.7-5.

TABLE 19.7-4 **WHO-HAEM5 Diagnostic Criteria for LBCL-IRF4r**

Essential

- **Morphology:** intermediate/large-cell morphology with follicular and/or diffuse growth pattern
- **Immunophenotype:** mature B-cell phenotype with co-expression of BCL6 and MUM1
- **Genetics:** *IRF4* translocation[a]

Desirable

- Evidence of the *IG::IRF4* translocation
- Absence of *BCL2* and *MYC* rearrangement

Based on the WHO Classification of Tumours Editorial Board. Haematolymphoid tumours [Internet]. Lyon (France): International Agency for Research on Cancer; 2024 (WHO classification of tumours series, 5th ed.; vol. 11). Available from: https://tumourclassification.iarc.who.int/chapters/63.

[a]Per the WHO-HAEM5, if *IRF4* rearrangement cannot be confirmed, a presumed diagnosis ("as not molecularly confirmed") can be made in the appropriate clinico-pathologic setting.

TABLE 19.7-5 WHO-HAEM5 Diagnostic Criteria for HGBLs

DLBCL/HGBL-MYC/BCL2

Essential
- **Morphology and immunophenotype:** consistent with aggressive BCL
- **Genetics:** detection of dual *MYC* and *BCL2* rearrangements (+/−BCL6 rearrangement)

Desirable
GCB phenotype
TdT protein expression status
Identification of the *MYC* fusion partner

HGBL with 11q aberrations

Essential
- **Morphology:** intermediate/blastoid or BL-like
- **Immunophenotype:** CD10$^+$, BCL6$^+$, BCL2$^-$
- **Genetics:** chromosome 11q: gain/loss, telomeric loss or telomeric LOH pattern

Desirable
Flow cytometry: expression of CD56 and lack of CD38^{high}

HGBL-NOS

Essential
- **Morphology:** intermediate or blastoid (does not fit DLBCL or BL)
- **Immunophenotype:** lack of TdT, CD34 and cyclin D1
- **Genetics:** lack of dual MYC and BCL2 rearrangements and the 11q aberration pattern seen in HGBL-11q

Desirable
- "Double-hit" gene expression profile
- Detection of *KMT2D* and *TP53* mutations

BCL, B-cell lymphoma; GCB, germinal center B cell; HGBL, high-grade B-cell lymphomas; LOH, loss of heterozygosity.
Based on the WHO Classification of Tumours Editorial Board. Haematolymphoid tumours [Internet]. Lyon (France): International Agency for Research on Cancer; 2024 (WHO classification of tumours series, 5th ed.; vol. 11). Available from: https://tumourclassification.iarc.who.int/chapters/63.

A. DLBCL/HGBL with *MYC* and *BCL2* rearrangements (DLBCL/HGBL-MYC/BCL2)

Introduction: DLBCL/HGBL-MYC/BCL2 is a genetically defined mature B-cell lymphoma characterized by dual rearrangements involving *MYC* (8q24) and *BCL2* (18q21). The latter usually involves the translocation of *BCL2* to the *IGH* locus (14q32). MYC translocation may involve *IG* loci (*IGH* most commonly) or non–IG partners.

Morphology, immunophenotype, and genetic features: The morphology may resemble DLBCL or HGBL (blastoid or BL-like), and immunophenotypic studies demonstrate the expression of mature B-cell markers, most often with GCB phenotype (e-Figure 19.7-3). IHC studies often show overexpression of MYC and BCL2 proteins; however, this is not a reliable marker for the presence of *MYC* and *BCL2* rearrangements, and FISH studies are recommended to establish the diagnosis. TdT expression is rare, and such cases should be differentiated from B-lymphoblastic leukemia/lymphoma (B-ALL). B-ALL may also have dual *MYC* and *BCL2* rearrangements. FC can help distinguish between mature and precursor phenotypes. Some studies have shown that the mutational landscape of TdT+ LBCL is different from that of B-ALL (*Am J Surg Pathol.* 2022;46:71-82). Follicular lymphoma (FL) with *MYC* and *BCL2* rearrangements is excluded from this category.

Prognosis and treatment: DLBCL/HGBL-MYC/BCL2 is an aggressive disease. Patients usually present with advanced-stage disease. Some patients have a previous history of follicular lymphoma. Standard R-CHOP therapy is usually not very effective; dose-adjusted R-EPOCH may be more effective. Other treatment options include anti-CD19 CAR–T-cell therapy.

B. HGBL with 11q aberrations (HGBL-11q)

Introduction: HGBL with 11q aberrations (HGBL-11q) is a rare and aggressive mature B-cell lymphoma characterized by a distinct complex abnormality (gain/loss pattern) involving the long arm of chromosome 11 (11q). The disease usually affects children and young adults. Lymph nodes (head and neck region most commonly) and extranodal sites can be involved.

Morphology, immunophenotype, and genetic features: The tumor morphology and immunophenotype typically resemble BL (previously known as BL-like lymphoma with 11q aberration), and *MYC* rearrangement is absent. Although the morphology is usually BL-like, intermediate blastoid and DLBCL-like morphology have also been described (*Virchows Arch.* 2023;483:281-298). Most cases show GCB phenotype by Han's algorithm (CD10 and BCL6$^+$), BCL2 is usually negative, and Ki-67 is 90% to 100% (features similar to BL). A recent study identified distinct immunophenotypic features associated with BL and HGBL-11q by FC (*Mod Pathol.* 2018;31:732-743). Co-expression of CD16 and CD56/expression of CD8, without CD38^{high}, was a characteristic finding in HGBL-11q cases. In contrast, BL cases were negative for CD16/CD56 and CD8 and showed CD38^{high}.

Studies have also shown genetic differences between the two entities. HGBL-11q cases usually lack the recurrent mutations associated with BL (*ID3, TCF3, CCND3*) (*Haematologica.* 2019;104:1822-1829). HGBL-11q is usually suspected when a case shows BL-like morphology and immunophenotype but lacks *MYC* rearrangement. The definite diagnosis relies on identifying the complex genomic abnormality, which involves gains of 11q23 and losses of 11q24-ter/telomeric loss of heterozygosity (LOH); some cases may only show the latter finding, which is more specific. According to the WHO-HAEM5, next-generation sequencing assays and high-resolution array-based comparative genomic hybridization tests are the most reliable techniques.

Prognosis and treatment: There is limited data on the optimal treatment approach. Dose-intensified chemotherapy protocols (similar to BL) have shown good response rates and favorable outcomes (*Haematol.* 2020;190:753-763).

C. High-Grade B-cell Lymphoma, Not Otherwise Specified (HGBL-NOS)

HGBL-NOS is a rare, aggressive disease with a mature B-cell phenotype and high-grade morphology (BL-like or blastoid) that does not meet the diagnostic criteria of other B-cell lymphomas. Given its rarity, data regarding this entity are limited. It is usually diagnosed in older adults and is often widespread at diagnosis. Most cases show GCB phenotype by Han's algorithm and GEP. *MYC* rearrangements (single hit) are common; some cases show *BCL2* and/or *BCL6* rearrangements. *KMT2D* and *TP53* are the most frequently mutated genes (*Blood.* 2022;140:943-954). Depending on the patient's age and comorbidities, dose-intensified chemotherapy protocols (similar to BL) may be appropriate.

IV. LARGE B-CELL LYMPHOMAS WITH POLYMORPHIC PATTERN

T-cell histiocyte-rich large B-cell lymphoma (THRLBCL), Epstein-Barr virus (EBV)–positive diffuse large B-cell lymphoma (EBV+ DLBCL), and lymphomatoid granulomatosis (LYG) are discussed together in this group due to their shared histologic feature, namely a polymorphic appearance with scattered large B cells in an inflammatory background (although it is important to note that EBV+ DLBCL can be polymorphic or monomorphic).

A. T cell histiocyte-rich large B cell lymphoma (THRLBCL)

Introduction: THRLBCL is a distinct mature B-cell neoplasm derived from GCBs and characterized by scattered large neoplastic B cells in a T-cell/histiocyte-rich background. The large B cells are usually in the distinct minority (1%-10% of the cells) and do not form diffuse or confluent sheets (*Haematologica*. 2010;95:352-356). THRLBCL usually presents with systemic involvement (stage III-IV), and it most often affects middle-aged and older adults with male predominance (*J Clin Oncol*. 2002;20:1269-1277). It may arise *de novo* or progress from nodular lymphocyte-predominant Hodgkin lymphoma (NLPHL). Lymph nodes, bone marrow, liver, and spleen are commonly involved. The diagnostic criteria for THRLBCL are summarized in Table 19.7-6.

Morphology and immunophenotype: The tissue architecture is effaced by a diffuse polymorphic infiltrate (e-Figure 19.7-4). Large neoplastic cells are usually individually scattered in a background rich in histiocytes and T cells, may resemble LP or Hodgkin Reed-Sternberg (HRS) cells, or show centroblastic or immunoblastic morphology. The histiocyte-rich background imparts a dense eosinophilic appearance at low power. The inflammatory background usually lacks plasma cells and eosinophils. Foci of necrosis may be present. The large cells are positive for pan B-cell markers and BCL6. CD10 is positive in a minor subset, and CD30 and CD15 are usually negative. MUM1 expression is variable. EBV is negative. CD21

TABLE 19.7-6 WHO-HAEM5 Diagnostic Criteria for THRLBCL

Essential

- Diffuse effacement of lymph node architecture: scattered large B cells (not forming sheets), reactive background infiltrate composed of histiocytes and small T cells, few/rare small B cells, and absence of FDC meshworks (by CD21/23)
- NLPHL is absent.

Desirable

- EBV-negative
- Diagnosis made on lymph node excision

EBV, Epstein-Barr virus; FDC, follicular dendritic cell; NLPHL, nodular lymphocyte-predominant Hodgkin lymphoma; THRLBCL, T-cell histiocyte-rich large B-cell lymphoma.
Based on the WHO Classification of Tumours Editorial Board. Haematolymphoid tumours [Internet]. Lyon (France): International Agency for Research on Cancer; 2024 (WHO classification of tumours series, 5th ed.; vol. 11). Available from: https://tumourclassification.iarc.who.int/chapters/63.

and CD23 show a lack of follicular dendritic cell (FDC) meshworks. CD3 and CD68/CD163 highlight the T-cell/histiocyte-rich background. Some studies show that CD8$^+$ T cells predominate in the background using IHC; others have shown a predominance of CD4$^+$ T cells using FC (*Pathology.* 2020;52:53-67).

Differential diagnosis: Features overlap with NLPHL, and some patients have a known history of NLPHL. The large cells in NLPHL and THRLBCL have similar morphologic and immunophenotypic features; the two can be distinguished by the overall architecture and the tumor microenvironment. In NLPHL, the morphology is at least focally nodular, small B cells are more abundant, and PD-1$^+$ T cells often form rosettes around neoplastic cells. In contrast, THRLBCL shows a diffuse growth pattern lacking FDC meshworks, and small B cells are not abundant, or even rare. PD-1$^+$ T cells may be present but do not form rosettes around the neoplastic cells (*Pathology.* 2020;52:53-67). The distinction may be challenging on small biopsies. NLPHL and THRLBCL share similar recurrent genetic mutations, suggesting a close relationship (*Haematologica.* 2019;104:330-337). The differential diagnosis includes classic Hodgkin lymphoma (CHL), EBV+ DLBCL, and T-cell lymphomas, which can show overlapping histologic features (see Table 19.7-15).

Prognosis and treatment: R-CHOP is the standard therapy, and the reported overall 5-year survival rate is 66% (*Leuk Lymphoma.* 2019;60:3426-3433).

B. **Epstein Bar virus-positive diffuse large B cell lymphoma (EBV+ DLBCL)**
Introduction: EBV+ DLBCL is an EBV-driven B-cell lymphoma that usually affects older adults (>50 years) without known immunodeficiency, and the majority of the neoplastic B cells are EBV-positive (ie, demonstrate nuclear positivity for EBV-encoded RNA [EBER] by in situ hybridization). However, the disease has also been reported in young adults (*Clin Lymphoma Myeloma Leuk.* 2011;11:512-516). The prevalence is higher in Asia and South America than in Western countries (*Cancers (Basel).* 2021;13:1785). Nodal and/or extranodal sites may be involved, and the frequency varies with age; older patients usually present with extranodal disease, and nodal disease is more common in young patients (*Blood Adv.* 2021;5:3227-3239). The diagnostic criteria for EBV+ DLBCL are summarized in Table 19.7-7.

Morphology, immunophenotype, and genetic features: Two morphologic patterns, polymorphic and monomorphic, have been described (*Am J Hematol.* 2022;97:951-965). The polymorphic pattern (CHL-like or THRLBCL-like) is more common and consists of scattered large EBV+ B cells (e-Figure 19.7-5) in a rich inflammatory background consisting of small lymphocytes, plasma cells, eosinophils, neutrophils, and histiocytes. The large cells may resemble HRS cells, LP cells, or immunoblasts. The monomorphic pattern comprises sheets of EBV+ large B cells (e-Figure 19.7-6) and a less prominent inflammatory background (resembling DLBCL-NOS). However, it is important to note that the two patterns may coexist.

Increased mitosis, apoptosis, necrosis, and angiodestructive growth may be present. The neoplastic larger cells are usually positive for pan B-cell markers and show non–GCB phenotype: CD10$^-$, BCL6$^{-/+}$, and MUM1$^+$. CD30 is variably positive in most cases. EBER is positive in the majority of tumor cells. The genetic landscape of EBV+ DLBCL differs from that of DLBCL-NOS (*Front Oncol.* 2019;9:683); recurrent genetic abnormalities include 6p deletions and mutations involving *CCR6, DAPK1, TNFRSF21, CCR7,* and *YY1* genes (*Blood Cancer J.* 2021;11:102).

TABLE 19.7-7 WHO-HAEM5 Diagnostic Criteria for EBV+ DLBCL

Essential

- **Clinical:** absence of inherited or acquired immunodeficiency or history of lymphoma
- **Morphology:** partial/complete effacement of architecture. Large neoplastic cells are scattered or in sheets. The background is rich in reactive cells. Necrosis often present
- **Phenotype of large B cells:** B-cell lineage, EBV+ (in majority of the tumor cells)
- Exclusion of other EBV-related lymphoproliferative disorders/lymphomas

Desirable

Detection of circulating EBV DNA (select cases)

EBV, Epstein-Barr virus; DLBCL, diffuse large B-cell lymphoma.
Based on the WHO Classification of Tumours Editorial Board. Haematolymphoid tumours [Internet]. Lyon (France): International Agency for Research on Cancer; 2024 (WHO classification of tumours series, 5th ed.; vol. 11). Available from: https://tumourclassification.iarc.who.int/chapters/63.

Differential diagnosis: The differential diagnosis includes other EBV+ lymphoproliferative disorders (LPDs) and lymphomas, and there is significant histologic overlap between these disorders which makes the distinction challenging. Clinical features and history are critical when considering the diagnosis. Patients with a known clinical history of immune deficiency/dysfunction (IDD) can present with a spectrum of EBV+ LPDs and lymphomas (discussed in Chapter 23), and the diagnosis of EBV+ DLBCL requires the exclusion of IDD (with the exception of age-related immune senescence). Other EBV+ LPDs/lymphomas in the differential diagnosis include those that occur in immunocompetent patients: LYG, CHL, nodal TFH cell lymphoma angioimmunoblastic type (nTFHL-AI). LYG (discussed later) usually involves the lungs and other extranodal sites; nodal disease is rare. HRS cells in CHL can be EBV+; however, unlike CHL, large cells in EBV+ DLBCL express pan B-cell markers. While nTFHL-AI also shows a polymorphic pattern with scattered EBV+ B cells, other features help distinguish it from EBV+ DLBCL. The presence of expanded FDC meshworks, vascular proliferation, and atypical/aberrant CD4$^+$ T-cell proliferation is typical for nTFHL-AI.

Prognosis and treatment: R-CHOP is the standard therapy. Data on prognosis are variable, with some studies reporting inferior outcomes compared to DLBCL-NOS, while other studies have reported similar outcomes in EBV+ and EBV− DLBCL treated with R-CHOP (*Am J Hematol.* 2022;97:951-965; *Hematol Oncol.* 2018;36:93-97).

C. Lymphomatoid granulomatosis (LYG)

Introduction: LYG is a rare EBV-associated extranodal B-cell LPD that almost always involves the lungs. The diagnosis of LYG requires the exclusion of inherited and acquired immunodeficiency disorders (with the exception of age-related immune senescence). Although an overt immune disorder should not be present, an association with immune dysfunction involving defective surveillance of EBV has been proposed (*Blood*. 1996;87:4531-4537; *Blood*. 2020;135:1344-1352). Patients may present with respiratory symptoms or manifestations related to the involvement of other extranodal sites such as skin and central nervous system (CNS). Imaging studies typically show bilateral nodular pulmonary lesions. LYG is a rare disease, with limited data on prevalence and demographics. The disease has mostly been reported in adults with a male predominance (*Blood*. 2020;135:1344-1352). The diagnostic criteria for LYG are summarized in Table 19.7-8.

Morphology, immunophenotype, and genetic features: LYG is characterized by a polymorphic infiltrate with an angiodestructive growth pattern (e-Figure 19.7-7) affecting small and large vessels, and necrosis is common. The infiltrate consists of large, atypical lymphoid cells in an inflammatory background (small lymphocytes—mainly T cells, plasma cells, and histiocytes). Granulocytes are infrequent. The large, atypical cells express pan B-cell markers, $CD30^{variable}$, and EBV. CD3-positive T cells are frequent in the background and angiocentric/angiodestructive foci ($CD4^+$ T cells usually predominate). Three histologic grades are recognized, and the grading is based on the proportion of EBV+ B cells (*Blood*. 2020;135:1344-1352, WHO-HAEM5).

- **Grade 1:** EBV+ large B cells are sparse, with minimal or absent necrosis.
- **Grade 2:** EBV+ large B cells are more frequent (5-50/HPF). Necrosis is common.
- **Grade 3:** EBV+ large B cells are abundant (>50/HPF) and may form clusters. Necrosis is present and may be extensive.

Clonal *IG* gene rearrangements are often detected with a higher frequency in higher-grade lesions; grade 1 lesions often show a polyclonal pattern (*Am J Surg Pathol*. 2015;39:141-156).

Differential diagnosis: The differential diagnosis includes other EBV+ LPDs and lymphomas (see discussion in EBV+ DLBCL). LYG is a rare disease that almost always presents with pulmonary disease in patients without overt immune deficiency. The clinical context is essential in establishing the diagnosis.

Prognosis and treatment: The clinical course is variable. Some patients with low-grade lesions have an indolent clinical course with spontaneous remission, but most require treatment. High-grade lesions are more likely to behave as lymphoma.

TABLE 19.7-8 WHO-HAEM5 Diagnostic Criteria for Lymphomatoid Granulomatosis

Essential

- **Clinical:** extranodal disease, exclusion of immunodeficiency (other than immune senescence)
- **Morphology and phenotype:** polymorphous lymphoid infiltrate, angiocentric and angiodestructive growth pattern. Large EBV+ B cells intermixed with small T cells

EBV, Epstein-Barr virus.
Based on the WHO Classification of Tumours Editorial Board. Haematolymphoid tumours [Internet]. Lyon (France): International Agency for Research on Cancer; 2024 (WHO classification of tumours series, 5th ed.; vol. 11). Available from: https://tumourclassification.iarc.who.int/chapters/63.

Treatment approaches include immune modulators (interferon [IFN]-α) for low-grade lesions and combination immunochemotherapy for high-grade lesions (*Blood.* 2020;135:1344-1352).

V. LARGE B CELL LYMPHOMAS ASSOCIATED WITH SPECIFIC ANATOMIC SITES

A unique feature of certain LBCL types is their association and/or confinement to specific anatomic sites/regions.

A. Large B cell lymphoma of immune-privileged sites (IP-LBCL)

Introduction: Large B-cell lymphoma of immune-privileged sites (IP-LBCL) is an umbrella term encompassing LBCLs confined to the CNS, vitreoretina (VR), and testis in immunocompetent patients. The diagnostic criteria for IP-LBCL are summarized in Table 19.7-9.

Morphology, immunophenotype, and genetic features: The three subtypes mentioned earlier have similar morphologic, immunophenotypic, and genetic features. The morphology is indistinguishable from systemic DLBCL-NOS. The tumor cells usually express pan B-cell markers and BCL2, and show a non–GCB phenotype: $CD10^-$, $BCL6^+$, $MUM1^+$. GCB phenotype ($CD10^+$) is uncommon and should prompt careful exclusion of systemic DLBCL. EBV is usually negative, and EBV positivity raises concern for an underlying immune deficiency. *MYD88* (p.L265P) and *CD79B* mutations are frequent (*Blood.* 2016;127:869-881).

Differential diagnosis: The main differential diagnosis is systemic LBCL, which requires correlation with clinical and imaging findings.

Prognosis and treatment: The prognosis of primary LBCL of CNS and VR is generally poor. Treatment includes methotrexate, rituximab-based regimens, and radiotherapy. Primary LBCL of testis is also an aggressive disease, and disease relapse involving the CNS can occur. The outcomes have improved with a combination of rituximab-based chemotherapy, radiation therapy, and CNS prophylaxis (*Int J Hematol.* 2014;100:370-378).

TABLE 19.7-9 WHO-HAEM5 Diagnostic Criteria for IP-LBCL

Essential	Desirable
- **Clinical:** disease confined to the CNS, VR, or testis at presentation. Exclusion of secondary involvement by other LBCLs and exclusion of immunodeficiency - **Morphology and immunophenotype:** consistent with LBCL	- Non–GCB phenotype - EBV is absent (>97% of cases). - If histology is not definitive: detection of clonal B-cell population or *MYD88* and/or *CD79b* hotspot mutations

CNS, central nervous system; IP, immune-privileged; LBCL, large B-cell lymphoma; VR, vitreoretina.
Based on the WHO Classification of Tumours Editorial Board. Haematolymphoid tumours [Internet]. Lyon (France): International Agency for Research on Cancer; 2024 (WHO classification of tumours series, 5th ed.; vol. 11). Available from: https://tumourclassification.iarc.who.int/chapters/63.

B. Primary mediastinal large B cell lymphoma (PMBL)

Introduction: Primary mediastinal large B-cell lymphoma (PMBL) arises in the anterior mediastinum. Local extension may occur, and regional lymph node involvement is frequent. Involvement of distant sites is not common at initial presentation but may occur with disease progression or relapse. PMBL mainly affects young adults with a female predominance. The diagnostic criteria for PMBL are summarized in Table 19.7-10.

Morphology, immunophenotype, and genetic features: The characteristic morphologic feature is the proliferation of large atypical cells in a background of dense fibrosis (e-Figure 19.7-8); the fibrosis may result in compartmentalization of the neoplastic cells. The large cells show variable cytologic features and may resemble HRS cells. The large cells are positive for pan B-cell markers and CD45 and typically lack surface and cytoplasmic immunoglobulin. MUM1, CD30, and CD23 are positive in most cases. CD30 expression is often heterogeneous, and CD15 is typically negative. BCL6 and BCL2 are variably expressed. Expression of other markers that can be helpful in the diagnosis of PMBL include CD200, MAL, PD-L1, and PD-L2 (WHO-HAEM5). Rearrangements involving *MYC*, *BCL2*, and *BCL6* are typically absent; testing for these is not required. Recurrent genetic abnormalities include structural changes involving 9p24.1 (*CD274/PDCD1LG12*) and structural variants of *CIITA* (*Blood*. 2022;140:955-970).

Differential diagnosis: The diagnosis of PMBL may be challenging due to the difficulty in obtaining adequate samples from lesions limited to the mediastinum with dense fibrosis. The differential diagnosis includes DLBCL-NOS and CHL. DLBCL-NOS is usually not primarily located in the mediastinum. Although CHL is also common in young adults and usually involves mediastinum, the large cells in PMBL show expression of pan B-cell markers, CD30 expression is variable/weak, and CD15 is usually absent.

Prognosis and treatment: The prognosis is usually favorable. Treatment options include R-CHOP and dose-adjusted R-EPOCH (*Blood*. 2022;140:955-970).

TABLE 19.7-10 WHO-HAEM5 Diagnostic Criteria for PMBL

Essential	Desirable
• **Clinical:** location—anterior mediastinum • **Morphology and immunophenotype:** LBCL with mature B-cell phenotype, with at least partial expression of CD23 and CD30	• Distinctive stromal sclerosis • Expression of at least one of the following markers: MAL, CD200, PD-L1, and PD-L2 • Copy gain or rearrangement of CD274/PDCD1LG2 locus and/or rearrangement involving *CIITA* (*C2TA*)

PMBL, primary mediastinal large B-cell lymphoma.
Based on the WHO Classification of Tumours Editorial Board. Haematolymphoid tumours [Internet]. Lyon (France): International Agency for Research on Cancer; 2024 (WHO classification of tumours series, 5th ed.; vol. 11). Available from: https://tumourclassification.iarc.who.int/chapters/63.

C. Mediastinal grey zone lymphoma (MGZL)
Mediastinal gray zone lymphoma (MGZL) is a B-cell neoplasm with features intermediate between PMBL and CHL (e-Figure 19.7-9). The disease is usually localized to the mediastinum; local extension and regional lymph node involvement are common. The diagnosis of MGZL is challenging and should be considered when the morphologic and immunophenotypic features do not fit either PMBL or CHL. The WHO-HAEM5 recognizes two spectrums based on morphologic and immunophenotypic features: "CHL-like" and "PMBL-like." The diagnostic criteria for MGZL are summarized in Table 19.7-11.

D. Intra-vascular large B cell lymphoma (IVLBCL)
Intravascular large B-cell lymphoma (IVLBCL) is a rare B-cell lymphoma confined to vascular lumens, especially capillaries (e-Figure 19.7-10). Vessels of any site may be involved. Three clinical subtypes are recognized by the WHO-HAEM5 (classic, cutaneous, and hemophagocytic). The classic subtype presents with skin manifestations and involvement of other organs, which may lead to multiorgan failure. The cutaneous subtype is confined to the skin, and the hemophagocytic subtype presents with rapid disease onset and progression and is associated with hemophagocytic syndrome. The large neoplastic cells are positive for pan B-cell markers and often show co-expression of CD5. Non–GCB phenotype is more common: $CD10^-$ and $MUM1^+$. The diagnostic criteria for IVLBCL are summarized in Table 19.7-12. IVLBCL is an aggressive disease. Rituximab-based chemotherapy regimens have improved survival (*Cancer Med.* 2022;11:3602-3611).

TABLE 19.7-11 WHO-HAEM5 Diagnostic Criteria for MGZL

Essential

CHL-like:
- **Morphology:** confluent growth of pleomorphic cells within a variably abundant microenvironment and dense fibrotic stroma
- **Immunophenotype:** uniform strong expression of CD20, PAX5, and at least more than one additional B-cell marker (CD19, CD79a, BOB1, OCT2)
- CD30 expression (variable intensity)

PMBL-like:
- **Morphology:** monomorphic sheets of medium-to-large neoplastic cells within a variably dense fibrotic stroma
- **Immunophenotype:** uniform strong expression of CD30 and partial/complete loss of B-cell markers or strong CD15 expression

Desirable
- Larger biopsy preferred as features on a needle core biopsy may not be reliable/limited.
- Absence of EBV

CHL, classic Hodgkin lymphoma; EBV, Epstein-Barr virus; MGZL, mediastinal gray zone lymphoma; PMBL, primary mediastinal large B-cell lymphoma.
Based on the WHO Classification of Tumours Editorial Board. Haematolymphoid tumours [Internet]. Lyon (France): International Agency for Research on Cancer; 2024 (WHO classification of tumours series, 5th ed.; vol. 11). Available from: https://tumourclassification.iarc.who.int/chapters/63.

TABLE 19.7-12 WHO-HAEM5 Diagnostic Criteria for IVLBCL

Essential

- Large lymphoid cells restricted to intravascular spaces, especially capillaries (a minimal extravascular component is acceptable)
- Pan B-cell markers-positive

Desirable

- KSHV/HHV8 and EBV-negative (by IHC and EBER in situ hybridization, respectively)

EBER, EBV-encoded RNA; IHC, immunohistochemical; IVLBCL, intravascular large B-cell lymphoma.
Based on the WHO Classification of Tumours Editorial Board. Haematolymphoid tumours [Internet]. Lyon (France): International Agency for Research on Cancer; 2024 (WHO classification of tumours series, 5th ed.; vol. 11). Available from: https://tumourclassification.iarc.who.int/chapters/63.

VI. LARGE B-CELL LYMPHOMAS WITH PLASMABLASTIC FEATURES

LBCLs that typically show plasmablastic features include plasmablastic lymphoma (PBL), ALK-positive large B-cell lymphoma (ALK+ LBCL), primary effusion lymphoma (PEL), and KSHV/HHV8-positive diffuse large B-cell lymphoma (KSHV/HHV8+ DLBCL). The first two are discussed next and the latter are discussed in Chapter 19.9. Occasionally, other lymphomas, such as DLBCL-NOS and EBV+ DLBCL, may show plasmablastic/immunoblastic morphology; however, they express pan B-cell markers. Plasma cell neoplasms may also show plasmablastic morphology, and the distinction from PBL may be challenging (see later).

A. Plasmablastic lymphoma (PBL)

Introduction: PBL usually arises *de novo* in the context of known IDD and is often diagnosed in patients with human immunodeficiency virus (HIV). Rarely, low-grade B-cell lymphomas can transform into PBL (*Hum Pathol.* 2013;44:2139-2148). The disease is often extranodal; the oral cavity and gastrointestinal (GI) tract are the most common sites. The diagnostic criteria for PBL are summarized in Table 19.7-13.

Morphology, immunophenotype, and genetic features: Histologic evaluation of involved tissues shows diffuse proliferation of large cells with plasmablastic (eccentric nucleus with moderate-to-abundant cytoplasm) or immunoblastic (central nucleus with central prominent nucleolus) cytomorphology. Increased mitosis and a "starry sky" pattern may be present. Necrosis is common. Neoplastic cells demonstrate terminal B-cell differentiation. Plasma cell markers (CD138, MUM1) are positive (e-Figure 19.7-11), and immunoglobulin light chain restriction can be identified in most cases. Most B-cell markers (CD19, CD20, PAX5) are usually negative. CD79a is expressed in almost half of the cases. CD45 is often negative, weak, or variable. Ki-67 is usually very high (>90%). EBV (EBER) is positive in most cases. HHV8 and ALK-1 are negative. IHC frequently shows MYC protein overexpression, and *MYC* translocation is detected in two-thirds of cases (*J Hematol Oncol.* 2015;8:65). *BCL2* and *BCL6* rearrangements are rare.

TABLE 19.7-13 WHO-HAEM5 Diagnostic Criteria for PBL

Essential
- **Morphology:** plasmablastic/immunoblastic
- **Immunophenotype:** plasma cell markers-positive (CD138, MUM1). CD20, PAX5, ALK, and KSHV/HHV8-negative

Desirable
- EBV (EBER)-positive in ~60% of cases
- Detection of *MYC* rearrangements
- Detection of monoclonal *IG* rearrangements

PBL, plasmablastic lymphoma.
Based on the WHO Classification of Tumours Editorial Board. Haematolymphoid tumours [Internet]. Lyon (France): International Agency for Research on Cancer; 2024 (WHO classification of tumours series, 5th ed.; vol. 11). Available from: https://tumourclassification.iarc.who.int/chapters/63.

Differential diagnosis: Other LBCLs can show plasmablastic/immunoblastic features, but a comprehensive immunophenotypic panel helps exclude other LBCLs. Plasmablastic plasma cell myeloma (PCM) and EBV+ plasmacytoma may pose a diagnostic challenge due to similar immunophenotypic features; the distinction is important as the treatment for plasma cell neoplasms differs from PBL. Features that favor PCM include a previous history of PCM, clinical findings CRAB (hyperCalcemia, Renal failure, Anemia, and Bone lesions), and detection of translocations associated with PCM. EBV+ plasmacytoma usually has mature plasma cell morphology, although cases with plasmablastic morphology have been reported. A criterion based on morphologic and immunophenotypic features has been proposed to distinguish between EBV+ plasmacytoma and PBL (*Am J Surg Pathol*. 2022;46:1364-1379).

Prognosis and treatment: PBL is an aggressive disease with generally a poor prognosis. Patients are usually treated with systemic chemotherapy (CHOP or more intensive regimens such as dose-adjusted EPOCH) (*Int J Lab Hematol*. 2022;44(suppl 1):54-63).

B. ALK-positive large B cell lymphoma (ALK+ LBCL)

ALK protein expression and *ALK* gene alterations can be seen in hematologic and nonhematologic neoplasms. Historically in hematopathology, ALK expression was primarily associated with T-cell lymphoma (anaplastic large-cell lymphoma) until 1997, when a series of B-cell lymphomas with distinct features and ALK expression were reported (*Blood*. 1997;89:1483-1490). ALK+ LBCL is a rare lymphoma characterized by plasmablastic differentiation and ALK expression (e-Figure 19.7-12). ALK+ LBCL has morphologic features similar to PBL (see earlier), and its immunophenotype also overlaps with PBL (positive for plasma cell markers and usually negative for most B-cell markers). However, the expression of ALK distinguishes ALK+ LBCL from other plasmablastic LBCLs. EBV and HHV8 are negative. Genetic alterations (usually translocations) involving the *ALK* gene (2p23) are detected in most cases. The diagnostic criteria for ALK+ LBCL are summarized in Table 19.7-14. The prognosis is poor, and standard treatment protocols are lacking due to the rarity of the disease. CHOP, CHOEP, and dose-adjusted EPOCH regimens have been used (*Leuk Lymphoma*. 2021;62:2845-2853).

TABLE 19.7-14 WHO-HAEM5 Diagnostic Criteria for ALK+ LBCL

Essential	Desirable
• **Morphology:** large neoplastic cells • **Immunophenotype:** ALK-positive and plasmablastic phenotype (plasma cells markers such as CD138 and MUM1$^+$ and CD20$^-$/variable/weak)	• *ALK* gene alterations (usually translocations) • No EBV association

ALK+ LBCL, ALK-positive large B-cell lymphoma; EBV, Epstein-Barr virus.
Based on the WHO Classification of Tumours Editorial Board. Haematolymphoid tumours [Internet]. Lyon (France): International Agency for Research on Cancer; 2024 (WHO classification of tumours series, 5th ed.; vol. 11). Available from: https://tumourclassification.iarc.who.int/chapters/63.

VII. LARGE B-CELL LYMPHOMAS CONFINED TO NATURAL OR ACQUIRED BODY SPACES

Diffuse large B-cell lymphoma associated with chronic inflammation (CI-DLBCL), fibrin-associated large B-cell lymphoma (FA-LBCL), and fluid overload–associated large B-cell lymphoma (FO-LBCL) arise in natural or acquired body spaces and do not infiltrate tissues. While a tumor mass is usually identified in CI-DLBCL, the other two do not form mass lesions. The key features of these entities are listed in Table 19.7-15.

A. Diffuse large B cell lymphoma associated with chronic inflammation (CI-DLBCL)
CI-DLBCL is also known as pyothorax-associated lymphoma (PAL). It most often arises in the pleural cavity following longstanding pyothorax and is associated with EBV infection. Patients are usually older adults (median age >60 years), and a tumor mass is identified in the majority. Most patients do not have established immunodeficiency; immune senescence in older patients may play a role. The prognosis is poor, with a reported overall 5-year survival of less than 50% (*Ann Oncol.* 2007;18:122-128; *J Clin Oncol.* 2002;20:4255-4260).

B. Fibrin-associated large B cell lymphoma (FA-LBCL)
FA-LBCL is confined to sites of chronic fibrin deposition and is usually an incidental finding. It has been reported in association with cardiac myxomas, cardiac prostheses, chronic hematomas, breast implants, and pseudocysts (*BMC Cancer.* 2019;19:916; *Haematologica.* 2020;105:e412-e414). The large cells are usually confined to fibrinous material and do not infiltrate normal tissues. Most cases are EBV+, but rare EBV(−) cases have been reported (*Int J Surg Pathol.* 2022;30:39-45). Unlike CI-DLBCL, FA-LBCL does not form a mass lesion and is an indolent disease (*Am J Surg Pathol.* 2017;41:299-312).

C. Fluid overload-associated large B cell lymphoma (FO-LBCL)
FO-LBCL is a new entity introduced in the WHO-HAEM5; a similar entity with slightly different diagnostic criteria is discussed in the ICC (see Table 19.7-1). FO-LBCL is confined to serous effusions and should be distinguished from PEL. Unlike PEL, FO-LBCL is negative for HHV8, and patients are usually not immunocompromised. Since the disease is mostly diagnosed in older adults, immune senescence may play a role. An association with hepatitis C has been reported (*Am J Clin Pathol.* 2013;140:258-273). Treatment options include CHOP/CHOP-like regimens, and the prognosis is usually favorable (Blood *Adv.* 2020;4:4442-4450).

TABLE 19.7-15 Key Features of Large B-Cell Lymphomas

LBCL	Key Features[a]	Differential Diagnoses/Diagnostic Caveats
DLBCL-NOS	The most common NHL. Diffuse sheets of LBCs positive for pan BCMs and CD45. May lose some BCMs and CD45 expression. GCB or non–GCB phenotype.[b] CD5+ in a small subset. *MYC*, *BCL2*, and *BCL6* R may be detected.[c] NGS studies show high molecular heterogeneity.	High-grade FL (FLBCL): follicular growth pattern MCL (blastoid and pleomorphic variants): cyclin D1+ and SOX11+ Other LBCLs should be excluded.
LBCL-*IRF4*	Young adults with localized head and neck disease. Proliferation of LBCs in a follicular, diffuse, or mixed pattern resembling FLBCL and/or DLBCL. BCMs-positive, strong expression of MUM1 and BCL6. CD10, BCL2, and CD5 are positive in a subset. *IRF4* R is detected. *MYC* and *BCL2* R are not present.	PTFL, FLBCL, and DLBCL can have overlapping morphology and/or immunophenotype but do not harbor *IRF4* R. If *IRF4* R cannot be confirmed, the diagnosis may be proposed in the appropriate clinicopathologic context.
HGBLs		
BL[d]	Monomorphic medium-sized cells. "Starry sky" appearance. BCMs-positive, CD10+, BCL6+, BCL2−. Ki-67 is ~100%. Positive for *MYC* R	The typical morphology, immunophenotype, and FISH findings distinguish BL from other HGBLs
DLBCL/HGBL with *MYC* and *BCL2* R	DLBCL-like or high-grade morphology[e] BCMs-positive, GCB phenotype[b] (majority). *MYC* and *BCL2* R should be detected.	BL and other HGBLs: IHC and FISH studies distinguish this entity from other HGBLs.

(continued)

TABLE 19.7-15 Key Features of Large B-Cell Lymphomas (continued)

LBCL	Key Features[a]	Differential Diagnoses/Diagnostic Caveats
HGBL with 11q aberrations	BL-like morphology and immunophenotype[f]. Characteristic FC findings[g]: CD16/CD56+/CD8+ and lack of CD38[high]. Lack of MYC R. Defining genetic feature: chromosome 11q-gain/loss, pattern	BL and HGBLs: Appropriate morphology, immunophenotype, and genetic studies are required to establish this diagnosis.
HGBL-NOS	High-grade/BL-like morphology. BCMs+, GCB phenotype[b] (majority). May express BCL2 and MYC. Lack of dual MYC and BCL2 R, 11q aberrations, and CCND1 R. Recurrent somatic mutations: KMT2D and TP53	Diagnosis of exclusion. Other B-cell lymphomas with high-grade morphology should be excluded.

LBCLs with polymorphic pattern

THRLBCL	Scattered LBCs resembling centroblasts, immunoblasts, LP cells, or HRS-like cells in a T-cell/histiocyte-rich background. BCMs-positive, CD45+, BCL6+, CD30−, CD15−, EBV−. Small B cells are few or rare. Absence of FDC meshworks by CD21/CD23. NGS studies show somatic mutations similar to NLPHL.	NLPHL[h]: Features that favor NLPHL include B-cell nodules with residual FDC meshworks and PD-1+ rosettes. CHL: HRS cells are usually CD45 and CD20−/partial, PAX5[weak], CD30+, and CD15+/−. EBV+ DLBCL: LBCs are EBV+. TCLs: atypical/aberrant T-cell infiltrate.
EBV+ DLBCL	Older adults (usually) without known IEI/IDD. Monomorphic or polymorphic pattern. BCMs (+) and EBV (+) in majority LBCs. Usually positive for CD30 and MUM1 and negative for CD10 and BCL6. CD15−/+	Features overlap with LYG and EBV+ LPDs associated with IEI/IDD. The diagnosis requires appropriate clinicopathologic context.

LYG	Lungs are almost always involved. No history of IEI/IDD. Polymorphic lymphoid infiltrate with scattered LBCs. Angiodestructive growth and frequent necrosis. BCMs⁺, CD30ᵛᵃʳⁱᵃᵇˡᵉ, EBV⁺; the proportion of EBV+ cells determines the histologic grade.	Features overlap with other EBV+ B-cell LPDs/lymphomas. Clinical history/evidence of IEI and/or IDD excludes this diagnosis.

LBCLs associated with specific anatomic sites

IP-LBCL	Diffuse proliferation of LBCs confined to CNS, VR, or testis. Necrosis and inflammatory cells are often present. BCMs⁺, non–GCB phenotype.[b] EBV⁻. *MYC* and *BCL2* R⁻. Recurrent mutations: *MYD88* and *CD79B*	Inflammatory conditions: Demonstration of B-cell clonality is helpful. Involvement by systemic LBCL should be excluded.
PMBL	Diffuse proliferation of LBCs in a f brotic background. The LBCs usually express CD45, pan BCMs, CD30ᵛᵃʳⁱᵃᵇˡᵉ, MUM1, and CD23. BCL2 and BCL6 expression is variable. *MYC*, *BCL2*, and *BCL6* R are absent.	CHL: Unlike CHL, LBCs in PMBL show a diffuse growth pattern and expression of pan BCMs. MGZL: See later.
MGZL	Morphology and immunophenotype overlap with CHL and PMBL. Genetic studies show shared phenotype with PMBL and CHL.	Diagnosis of exclusion. Location is almost always mediastinum, and features are intermediate between CHL and PMBL.
IVLBCL	Proliferation of LBCs, usually restricted to the lumens of small blood vessels. Pan BCMs-positive, usually non–GCB phenotype,[b] EBV⁻, HHV8⁻. *MYD88* and *CD79B* mutations are common.	Other large-cell lymphomas involving vessels should be excluded.

(continued)

TABLE 19.7-15 Key Features of Large B-Cell Lymphomas (*continued*)

LBCL	Key Features[a]	Differential Diagnoses/Diagnostic Caveats
LBCLs with plasmablastic features		
PBL	Diffuse proliferation of LBCs resembling immunoblasts or plasmablasts. Plasmablastic immunophenotype,[i] MYC and EBV (+) in the majority, ALK−, HHV8−, *MYC* R is common (>50%).	PCM with plasmablastic features: Clinical findings such as CRAB and genetic translocations associated with PCM (not seen in PBL) can help to distinguish between PCM and PBL.
ALK+ LBCL	Diffuse proliferation of LBCs resembling immunoblasts or plasmablasts. Plasmablastic immunophenotype,[i] ALK+, negative for CD19, CD22, BCL2, cyclin D1, and EBV. *ALK* alterations (usually *ALK* R). Gains and amplifications of *MYC* are common.	Other neoplasms with plasmablastic phenotype or ALK expression: Plasmablastic phenotype with ALK expression are unique to this lymphoma.
LBCLs confined to natural or acquired body spaces		
CI-DLBCL	Proliferation of LBCs usually with centroblastic or immunoblastic morphology in a confined space. Angiocentric growth pattern and prominent necrosis may be present. BCMs-positive and non-GCB phenotype (majority). Some may show plasmablastic features.[i] EBV+. Complex karyotype and *TP53* mutations are common.	The diagnosis requires appropriate clinicopathologic context. CI-DLBCL occurs in the setting of local longstanding CI. The most common location is the pleural cavity. Most patients do not have an overt immune deficiency.
FA-LBCL	LBCs are surrounded by fibrin and debris. BCMs-positive and non-GCB phenotype (majority). Some may show plasmablastic features.[i] EBV+. Usually negative for *MYC*, *BCL2*, and *BCL6* R.	The diagnosis requires appropriate clinicopathologic context. The lesion is confined to fibrinous debris and does not form a mass or infiltrate tissues.

LBCL	Key Features[a]	Differential Diagnoses/Diagnostic Caveats
FO-LBCL	LBCs in fluid (restricted to body cavity effusions) BCMs-positive and non-GCB phenotype (majority). HHV8−. High frequency of *MYC* R	PEL and secondary involvement by systemic LBCL should be excluded.

BCMs, B-cell markers; BL, Burkitt lymphoma; CHL, classic Hodgkin lymphoma; CI-DLBCL, DLBCL associated with chronic inflammation; DLBCL-NOS, diffuse LBCL, not otherwise specified; FA-LBCL, fibrin-associated LBCL; FC, flow cytometry; FL, follicular lymphoma; FLBCL, follicular LBCL; FO-LBCL, fluid overload–associated large B-cell lymphoma; GCB, germinal center B cell; HGBL, high-grade B-cell lymphoma; HRS, Hodgkin Reed-Sternberg; IDD, immune deficiency/dysregulation; IEI, inborn error of immunity; IP-LBCL, primary LBCL of immune-privileged sites; IVLBCL, intravascular large B-cell lymphoma; LBCL-*IRF4*r, LBCL with *IRF4* rearrangement; LBCs, large B cells; LN, lymph node; LP, lymphocyte predominant; LPD, lymphoproliferative disorder; LYG, lymphomatoid granulomatosis; MCL, mantle cell lymphoma; MCU, mucocutaneous ulcer; MGZL, mediastinal gray zone lymphoma; NHL, non-Hodgkin lymphoma; NLPHL, nodular lymphocyte-predominant Hodgkin lymphoma; PBL, plasmablastic lymphoma; PCM, plasma cell myeloma; PEL, primary effusion lymphoma; PMBL, primary mediastinal LBCL; PTFL, pediatric-type follicular lymphoma; R, rearrangement(s); THRLBCL, T-cell histiocyte-rich LBCL.

[a] All LBCLs show mature B-cell or plasmablastic phenotype. The key features listed here represent most cases, but there are exceptions.
[b] See Figure 19.7-1.
[c] If both *MYC* and *BCL2* R are detected, these cases are classified as DLBCL/HGBL with *MYC* and *BCL2* R.
[d] Discussed here for comparison, details in Chapter 19.8.
[e] The morphology may resemble DLBCL-NOS or can be of higher grade, resembling BL.
[f] BL immunophenotype: mature B-cell phenotype; positive for CD10 and BCL6 and negative for BCL2.
[g] Reference: *Mod Pathol.* 2018;31(5):732-743.
[h] The distinction between NLPHL and THRLBCL is challenging in small biopsies.
[i] Positive for CD138 and MUM1 and dim to negative expression of CD45, CD20, and PAX5.

SUGGESTED READINGS

Alduaij W, Collinge B, Ben-Neriah S, et al. Molecular determinants of clinical outcomes in a real-world diffuse large B-cell lymphoma population. *Blood*. 2023;141(20):2493-2507.

Kurz KS, Ott M, Kalmbach S, et al. Large B-cell lymphomas in the 5th edition of the WHO-classification of haematolymphoid neoplasms-updated classification and new concepts. *Cancers (Basel)*. 2023;15(8):2285.

Malpica L, Marques-Piubelli ML, Beltran BE, et al. EBV-positive diffuse large B-cell lymphoma, not otherwise specified: 2022 update on diagnosis, risk-stratification, and management. *Am J Hematol*. 2022;97(7):951-965.

Melani C, Jaffe ES, Wilson WH. Pathobiology and treatment of lymphomatoid granulomatosis, a rare EBV-driven disorder. *Blood*. 2020;135(16):1344-1352.

Quintanilla-Martinez L, Laurent C, Soma L, et al. Emerging entities: high-grade/large B-cell lymphoma with 11q aberration, large B-cell lymphoma with IRF4 rearrangement, and new molecular subgroups in large B-cell lymphomas: a report of the 2022 EA4HP/SH lymphoma workshop. *Virchows Arch*. 2023;483(3):281-298.

Savage KJ. Primary mediastinal large B-cell lymphoma. *Blood*. 2022;140(9):955-970.

Sehn LH, Salles G. Diffuse large B-cell lymphoma. *N Engl J Med*. 2021;384(9):842-858.

Sukswai N, Lyapichev K, Khoury JD, Medeiros LJ. Diffuse large B-cell lymphoma variants: an update. *Pathology*. 2020;52(1):53-67.

19.8 Burkitt Lymphoma

Anurag Khanna and Brooj Abro

Burkitt lymphoma (BL) is an aggressive mature B-cell lymphoma characterized by a uniform proliferation of monomorphic medium-sized B cells with a very high proliferation index, germinal center phenotype, negative BCL2 expression, and the presence of *IG::MYC* rearrangement. BL classically shows a "starry-sky appearance" on tissue sections, although this feature is not specific to BL. Traditionally, BL has been divided into the following subtypes: endemic, sporadic, and immunodeficiency associated. However, the recent WHO-HAEM5 recommends subtyping BL based on Epstein-Barr virus (EBV) status into EBV-associated BL and EBV-negative BL. This recommendation is based on data from recent studies showing distinct biologic features associated with EBV status in BL (*Mol Cancer Res*. 2017;15:563; *Br J Haematol*. 2022;196:468). BL is more common in males, and studies have shown multimodal incidence peaks at various ages, with peaks observed in children around the age of 10 and in adults around the ages of 40 and 70 (*Int J Cancer*. 2010;126:1732; *Am J Hematol*. 2012;87:573). The diagnostic criteria of BL are summarized in Table 19.8-1.

Clinical Features

- **Clinical Presentation:** Patients usually present with rapidly progressing disease due to the highly proliferative nature of the tumor. Symptoms may vary depending on the disease location.
- **Sites of Involvement:** BL most commonly involves extranodal sites. Lymphadenopathy, peripheral blood, and bone marrow involvement can be present and are

TABLE 19.8-1 WHO-HAEM5 Diagnostic Criteria for Burkitt Lymphoma

Essential
- **Morphology:** Uniform, medium-sized cells with basophilic cytoplasm and multiple nucleoli
- **Immunophenotype:** CD20$^+$, CD10$^+$, BCL2$^-$, MYC (usually strongly + in >80% of the cells). Rarely, weak expression of BCL2
- Presence of MYC breakage or *IG::MYC* translocation

Desirable
- **Morphology:** Starry-sky appearance, cohesive growth pattern
- **Immunophenotype:** BCL6$^+$, CD38$^+$, TdT$^-$
- Absence of *BCL2* and *BCL6* rearrangements (usually required in adults)

Based on the WHO Classification of Tumours Editorial Board. Haematolymphoid tumours [Internet]. Lyon (France): International Agency for Research on Cancer; 2024 (WHO classification of tumours series, 5th ed.; vol. 11). Available from: https://tumourclassification.iarc.who.int/chapters/63.

more common in the setting of immunodeficiency/dysregulation (*Ann Hematol.* 2020;99:571). Facial bones are commonly involved in endemic BL. Sporadic BL can present at various locations, most commonly in the abdomen and head and neck regions. Central nervous system (CNS) involvement is not uncommon.

Morphology

In tissue sections, a "starry-sky" pattern is often present, which is not entirely specific to BL (e-Figure 19.8-1). This pattern is formed by tingible-body macrophages scattered in a background of neoplastic basophilic lymphoid cells (macrophages are the "stars" and the blue lymphoid cells are the "sky"). The neoplastic lymphoid cells are uniformly medium-sized with round nuclei, finely dispersed chromatin, multiple nucleoli, and show a somewhat cohesive growth pattern. The tumor is highly proliferative with abundant mitosis and apoptosis, and prominent necrosis may be present. In fine needle aspirate smears, peripheral blood, and bone marrow aspirate smears, BL cells show basophilic cytoplasm and often have cytoplasmic vacuoles (e-Figure 19.8-2). While cytoplasmic vacuoles are not a specific feature of BL, this finding, along with other typical morphologic features, raises suspicion of BL.

Occasionally, variant morphologic features such as pleomorphism and plasmacytoid differentiation can be present. Plasmacytoid differentiation is associated with immunodeficiency (*Ann Oncol.* 1991;2:289). A florid granulomatous reaction has been reported in EBV-positive BL, and this feature is associated with a favorable prognosis (*Histopathology.* 2022;80:430).

Immunophenotype

The characteristic immunophenotype of BL includes expression of pan B-cell antigens (CD19, CD20, PAX5, etc), germinal center markers such as CD10 (usually strong) and BCL6, MYC (usually strong and positive in more than 80% of the cells), very high Ki-67 (95%-100%), monotypic surface κ or λ light chain expression, and negative BCL2. Occasionally, weak BCL2 expression can be present. The tumor cells are negative for cyclin D1, CD5, CD34, and TdT (helpful in excluding blastoid mantle cell lymphoma and acute lymphoblastic leukemia).

Genetic Features

BL is defined by *IG::MYC* translocation, involving t(8;14)(q24;q32), t(8;22)(q24;q11), or t(2;8)(p12;q24). The presence of *BCL2* and/or *BCL6* translocations excludes the diagnosis of BL. Karyotype analysis usually shows a simple karyotype. A complex karyotype should raise the possibility of other diagnoses such as high-grade B-cell lymphoma. Recurrently mutated genes include *TCF3, ID3, CCND3, GNA13, IGLL5, BACH2, SIN3A, DNMT1, RET, PIK3R1, ARID1A,* and *TP53* (*Nat Genet.* 2012;44:1321; *Nature.* 2012;490:116; *Blood* 2019;134:1598). Recent studies have demonstrated distinct molecular features in EBV-associated BL, including fewer driver mutations compared to EBV-negative BL, justifying the subtyping of BL based on EBV status (*Blood.* 2019;133:1313).

Prognosis and Treatment

BL is very sensitive to chemotherapy due to its highly proliferative nature. The prognosis is usually excellent with standard immunochemotherapy regimens (*Blood.* 2021;137:743).

Differential Diagnosis

- **B-lymphoblastic leukemia/lymphoma:** TdT$^+$, CD34$^+$, no light chain expression
- **High-grade B-cell lymphoma (HGBCL):** HGBCL subtypes can have overlapping morphologic features with BL. HGBCL with *MYC* and *BCL2* translocations by definition requires the presence of both, which excludes BL. HGBCL with 11q aberration is negative for *MYC* translocation. HGBCL, NOS does not have defining genetic features, and *MYC* translocation may be present; however, these cases are usually positive for BCL2 and negative for CD10.

> ### Key Points
>
> - BL is an aggressive mature B-cell neoplasm characterized by strong MYC expression, a high Ki-67 index (>95%), a germinal center phenotype, and absent (rarely weak) BCL2 expression.
> - *IG::MYC* translocation with the absence of *BCL2* and *BCL6* translocation helps support a diagnosis of BL.
> - The recent WHO-HAEM5 recommends subtyping BL based on EBV status into EBV-associated BL and EBV-negative BL.
>
> #### Diagnostic Caveats
>
> - B-lymphoblastic leukemia/lymphoma and HGBCL subtypes can show similar morphologic features to BL.
> - Evaluation of *BCL2* and *BCL6* translocations, as well as markers of immaturity (TdT, CD34, light chain expression), is helpful in the initial diagnosis.

SUGGESTED READINGS

King RL, Hsi ED, Chan WC, et al. Diagnostic approaches and future directions in Burkitt lymphoma and high-grade B-cell lymphoma. *Virchows Arch.* 2023;482(1):193-205.

Thomas N, Dreval K, Gerhard DS, et al. Genetic subgroups inform on pathobiology in adult and pediatric Burkitt lymphoma. *Blood.* 2023;141(8):904-916.

19.9 Kaposi Sarcoma Associated Herpes Virus (KSHV)/Human Herpesvirus 8 (HHV8) Associated B-Cell Proliferations and Lymphomas

Barina Aqil and Anjum Hassan

Kaposi sarcoma (KS) was first described by Moritz Kaposi in 1872. The discovery of human herpesvirus-8 (HHV8), also known as Kaposi sarcoma–associated herpesvirus (KSHV), as the causative agent of KS (*Science.* 1994;266:1865-1869) occurred in the setting of the human immunodeficiency virus (HIV) epidemic in North America. Since then, HHV8 has been associated with several lymphoproliferative disorders (LPDs), including HHV8-positive multicentric Castleman disease (MCD), primary effusion lymphoma (PEL)/extracavitary primary effusion lymphoma (EC-PEL), KSHV/HHV8–positive germinotropic lymphoproliferative disorder (KSHV/HHV8+ GLPD), and KSHV/HHV8–positive diffuse large B-cell lymphoma (KSHV/HHV8+ DLBCL). These disorders can usually be distinguished based on clinical presentation, localization, histology, immunophenotype, genetic profile, and the presence of Epstein-Barr virus (EBV) co-infection.

An important factor in the development of KSHV/HHV8–associated LPDs is the activation of the interleukin-6 receptor (IL-6R) signaling pathway, which promotes lymphoid proliferation and angiogenesis. KSHV/HHV8-infected plasmablasts can be identified by their expression of the HHV8 gene product known as LANA (latency-associated nuclear antigen), a protein that may also function to increase the expression of human IL-6 (huIL-6) (*Blood.* 2002;99:649-654). KSHV/HHV8 also encodes a functional homolog of huIL-6 called viral interleukin-6 (vIL-6), which can activate the IL-6R by bypassing the gp80 regulatory checkpoint (*Science.* 2002;298:1432-1435).

I. KAPOSI SARCOMA–ASSOCIATED HERPESVIRUS/HUMAN HERPESVIRUS-8–ASSOCIATED MULTICENTRIC CASTLEMAN DISEASE

Kaposi sarcoma–associated herpesvirus/human herpesvirus-8–associated multicentric Castleman disease (KSHV/HHV8-MCD) is an LPD characterized by idiopathic Castleman disease-like morphology, KSHV/HHV8-infected plasmablasts (LANA-positive), and systemic inflammatory symptoms. The majority of patients with KSHV/HHV8-MCD are HIV-positive (~80%). The connection between KSHV/HHV8 susceptibility and host genetic factors is related to host immunity to viral infection (perforin-granzyme pathway, MBL-mannose binding ligand, natural killer [NK] cell activation) (*Retrovirology.* 2018;15:1-9) or viral access to host cells via entry mechanisms (ephrin type-A receptor 2 [EPHA2] entry receptor) (*Cancer Epidemiol.* 2018;56:133-139). The diagnostic criteria for KSHV/HHV8-MCD are summarized in Table 19.9-1.

Clinical Features

- **Clinical presentation:** Fever, myalgia, and weight loss are common presenting symptoms. Physical examination and laboratory evaluation show elevated

TABLE 19.9-1 WHO-HAEM5 Diagnostic Criteria for KSHV/HHV8+ MCD

Major Criteria

- Lymphadenopathy involving two or more LN stations
- Grade 2-3 RGCs and/or Grade 2-3 plasmacytosis
- KSHV/HHV8-LANA+ plasmablasts

Minor Criteria

- Fever and CRP >2 mg/dL and at least three laboratory/clinical criterion not related to other HIV complications

Criteria

- Anemia
- Thrombocytopenia
- Hyponatremia
- Hypoalbuminemia

For flares (after original diagnosis): KSHV viral load

Criteria

- Splenomegaly
- Fatigue
- Weight loss
- Respiratory symptoms
- Gastrointestinal symptoms
- Neuropathy
- Headache
- Edema
- Rash
- Myalgia
- Fluid accumulation (edema, effusions)

Additional supportive histopathologic features (not required)

- Plasmablasts express monotypic λ light chain
- Prominent vascularity
- Kaposi sarcoma often present

Other supportive features; not required

- Elevated KSHV/HHV8 viral load
- Positive DAT
- Elevated interleukins (vIL6, IL6, IL10)
- Hemophagocytic lymphohistiocytosis

CRP, C-reactive protein; DAT, direct antiglobulin test; HHV8, human herpesvirus-8; KSHV, Kaposi sarcoma–associated herpesvirus; LANA, latency-associated nuclear antigen; LN, lymph node; MCD, multicentric Castleman disease; RGC, regressed germinal center.
Based on the WHO Classification of Tumours Editorial Board. Haematolymphoid tumours [Internet]. Lyon (France): International Agency for Research on Cancer; 2024 (WHO classification of tumours series, 5th ed.; vol. 11). Available from: https://tumourclassification.iarc.who.int/chapters/63.

C-reactive protein (CRP), cytopenias, hypoalbuminemia, effusions, diffuse lymphadenopathy, and hepatosplenomegaly.
- **Sites of involvement:** Involves the lymph node, spleen, and less frequently the bone marrow

Morphology

The following histopathologic features in Castleman disease are graded using a scale of 0 to 3 (Table 19.9-2): regressed germinal centers (RGCs), follicular dendritic cell (FDC) prominence, vascular proliferation, plasmacytosis, and hyperplastic germinal centers (GCs) (*Blood.* 2017;129:1646-1657).

KSHV/HHV8-MCD is characterized by Grade 2 to 3 RFGs and/or Grade 2 to 3 plasmacytosis. Most cases are of the plasmacytic subtype with hyperplastic GCs and profuse plasmacytosis or the mixed subtype with a combination of hypervascular and plasmacytic features. Plasmablasts, which are medium to large cells with 1 to 2 nucleoli and a moderate amount of amphophilic cytoplasm, are present, either scattered or forming aggregates, usually within the mantle zones of the follicles (e-Figure 19.9-1A-D).

Immunophenotype

Plasmablasts are negative to dim for CD20, positive for CD79a, and positive for MUM1, LANA (HHV8), and IgM λ, but negative for CD138 and EBER. They are also usually negative for other B-cell markers (e-Figure 19.9-1 E-K). The RGCs are positive for CD10 and BCL6 but negative for BCL2. Interfollicular plasma cells are polytypic and usually IgM-negative.

TABLE 19.9-2 Pathologic Grading in Multicentric Castleman Disease

Grade	0	1	2	3
RGCs	No regressed GCs	Few regressed GCs	Many regressed GCs	Most GCs regressed
FDC prominence	No FDC prominence	Mild FDC prominence	Moderate FDC prominence	Very prominent FDCs
Vascularity	Normal	Mildly increased	Moderately increased	Very prominent
Hyperplastic GCs	No hyperplastic GCs	Few hyperplastic GCs	Many hyperplastic GCs	Most GCs hyperplastic
Plasmacytosis	None	Mildly increased	Moderately increased	Very increased

FDC, follicular dendritic cell; GCs, germinal centers; RGCs, regressed germinal centers.
Modified from *Blood.* 2017;129(12):1646-1657.

Genetic Features

Plasmablasts are polyclonal B cells based on molecular studies (*Blood*. 2001;97: 2130-2136) and lack somatic hypermutation.

Prognosis and Treatment

KSHV/HHV8-MCD is a relapsing and remitting disease with an increased propensity for the development of lymphoma and other KSHV/HHV8–associated diseases (*Blood Adv*. 2021;5:1660-1670). Overall survival has improved with the use of rituximab and antiretroviral therapy (ART) for patients who are HIV-positive (*Blood*. 2014;124:3544-3552).

Differential Diagnosis

- **Idiopathic MCD:** Similar to KSHV/HHV-MCD, Grade 2 or 3 RGCs or plasmacytosis is required for diagnosis. No LANA (KSHV/HHV8)-positive cells are seen.
- **HIV-associated lymphadenopathy:** Different stages of follicular hyperplasia and follicular involution can be seen in HIV cases, but no LANA-positive plasmablasts are present.
- **Autoimmune disorder–associated lymphadenopathy:** Autoimmune diseases such as systemic lupus erythematosus (SLE), Sjogren syndrome, and rheumatoid arthritis, depending on the site of involvement, would have reactive follicles and paracortical expansion by a polymorphous infiltrate including immunoblasts, histiocytes, and prominent plasma cells. Lymphoepithelial lesions can also be seen. The presence of apoptotic and amorphous debris is seen in SLE; however, no prominent RGCs or LANA-positive plasmablasts are noted.
- **IgG4-related disease:** This disease can have some morphologic overlap with CD but usually has lymphoplasmacytic infiltrate with increased IgG4 positive plasma cells, an elevated IgG4/IgG ratio greater than 40%, and obliterative phlebitis in a setting of fibrosis and an increased serum IgG4 titer. The plasma cells are polytypic in this entity with no LANA-positive cells.
- **Follicular lymphoma (FL):** Some cases of FL may have foci of sclerosis or hyalinosis within the neoplastic follicles resembling the hyaline-vascular follicles of Castleman disease. However, the small neoplastic follicles are more cellular than lymphocyte-depleted follicles of true hyaline-vascular CD, and the interface between GCs and mantle zones is ill-defined. Immunohistochemistry for BCL-2 is positive, and flow cytometry should show a monotypic B-cell population. Fluorescence in situ

---

Key Points

- Characterized by Grade 2 to 3 regressed follicles and/or Grade 2 to 3 plasmacytosis.
- The presence of LANA (HHV8)-positive plasmablasts is characteristic.
- KSHV/HHV8-MCD is a relapsing and remitting disease with an increased incidence of lymphoma and other KSHV/HHV8–associated diseases.

Diagnostic Caveats

- Plasmablasts are positive for MUM1, LANA (HHV8), and IgM λ, but negative for CD20, CD138, and EBER.

hybridization (FISH) positivity for t(14;18)(q32;q21) or IGH-BCL2 can help establish the diagnosis in challenging cases.

II. PRIMARY EFFUSION LYMPHOMA

PEL is a rare large B-cell lymphoma that most often occurs in immunocompromised patients, such as the older population, those with HIV infection, and solid organ transplant recipients. Patients classically present with malignant effusions in body cavities without detectable tumor masses. A much rarer extracavitary form (EC-PEL) can present as nodal or extranodal tumor masses in the gastrointestinal tract, skin, lung, and rarely in the central nervous system or bone marrow.

PEL accounts for approximately 4% of HIV-associated non-Hodgkin lymphoma and less than 1% of non-HIV–related lymphomas (*Cancer Cytopathol.* 2021;129:62-74). Most cases harbor EBV in addition to HHV8, the latter of which is present in virtually all cases (*Blood.* 1996;88:645-656). The diagnostic criteria for PEL are summarized in Table 19.9-3.

Morphology

PEL cells have varied morphology, including round or irregular nuclear contours, variably prominent nucleoli, and moderately abundant agranular basophilic to occasionally vacuolated cytoplasm. EC-PEL shows similar morphologic features with diffuse or sinusoidal growth patterns.

Immunophenotype

The neoplastic cells are positive for MUM1, CD138, CD38, CD30, EMA, LANA, and EBER. They lack CD45 and most B-cell markers (CD20, CD19, CD22, Pax-5,

TABLE 19.9-3 WHO-HAEM5 Diagnostic Criteria for PEL/EC-PEL

Essential	Desirable
PEL • Large B-cell lymphoma, involving serous cavities • No involvement of LN or other extranodal site (tumor mass directly associated with the effusion is acceptable) • Neoplastic cells positive for terminally differentiated B cells (HLA-DR, CD30, EMA, CD38, Vs38c, CD138, MUM1, and BLIMP1) • KSHV/HHV8 (LANA-positive)	• Presence of EBV
EC-PEL • Nodal or extranodal site involvement without effusion with the above diagnostic findings	

EBV, Epstein-Barr virus; EC-PEL, extracavitary primary effusion lymphoma; LN, lymph node.
Based on the WHO Classification of Tumours Editorial Board. Haematolymphoid tumours [Internet]. Lyon (France): International Agency for Research on Cancer; 2024 (WHO classification of tumours series, 5th ed.; vol. 11). Available from: https://tumourclassification.iarc.who.int/chapters/63.

CD79a, OCT2, and BOB.1), as well as surface and cytoplasmic immunoglobulins, CD10, and BCL6. Aberrant expression of T-cell markers has been reported. EC-PELs are reported to have a slightly higher proportion expressing B-cell–associated antigens (25%) and immunoglobulin (25%) compared to PELs (<5% and 15%, respectively) (e-Figure 19.9-2A-K).

Genetic Features

Clonal *IGH* gene rearrangement is present usually with somatic hypermutation. In some cases, polymerase chain reaction (PCR) testing for the presence of KSHV and EBV may be required to establish the diagnosis.

Prognosis and Treatment

PEL and EC-PEL are aggressive lymphomas with a poor prognosis (*Cancers* (*Basel*). 2021;13:878), though the prognosis of EC-PEL is slightly more favorable. EBV-positive PEL also tends to exhibit better overall outcomes. Notably, high-dose chemotherapy with autologous stem cell support (HDCT/ASCT) has not been successful as a treatment option (*Br J Haematol.* 2021;194:642-646). The site of effusion and serum LDH levels are considered potential prognostic factors in patients with PEL (*Leuk Lymphoma.* 2020;61:2093-2102). The effect of highly active antiretroviral therapy (HAART) on HIV-associated malignancies is well-known, with some patients attaining and maintaining remission after chemotherapy combined with HAART (*Hemasphere.* 2018;2:e143).

Differential Diagnosis

- **KSHV/HHV8+ DLBCL:** The morphology of this entity is similar with effacement of tissue architecture, but the neoplastic cells are IgM λ^+, CD138$^-$, and more often CD20$^+$. EBER is also usually negative.
- **KSHV/HHV8+ GLPD:** Although the morphology of neoplastic cells and immunophenotypic findings (negative B-cell markers, MUM1$^+$, CD138$^{+/-}$, HHV8$^+$, and EBER$^+$) resemble those of PEL/EC-PEL, this entity is seen in immunocompetent individuals who are HIV-negative and exhibits relatively preserved nodal architecture.
- **Fluid overload–associated large B-cell lymphoma:** Similar to PEL in presentation, this disease is seen in patients with fluid overload. The neoplastic cells express pan B-cell markers and are negative for LANA (HHV8).
- **Anaplastic lymphoma kinase (ALK)–positive large B-cell lymphoma:** ALK-positive large B-cell lymphomas do not have an association with

---

Key Points

- A large B-cell lymphoma that involves serous cavities, including the pleura, pericardium, and peritoneum
- Seen in immunosuppressed patients
- The cells lack pan B-cell markers but are positive for markers associated with terminally differentiated B cells.

Diagnostic Caveats

- Histologically, there is complete effacement of tissue architecture with expression of both EBER and LANA (HHV8).
- If a tumor mass is present, it must be directly associated with the effusion, with no nodal or extranodal involvement.

immunosuppression and have an immunoblastic or plasmablastic morphology. They express EMA, CD138, VS38, and MUM1, but are negative for CD30 and LANA. Strong ALK1 positivity is observed, often with a restricted granular cytoplasm staining pattern indicative of t(2;17)(p23;q23) or *CLTC::ALK* fusion. ALK-positive large B-cell lymphomas also express cytoplasmic immunoglobulins.

III. KSHV/HHV8–POSITIVE DIFFUSE LARGE B-CELL LYMPHOMA

KSHV/HHV8+ DLBCL characteristically arises in association with MCD and HIV infection, although cases have been described in the absence of MCD (*Mod Pathol.* 2003;16:424-429). The diagnostic criteria for KSHV/HHV8+ DLBCL are summarized in Table 19.9-4.

Clinical Features

- **Clinical presentation:** KSHV/HHV8+ DLBCL usually arises in a background of KSHV/HHV8+ MCD, particularly in patients who are HIV-positive. However, similar lymphomas have been reported in patients with KSHV/HHV8+ GLPD or in immunocompetent patients (*Am J Clin Pathol.* 2014;142:816-829; *Mod Pathol.* 2017;30:745-760). The most common presentation is diffuse lymphadenopathy or splenomegaly.
- **Sites of involvement:** Lymph nodes and spleen are most commonly involved, but extranodal sites may also be involved.

Morphology

The lymphoma is characterized by effacement of tissue architecture, with sheets or confluent clusters of large monomorphic cells resembling plasmablasts or immunoblasts. These cells exhibit an eccentric nucleus, vesicular chromatin, single or multiple prominent nucleoli, and moderate to abundant amphophilic cytoplasm.

Immunophenotype

The neoplastic cells are variably positive for CD45 and CD20; they are positive for MUM1, cytoplasmic IgM (usually λ light chain), and LANA but often negative for CD79a, CD38, CD138, and EBER. In rare cases, they are positive for EBER.

TABLE 19.9-4 WHO-HAEM5 Diagnostic Criteria for KSHV/HHV8+ DLBCL

Essential	Desirable
- Nodal and/or splenic involvement - Effacement of architecture by large B cells (plasmablasts, immunoblasts, or anaplastic morphology) - Positive for IgM and LANA	- Usually negative for EBER (rare cases may be positive) - Presence of immunoglobulin somatic hypermutation

KSHV/HHV8+ DLBCL, KSHV/HHV8–positive diffuse large B-cell lymphoma; LANA, latency-associated nuclear antigen.
Based on the WHO Classification of Tumours Editorial Board. Haematolymphoid tumours [Internet]. Lyon (France): International Agency for Research on Cancer; 2024 (WHO classification of tumours series, 5th ed.; vol. 11). Available from: https://tumourclassification.iarc.who.int/chapters/63.

Genetic Features

Molecular studies usually reveal a monoclonal *IGH* gene rearrangement, along with the absence of somatic mutations in the *IGH* variable regions.

Prognosis and Treatment

KSHV/HHV8+ DLBCL is an aggressive lymphoma, and there is no consensus regarding its optimal treatment. Prognosis is generally poor (*Blood Adv.* 2021;5:1660-1670).

Differential Diagnosis

- **Diffuse large B-cell lymphoma, not otherwise specified (DLBCL, NOS):** DLBCL, NOS is negative for IgM, λ light chains, and LANA.
- **KSHV/HHV8+ MCD with clusters of plasmablasts:** The characteristic lesions were previously referred to as "microlymphomas" arising in the setting of KSHV/HHV8+ MCD, but this entity has now been eliminated since the characteristic lesions are not clonal neoplasms and do not necessarily progress to lymphoma. HHV8+ DLBCL differs from these plasmablastic aggregates as there are sheets of clonal lymphoma cells that efface the tissue architecture.
- **KSHV/HHV8+ GLPD:** See description later.
- **EC-PEL:** The morphology and presentation are similar to KSHV/HHV8+ DLBCL, but the immunophenotype is different with a lack of IgM, λ light chain, and EBER, but with expression of CD30.

Key Points

- Seen in association with HIV and KSHV/HHV8+ MCD
- Characterized by sheets of large cells with effacement of tissue architecture
- Variably positive for CD20 and express IgM, λ light chain, MUM1, EBER, and LANA

Diagnostic Caveats

- Difficult to differentiate from KSHV/HHV8+ GLPD by needle core biopsy, especially in patients with HIV, so excisional biopsy is required.

IV. KAPOSI SARCOMA–ASSOCIATED HERPESVIRUS/HUMAN HERPESVIRUS-8–POSITIVE GERMINOTROPIC LYMPHOPROLIFERATIVE DISORDER

GLPD is a rare lymphoproliferative disorder, with only a few cases described in the literature. It presents mostly in patients who are HIV-negative, although it is occasionally seen in patients with HIV who present with diffuse lymphadenopathy (*Mod Pathol.* 2017;30:745-760). The diagnostic criteria for GLPD are summarized in Table 19.9-5.

Clinical Features

- **Clinical presentation:** Lymphadenopathy is present in almost all of cases, which is generally localized. Most patients do not have many constitutional symptoms, and most of those who do are patients living with HIV (PLWH).
- **Sites of involvement:** Lymph nodes, most frequently in the neck

TABLE 19.9-5 WHO-HAEM5 Diagnostic Criteria for KSHV/HHV8+ GLPD

Essential
- Lymph node architecture retention with partial or complete GCs replacement by clusters or sheets of large B cells
- LANA+

Desirable
- EBER-positive
- Polyclonal *IGH* gene rearrangement

EBER, EBV-encoded RNA; GCs, germinal centers; IGH, immunoglobulin heavy chain; KSHV/HHV8+ GLPD, KSHV/HHV8–positive germinotropic lymphoproliferative disorder. Based on the WHO Classification of Tumours Editorial Board. Haematolymphoid tumours [Internet]. Lyon (France): International Agency for Research on Cancer; 2024 (WHO classification of tumours series, 5th ed.; vol. 11). Available from: https://tumourclassification.iarc.who.int/chapters/63.

Morphology

Lymph nodes show retention of the nodal architecture with clusters or sheets of large atypical cells with immunoblastic, anaplastic, or plasmablastic features. These cells infiltrate and partially or completely replace GCs. These atypical cells are seen in mantle zones, interfollicular areas, or sinuses. Polytypic plasmacytosis may also be seen.

Immunophenotype

The atypical cells are variably positive for MUM1, CD138, LANA, and EBER. They are positive for monotypic immunoglobulin (rarely); show variable expression of CD38 and EMA; and are negative for B-cell markers, CD45, and CD30. Follicular dendritic meshworks are highlighted with CD21, with associated atypical cells.

Genetic Features

Molecular studies are not essential for diagnostic purposes, but the polyclonal nature of KSVH/HHV8+ GLPD is helpful in distinguishing this entity from EC-PEL (although monoclonality has been described in rare cases). To date, no deleterious driver mutations have been demonstrated.

Prognosis and Treatment

KSHV/HHV8+ GLPD is a very rare disease with an indolent clinical course (*Pathology.* 2017;49:430-435). Therapeutic approaches have been extremely variable, ranging from no treatment to surgery alone, or with radiotherapy and/or chemotherapy with or without rituximab (*Am J Surg Pathol.* 2017;41:795-800). In rare instances, patients have developed aggressive lymphomas, such as KSHV/HHV8+ and EBV+ DLBCL (*Am J Surg Pathol.* 2017;41:795-800).

Differential Diagnosis

- **Intrafollicular EBV+ LBCL:** Some EBV-positive DLBCL with exclusive intrafollicular localization have been described in patients without immunodeficiency. These are LANA-negative.
- Refer to Table 19.9-5 for other KSHV/HHV8+ LPD.

> **Key Points**
>
> - The disease is seen as mostly localized disease in HIV-negative cases; multifocal presentation is common in PLWH.
> - There is retention of LN architecture, with variable particle or complete replacement of GCs by atypical large B cells.
> - The cells are positive for MUM1, CD138, LANA, and EBER; show monotypic immunoglobulin expression; are variable for CD38 and EMA; and are negative for B-cell markers, CD45, and CD30.
>
> **Diagnostic Caveats**
>
> - Retention of tissue architecture along with polyclonal nature of KSVH/HHV8+ GLPD is helpful in distinguishing it from EC-PEL.

19.10 Primary Cutaneous B-Cell Lymphoproliferative Disorders/Lymphomas

Carina A. Dehner and Leigh A. Compton

I. PRIMARY CUTANEOUS MARGINAL ZONE LYMPHOMA

Primary cutaneous marginal zone lymphoma (PCMZL) is a low-grade B-cell lymphoma composed of marginal zone B cells, lymphoplasmacytoid cells, and plasma cells. There are multiple proposed histopathologic subtypes, but the so-called conventional type is by far the most common and will be discussed here. The International Consensus Classification (ICC) suggests referring to this as primary cutaneous marginal zone lymphoproliferative disorder given its very indolent clinical course. The diagnostic criteria for PCMZL are summarized in Table 19.10-1.

TABLE 19.10-1 Diagnostic Criteria for PCMZL

Essential	Desirable
• Morphology and immunophenotype of MZL (negative for CD5 and CD10)	• Involvement of trunk and arms
• Demonstration of clonality (B cells and/or plasma cells)	• Presence of reactive follicles within the lesion
• Exclusion of extracutaneous disease and other cutaneous lymphomas	

MZL, marginal zone lymphoma; PCMZL, primary cutaneous marginal zone lymphoma. Based on the WHO Classification of Tumours Editorial Board. Haematolymphoid tumours [Internet]. Lyon (France): International Agency for Research on Cancer; 2024 (WHO classification of tumours series, 5th ed.; vol. 11). Available from: https://tumourclassification.iarc.who.int/chapters/63.

Clinical Features

- **Clinical presentation:** Patients present with one or multiple red to red-brown papules, plaques, or nodules that may appear and disappear (and possibly even undergo spontaneous regression) (*J Cutan Pathol.* 2011;38:342-345). It is one of the lymphomas that may be associated with anetoderma (ie, loss of elastic tissue) (*Arch Dermatol.* 2010;146:175-182) subsequent to spontaneous involution. Additionally, it is also associated with gastrointestinal disorders and autoimmune conditions (*JAMA Dermatol.* 2014;150:412-418). The etiology of PCMZL is unclear; however, chronic antigen stimulation is suggested as one mechanism (*Br J Haematol.* 2006;132:571-575), while other studies associate the herpes viruses Epstein-Barr virus (EBV) and human herpesvirus type 8 (HHV8) with the disease (*Blood.* 2009;113:1213-1224). Interestingly, the presence of *Borrelia burgdorferi* DNA was found in the skin of some European patients (*Dermatology.* 2007;215:229-232).
- **Sites of involvement:** PCMZL most commonly presents on the upper extremities and upper trunk. The second most common site is the head and neck region.

Morphology

There is a multinodular to diffuse lymphoid infiltrate that spares the epidermis and papillary dermis (grenz zone) and may extend to the subcutis (e-Figure 19.10-1A and B). The infiltrate comprises small- to medium-sized lymphocytes, plasmacytoid lymphocytes, plasma cells, and a variably mixed reactive inflammatory infiltrate of histiocytes, eosinophils, and neutrophils. Dutcher bodies may be present. Reactive germinal centers may also be present and colonized by neoplastic cells, possibly causing confusion with follicular center cell lymphoma; however, reactive germinal centers retain their tingible body macrophages and should not be expansile.

Immunophenotype

Lesional infiltrates express B-cell markers CD20 and Pax5 and show Bcl-2 expression (e-Figure 19.10-1C and D). CD10, Bcl-6, CD21, CD23, and CD5 are negative. Of note, reactive germinal centers will be highlighted by Bcl-6 but may also be colonized by Bcl-2–positive neoplastic marginal zone cells. CD43 expression is variable. A monotypic light chain–restricted population of plasma cells may be detected by immunohistochemistry or in situ hybridization studies; this is a particularly useful diagnostic finding given the population of neoplastic B cells can be variable and obscured by a reactive infiltrate.

Genetic Features

Clonal *IGH* gene rearrangements can be detected. Studies have identified recurrent *FAS* mutations in PCMZL (*J Invest Dermatol.* 2018;138(7):1573-1581).

Prognosis and Treatment

PCMZL has an excellent prognosis with a 5-year overall survival of over 98%. Local recurrence is common, but extracutaneous spread is very rare.

Differential Diagnosis

- **Secondary involvement by systemic marginal zone lymphoma:** Immunophenotype and morphology may be identical to PCMZL, however, more commonly IgM and IgD+; patients are older; t(11:18) may be positive.

- **Primary cutaneous follicle center cell lymphoma:** Follicles are neoplastic (expansile and lack tingible body macrophages), not reactive.
- **Primary cutaneous diffuse large B-cell lymphoma, leg type (PCDLBCL-LT):** Significantly worse prognosis; presents more commonly on legs; co-expression of BCL2 and BCL6 with often strong/diffuse MUM1

Key Points

- PCMZL most commonly presents on the trunk and upper extremities.
- Composed of small B cells, plasmacytoid forms, and plasma cells in clusters with reactive germinal center that may be colonized by tumor cells
- Neoplastic lymphocytes show expression of B-cell markers and Bcl-2 and are negative for CD5, cyclin D1, CD10, and Bcl-6. Light chain restriction of plasma cells is helpful for this diagnosis.

Diagnostic Caveats

- Secondary MZL may be morphologically and immunophenotypically identical to PCMZL; clinical correlation is key.

II. PRIMARY CUTANEOUS DIFFUSE LARGE B-CELL LYMPHOMA, LEG TYPE

PCDLBCL-LT is an aggressive lymphoma with a disease survival comparable to systemic diffuse large B-cell lymphoma (DLBCL), most commonly presenting on the legs of older patients. The molecular workup required for subclassification of DLBCL is not commonly employed in PCDLBCL-LT, as "double-hit" and "triple-hit" variants are not frequently encountered and do not appear to affect prognosis. MYC rearrangements may be associated with disease relapse but do not affect overall survival. Furthermore, the HANS criteria are not typically used in skin-limited disease (*Mod Pathol.* 2014;27:402-411). The diagnostic criteria for PCDLBCL-LT are summarized in Table 19.10-2.

TABLE 19.10-2 Diagnostic Criteria for PCDLBCL-LT

Essential	Desirable
- Sheets of large B cells with mature phenotype infiltrating the dermis/subcutaneous tissue - Diffuse growth pattern - Exclusion of extracutaneous disease at presentation	- Expression of BCL2 (strong), IgM and MUM1 (nongerminal center phenotype)

PCDLBCL-LT, primary cutaneous diffuse large B-cell lymphoma, leg type.
Based on the WHO Classification of Tumours Editorial Board. Haematolymphoid tumours [Internet]. Lyon (France): International Agency for Research on Cancer; 2024 (WHO classification of tumours series, 5th ed.; vol. 11). Available from: https://tumourclassification.iarc.who.int/chapters/63.

Clinical Features

- **Clinical presentation and sites of involvement:** Patients present with rapidly growing lesions on one or both legs, often with a high likelihood of spread to extracutaneous sites. There is a predilection for older females. Superficial ulceration is common.

Morphology

Lesions are composed of diffuse sheets of monotonous large, atypical immunoblasts or centroblasts with only occasional reactive T cells in the background (e-Figure 19.10-2A-C). Similar to other B-cell lymphomas, there is sparing of the epidermis and papillary dermis ("grenz zone"). Mitotic figures are commonly encountered. Small B lymphocytes and follicular dendritic cell meshworks are not apparent, compared to other indolent cutaneous B-cell lymphomas.

Immunophenotype

Cells express pan-B-cell antigens such as CD20, PAX-5, and CD79a. Lesional cells typically show strong diffuse positivity for Bcl-2, Mum-1, and FOX-P1 (e-Figure 19.10-2D-F). Bcl-6 is often positive, while CD10 is negative, but there is variability in the expression of these germinal center cell markers. MYC may be positive. There is cytoplasmic IgM, with about half of cases showing co-expression of IgD (*Am J Surg Pathol*. 2003;27:1538-1545; *Am J Surg Pathol*. 2010;34:1043-1048). The tumors usually display a very high proliferation rate.

Genetic Features

Monoclonal *IGH* gene rearrangements are common. The *MYC* translocation is identified in about 30% of cases. Other findings include mutations in *MYD88 L265P, CARD11, CD79B,* and *TNFAIP3*.

Prognosis and Treatment

Historically, the prognosis has been quite poor, with a 40% to 50% survival rate. The use of rituximab with a multiagent chemotherapeutic regiment has significantly improved outcomes (*Int J Radiat Oncol Biol Phys*. 2013;87:719-725). The presence of multiple lesions and loss of *CDKN2A*, along with *MYD88* L265P mutations, seem to go along with a worse prognosis (*J Clin Oncol*. 2001;19:3602-3610).

Differential Diagnosis

- **Systemic DLBCL involving the skin:** It may be difficult to differentiate based on histopathologic features alone and requires clinical history and an appropriate staging workup to evaluate for systemic disease. Large tumors on the leg favor PCDLBCL-LT.
- **Primary cutaneous follicle center cell lymphoma:** The presence of a follicular growth pattern is helpful to differentiate morphologically. Diffuse growth patterns may be difficult to differentiate based on morphology alone but are typically negative for Bcl-2 and MUM-1. Most commonly has a follicular pattern which helps distinguish, while diffuse pattern is harder; usually involves head, neck, trunk and arms; typically negative for Bcl-2 and MUM-1.

> **Key Points**
>
> - PCDLBCL-LT is the most aggressive primary cutaneous B-cell lymphoma.
> - It commonly presents on the legs of older patients with a female predominance.
> - HANS criteria are not used for PCDLBCL-LT.
> - The histopathologic features and immunophenotype may be identical to systemic DLBCL; clinical history and full staging are required for definitive diagnosis.
>
> **Diagnostic Caveats**
>
> - PCDLBCL-LT and PCFCL with a diffuse growth pattern may be morphologically identical but have significantly different treatment and outcomes; clinical presentation and a complete immunohistochemical profile will aid accurate diagnosis.

III. PRIMARY CUTANEOUS FOLLICLE CENTER TYPE LYMPHOMA

Primary cutaneous follicle center type lymphoma (PCFCL) is a skin-limited mature B-cell lymphoma composed of germinal center cells (centrocytes and centroblasts). Like systemic follicle center lymphoma (FCL), lesions may show follicular, diffuse, or mixed growth patterns. However, PCFCL behaves in an indolent fashion irrespective of the growth pattern, and a grading scheme is not commonly used (*Histopathology*. 2012;60:774-784). The diagnostic criteria for PCFCL are summarized in Table 19.10-3.

Clinical Features

- **Clinical presentation and sites of involvement**: Lesions present as solitary or clustered, firm papules, plaques, and nodules of variable size, commonly observed on the head and neck, particularly the scalp, or trunk. A small number of cases (~5%) may present with multifocal skin disease (~15%) (*Blood*. 2005;106:2491-2497; *J Clin Oncol*. 2007;25:1581-1587). Ulceration is uncommon.

TABLE 19.10-3 Diagnostic Criteria for PCFCL

Essential	Desirable
- Cutaneous lymphoid infiltrate consisting of admixed centrocytes and centroblasts with follicular or diffuse growth pattern - Germinal center phenotype - Exclusion of extracutaneous disease	- Location: head or trunk - Negative for MUM1 and negative to weak for BCL2 - Lack of BCL2 rearrangement - Demonstration of monoclonal B cells

PCFCL, primary cutaneous follicle center type lymphoma.
Based on the WHO Classification of Tumours Editorial Board. Haematolymphoid tumours [Internet]. Lyon (France): International Agency for Research on Cancer; 2024 (WHO classification of tumours series, 5th ed.; vol. 11). Available from: https://tumourclassification.iarc.who.int/chapters/63.

Morphology

As previously alluded, growth patterns are important for histopathologic recognition and are not of prognostic value for PCFCL (*Cancer*. 1991;67:2311-2326; *Blood*. 2005;105:3768-3785). Regardless of the growth pattern, infiltrates are dermal-based with sparing of the epidermis and papillary dermis ("grenz zone") and frequently extend into the subcutaneous tissue (e-Figure 19.10-3A and B). Tumors with a follicular growth pattern show numerous and/or expansile nodules of small and large cleaved centrocytes and scattered centroblasts. These nodules lack tingible body macrophages, a feature that may help in distinguishing PCFCL from reactive germinal centers found in inflammatory conditions and other B-cell lymphomas such as PCMZL. There may be a so-called inverted growth pattern where a band of tumor cells encircle a nodule of reactive lymphocytes. A diffuse growth pattern is defined as sheets of medium to large cleaved centrocytes and scattered centroblasts. There are admixed small reactive lymphocytes. In cases of diffuse growth patterns, large centrocytes may be present, some of which may appear spindled in rare cases (*Am J Dermatopathol*. 2000;22:299-304). These diffuse cases usually have a much higher proliferation index using Ki-67. Mixed follicular and diffuse patterns may be observed within a single lesion.

Immunophenotype

The neoplastic cells are positive for B-cell markers such as CD20 (e-Figure 19.10-3C), CD19, CD79a, and PAX5, with co-expression of the follicle center marker BCL6, while CD10 expression is variable. Most cases are negative for co-expression of Bcl-2, or there is only weak, focal positivity compared with the diffuse positivity seen in systemic follicular lymphoma (*J Invest Dermatol*. 1994;102:231-235; *Br J Dermatol*. 2003;149:1183-1191). Bcl-2 positivity may be associated with a follicular growth pattern. Therefore, co-expression of Bcl-2 does not serve as a definitive diagnostic marker for cutaneous involvement by systemic follicular lymphoma but should prompt further clinical, laboratory, and radiologic investigation for systemic disease (*J Cutan Pathol*. 2019;46:182-189). IRF4/MUM1 and FOXP1 are usually negative, which helps in differentiation from PCDLBCL-LT. CD5 and CD43 are essentially always negative. CD21-positive follicular dendritic cells are present in all cases with a follicular growth pattern, although they may also sometimes be present in diffuse cases as scattered clusters.

Genetic Features

According to several studies, PCFCL does not show BCL2 rearrangements (*J Am Acad Dermatol*. 2011;65:991-1000; *Am J Surg Pathol*. 2004;28:748-755). However, other studies using techniques such as fluorescence in situ hybridization (FISH) or polymerase chain reaction (PCR) have found a higher incidence of t(14;18)IGH/BCL-2 translocations, as seen in systemic FCL (*J Clin Oncol*. 2002;20:647-655). Clonal *IGH* gene rearrangements are detected in about 45% of cases. Inactivation of *CDKN2A* and *CDKN2B* is identified only rarely (*J Clin Oncol*. 2006;24:296-305).

Prognosis and Treatment

The prognosis for PCFCL is very good, and factors such as growth pattern, number of lesions, and presence of tumor nodules (versus papules and plaques) do not appear to affect the outcome (*J Clin Oncol*. 2001;19:3602-3610; *J Clin Oncol*. 2007;25:1581-1587). Local recurrence is common, while distant spread is rare. However, locally aggressive growth, though rare, may occur and result in bony erosion and related sequelae (*Am J Dermatopathol.* 2013;35:319-326). Standard treatment varies depending on the clinical course, ranging from observation to surgical removal or local radiation therapy. If the skin is extensively involved, treatment with rituximab alone or in combination with chemotherapy may be required (*Br J Dermatol.* 2005;153:167-173; *Ann Oncol.* 2009;20:326-330).

Differential Diagnosis

- **PCDLBCL-LT:** May be difficult to differentiate from diffuse pattern PCFCL as both show sheets of large B cells. However, PCDLBCL-L shows round cells instead of cleaved centrocytes. Cells may similarly be positive for follicular center cell markers (CD10 and Bcl-6) but are also positive for MUM1/IRF4 and Bcl-2, which helps distinguish it from PCFCL.
- **Reactive lymphoid hyperplasia (pseudolymphoma):** Composed of mixed inflammatory infiltrates with well-formed follicles showing polarization and tingible body macrophages

Key Points

- Indolent B-cell lymphoma confined to the skin with a predilection for the head and neck
- Displays follicular, diffuse, and mixed growth patterns that are important for diagnostic recognition but are not of diagnostic utility
- CD20$^+$, Bcl-6$^+$, CD10$^{+/-}$. Bcl-2 is typically negative or shows weak/focal positivity, and positive staining should prompt investigations for systemic lymphoma.

Diagnostic Caveats

- Accurate distinction between PCDLBCL and PCFCL is essential due to morphologic overlap and significant differences in treatment and prognosis.
- BCL2 may be a useful marker to differentiate between PCFCL (typically negative or weak/focal) and cutaneous involvement by systemic FCL (diffusely positive), but it should not be the sole criterion.

IV. EPSTEIN-BARR VIRUS–POSITIVE MUCOCUTANEOUS ULCER

Epstein-Barr virus–positive mucocutaneous ulcer (EBVMCU) is a fairly new entity described in older and immunosuppressed patients. The diagnostic criteria for EBVMCU are summarized in Table 19.10-4.

Clinical Features

- **Clinical presentation and sites of involvement**: Patients present with demarcated ulcers, typically involving the oral mucosa, although the skin or other mucosal site may be affected (*Exp Hematol Oncol.* 2015;5:13). Lesions may occur in patients over a broad age range, but the older patients are more affected, with a slight female predominance (*J Clin Exp Hematol.* 2019;59:64-71). There is a strong association with EBV infection, likely due to a lapse in immunosurveillance (*Am J Surg Pathol.* 2010;34:405-417), such as a reduction in the T-cell repertoire (*Blood.* 2011;117:4726-4735).

TABLE 19.10-4 Diagnostic Criteria for EBVMCU

Essential
- Clinical evidence or high suspicion of immune deficiency/dysregulation
- Involvement of cutaneous/mucosal sites
- Well-circumscribed ulcer with a polymorphous lymphoid infiltrate
- Atypical large cells positive for PAX5 and with variable expression of CD20 and CD30
- EBV infection (EBV+ in tissue)

Desirable
- CD3-positive T cells at the periphery

EBVMCU, Epstein-Barr virus–positive mucocutaneous ulcer.
Based on the WHO Classification of Tumours Editorial Board. Haematolymphoid tumours [Internet]. Lyon (France): International Agency for Research on Cancer; 2024 (WHO classification of tumours series, 5th ed.; vol. 11). Available from: https://tumourclassification.iarc.who.int/chapters/63.

Morphology

Beneath an ulcerated epidermis, there is a dense lymphoid infiltrate containing large atypical, Reed-Sternberg (RS)–like cells in a background of lymphocytes, plasma cells, histiocytes, and eosinophils (e-Figure 19.10-4A). Dispersed plasmacytoid apoptotic cells are frequent (*Am J Surg Pathol*. 2010;34:405-417). Necrosis may be present, and angioinvasion with associated thrombosis has been described in several cases.

Immunophenotype

The large RS-like cells stain positive for CD30 and Pax5. CD20 expression may be dim or reduced. CD15 expression is variable. Otherwise, the cells stain with a nongerminal center cell immunophenotype (IRF4/MUM1$^+$, CD10$^-$, BCL6$^-$). EBV is detected by in situ hybridization studies within the RS-like cells and within background lymphocytes (e-Figure 19.10-4B).

Genetic Features

Monoclonal IGH and T-cell receptor gene rearrangements are detected in a subset of cases (*Am J Surg Pathol*. 2010;34(3):405-417).

Prognosis and Treatment

The clinical course is typically benign, and treatment serves to heal symptomatic ulcer. Reduction of immunosuppression, when possible, may be curative. Otherwise, localized radiotherapy or rituximab may be used.

Differential Diagnosis

- **Polymorphic posttransplant lymphoproliferative disorder:** Usually no cutaneous ulceration present
- **EBV-positive DLBCL; not otherwise specified (NOS):** Will usually not present as an isolated cutaneous/mucosal lesion

> **Key Points**
>
> - Benign mucocutaneous B-cell proliferation with ulceration seen in the older and immunosuppressed individuals, associated with EBV infection
> - Presence of large RS-like cells in a dense background of lymphocytes, histiocytes, plasma cells, and eosinophils
> - PAX5$^+$, CD30$^+$, CD15$^{+/-}$, EBER$^+$, CD10$^-$, Bcl-6$^-$
>
> **Diagnostic Caveats**
>
> - Avoid confusion with EBV-positive DLBCL, NOS, due to significant difference in outcome and treatment. Clinical context is crucial.

SUGGESTED READINGS

Willemze R, Cerroni L, Kempf W, et al. The 2018 update of the WHO-EORTC classification for primary cutaneous lymphomas [published correction appears in *Blood*. 2019;134(13):1112]. *Blood.* 2019;133(16):1703-1714.

19.11 Plasma Cell Neoplasms and Other Diseases Associated With Paraproteins

Barina Aqil, Anjum Hassan, and David L. Jaye

Plasma cell neoplasms (PCNs) and a subset of mature B-lineage disorders produce intact monoclonal immunoglobulins, light chains, heavy chains, and class-switched immunoglobulins, collectively referred to as M-protein, paraprotein, or misfolded immunoglobulins. These conditions range from asymptomatic conditions such as monoclonal gammopathy of undetermined significance (MGUS) to symptomatic conditions such as plasma cell (multiple) myeloma (PCM/MM).

I. MONOCLONAL GAMMOPATHIES

Nonmalignant monoclonal gammopathies include conditions such as cold agglutinin disease (CAD), IgM monoclonal gammopathy of undetermined significance (IgM MGUS), non-IgM monoclonal gammopathy of undetermined significance (non-IgM MGUS), and monoclonal gammopathy of renal significance (MGRS).

i. Cold Agglutinin Disease

Idiopathic CAD is an autoimmune hemolytic anemia marked by clonal B-cell proliferation in the bone marrow (BM) and agglutination of red blood cells (RBC) at temperatures ranging from 0 to 4 °C, driven by monoclonal antibodies in the

TABLE 19.11-1   WHO-HAEM5 Diagnostic Criteria for CAD

Essential
- Chronic hemolysis
- Monospecific DAT strongly positive for C3d
- Cold agglutinin titer >64 at 4 °C
- No overt malignant disease or relevant infection
- Evidence of a clonal B-cell disorder

Desirable
- Monoclonal IgM-κ in plasma/serum (or, rarely, IgG or λ phenotype)
- Ratio between κ and λ positive B cells >3.5 (or, rarely, <0.9)
- Cold agglutinin–associated lymphoproliferative disorder by histopathology
- *MYD88* L265P mutation not found

CAD, cold agglutinin disease; DAT, direct antiglobulin test.
Based on the WHO Classification of Tumours Editorial Board. Haematolymphoid tumours [Internet]. Lyon (France): International Agency for Research on Cancer; 2024 (WHO classification of tumours series, 5th ed.; vol. 11). Available from: https://tumourclassification.iarc.who.int/chapters/63

absence of malignancies or infections. It accounts for about 15% of autoimmune hemolytic anemias (*Br Med J Clin Res Ed*. 1981;282(6281):2023-2027). These antibodies bind the I antigen on RBCs and activate the classical complement pathway, initiating extravascular hemolysis. The diagnostic criteria for CAD are summarized in Table 19.11-1.

Clinical Features

Patients show anemia and cold-induced circulatory symptoms, ranging from mild acrocyanosis to Raynaud phenomena. Monoclonal IgM is more common than IgG and IgA.

Morphology and Immunophenotype

The blood smear displays RBC agglutination (e-Figure 19.11-1). BM examination shows erythroid predominance with interstitial or aggregated small lymphoid cells, generally without increased plasma cells. The lymphocytes express pan B-cell markers (CD19, CD20, PAX5, CD79a, CD22, CD79b) and a monotypic surface light chain. Plasma cells express CD138, IgM, and a monotypic light chain.

Genetic Features

Somatic mutations in *KMT2D* and *CARD11* are frequently detected, while the *MYD88* L265P mutation is not found (*Br J Haematol*. 2018;183(5):838-842; *Haematologica*. 2014;99(3):497-504).

Prognosis and Treatment

Patients with mild anemia and mild symptoms can be observed. About 75% of patients receive therapy targeting the B-cell clone. Progression to lymphoma is rare (*Blood*. 2020;136(4):480-488).

Differential Diagnosis

- **Lymphoplasmacytic lymphoma (LPL):** LPL shows paratrabecular lymphoid aggregates, lymphoplasmacytoid morphology, and *MYD88* L265P mutation.

TABLE 19.11-2 WHO-HAEM5 Diagnostic Criteria for IgM MGUS

Diagnostic Criteria

- Serum IgM M-protein present but <3 g/dL
- BM minor lymphoplasmacytic infiltration <10%
- Lack of anemia, constitutional symptoms, hyperviscosity, lymphadenopathy, or hepatosplenomegaly that can be attributed to the underlying lymphoproliferation

---

BM, bone marrow; IgM MGUS, IgM monoclonal gammopathy of undetermined significance.
Based on the WHO Classification of Tumours Editorial Board. Haematolymphoid tumours [Internet]. Lyon (France): International Agency for Research on Cancer; 2024 (WHO classification of tumours series, 5th ed.; vol. 11). Available from: https://tumourclassification.iarc.who.int/chapters/63

- **Marginal zone lymphoma (MZL):** MZL often displays extramedullary disease with diffuse and/or intrasinusoidal infiltrates, typically in BM.

ii. IgM Monoclonal Gammopathy of Undetermined Significance

Patients with MGUS demonstrate paraproteinemia but do not meet the criteria for lymphoma, amyloidosis, or myeloma. IgM MGUS accounts for about 15% of patients with MGUS and 30% of patients with an IgM monoclonal protein (*Clin Cancer Res.* 2005;11:1786-1790). The diagnostic criteria for IgM MGUS are summarized in Table 19.11-2.

Clinical Features

Most patients are asymptomatic, with the diagnosis often made incidentally during evaluation for other conditions. They lack anemia, hyperviscosity, lymphadenopathy, and hepatosplenomegaly. Rarely, IgM MGUS may be associated with neuropathy, cryoglobulinemia, Raynaud phenomenon, vasculitis, or urticarial rash (*Mayo Clin Proc.* 2017;92(5):838-850; *Lancet.* 2012;379(9813):348-360). BM is typically involved.

Morphology and Immunophenotype

In BM, low-level to inconspicuous lymphoplasmacytic infiltrates account for less than 10% of the marrow cellularity. Typically, a clonal population of CD5-/CD10-negative B-cell and/or plasma cells expressing IgM with light chain restriction are detected.

Genetic Features

MYD88 L265P mutation is found in about 50% of patients (*Blood.* 2013;13(121):2522-2528).

Prognosis and Treatment

Asymptomatic patients are observed, with about 1.5% progressing annually to conditions such as LPL/Waldenström macroglobulinemia (WM), chronic lymphocytic leukemia/small lymphocytic lymphoma (CLL/SLL), smoldering multiple myeloma (SMM), PCM/MM, or amyloidosis (*Clin Lymphoma Myeloma Leuk.* 2011;11(1):74-76). Intravenous immunoglobulin G (IVIG) and rituximab have been used for neuropathy.

Differential Diagnosis
- **LPL/WM:** LPL has larger BM lymphoplasmacytic infiltrates and higher levels of IgM M-protein, B-cell and plasma cell clones, blood hyperviscosity, lymphadenopathy, and splenomegaly.
- **SMM:** In SMM, clonal plasma cells constitute 10% to 59% of marrow cellularity. IgM myeloma is exceptionally rare.
- **CLL/SLL, mantle cell lymphoma:** While the expression of CD5 may be seen in IgM MGUS, the expression of LEF1, BCL1, and SOX11 is not.

iii. Non-IgM Monoclonal Gammopathy of Undetermined Significance

Non-IgM MGUS represents about 85% of all MGUS cases. The majority of cases express IgG, followed by IgA, with IgE, IgD, or light chain–only cases being rare (*Lancet Oncol.* 2014;15(12):e538-e548). The risk of progression to MM is approximately 1% per year for MGUS, while light chain MGUS display 0.3% annual progression (*Br J Haematol.* 2006;134(6):573-589; *Lancet.* 2010;375(9727):1721-1728). Diagnostic criteria for non-IgM MGUS are summarized in Table 19.11-3.

Clinical Features
Most patients with MGUS lack symptoms, and the diagnosis is often incidental. Neither end-organ damage (anemia, hypercalcemia, renal injury, bone lesions) nor amyloid deposition are present. Serum M-protein levels are less than 3 g/dL, the free

TABLE 19.11-3 WHO-HAEM5 Diagnostic Criteria for Non-IgM MGUS and LC-MGUS

Diagnostic Criteria

Non-IgM MGUS	LC-MGUS
All three criteria must be met:	**All criteria must be met:**
• Serum M-protein (non-IgM type) <3 g/dL	• Abnormal FLC ratio (<0.26 or >1.65)
• Clonal BM plasma cells <10%	• Increased level of the appropriate involved light chain (increased κ FLC with ratio >1.65 or increased λ FLC with ratio <0.26)
• Absence of end-organ damage such as hypercalcemia, renal insufficiency, anemia, and bone lesions (CRAB) that can be attributed to the plasma cell proliferative disorder	• No immunoglobulin heavy chain detected on IFE
	• Absence of end-organ damage that can be attributed to the plasma cell proliferative disorder
	• Clonal BM plasma cells <10%
	• Urinary M-protein <500 mg/24 h

BM, bone marrow; FLC, free light chain; IFE, immunofixation electrophoresis; LC-MGUS, light chain monoclonal gammopathy of undetermined significance; non-IgM MGUS, non-IgM monoclonal gammopathy of undetermined significance.
Based on the WHO Classification of Tumours Editorial Board. Haematolymphoid tumours [Internet]. Lyon (France): International Agency for Research on Cancer; 2024 (WHO classification of tumours series, 5th ed.; vol. 11). Available from: https://tumourclassification.iarc.who.int/chapters/63

light chain ratio is less than 100:1, and fewer than two focal bone lesions are found on magnetic resonance imaging (MRI).

Morphology and Immunophenotype
Plasma cells comprise less than 10% of the marrow cellularity (e-Figure 19.11-2). Clonal plasma cells express CD38, CD138, CD45 (weak), and CD19 (negative in a subset).

Genetic Features
Chromosomal abnormalities typical of PCM/MM, such as t(11;14), t(4;14), t(14;16), and hyperdiploidy with trisomies of chromosomes 7, 9, 11, 15, and 19, can be identified.

Prognosis and Treatment
The risk of progression to PCM/MM increases with three factors: having a non-IgG paraprotein, M-protein levels greater than 1.5 g/dL, and an abnormal free light chain ratio. The 20-year risk of progression to PCM/MM is 58% when all three factors are present, 5% when none are present, and falls between these percentages when one and two factors are present (*Blood*. 2005;106(3):812-817). Most patients are observed. However, a subset may develop demyelinating neuropathy, with 80% of cases showing a positive response to IVIG, steroids, and/or plasmapheresis (*Lancet Neurol*. 2019;18(8):784-794).

Differential Diagnosis
- **SMM, PCM/MM:** See "Plasma Cell Neoplasms" section.
- **LPL/WM:** See "Differential Diagnosis" section for IgM MGUS.

iv. Monoclonal Gammopathy of Renal Significance
MGRS represents MGUS characterized by kidney injury due to M-protein toxic effects and autoantibody activity, with complement activation in a subset. The diagnostic criteria for PCM/MM or lymphoid malignancy are not met. MGRS includes glomerulopathies with immunoglobulin deposits, such as those with amyloid (light chain [AL], heavy chain [AH], and combined light and heavy chain [ALH] amyloidosis), microtubular disorders (cryoglobulinemias and immunotactoid glomerulopathy), and nonorganized deposits (monoclonal immunoglobulin deposition disease [MIDD]). Light chain cast nephropathy accompanies PCM/MM, precluding MGRS (*Blood*. 2013;122(22):3583-3590). Diagnostic criteria for MGRS are summarized in Table 19.11-4.

Clinical Features
Patients present with progressive decline in kidney function, along with symptoms such as hematuria, proteinuria, and/or proximal tubular dysfunction. Patients with amyloidosis, MIDD, or cryoglobulinemia often have extrarenal involvement, with congestive heart failure, liver failure, neuropathies, and skin rash/purpura (*N Engl J Med*. 2021;384(20):1931-1941).

Morphology, Immunophenotype, and Genetic Features
The findings are similar to other MGUS. Amyloid is demonstrable in a subset.

Prognosis and Treatment
Treatment is focused on preserving kidney function by targeting the B-cell or plasma cell clone producing the M-protein. Progression to end-stage renal disease occurs in the majority of cases (*Am J Kidney Dis*. 1992;20(1):34-41). MGRS often recurs after

TABLE 19.11-4 WHO-HAEM5 Diagnostic Criteria for MGRS

Essential	Desirable
• Kidney biopsy demonstrating injury as a result of an M-protein • Proteinuria >1 g/d composed mostly of albuminuria • Progressive acute or subacute kidney injury	• Lack of lytic bone lesions • No extramedullary plasmacytoma • No hypercalcemia secondary to bone lesions • No anemia with hemoglobin <10 g/dL • BM plasma cells <60% • Involved to uninvolved free light chain ratio <100 • No hyperviscosity • No bulky lymphadenopathy • No thrombocytopenia (<100 × 10^9/L)

BM, bone marrow; MGRS, monoclonal gammopathy of renal significance.
Based on the WHO Classification of Tumours Editorial Board. Haematolymphoid tumours [Internet]. Lyon (France): International Agency for Research on Cancer; 2024 (WHO classification of tumours series, 5th ed.; vol. 11). Available from: https://tumourclassification.iarc.who.int/chapters/63

renal transplant with allograft loss (*Kidney Int*. 2018;94(1):159-169); complete hematologic response enhances allograft survival.

Differential Diagnosis
- **PCM/MM, SMM:** These disorders display non-IgM serum monoclonal protein levels exceeding 3 g/dL and/or 10% or more BM clonal plasma cells. PCM/MM typically displays end-organ damage.
- **LPL/WM:** Refer to "IgM Monoclonal Gammopathy of Undetermined Significance" section.

II. DISEASES WITH MONOCLONAL IMMUNOGLOBULIN DEPOSITION

i. Immunoglobulin Light Chain Amyloidosis

Systemic light chain (AL) amyloidosis is a protein misfolding disorder characterized by deposition of abnormal immunoglobulin light chains in fibrillary aggregates (β-pleated sheet biochemical structure), causing end-organ damage. These abnormal light chains are produced by clonal plasma cells and rarely by clonal B cells (*Biochim Biophys Acta*. 2020;1753:11-22). Often more than one organ is involved at diagnosis. Early diagnosis and treatment targeting the M-protein producing clone are imperative to minimize organ damage. Diagnostic criteria for AL amyloidosis are summarized in Table 19.11-5.

Clinical Features
Depending on the site(s) of amyloid deposition, presenting symptoms are varied and nonspecific, including weight loss, edema, fatigue, macroglossia, periorbital purpura, peripheral neuropathy, and cardiac failure. Nearly 100% of patients have an elevated

TABLE 19.11-5 WHO-HAEM5 Diagnostic Criteria for AL Amyloidosis

Essential

- End-organ dysfunction related to amyloid by clinical examination, which is supported by abnormality on tests for organ function
- M-protein in serum or urine or abnormal serum free light chains
- Demonstration of amyloid deposition on tissue biopsy (abdominal fat or BM or salivary gland or affected organ biopsy) by Congo red (or similar thioflavin) stain or typical fibrils on electron microscopy

Desirable

- Typing of amyloid fibril protein by laser capture followed by mass spectrometry or immunohistochemistry/ immunoelectron microscopy
- Confirmation of organ involvement by imaging (echocardiography or cardiac magnetic resonance imaging for the heart)
- Mutation of one or more genes associated with hereditary amyloidosis (especially when typing by mass spectrometry unavailable or inconclusive)

Based on the WHO Classification of Tumours Editorial Board. Haematolymphoid tumours [Internet]. Lyon (France): International Agency for Research on Cancer; 2024 (WHO classification of tumours series, 5th ed.; vol. 11). Available from: https://tumourclassification.iarc.who.int/chapters/63

serum free light chain (FLC) ratio. The kidney, heart, gastrointestinal (GI) tract, liver, and nervous system are typically involved.

Morphology

Amyloid deposits appear as pink amorphous material in the blood vessel walls, basement membranes, and tissue interstitia. These deposits are observed in up to 60% of BM biopsy cores (*Am J Clin Pathol.* 2003;120(4):610-616), sometimes with adjacent foreign body giant cell reaction and increased plasma cells. BM biopsy findings vary from no pathology to PCNs (MGUS, PCM/MM), and rarely LPL. Congo red stains AL amyloid orange/pink, yielding apple-green birefringence upon polarization (e-Figure 19.11-3).

Immunophenotype

Clonal plasma cells are identified by techniques such as immunohistochemistry (IHC), in situ hybridization, and/or flow cytometry (FC). Aberrant expression of CD56 and CD117 is common. Lambda light chain restriction is observed in over 80% of cases (*Am J Clin Pathol.* 2003;120(4):610-616). Mass spectrometry can be employed to confirm AL amyloidosis and differentiate it from secondary amyloidoses.

Genetic Features

There are no specific molecular tests for AL amyloidosis. Testing for mutations associated with familial forms of non-AL types of amyloidosis can be considered.

Prognosis and Treatment

Multiple factors and biomarkers at diagnosis portend adverse prognosis, including marrow plasmacytosis, increased FLCs, presence of t(11;14), 1q+, del(17p), trisomies, and biomarkers such as NT-proBNP, eGFR, albumin, uric acid, and proteinuria (*Acta*

Haematol. 2020;143:388-399). Cardiac involvement severity is the major determinant of morbidity and mortality (*Br J Haematol.* 2019;185(4):701-707). Survival improves with early diagnosis and plasma and/or B-cell–targeted therapy (*Blood Cancer J.* 2021;11(5):97).

Differential Diagnosis

- **Secondary amyloidosis:** These encompass over 35 subtypes that vary in their ability to stain with Congo red, systemic versus localized forms, and hereditary versus acquired forms. More common subtypes include transthyretin-associated (ATTR) and serum amyloid A–associated (AA) amyloidosis. Mass spectroscopy of deposits identifies specific abnormal amyloidogenic proteins, differentiating among primary AL and many secondary forms.
- **MIDD:** The presence of M-protein, clonal plasma cells, and monotypic light chains with abnormal tissue deposits are identified, although Congo red stain is negative.
- **MGUS, PCM/MM, LPL:** Refer to the specific sections for these topics.

ii. Monoclonal Immunoglobulin Deposition Disease

MIDDs are rare disorders characterized by nonorganized deposits of intact or fragmented immunoglobulins that lead to organ damage. These deposits lack β-pleated sheets and fibrillary structure of AL amyloidosis. The abnormal immunoglobulin is produced by a neoplasm of plasma cells or, rarely, by B cells (CLL, LPL). The diagnostic criteria for MIDD are summarized in Table 19.11-6.

MIDDs are subdivided based on the content of immunoglobulin chains. Light chain deposition disease (LCDD), about 80% of cases, has light chain–only deposits, mostly being κ light chain. Heavy chain deposition disease (HCDD), about 10% of cases, has heavy chain–only deposits, typically formed of truncated γ chain. Light and heavy chain deposition disease (LHCDD), about 10% of cases, has light and heavy chain deposits.

TABLE 19.11-6   WHO-HAEM5 Diagnostic Criteria for MIDD

Essential

- Demonstration of monoclonal immunoglobulin deposition in tissue
  - In the kidney, this should be demonstrated by immunohistochemistry and electron microscopy.
  - In cases where there is coexistence of light chain cast nephropathy, MIDD may be demonstrated by immunohistochemistry only.
  - Diagnosis in other tissues relies on immunohistochemistry, as electron microscopy is not commonly used. Besides light chain cast nephropathy, AL amyloidosis and light chain proximal tubulopathy have been found to coexist with MIDD in the same kidney.

MIDD, monoclonal immunoglobulin deposition disease.
Based on the WHO Classification of Tumours Editorial Board. Haematolymphoid tumours [Internet]. Lyon (France): International Agency for Research on Cancer; 2024 (WHO classification of tumours series, 5th ed.; vol. 11). Available from: https://tumourclassification.iarc.who.int/chapters/63

Clinical Features

MIDDs are rare systemic disorders with variable findings related to deposition sites, including renal disease, cardiomyopathy, hepatomegaly, and peripheral neuropathy (*Blood.* 2019;133(6):576-587). The kidneys, heart, liver, peripheral nerves, salivary glands, GI tract, and skin can all be involved.

Morphology and Immunophenotype

Deposits in MIDD accumulate in renal tubular and glomerular basement membranes, vessel walls, interstitium, endocardium, and epicardium. These eosinophilic deposits stain positively with periodic acid-Schiff, trichrome, and silver stains but are negative for Congo red. Deposits show distinctive findings on immunofluorescence during renal biopsy. MIDD sometimes coexist with light chain cast nephropathy, in which distal tubules have geometric, PAS-negative, fractured casts that stain for pathogenic light chain (*J Am Soc Nephrol.* 2001;12:1482-1492). B-cell and/or plasma cell markers, with light chain restriction, are detected depending on the specific neoplastic process.

Genetic Features

There are no specific genetic abnormalities.

Prognosis and Treatment

Similar to AL amyloidosis, the prognoses of MIDDs vary considerably depending on the extent of organ involvement, patient age, presence of renal insufficiency, and the type of underlying hematologic disorder (*Am J Kidney Dis.* 2003;42(6):1154-1163). Treatment may include chemotherapy, immunotherapy, and stem cell transplant, targeting the specific B-cell or plasma cell clonal process with the goal of preserving function of involved organs (*Blood Adv.* 2020;4(7):1321-1324).

Differential Diagnosis

- **AL amyloidosis:** Unlike MIDDs, Congo red and thioflavin-T is positive in deposits, and electron microscopy demonstrates a fibrillar structure.
- **Nodular glomerulosclerosis:** In MIDD, glomeruli characteristically show nodule formation (nodular glomerulosclerosis), which can also be observed in diabetes, systemic lupus erythematosus (SLE), and chronic thrombotic microangiopathy. However, kidney electron microscopy and immunofluorescence findings in MIDD are distinctive.

III. HEAVY CHAIN DISEASES

HCDs are a group of clinically and morphologically distinct B-cell neoplasms that produce an abnormal immunoglobulin heavy chain incapable of binding light chain. Heavy chain abnormalities result from a variety of genetic mutations acquired during somatic hypermutation that most often lead to loss of a large portion of the heavy chain constant-1 domain (*Hematol Oncol Clin North Am.* 1999;13:1281-1294). Altered clonal heavy chains without light chains are in serum and/or urine. Detection generally requires immunofixation electrophoresis (IFE) (*Oncology.* 2014;28:45-53). Defective μ, α, and γ heavy chain forms display distinct clinicopathologies.

i. Mu Heavy chain disease

Mu heavy chain disease (MHCD) is very rare and the least common HCD. Most patients have a lymphoid neoplasm resembling CLL/SLL (*Am J Hematol*. 1992;40:56-60). IFE shows anti-mu reactivity with polymers of diverse sizes, without associated light chains. Diagnostic criteria for MHCD are summarized in Table 19.11-7.

Clinical Features

Hepatomegaly, splenomegaly, and lymphadenopathy are common at presentation. MHCD has been associated with SLE, recurrent pulmonary infections, portal hypertension, pancytopenia, myelodysplastic syndrome, and amyloid arthropathy (*Ann Hematol*. 1998;77:231-234; *Hematology*. 2004;9:135-137). Lytic bone lesions occur in a minority of cases.

Morphology and Immunophenotype

Infiltrated tissues usually show small, round lymphoid cells resembling those seen in CLL/SLL, along with atypical plasma cells with cytoplasmic vacuoles. Neoplastic cells express cytoplasmic IgM but lack light chain staining by IHC. FC demonstrates CD19, CD20, and CD38 expression, with minimal or no light chain detected (*Int J Hematol*. 2006;84:286-287).

Genetic Features

Clonal *IG* gene rearrangements may be detected in MHCD. Recurrent genetic mutations have not been described.

Prognosis and Treatment

The prognosis and optimal treatment are uncertain. Asymptomatic patients with low-level M-protein have been observed, whereas symptomatic patients have received chemotherapy. Variable survival is reported (*Curr Treat Options Oncol*. 2002;3:247-254).

Differential Diagnosis

- **CLL/SLL:** Differentiation can be challenging. CLL/SLL generally would not include vacuolated plasma cells, whereas monoclonal proteins on IFE are noted.
- **LPL:** Lymphoplasmacytic cells stain for cytoplasmic heavy and light chains.

TABLE 19.11-7 WHO-HAEM5 Diagnostic Criteria for MHCD

Essential	Desirable
• Anti-mu reactivity seen on IFE without associated light chain • BM or tissue involvement by small, round lymphocytes and vacuolated plasma cells	• Frequent κ Bence-Jones proteinuria; B cells with cytoplasmic IgM staining that are negative for light chains

IFE, immunofixation electrophoresis; MHCD, mu heavy chain disease.
Based on the WHO Classification of Tumours Editorial Board. Haematolymphoid tumours [Internet]. Lyon (France): International Agency for Research on Cancer; 2024 (WHO classification of tumours series, 5th ed.; vol. 11). Available from: https://tumourclassification.iarc.who.int/chapters/63

- **MGUS, PCM/MM:** Monoclonal peaks are detected on serum protein electrophoresis (SPEP), and IFE shows complete immunoglobulins rather than solely heavy chains.

ii. Gamma Heavy Chain Disease

Gamma heavy chain disease (GHCD) displays a female predominance, with the median age of presentation in the sixties (*Am J Med.* 1964;37:332-350). The detection of a clonal γ heavy chain in serum and/or urine, without associated light chains, is a hallmark feature. Associations with various autoimmune diseases have been reported. Diagnostic criteria for GHCD are summarized in Table 19.11-8.

Clinical Features

GHCD has diverse clinical presentations grouped into three categories. The first category is disseminated lymphoproliferative disease, which is seen in most patients. These patients usually present with B symptoms, anemia, lymphadenopathy, splenomegaly, and hepatomegaly. The second category is localized lymphoproliferative disease, which is observed in a subset of patients who have BM involvement or limited extranodal disease. The third category comprise patients without identified lymphoproliferative disease but with underlying autoimmune conditions (*Best Pract Res Clin Haematol.* 2005;18:729-746; *Medicine (Baltimore).* 2003;82:236-250). Common sites of involvement include lymph nodes (LNs), BM, and extranodal sites such as the skin, thyroid, and parotid gland.

Morphology

There is no specific associated morphology for GCHD, with cases displaying diverse findings reminiscent of any of a spectrum of known lymphoid malignancies (eg, MZL, CLL/SLL, DLBCL, Hodgkin lymphoma) to reactive infiltrates, often with plasmacytoid differentiation. Described patterns include pleomorphic lymphoplasmacytic infiltrates with immunoblasts, eosinophils, and histiocytes, as well as plasma cell infiltrates and small lymphoid proliferations. Rarely, Reed-Sternberg (RS)–like cells are found. MZL-like patterns are described at extranodal sites (*Medicine (Baltimore).* 2003;82:236-250; *Am J Surg Pathol.* 2012;36:534-543).

Immunophenotype

GHCD lacks demonstrable light chains but are positive for γ heavy chain by immunostaining. Immunophenotypes vary, but lymphoid cells commonly express CD19

TABLE 19.11-8 WHO-HAEM5 Diagnostic Criteria for GHCD

Essential	Desirable
• Serum or urine IFE demonstrates γ monoclonal band without associated light chain, which may be the only manifestation in patients with autoimmune disease	• FNA or tissue biopsy demonstrating atypical lymphoplasmacytic proliferation expressing IgG without light chains

GHCD, gamma heavy chain disease; IFE, immunofixation electrophoresis.
Based on the WHO Classification of Tumours Editorial Board. Haematolymphoid tumours [Internet]. Lyon (France): International Agency for Research on Cancer; 2024 (WHO classification of tumours series, 5th ed.; vol. 11). Available from: https://tumourclassification.iarc.who.int/chapters/63

and CD20, while being negative for CD5 and CD10. In addition, MUM1, CD38, and CD138 can be found with plasmacytic differentiation.

Genetic Features

Cases test negative for the *MYD88* L265P mutation (*Haematologica*. 2014;99(9): e154-e155) and recurrent somatic mutations. However, clonal *IG* gene rearrangements can be detected.

Prognosis and Treatment

The clinical behavior of GHCD varies from indolent to rapidly progressive. Patients with no lymphoproliferation have prolonged survival, while those with disseminated lymphoma display a poorer prognosis. Median survival is reported at 7 years (*Medicine (Baltimore)*. 2003;82:236-250). Treatments are based on underlying clinicopathologic features and may include observation, chemoimmunotherapy, surgery, and/or radiation. Autoimmune diseases are treated according to usual guidelines (*Acta Haematol.* 2012;128:139-143).

Differential Diagnosis

- **Infection, inflammation:** GHCD is commonly associated with autoimmunity and abnormal plasma cells devoid of light chains. Infectious agents should be excluded.
- **MGUS:** Cases with no lymphoplasmacytic proliferation may mimic MGUS. IFE shows clonal γ heavy chain without light chains.
- **PCM/MM, MZL, LPL:** These conditions are considered when monomorphic lymphoid or plasmacytoid infiltrates are present. Staining for light chains and testing for *MYD88* mutation can help in differentiation.
- **Hodgkin lymphoma, T-cell lymphoma:** While polymorphous background cells and RS-like cells are rare in GHCD, GCHD cells display B-cell markers CD20, Pax5, OCT2, and BOB1, with variable CD30 expression and negativity for CD15, distinguishing them from classic Hodgkin lymphoma. In rare cases, GHCD may show vascular proliferation with prominent eosinophils, mimicking features of angioimmunoblastic T-cell lymphoma.

iii. Alpha Heavy Chain Disease

Alpha heavy chain disease (AHCD), the most common form of HCD, primarily affects individuals of Mediterranean, Northern African, and Middle Eastern descent, particularly males in their second to third decades of life. A defective truncated α heavy chains without light chains is characteristic. An association between immunoproliferative small intestinal disease (IPSID), an MZL-like lymphoma generally found in AHCD, and *Campylobacter jejuni* and parasitic infections is recognized (*Curr Gastroenterol Rep*. 2018;20(1):3). Diagnostic criteria for AHCD are summarized in Table 19.11-9.

Clinical Features

GI and nonspecific symptoms are most common in AHCD, including nausea, vomiting, diarrhea, weight loss, fever, and growth retardation, often associated with profound malabsorption (*Pathol Res Pract*. 1988;183:717-723; *Blood*. 2005;105:2274-2280). The small intestine is frequently affected, with the duodenum being affected more frequently than the jejunum and ileum. However, overall involvement can be extensive. Rarely, other sites such as the stomach, colon, respiratory tract, spleen, BM, LNs outside GI tract, and thyroid may also be affected.

TABLE 19.11-9 WHO-HAEM5 Diagnostic Criteria for AHCD

Essential	Desirable
• Tissue biopsy with features of extra-nodal MZL with extensive plasmacytic differentiation expressing IgA without light chains	• Serum IFE demonstrating anti-alpha reactivity without associated light chain

AHCD, alpha heavy chain disease; IFE, immunofixation electrophoresis, MZL, marginal zone lymphoma.
Based on the WHO Classification of Tumours Editorial Board. Haematolymphoid tumours [Internet]. Lyon (France): International Agency for Research on Cancer; 2024 (WHO classification of tumours series, 5th ed.; vol. 11). Available from: https://tumourclassification.iarc.who.int/chapters/63

Morphology

Lymphoproliferations associated with IPSID/AHCD have a range of features ranging from MALT-type MZL characteristics, including lymphoepithelial lesions and plasmacytoid differentiation, to large B-cell lymphoma. A three-tier morphologic staging system has prognostic and therapeutic implications (*Cancer.* 1977;39:2081-2101).

- **Stage A:**
  Small intestine: Plasmacytic or lymphoplasmacytic infiltrate in the lamina propria with or without villous broadening and atrophy
  LN: Preserved architecture with plasmacytic infiltrate
- **Stage B:**
  Small intestine: Atypical lymphoplasmacytic infiltrate or cells with a more immunoblastic appearance extending beyond the lamina propria into the submucosa, with subtotal or total villous atrophy
  LN: Atypical plasmacytic infiltrate with immunoblast-like cells, leading to subtotal or total effacement of nodal architecture
- **Stage C:**
  Small intestine: Extension through muscularis propria
  LN: Complete effacement of LN architecture by lymphoma

Immunophenotype

Neoplastic B cells are negative for CD5 and CD10, while the plasma cells are positive for CD38 and CD138. The lymphoplasmacytic infiltrates express α heavy chain without associated light chains.

Genetic Features

Clonal *IG* gene rearrangements are detected. While IPSID/AHCD lacks the t(11;18) translocation seen in typical MZL, translocations involving heavy and light chain gene loci have been reported.

Prognosis and Treatment

The prognosis of IPSID/AHCD depends on complications arising from bowel involvement, infection, and malnutrition. Chemotherapy, radiotherapy, and autologous stem cell transplantation have been employed (*Cancer.* 1997;80:8-14; *Cancer.*

2005;11:374-382). Remission postchemotherapy in a majority results in a reported 5-year overall survival rate of 67% (*Am J Gastroenterol.* 1999;94:1139-1152).

Differential Diagnosis

- **MZL, MALT type:** Knowledge of clinical and demographic data associated with IPSID/AHCD is helpful. Infiltrates tend to be more extensive than MZL in intestine and immunostains show α heavy chain without light chains in the plasmacytoid component.
- **Chronic inflammation, celiac sprue:** Differentiation can be difficult on small biopsies. Celiac sprue has more extensive villous atrophy, intraepithelial T cells, and eventuates in T-cell lymphoma more typically.

IV. PLASMA CELL NEOPLASMS

PCNs result from the expansion of neoplastic, terminally differentiated B cells that generally produce M-proteins. PCM/MM, the most common PCN, comprises about 1% of all malignancies and 10% to 15% of hematolymphoid neoplasms. Most patients with PCN are over 50 years old, with a median age of 66 years at diagnosis. Male sex and African ancestry confer increased disease risk.

i. Plasmacytoma

Plasmacytoma is a type of PCN characterized by a localized medullary or extramedullary plasma cell mass. Several subtypes of plasmacytoma are recognized (*Br J Haematol.* 2003;121(5):749-757). Solitary plasmacytoma (SP) includes solitary plasmacytoma of bone (SPB) and extramedullary plasmacytoma (EMP), each comprising about 4% of all PCN cases. SPB is subdivided based on clonal plasma cell content on random BM biopsy into a form with minimal (<10%) and one with no involvement (*Cancer.* 2018;9(21):3894-3897). The risk factors for EMP include chemical exposure, radiation, and viral infection. Multiple plasmacytoma (MP) is less common. Diagnostic criteria for plasmacytoma are summarized in Table 19.11-10.

TABLE 19.11-10 WHO-HAEM5 Diagnostic Criteria for Plasmacytoma

Essential

- Biopsy-proven clonal PCN of bone or extramedullary site
- No clonal B cells
- No other lesions on physical examination or imaging studies
- No end-organ damage (CRAB): hypercalcemia, renal insufficiency, anemia, or bone lesions due to PCN
- <10% clonal plasma cells on nontargeted BM sampling. Plasmacytomas with no BM involvement must be distinguished from those with minimal (<10%) BM involvement.

BM, bone marrow; PCN, plasma cell neoplasm.
Based on the WHO Classification of Tumours Editorial Board. Haematolymphoid tumours [Internet]. Lyon (France): International Agency for Research on Cancer; 2024 (WHO classification of tumours series, 5th ed.; vol. 11). Available from: https://tumourclassification.iarc.who.int/chapters/63

Clinical Features

- **Clinical presentation:** SPB symptoms correlate with the anatomic location of the tumor. Patients present with pain, swelling, fractures, and spinal cord compression, and present with uncommon symptoms such as headaches, strabismus, dizziness, and otalgia with skull-based disease (*Otol Neurotol.* 2017;38(3):400-407). In contrast, EMP presents with respiratory and digestive symptoms, including nasal discharge, dysphagia, sore throat, epistaxis, hoarseness, dyspnea, and hemoptysis. Rarely, patients may display paraneoplastic syndromes such as POEMS, TEMPI, and AESCOP, which are discussed later.
- **Sites of involvement:** Axial skeleton (spine, pelvis, ribs, skull and long bones) is the most commonly involved. EMP occurs more frequently in the upper respiratory tract and less commonly in the digestive system (oral cavity, tonsillar fossa), lungs, LNs, and skin.

Morphology

Affected sites display sheets of plasma cells, with cytologies ranging from normal-appearing to atypical forms with plasmablastic or anaplastic features (e-Figure 19.11-4).

Immunophenotype

Plasma cells express CD138 and CD38, with subsets positive for of CD56, CD117, and cyclin D1. The most commonly expressed isotype is IgG, followed by IgA. Epstein-Barr virus (EBV) is generally negative.

Genetic Features

Clonal *IG* gene rearrangements and cytogenetic abnormalities similar to those observed in PCM/MM are found.

Prognosis and Treatment

Increased age, tumor size, presence of plasmablastic/anaplastic cytology, bone-based disease, regional LN involvement, and higher serum M-protein levels are adverse prognosticators (*Sci World J.* 2012;2012:895765). Spontaneous bacterial peritonitis (SBP) demonstrates a poorer prognosis compared to EMP, with increased progression to PCM/MM within a median of 2 to 3 years. Radiotherapy is administered for SPB and EMP. In some cases, surgical resection can facilitate diagnosis and provide symptomatic relief.

Differential Diagnosis

- **B-cell lymphomas with extensive plasmacytic differentiation (MZL, LPL):** MZL and LPL show a B-cell lymphoid component with plasma cells that usually express CD19, without CD56 and CD117.
- **PCM/MM:** A systemic disease generally containing over 10% plasma cells on BM biopsy.
- **Plasmablastic lymphoma (PL):** PL shows plasmablastic morphology, is more common with immune dysregulation, and is typically EBV-positive.
- **Neuroendocrine neoplasm:** Morphology and expression of CD138 and CD56 can mimic PCN, but, in contrast, expresses pancytokeratin, synaptophysin, and chromogranin.

> **Key Points**
> - SP and multiple solitary plasmacytoma (MSP) are the two types of plasmacytomas, most common to the head and neck.
> - SP consists of SBP and EMP, with SBP having a poor prognosis.
>
> **Diagnostic Caveats**
> - Differentiation from MZL with extensive plasmacytoid differentiation is challenging.
> - EBV is typically negative in plasmacytoma with rare exceptions.

ii. Plasma Cell Myeloma/Multiple Myeloma (PCM/MM)

PCM/MM is a systemic PCN involving multiple sites in the BM and generally produces an intact or fragmented M-protein. A small subset, about 3%, are nonsecretory, wherein no serum M-protein is detected. Plasma cell leukemia (PCL) represents aggressive disease in cases where 5% or more plasma cells are observed on the blood smear in patients otherwise diagnosed with PCM/MM. SMM serves as an asymptomatic precursor to PCM/MM, characterized by plasma cells comprising 10% to 59% on BM biopsy, and neither end-organ damage nor other PCM/MM-defining events are demonstrable. Diagnostic criteria incorporate clinical, radiographic, laboratory, and pathologic findings (*Lancet Oncol.* 2014;15(12):e538-e548). The diagnostic criteria for PCM/MM are summarized in Tables 19.11-11 and 19.11-12.

The International Consensus Classification (ICC) classifies MM into two groups on the basis of cytogenetic features: MM, NOS (not otherwise specified) and MM with recurrent genetic abnormalities. The latter group includes various genetic subtypes, including MM with *CCND* family translocation, MM with *MAF* family translocation, MM with *NSD2* translocation, and MM with hyperdiploidy. These genetic abnormalities hold therapeutic and prognostic significance and may also be associated with distinct phenotypic features.

Clinical Features

- **Clinical presentation:** Patients with PCM/MM display signs and symptoms (fatigue, pallor, bleeding, and susceptibility to infections) largely due to the impact of disease on BM function and the effects of the M-protein on other organs. Findings demonstrative of "symptomatic" disease and indicative of end-organ damage

TABLE 19.11-11 WHO-HAEM5 Diagnostic Criteria for SMM

Diagnostic Criteria

- Serum monoclonal protein (IgG or IgA) ≥3 g/dL or urinary monoclonal protein ≥500 mg/24 h and/or clonal BM plasma cells 10%-59%
- Absence of myeloma-defining events or amyloidosis

BM, bone marrow; SMM, smoldering multiple myeloma.
Based on the WHO Classification of Tumours Editorial Board. Haematolymphoid tumours [Internet]. Lyon (France): International Agency for Research on Cancer; 2024 (WHO classification of tumours series, 5th ed.; vol. 11). Available from: https://tumourclassification.iarc.who.int/chapters/63

TABLE 19.11-12 WHO-HAEM5 Diagnostic Criteria for PCM/MM

Diagnostic Criteria

- Clonal BM plasma cells ≥10% or biopsy-proven bony or extramedullary plasmacytoma
- And, any one or more of the following myeloma-defining events:
  - Evidence of end-organ damage that can be attributed to the underlying plasma cell proliferative disorder, specifically:
    - Hypercalcemia: Serum calcium >0.25 mmol/L (>1 mg/dL) higher than the upper limit of normal or >2.75 mmol/L (>11 mg/dL)
    - Renal insufficiency: Creatinine clearance <40 mL/min or serum creatinine >177 µmol/L (>2 mg/dL)
    - Anemia: Hemoglobin value of >2 g/dL below the lower limit of normal or a hemoglobin value <10 g/dL
    - Bone lesions: One or more osteolytic lesions on skeletal radiography, CT, or PET-CT
  - Clonal BM plasma cell percentage ≥60%
  - Involved: Uninvolved serum FLC ratio ≥100 (involved free light chain level must be ≥100 mg/L)
  - >One focal lesions on MRI studies (≥5 mm)

BM, bone marrow; CT, computed tomography; FLC, free light chain; MRI, magnetic resonance imaging; PCM/MM, plasma cell (multiple) myeloma; PET, positron emission tomography.
Based on the WHO Classification of Tumours Editorial Board. Haematolymphoid tumours [Internet]. Lyon (France): International Agency for Research on Cancer; 2024 (WHO classification of tumours series, 5th ed.; vol. 11). Available from: https://tumourclassification.iarc.who.int/chapters/63

meet the "CRAB" criteria, which include hyper**c**alcemia, **r**enal insufficiency, **a**nemia, and lytic **b**one lesions. Additionally, extramedullary disease may present as lymphadenopathy, hepatomegaly, and splenomegaly.
- **Sites of involvement:** Bone, BM, and less commonly blood and various extramedullary sites including soft tissues

Morphology

Plasma cell cytomorphology in PCM/MM varies from unremarkable to plasmablastic/anaplastic (e-Figures 19.11-5 and 19.11-6). A subset of cases demonstrate rouleaux formation, leukoerythroblastosis, and/or plasma cells on blood smear (e-Figures 19.11-7 and 19.11-8). BM shows greater than 10% clonal plasma cells, sometimes with amyloid. Light chain casts are seen in kidney tubules in some patients.

Immunophenotype

Light chain–restricted plasma cells express CD38 and CD138, and may occasionally show aberrant expression of CD20, CD56, and/or CD117. However, they are often negative for CD19 and CD45.

Genetic Features

Recurrent chromosomal abnormalities detected by fluorescence in situ hybridization (FISH) and karyotyping in PCM/MM include t(11;14), t(4;14), t(14;16), and hyperdiploidy with multiple trisomies of odd-numbered chromosomes, including 7, 9, 11, 15, and 19. Recurrent secondary genetic changes are more common in PCM/MM than in SMM and include 1q+, del(13q)/monosomy 13, del(17p), and del(1p). Recurrent mutations of *KRAS*, *NRAS*, *TP53*, and *MYC*, among others, have also been described (*Blood*. 2005;106(1):296-230; *Nat Commun*. 2021;12(1):293).

Prognosis and Treatment

Prognostic factors for PCM/MM include disease stage, genetics, age, performance status, co-morbidities, and response to therapy. The revised international staging system (R-ISS) employs serum β_2-microglobulin, albumin, LDH levels, and genetic risk to predict survival (*J Clin Oncol*. 2015;33(26):2863-2869). High-risk genetic abnormalities by FISH include t(4;14), t(14;16), del(17p), and 1q+. Biallelic *TP53* mutation/loss is associated with poor outcome. Available treatments for PCM/MM include chemotherapy, immunotherapies, immunomodulatory drugs, radiation therapy, and autologous stem cell transplant. However, PCM/MM is an incurable disease marked by eventual relapses. Therapy depends on prognostic and risk stratification and may vary with disease recurrence.

Differential Diagnosis

- **Amyloidosis, MGUS, LCDD, plasmacytoma, LPL, MZL:** Refer to separate sections covering these disorders.

iii. Plasma Cell Neoplasms with Associated Paraneoplastic Syndrome

PCNs can manifest as three rare paraneoplastic syndromes with poorly understood etiologies: POEMS syndrome (**p**olyneuropathy, **o**rganomegaly, **e**ndocrinopathy, **m**onoclonal gammopathy, **s**kin changes), TEMPI syndrome (**t**elangiectasia, **e**levated erythropoietin and erythrocytosis, **m**onoclonal gammopathy, **p**erinephric fluid collection, **i**ntrapulmonary shunting), and AESOP syndrome (**a**denopathy and **e**xtensive **s**kin patch **o**verlying **p**lasmacytoma). POEMS and AESOP syndromes appear to result from imbalanced proinflammatory cytokines (*Lancet*. 1996;347(9002):702). The pathogenesis of TEMPI syndrome remains unclear. Diagnostic criteria for TEMPI are summarized in Tables 19.11-13 and 19.11-14.

Key Points

- Diagnostic criteria for PCM/MM and SMM incorporate clinical, radiographic, laboratory, and pathology data.
- t(4;14), t(14;16), del(17p), and 1q+ FISH abnormalities portend poor prognosis.

Diagnostic Caveats

- Differential diagnosis among PCM/MM, SMM, and MGUS includes morphologic assessment of plasma cell percentages in BM, which can show interobserver variation introducing possible diagnostic error.

TABLE 19.11-13 WHO-HAEM5 Diagnostic Criteria for POEMS Syndrome

Mandatory Major Criteria	Major Criteria	Minor Criteria
- Polyneuropathy (typically demyelinating) - Monoclonal plasma cell proliferative disorder (almost always λ)	- Castleman disease - Sclerotic bone lesions - VEGF elevation	- Organomegaly (splenomegaly, hepatomegaly, or lymphadenopathy) - Extravascular volume overload (edema, pleural effusion, or ascites) - Endocrinopathy (adrenal, thyroid, pituitary, gonadal, parathyroid, pancreatic) - Skin changes - Papilledema - Thrombocytosis/polycythemia

VEGF, vascular endothelial growth factor.
The diagnosis requires one major and one or more minor criteria in addition to the two mandatory criteria.
Based on the WHO Classification of Tumours Editorial Board. Haematolymphoid tumours [Internet]. Lyon (France): International Agency for Research on Cancer; 2024 (WHO classification of tumours series, 5th ed.; vol. 11). Available from: https://tumourclassification.iarc.who.int/chapters/63

Clinical Features

- **Clinical presentation:**
  POEMS syndrome: Polyneuropathy is the dominant feature. Peripheral edema, papilledema, ascites, and effusions are reported. Organomegaly involves the liver, spleen, and LNs. Diabetes mellitus and hypothyroidism are the common endocrine abnormalities. Skin changes include hyperpigmentation, acrocyanosis, hypertrichosis, and plethora (*Blood*. 2003;101(7):2496-2506).
  TEMPI syndrome: Telangiectasias are seen on the upper body, with frequent involvement of the hands but sparing the lower extremities. Patients show monoclonal gammopathy without heavy or light chain specificity. Vascular endothelial growth factor (VEGF) levels are not elevated. Elevated erythropoietin levels and erythrocytosis, in the absence of *JAK2* mutations, precede the development of intrapulmonary shunting and perinephric fluid collections.

TABLE 19.11-14 WHO-HAEM5 Diagnostic Criteria for TEMPI Syndrome

Major Criteria	Minor Criteria	Other
- Telangiectasias - Elevated erythropoietin and erythrocytosis - Monoclonal gammopathy (IgG κ)	- Perinephric fluid - Intrapulmonary shunting	- Venous thrombosis

The diagnosis requires fulfillment of all the major and one or more minor criteria.
Based on the WHO Classification of Tumours Editorial Board. Haematolymphoid tumours [Internet]. Lyon (France): International Agency for Research on Cancer; 2024 (WHO classification of tumours series, 5th ed.; vol. 11). Available from: https://tumourclassification.iarc.who.int/chapters/63

AESOP syndrome: It is associated with SP. This syndrome presents with violaceous skin patches with visible vessels present on the thorax. Polyneuropathy and lymphadenopathy may develop after the appearance of skin lesions.
- **Sites of involvement:** PCNs involve the BM in POEMS. SBP and overlying skin patches are noted in AESOP syndrome.

Morphology

Clonal marrow plasma cells in POEMS syndrome display λ light chain restriction and comprise less than 5% of the total marrow cellularity. Some patients have SP or MP with no BM disease. Reactive lymphoid aggregates are rimmed by plasma cells (*Blood.* 2011;117(24):6438-6444). Approximately 15% of patients have HHV8-negative multicentric Castleman disease or Castleman-like changes. In TEMPI syndrome, BM examination shows mildly increased plasma cells (5%-10%) (*Mod Pathol.* 2015;28(3):367-372). Erythrocytosis may prompt an evaluation for polycythemia vera, but BM findings do not support this diagnosis, showing erythroid hyperplasia without megakaryocyte clusters or fibrosis. Skin findings are nonspecific and may include increased mucin deposition and dermal vascular proliferation. LN histology shows lymphoid hyperplasia and prominent sinusoidal plasmacytosis.

Immunophenotype

Plasma cells in POEMS syndrome show λ light chain restriction, whereas IgG κ is typical for TEMPI syndrome.

Prognosis and Treatment

POEMS syndrome is chronic and progressive. VEGF blood levels correlate with disease severity (*Blood.* 2011;118(17):4663-4665). Therapies for POEMS, TEMPI, and AESOP are directed toward eradication of the plasma cell clone and can lead to clinical improvement (*Leukemia.* 2015;29(12):2414-2416; *Blood.* 2020;135(15):1199-1203).

Differential Diagnosis

- **MGUS, PCM/MM:** SPEP/IFE and BM evaluation alone are insufficient to exclude these rare syndromes. Close clinicopathologic correlation is required.
- **Myeloproliferative neoplasm (MPN):** Persistent erythrocytosis in TEMPI leads to consideration of polycythemia vera. Elevated erythropoietin and lack of most MPN-type BM morphologic abnormalities and MPN-associated gene mutations argue against MPN.

Key Points

- POEMS, TEMPI, and AESOP syndromes are very rare paraneoplastic syndromes associated with PCNs.
- M-proteins are IgA or IgG with λ light chain restriction in POEMS and predominantly IgG κ in TEMPI.
- The BM in POEMS and TEMPI syndromes shows clonal plasma cells <5%.

Diagnostic Caveats

- With the diversity of clinical signs and symptoms, close clinical, pathologic, radiologic, and laboratory correlation is required to arrive at the diagnosis.

Hodgkin Lymphomas

20.1 Nodular Lymphocyte-Predominant Hodgkin Lymphoma

Anne L. Chen and Brooj Abro

Nodular lymphocyte-predominant Hodgkin lymphoma (NLPHL) accounts for approximately 5% of Hodgkin lymphomas and typically presents in adult males (male:female ratio ~3:1). There is a wide age range with peak incidence in the fourth decade (*Adv Hematol.* 2011;2011:725219). The characteristic neoplastic cells known as lymphocyte-predominant (LP) cells are markedly enlarged with multilobate nuclei, prominent nucleoli, and pale chromatin (also referred to as popcorn cells). LP cells express multiple B-cell markers in contrast to neoplastic cells in classic Hodgkin lymphoma (CHL) (discussed in Chapter 20.2). The immunophenotypic differences between CHL and NLPHL are summarized in Table 20.1-1. The neoplastic LP cells are outnumbered by numerous reactive small lymphocytes, which tend to be a mixture of T and B cells, with B-cell predominance. As the name implies, the architecture is usually nodular; however, variant patterns without distinct nodular morphology can be seen. The diagnostic criteria are summarized in Table 20.1-2. Given the biologic and clinical differences from CHL, NLPHL has been recently renamed as "nodular lymphocyte-predominant B-cell lymphoma" by the International Consensus Classification (ICC; *Blood.* 2022;140:1229-1253).

Clinical Features

- **Clinical presentation:** Patients often present with chronic, painless lymphadenopathy and are usually diagnosed with early-stage disease (stages 1-2). B symptoms can be present in a subset of patients.
- **Sites of involvement:** Lymph nodes in the cervical and axillary regions are most commonly involved. Mediastinal and bone marrow involvement is rare.

Morphology

- **LP cells:** Large, atypical cells with multilobate nuclei, prominent nucleoli, and pale chromatin (also referred to as popcorn cells). LP cells are scattered in a background rich in nonneoplastic cells (e-Figure 20.1-1).
- **Background nonneoplastic cells:** The background cells are predominantly lymphocytes (e-Figure 20.1-1) rich in small B cells with intermixed T cells and

TABLE 20.1-1 Immunophenotypic Features of CHL Versus NLPHL

Antigen	CHL	NLPHL
	Most Common Expression	
CD30	+	−
CD15	+	−
PAX5	+ (dim to moderate)	+ (strong)
CD45	−	+
CD20	Variable (+/−)	+
OCT2	−	+
BOB-1	−	+
BCL6	−	+
EBV	+/−	−/(rarely +)
MUM1	+ (strong)	Variable (+/−)
Background infiltrate/architecture	Predominance of CD4+ T cells	Predominance of B cells
	Nodules with surrounding fibrosis (NSCHL subtype)	Nodules with CD21/CD23+ FDC meshworks (nodular patterns)
	NA	CD3+/PD-1+/CD57+ T cells form rosettes around LP cells.

CHL, classic Hodgkin lymphoma; FDC, follicular dendritic cell; NLPHL, nodular lymphocyte-predominant Hodgkin lymphoma; NSCHL, nodular sclerosis CHL.

TABLE 20.1-2 WHO-HAEM5 Diagnostic Criteria for NLPHL

Essential

- Nodular architecture (can be focal)
- Scattered large cells with with LP cell morphology and immunophenotype (express several B-cell markers)
- Background small lymphocytes, histiocytes, FDCs, and lack of eosinophils

Desirable

- Typical phenotype of LP cells (CD20+, BCL6+, OCT2+) and background PD-1+ TFH cells forming rosettes around LP cells
- Determination of growth pattern (excisional biopsy preferred)

FDC, follicular dendritic cell; LP, lymphocyte predominant; NLPHL, nodular lymphocyte-predominant Hodgkin lymphoma; TFH, T follicular helper.
Based on the WHO Classification of Tumours Editorial Board. Haematolymphoid tumours [Internet]. Lyon (France): International Agency for Research on Cancer; 2024 (WHO classification of tumours series, 5th ed.; vol. 11). Available from: https://tumourclassification.iarc.who.int/chapters/63.

TABLE 20.1-3 Growth Patterns in NLPHL

Pattern	Description	Key Features
A	B-cell-rich nodular	• Classic nodular pattern with FDC meshworks • Tumor cells predominantly within nodules • Nodules rich in B cells • PD-1+ rosettes usually present
B	Serpiginous-interconnected	• Irregular interconnected nodules with FDC meshworks • Tumor cells predominantly within nodules • Nodules rich in B cells • PD-1+ rosettes usually present
C	Prominent extranodular tumor cells	• Condensed nodules with FDC meshworks • Tumor cells frequently outside nodules • Nodules rich in B cells • PD-1+ rosettes present (can be few)
D	T-cell-rich nodular	• Nodules with FDC meshworks • Tumor cells usually within nodules • Nodules rich in TFH cells
E	Diffuse (THRLBCL like)	• Diffuse growth without FDC meshworks • At least focal nodular pattern required to classify as NLPHL • Background rich in T cells and histiocytes
F	Diffuse moth-eaten, B cell rich	• Diffuse growth without well-defined nodules and partial FDC meshworks • Areas with predominance of B cells and TFH cells

FDC, follicular dendritic cell; NLPHL, nodular lymphocyte-predominant Hodgkin lymphoma; TFH, T follicular helper; THRLBCL, T-cell/histiocyte-rich large B-cell lymphoma.

histiocytes. Neutrophils and eosinophils are not present. T cells may show clear cytoplasm. Histiocytes may form aggregates and granulomas.
- **Architectural patterns:** The overall architecture is usually nodular with or without diffuse areas (e-Figure 20.1-2A,B). Six growth patterns have been described in NLPHL (*Am J Surg Pathol.* 2003;27:1346-1356). The nodular, B-cell-rich growth patterns (A-B) are the most common and are associated with good prognosis. The key features of nodular and variant growth patterns are summarized in Table 20.1-3. Lymph nodes with partial involvement may show reactive follicular hyperplasia and progressive transformation of germinal centers (PTGC) in residual uninvolved areas.

Immunophenotype

- **Immunohistochemistry:** LP cells are positive for CD45 and multiple B-cell markers (CD20, PAX-5, CD79a, OCT-2, and BOB-1) (e-Figure 20.1-3) and usually negative for CD30 and CD15 (see Table 20.1-1). Background small B cells are positive for immunoglobulin D (IgD) and negative for germinal center markers (mantle zone type). CD21 and CD23 usually show expanded follicular dendritic cell (FDC) meshworks (e-Figure 20.1-2B). Background CD3+ T cells with T follicular helper (TFH) phenotype (PD-1+) form rosettes around LP cells (e-Figure 20.1-4).
- **Flow cytometry:** Limited utility in detecting the neoplastic cells but increased portions of double positive (CD4 and CD8 positive) reactive T cells is a clue to the diagnosis (*Am J Clin Pathol*. 2006;126(5):805-814).

Genetic Features

LP cells are germinal center–derived clonal B cells; however, routine molecular studies are usually unable to detect clonality due to the paucity of LP cells compared to background nonneoplastic cells. *BCL6* translocations are common (*Blood*. 2003; 101:706-710).

Progression and Transformation

NLPHL can transform into large B-cell lymphoma. Transformed areas show features of diffuse large B-cell lymphoma (DLBCL) and/or T-cell/histiocyte-rich large B-cell lymphoma (THRLBCL). The diagnosis of transformation may be challenging in small biopsies, and adequate tissue sampling is critical to distinguish variant patterns from THRLBCL transformation. Patients with transformation usually have advanced-stage disease.

Prognosis and Treatment

NLPHL is an indolent disease with an estimated overall 10-year survival greater than 90% and approximately 75% 10-year progression-free survival (*Ann Hematol*. 2016;95:417-423). The following features have been found to be associated with an increased risk of relapse: variant patterns, male gender, and low serum albumin (*Blood*. 2013;122:4246-4252). Treatment regimens vary and depend on the patient's age and disease stage. Therapeutic options include excision, chemotherapy, and radiation therapy. Systemic therapy is recommended in advanced disease (*Leuk Lymphoma*. 2021;62(5):1057-1065).

Differential Diagnosis

- **CHL:** Particularly the lymphocyte-rich variant subtype. The immunophenotype of neoplastic cells in CHL is different from that of LP cells. See Table 20.1-1. Recently, GATA3 and STAT6 have been reported to be negative in NLPHL and positive in 80% of CHL (*Appl Immunohistochem Mol Morphol*. 2019;27: 180-184, *Mod Pathol*. 2020;33:834-845.)
- **THRLBCL:** Usually advanced disease at presentation. Diffuse pattern with predominance of T cells and histiocytes.
- **Peripheral T-cell lymphoma (PTCL):** Systemic disease, aberrant T cells, clonal T-cell receptor gene rearrangements.
- **PTGC:** LP cells are not present.

> **Key Points**
> - The diagnosis of NLPHL requires both the appropriate overall morphology and the correct immunophenotypic profile of the neoplastic cells.
>
> **Diagnostic Caveats**
> - NLPHL has two associated entities, with overlapping morphologic features, that may precede, be found concurrently with, or develop after its diagnosis: PTGC and THRLBCL.
> - The diagnosis can be challenging on small biopsies and adequate tissue sampling is critical particularly for distinguishing variant patterns from THRLBCL.

SUGGESTED READINGS

Fan Z, Natkunam Y, Bair E, et al. Characterization of variant patterns of nodular lymphocyte predominant Hodgkin lymphoma with immunohistologic and clinical correlation. *Am J Surg Pathol.* 2003;27:1346-1356.

Hartmann S, Eichenauer DA, Plütschow A, et al. The prognostic impact of variant histology in nodular lymphocyte-predominant Hodgkin lymphoma: a report from the German Hodgkin Study Group (GHSG). *Blood.* 2013;122:4246-4252.

Momotow J, Borchmann S, Eichenauer DA, Engert A, Sasse S. Hodgkin lymphoma-review on pathogenesis, diagnosis, current and future treatment approaches for adult patients. *J Clin Med.* 2021;10(5):1125.

Wang HW, Balakrishna JP, Pittaluga S, Jaffe ES. Diagnosis of Hodgkin lymphoma in the modern era. *Br J Haematol.* 2019;184(1):45-59.

20.2 Classic Hodgkin Lymphoma

Anne L. Chen and Brooj Abro

Classic Hodgkin lymphoma (CHL) is characterized by neoplastic cells of B-cell origin with defective B-cell differentiation, known as Hodgkin Reed-Sternberg (HRS) cells, in a background of reactive inflammatory cells. Histologically, CHL can be subclassified into four types (see Table 20.2-1). The distinction between these subtypes is sometimes difficult, especially on core biopsies, and may not be relevant therapeutically. The age distribution is bimodal, with peaks in young adults (25-35 years) and older adults (>60 years) (*Cancer Med.* 2018;7(4):953-965). There is a slight male predilection except for the nodular sclerosis subtype (more common in females). The diagnostic criteria are summarized in Table 20.2-2.

Clinical Features

- **Clinical presentation:** Painless lymphadenopathy is the most common presentation. B symptoms are more common in patients with advanced-stage disease. Respiratory symptoms such as cough and shortness of breath can occur secondary to bulky mediastinal disease.
- **Sites of involvement:** CHL primarily involves the lymph nodes, with a predilection for sites above the diaphragm such as the axilla, neck, and mediastinum. Extranodal

TABLE 20.2-1 Subtypes of CHL

Subtype	Morphology	Frequency
NSCHL	Neoplastic nodules consisting of HRS cells in a background of mixed inflammatory cells, surrounded by sclerotic bands (e-Figure 20.2-3)	Most common, ~70% of CHL cases
MCCHL	Frequent HRS cells in a background of mixed inflammatory cells without significant sclerosis	~20%-25% of CHL cases
LRCHL	Nodular or diffuse infiltrate consisting of HRS cells in a background of predominantly small mature lymphocytes	~5% of CHL cases
LDCHL	Nodular or diffuse infiltrate consisting of frequent HRS cells in a background of scarce lymphocytes. Strongly associated with EBV	<1% of CHL cases

CHL, classic Hodgkin lymphoma; EBV, Epstein-Barr virus; HRS, Hodgkin Reed-Sternberg; LDCHL, lymphocyte-depleted CHL; LRCHL, lymphocyte-rich CHL; MCCHL, mixed-cellularity CHL; NSCHL, nodular sclerosis CHL.

involvement is seen in advanced-stage disease; however, primary extranodal disease is rare. Extranodal sites of disease include the lungs, bones, bone marrow, and liver. At mucosal sites, an important differential is Epstein-Barr virus (EBV)-associated mucocutaneous ulcer. At cutaneous sites, CD30+ lymphoproliferative disorders of the skin should be considered.

TABLE 20.2-2 WHO-HAEM5 Diagnostic Criteria for CHL

Essential	Desirable
• Nodal/mediastinal disease • HRS cells in a background of inflammatory cells • HRS cells with the appropriate immunophenotype: CD30+, PAX5+ (dim to moderate intensity) and variable CD20 (dim to negative)	• HRS cells: CD45−, CD15+, decreased/negative expression of B-cell markers OCT2 and BOB1 • EBV+ (subset of cases) • Histologic subtyping when possible • Exclusion of CHL mimics

CHL, classic Hodgkin lymphoma; EBV, Epstein-Barr virus; HRS, Hodgkin Reed-Sternberg.
Based on the WHO Classification of Tumours Editorial Board. Haematolymphoid tumours [Internet]. Lyon (France): International Agency for Research on Cancer; 2024 (WHO classification of tumours series, 5th ed.; vol. 11). Available from: https://tumourclassification.iarc.who.int/chapters/63.

Morphology

CHL consists of large atypical neoplastic cells in a background of variable proportions of nonneoplastic inflammatory cells. The large neoplastic cells are a mixture of mononuclear Hodgkin cells and classic HRS cells.

- **Hodgkin cells:** Hodgkin cells have variable morphology. They are usually much larger than background lymphocytes (4-5×), can be mono- or multinucleated, and show prominent eosinophilic nucleoli. The classic HRS cell shows binucleation, prominent eosinophilic nucleoli, and perinuclear halo (owl's eye appearance) (e-Figure 20.2-1). A special variant called the lacunar cell is characteristically seen in the nodular sclerosis subtype (e-Figure 20.2-2), which may have less prominent nucleoli and shows formalin fixation artifact causing nuclear shrinkage with spiderweb-like extensions to the cell membrane. Another variant is the lymphocyte-predominant (LP) cell, seen in nodular lymphocyte-predominant Hodgkin lymphoma (NLPHL) (discussed in Chapter 20.1); however, LP-like cells may appear in the lymphocyte-rich subtype of CHL. Degenerated HRS cells are known as "mummified cells." Hodgkin cells may be sparse and difficult to find in needle core biopsies. Excisional biopsy is usually recommended for the evaluation of CHL.
- **Background inflammatory cells:** The background inflammatory infiltrate varies with the histologic subtype (Table 20.2-1) and is usually composed of variable proportions of small lymphocytes, plasma cells, eosinophils, neutrophils, and histiocytes. Epithelioid granulomas may also be present. The background lymphocytes are a mixture of B and T cells with a predominance of CD4-positive T cells; however, abundant B cells (mantle cell type) may be seen in the lymphocyte-rich subtype.
- **Bone marrow:** Bone marrow involvement can be present in advanced-stage disease. The number of HRS is variable and may be accompanied by prominent eosinophilia and diffuse fibrosis.

Immunophenotype

- **Immunophenotype of HRS cells:** HRS cells are positive for CD30, CD15 (~70% of cases), PAX5 (dim to moderate), fascin, and MUM1. Variable CD20 expression can be seen, and EBV is positive in a subset of cases. HRS cells are negative for CD45 and show decreased to negative expression of B-cell markers such as OCT2 and BOB1. Rarely T-cell markers may be expressed by HRS cells (*Blood*. 2013;121:1795-1804).
- **Background nonneoplastic cells:** Majority of the background lymphocytes in CHL are CD4-positive T cells, which may form rosettes around HRS cells. B-cell-rich nodules can be seen in the lymphocyte-rich variant of CHL, mimicking NLPHL. CD15 also highlights background eosinophils and neutrophils.
- **Flow cytometry:** The neoplastic cells of CHL are not detectable by flow cytometry. Flow cytometry may show an increased CD4:CD8 ratio (*Cytometry B Clin Cytom*. 2016;90:424-432). Flow cytometry can be helpful in excluding T-cell lymphomas.

Genetic Features

In specialized single-cell analysis, HRS cells were found to have clonal *IGH* gene rearrangements demonstrating B-cell origin (*J Exp Med*. 1996;184:1495-1505). Gene expression profiling shows that B-cell antigens are downregulated. Studies have shown recurrent somatic mutations in genes regulating the nuclear factor kappa B (NF-κB) and JAK/STAT pathway (*Blood*. 2018;131:2454-2465).

In current clinical practice, cytogenetic and molecular testing are not required for the diagnosis of CHL. TCR clonality can be helpful to exclude T-cell lymphoma in some cases.

Prognosis and Treatment

Current chemotherapies in combination with radiation therapy can cure 80% to 90% of cases. Therapeutic options for relapsed CHL include brentuximab vedotin (anti-CD30) immune checkpoint inhibitors and autologous stem cell transplant (*J Clin Med*. 2021;10:1125).

Differential Diagnosis

It is critical to rule out nonneoplastic conditions and immune deficiency/dysregulation–associated lymphoproliferative disorders (IDD-LPDs) that can present with HRS-like CD30+ cells. Other lymphomas to consider in the differential diagnosis include NLPHL, T-cell-/histiocyte-rich large B-cell lymphoma (THRLBCL), EBV-positive diffuse large B-cell lymphoma (DLBCL), primary mediastinal large B-cell lymphoma (PMLBCL), peripheral T-cell lymphoma not otherwise specified (PTCL, NOS), and anaplastic large cell lymphoma (ALCL).

- **NLPHL:** Overlapping histologic features, particularly with the lymphocyte-rich CHL variant. The key difference is the immunophenotype of the neoplastic cells (see Chapter 20.1).
- **THRLBCL, PMLBCL, and EBV+ DLBCL:** Neoplastic cells typically show expression of CD45 and B-cell markers.
- **PTCL, NOS, and ALCL:** The neoplastic cells are T cells, and T-cell clonality can be demonstrated.
- **IDD-LPD:** Clinical history is important to differentiate from these disorders.
- **Infectious mononucleosis (IM):** A subset of CD30+ immunoblasts may resemble HRS cells; however, the overall immunophenotype is different from that of HRS cells (CD45 and CD20+, CD15−).
- **Methotrexate-associated CHL-like lesions:** Clinical history is important. The HRS-like cells are CD20+.

Key Points

- CHL is characterized by HRS cells, which may be sparse in a background of inflammatory cells.
- Clinical history and presence of HRS cells in appropriate histologic milieu are required for diagnosis.

Diagnostic Caveats

- Nonneoplastic conditions and other lymphomas may mimic CHL.
- HRS-like cells may be seen in non-Hodgkin B-cell lymphomas such as follicular lymphoma, marginal zone lymphoma, and chronic lymphocytic leukemia/small lymphocytic lymphoma.

SUGGESTED READINGS

Momotow J, Borchmann S, Eichenauer DA, Engert A, Sasse S. Hodgkin lymphoma—review on pathogenesis, diagnosis, current and future treatment approaches for adult patients. *J Clin Med*. 2021;10(5):1125.

Wang HW, Balakrishna JP, Pittaluga S, Jaffe ES. Diagnosis of Hodgkin lymphoma in the modern era. *Br J Haematol*. 2019;184(1):45-59.

21 Mature T/NK-cell Neoplasms

21.1 Mature T-/NK-Cell Leukemias

Cecilia C.S. Yeung, Mitra Afsharpad, Xi Zhang, and Anjum Hassan

This chapter covers entities with T- or natural killer (NK)-cell differentiation that present primarily as leukemic disease. The WHO-HAEM5 recognizes six distinct entities with leukemic presentation, whereas the International Consensus Classification (ICC) does not separate the entities with leukemic presentation and instead presents both T- and NK-cell neoplasms together. One other deviation between the WHO-HAEM5 and the ICC is the official naming of NK-large granular leukemia (WHO-HAEM5), which was based on evidence and the ability to detect monoclonal and oligoclonal NK-cell populations. The entity was previously known as "chronic lymphoproliferative disorder of NK cells (CLD-NK)," which remains a provisional entity in the ICC classification.

I. T-CELL PROLYMPHOCYTIC LEUKEMIA

T-cell prolymphocytic leukemia (T-PLL) is a T-cell leukemia characterized by a clonal proliferation of small- to medium-sized prolymphocytes with a mature post-thymic T-cell phenotype. T-PLL accounts for approximately 2% of mature lymphocytic leukemias with median age of 65 years at presentation and a male:female ratio of about 3, and an increased incidence in patients with ataxia telangiectasia due to germline mutations in the *ATM* gene (*Blood*. 1996;87:423-438). T-PLL includes the previous T-cell chronic lymphocytic leukemia (T-CLL), a now obsolete terminology, due to confusion with other entities. The diagnostic criteria are summarized in Table 21.1-1.

Clinical Features

T-PLL typically presents with profound leukocytosis (>100 × 10^9/L in 75%) with involvement of bone marrow, lymph nodes, and spleen. Skin infiltration and serous effusions may also occur in a subset of patients (20% and 15%, respectively); involvement of mucocutaneous and serosal sites is less common (*Am J Hematol*. 2023;98:913-921). Approximately 30% of patients have been reported to have an indolent and asymptomatic disease at the time of diagnosis, clinically termed "inactive T-PLL" (*Leuk Lymphoma*. 2015;57:942-944).

Morphology

- **Peripheral blood:** Prolymphocytes show a broad spectrum of morphology. In 75% of cases, the circulating neoplastic cells are small to medium sized with a nongranular basophilic cytoplasm and frequent cytoplasmic blebs or projections. The nuclei are irregular round to oval with mature chromatin and variably prominent nucleoli

TABLE 21.1-1 WHO-HAEM5 Diagnostic Criteria for T-PLL

Essential

- Atypical lymphocytosis >5 × 10^9/L in peripheral blood or bone marrow with T-PLL immunophenotype
- T-cell monoclonality (determined by T-cell receptor β/γ or flow cytometry)
- Detection of *TCL1A* or *MTCP1* rearrangement or TCL1 protein expression in neoplastic lymphocytes

Desirable

- Detection of a juxtaposition of the *TCL1A* or *MTCP1* gene next to a TCR locus mostly (commonly the TRA/TRD locus)
- Paracentric inversion of chromosome 14, inv(14)(q11q32) and t(14;14)(q11;q32)
- CD4+/CD8+ in a T-cell neoplasm with post-thymic T-cell phenotype is distinct for T-PLL.

T-PLL, T-cell prolymphocytic leukemia; TCR, T-cell receptor.
Based on the WHO Classification of Tumours Editorial Board. Haematolymphoid tumours [Internet]. Lyon (France): International Agency for Research on Cancer; 2024 (WHO classification of tumours series, 5th ed.; vol. 11). Available from: https://tumourclassification.iarc.who.int/chapters/63.

(e-Figure 21.1-1). Approximately 25% of T-PLL cases are the *"small cell variant,"* with smaller nuclei, condensed chromatin, and inconspicuous nucleoli. In about 5% of T-PLL cases, the circulating neoplastic cells may resemble the cerebriform cells of Sézary syndrome (SS).

- **Bone marrow:** Bone marrow aspirates show aggregates of atypical small- to medium-sized lymphocytes with mature round, oval, or sometimes irregular nuclear contours and a visible nucleolus. Core biopsy commonly shows effacement of architecture by diffuse interstitial infiltration of atypical small- to medium-sized lymphocytes (e-Figure 21.1-2). Myelofibrosis can be appreciated.
- **Spleen:** When T-PLL involves the spleen, there is typically red pulp expansion, with variable white pulp attenuation, with infiltration of the splenic capsule and the white pulp by predominantly medium-sized monotonous cells.
- **Lymph node:** Leukemic cells infiltrate the paracortical zones in early phases of involvement, leading to attenuation of the germinal centers. Complete architectural effacement is noted in advanced involvement (e-Figure 21.1-3).
- **Skin:** Skin is the most common extramedullary site of involvement by T-PLL. Cutaneous involvement is commonly seen as perivascular, periadnexal, and dermal infiltration without any evidence of epidermotropism. However, dense infiltrations can be associated with marked epidermotropism, histologically mimicking mycosis fungoides (*Blood*. 2019;134:1132-1143).

Immunophenotype

T-PLL generally shows a mature post-thymic T-helper phenotype, expressing CD3 (can be weak), CD4, CD2, CD5, and CD7 (40%-60% of cases); CD4−/CD8+ can be seen in 10% to 15% of the cases, and CD4+/CD8+ is present in 20% of cases. The double-positive cases tend to be more of the small cell variant type. Double expression of CD4 and CD8 is a unique finding in T-PLL since this coexpression is rarely seen in mature post-thymic T-cell neoplasms (*Blood*. 2019;134:1132-1143).

Approximately 70% to 80% of cases show overexpression of TCL1 by immunohistochemistry (IHC) and/or flow cytometry, a helpful marker for T-PLL, and can be both nuclear and cytoplasmic. Nuclear expression of TCL1 is associated with positive fluorescence in situ hybridization (FISH) for TCL1A rearrangement (*J Clin Pathol.* 2018;71:309-315.) T-PLL also shows a high level of positivity with CD52, often at a level suitable for targeted therapy (*Curr Hematol Malig Rep.* 2020;15:113-124).

Genetic Features

Certain cytogenetic abnormalities are characteristic of T-PLL, but are not specific for it. The most common recurrent abnormalities are a paracentric inversion of chromosome 14, inv(14) (q11q32) and t(14;14)(q11;q32), the latter of which involves juxtaposition of the *TCL1A* or *MTCP1* gene to the T-cell receptor (*TCR*) gene enhancer locus, usually *TRA/TRD* (*Front Oncol.* 2021;11:775363). Aberrant expression of TCL1 increases cell proliferation and survival by enhancing the AKT signaling pathway. In up to 75% of T-PLL cases, activating mutations of *IL2RG*, *JAK1/3*, and *STAT5B* genes are present (*Cancers (Basel).* 2019;11:1833). Approximately 70% to 80% of cases have a complex karyotype, with trisomy 8q seen in more than 70% of these cases.

Prognosis and Treatment

T-PLL is considered an aggressive neoplasm with a poor outcome (*Am J Hematol.* 2023;98:913-921). Alemtuzumab (also known as Campath-1H) remains the mainstay of therapy for treatment-naive patients as well as those with refractory or relapsed disease (*Cureus.* 2021;13:e13237). About 20% to 30% of patients have a more stable and slowly progressing disease (*Eur J Haematol.* 2015;94:265-269). Age above 65 years, hepatic or central nervous system (CNS) involvement, bulky lymphadenopathy, serous effusion, complex karyotype, very high absolute lymphocyte count, organ dysfunction, bone marrow suppression, high TCL1A and/or AKT1 protein expression, and JAK3 mutation are all variables that individually or collectively adversely affect outcomes (*Am J Hematol.* 2023;98:913-921; *Haematologica.* 2022;107:187-200).

Introduction of anti-CD52 monoclonal antibody (alemtuzumab) has significantly improved the outcomes in patients with T-PLL (*Am J Hematol.* 2023;98:913-921). Long-term disease survival post–hematopoietic stem cell transplant has been reported in some cases.

Differential Diagnosis

- **Mature T-cell neoplasms with leukemic presentation**
  - **T-cell large granular lymphocytic leukemia (T-LGLL):** Clinically T-LGLL is an indolent disease with reported spontaneous remission. It is associated with neutropenia and mild lymphocytosis with peripheral large granular lymphocytosis. T-LGLL shows strong CD3 positivity and is almost always CD8+/CD4− with coexpression of CD57.
  - **Sézary syndrome:** Circulating atypical lymphocytes are predominantly "giant" (monstrosity) cells with cerebriform nuclei and inconspicuous nucleoli, and immunophenotypically are characterized by loss of CD7 and CD26 expression.
  - **Adult T-cell leukemia/lymphoma (ATLL):** Epidemiologically, ATLL follows the endemic distribution of the human T-cell lymphotropic virus type 1 (HTLV-1), and consequently HTLV-1 polymerase chain reaction (PCR) and/or

serology is positive. Neoplastic T cells show nuclear lobulations (flower cells) and are positive for CD3, CD4, and CD25 but are CD7 negative and are negative for expression of TCL1.

- **Other lymphoid neoplasms with leukemic presentation**
  Other lymphoid neoplasms such as T- and B-cell lymphoblastic leukemia/lymphoma can have overlapping clinical features with T-PLL. A complete diagnostic workup and immunophenotyping helps differentiate T-PLL from immature B- and T-cell neoplasms.

> ### Key Points
>
> - The diagnosis requires the presence of lymphocytosis $>5 \times 10^9$/L, T-PLL immunophenotype, and clonal T cells showing *TCL1A* or *MTCP1* rearrangement or TCL1A protein expression.
> - The characteristic phenotype is post-thymic with coexpression of TCL-1 and CD52. The majority of cases are CD4+/CD8−; however, a CD4+/CD8+ and less commonly a CD4−/CD8+ immunophenotype can be seen.
> - CD4+/CD8+ in a T-cell neoplasm with post-thymic T-cell phenotype is distinct for T-PLL.
> - Very high expression of TCL-1, bone marrow failure, bulky lymphadenopathy, involvement of other organs and/or organ failure, and complex karyotype are associated with poor prognosis.
> - Introduction of anti-CD52 monoclonal antibody as first-line treatment in T-PLL has shown significant improvement in outcomes.
>
> #### Diagnostic Caveats
>
> - Approximately 5% of T-PLL cases show medium-sized nuclei with irregular nuclear contours resembling cerebriform cells of SS. However, in T-PLL, the neoplastic T cells have retained expression of CD7 and are TCL1 positive, whereas in SS CD7 and CD26 expression is aberrantly lost.
> - The T-PLL "small cell variant" can mimic other mature T-cell neoplasms with leukemic presentation. However, the expression of TCL1A in T-PLL, along with the post-thymic phenotype and TCL1A rearrangement, is helpful for diagnosis.
> - About 30% of the T-PLL cases will be in an "inactive" stage and asymptomatic. These cases usually have a more stable and slow-progressing disease.

II. T-CELL LARGE GRANULAR LYMPHOCYTIC LEUKEMIA

T-LGLL is an indolent neoplasm of clonal cytotoxic large granular T cells that clinically manifests with persistent peripheral large granular lymphocyte (LGL) expansion of $>0.5 \times 10^9$/L, associated with lymphocytosis (either relative [>50%] or absolute [$>2 \times 10^9$/L]), which compares with the absolute number of LGLs in the peripheral blood of normal subjects of 200 to 400/µL (*Am J Blood Res*. 2022;12:17-32). T-LGLL accounts for 2% to 5% of CLDs. The reported median age is 60 years with no gender predilection, and a higher prevalence in Asia. The diagnostic criteria are summarized in Table 21.1-2.

Clinical Features

Approximately a third of T-LGLL cases are found incidentally and are asymptomatic at the time of diagnosis. In symptomatic cases, the clinical features are mostly attributed to cytopenias (*Blood*. 2023;141:967-969). T-LGLL is typically not associated with thrombocytopenia and bleeding complications. Although fatigue can be seen in cases of severe anemia, B symptoms are very unlikely to be present.

TABLE 21.1-2 WHO-HAEM5 Diagnostic Criteria for T-LGLL

Essential

- Increase in circulating cytotoxic T cells, often >2,000 LGLs/μL, with a median value of 4,200 LGLs/μL (normal range 200-400 LGLs/μL); however, an absolute LGL count between 500 and 2,000 LGLs/μL may be consistent with the diagnosis if the LGLs are clonal and the patient has a typical clinical presentation.
- Aberrant T-cell population (usually CD8 positive) with downregulation of CD5 and/or CD7 and/or abnormal expression of CD16 and NK-cell-associated receptors
- Evidence of T-cell clonality (or oligoclonality)

Desirable

- Intrasinusoidal cytotoxic T-lymphocyitc infiltrates confirmed by immunohistochemistry
- Detection of *STAT3* mutation
- Detection of *STAT5b* mutation, which is more often seen in CD4-positive T-LGLL

Presence of all three essential or two essential and one desirable criterion is required for diagnosis.
LGL, large granular lymphocyte; NK, natural killer; T-LGLL, T-cell large granular lymphocytic leukemia.
Based on the WHO Classification of Tumours Editorial Board. Haematolymphoid tumours [Internet]. Lyon (France): International Agency for Research on Cancer; 2024 (WHO classification of tumours series, 5th ed.; vol. 11). Available from: https://tumourclassification.iarc.who.int/chapters/63.

Approximately 80% of T-LGLL cases have neutropenia with an absolute neutrophil count of $<1.5 \times 10^9$/L or severe neutropenia (absolute neutrophil count $<0.5 \times 10^9$/L). As a result, patients present with infections that typically involve the skin, oropharynx, and perirectal areas, but severe sepsis or pneumonia can also occur; opportunistic infections are uncommon. T-LGLL-associated anemia is present in 50% of cases and can lead to transfusion dependence in a minority of these. Pure red cell aplasia has been reported in rare cases.

An association with autoimmune disorders, mainly rheumatoid arthritis, Sjögren syndrome, and systemic lupus erythematosus (SLE) is present in 20% to 30% of cases. Concurrent hematologic malignancies including lymphoma and myelodysplastic neoplasms, as well as frequent seroreactivity to HTLV-1-related proteins, have also been reported. Abnormal serologies, including polyclonal hypergammaglobulinemia and positive antinuclear antibodies (ANAs) are reported in up to 30% of T-LGLL cases (*Br J Haematol.* 2021;192:484-493).

The etiology of T-LGLL is attributed to chronic antigen exposure (*Br J Haematol.* 2020;188:522-527), which is thought to lead to oligoclonal or clonal expansion of memory effector T cells causing an acquired resistance to activation-induced cell death. Secondary factors in pathogenesis include interleukin (IL)-15 stimulation, resistance to Fas/FasL-mediated cell death, autocrine platelet-derived growth factor (PDGF) stimulation, and abnormalities in cell signaling pathways (*Front Oncol.* 2022;12:854499).

Morphology

- **Peripheral blood:** Circulating neoplastic cells have abundant pale basophilic cytoplasm with variable amounts of azurophilic granules, slightly irregular nuclei, condensed chromatin, and inconspicuous nucleoli (e-Figure 21.1-4).
- **Bone marrow:** The extent of involvement varies. Although bone marrow examination is not required for diagnosis, it is helpful in the exclusion of other causes. Typically, a bone marrow aspirate shows left-shifted granulopoiesis, erythroid hypoplasia, and lymphocytosis (e-Figure 21.1-5). However, the cytologic features of the LGLs can be difficult to identify in an aspirate. The core biopsy may show a variably dense interstitial and/or intrasinusoidal small lymphocytic infiltrate with or without aggregates.
- **Spleen:** Splenic involvement by T-LGLL manifests as red pulp hyperplasia by linear arrays of lymphocytes.

Immunophenotype

T cells in T-LGLL are of cytotoxic CD8+ αβ T-cell lineage and express a mature effector memory T-cell phenotype (positive for CD3, CD2, CD5, CD7, and CD45RA). Cytotoxic granular markers including TIA-1, perforin, granzyme B, and granzyme A are usually positive. Aberrant expression of NK-cell markers such as CD57 and CD16 is frequently seen. In rare cases, bright expression of CD4 with dim expression of CD8 has been reported; these cases are categorized as CD4+ T-LGLL (*Blood Cancer J.* 2022;12:31).

Less than 10% of T-LGLL cases are of γ/δ T-cell lineage. These cases may exhibit dim CD8 expression (*Blood.* 2023;141:1036-1046).

Genetic Features

Identification of clonally rearranged *TCR* genes is a key factor in the diagnosis of T-LGLL. As noted earlier, most cases are αβ variants, while fewer than 10% are γ/δ variants. In T-LGLL, activation of STAT3, with or without a mutation, stimulates cellular survival. Cases of indolent CD4+ T-LGLL have recurrent *STAT5B* mutations; however, this mutation in CD8+ T-LGLL and T-γ/δ LGLL is associated with an aggressive disease (*Blood.* 2023;141:1036-1046). Other reported genetic findings include aberrations in the phosphoinositide 3-kinase (PI3K)/AKT and nuclear factor (NF)-κB signaling pathways, and mutations in *ET2*, *TNFAIP3*, *BCL11B*, *FLT3*, and *PTPN23*.

Differential Diagnosis

- **Reactive CD8+ T-cell expansion:** Suppressor T-cell expansions can be secondary to viral infections, chronic/sustained inflammatory conditions, and/or autoimmune diseases. These expansions are polyclonal.
- **CLD-NK cells:** The clinical picture in CLD-NK mimics T-LGLL and it is generally treated similarly. However, the cells in CLD-NK show aberrant loss of CD3 and CD5, and show strong positivity for NK-cell markers.
- **Mature T-cell neoplasm with leukemic presentation**
  - **NK-cell large granular lymphocytic leukemia (NK-LGLL):** NK-LGLL has similar clinical features to T-LGLL and may bear STAT3 and/or TET2 mutations. However, the neoplastic NK cells are negative for surface CD3, CD2, and CD7 expression. Expression of NK-cell markers CD16 and CD57 is strong.

- **ATLL:** By morphology, the atypical T cells in ATLL show nuclear lobulations, and IHC and flow cytometry show aberrant loss of CD7 expression.
- **Hepatosplenic T-cell lymphoma (HSTL):** This is a neoplasm of mature γ/δ T cells that infiltrate the sinusoids of the spleen, liver, and bone marrow, typically presenting with hepatosplenomegaly in young men. Lymphadenopathy or peripheral blood lymphocytosis is usually absent. Most cases of HSTL and T-LGLL express CD3 and CD16; however, HSTL shows CD56 and γ/δ TCR expression, in contrast to T-LGLL that is CD56 negative and usually expresses the $\alpha\beta$ TCR.
- **Aplastic anemia (AA):** Up to 5% of patients with T-LGLL will have pancytopenia and fulfill clinical criteria for AA. The distinction between idiopathic AA and T-LGLL with pancytopenia may be difficult in such cases; however, the presence of substantial numbers of clonal T cells in the peripheral blood or bone marrow is diagnostic of T-LGLL.

Prognosis and Treatment

T-LGLL is considered an indolent disease with an overall favorable prognosis. Poor prognostic factors include age greater than 60 years, presence of comorbidities, marked neutropenia, transfusion-dependent anemia, and *STAT3* mutation.

Given the association with poor prognosis, cases with cytopenia require treatment, and methotrexate, cyclophosphamide, and cyclosporin A are considered first-line single-agent therapy in these cases (*Br J Haematol.* 2021;192:484-493).

> **Key Points**
>
> - About two-thirds of cases of T-LGLL are symptomatic at diagnosis; when symptomatic, clinical finings can be attributed to anemia and neutropenia.
> - Etiology is ascribed to chronic antigen exposure due to autoimmunity, hematolymphoid malignancies, and viral infection, which leads to oligoclonal or clonal expansion of memory effector T cells causing an acquired resistance to activation-induced cell death.
> - Molecular genetic findings include *STAT3* and *STAT5B* mutations.
> - The majority of cases are of CD8+ $\alpha\beta$ T-cell origin with expression of CD3, CD2, CD5, CD7, CD56, CD16, and cytotoxic markers.
> - The majority have a favorable outcome with an indolent course. Poor prognostic factors include marked neutropenia, transfusion-dependent anemia, and STAT3 mutation.
>
> **Diagnostic Caveat**
>
> - Clinically and morphologically, T-LGLL overlaps with a variety of other entities including nonneoplastic, malignant, and aggressive entities. Close clinical correlation, established evidence of clonality, and the specific immunophenotype are required for definitive diagnosis.

III. NK-CELL LARGE GRANULAR LYMPHOCYTIC LEUKEMIA

NK-LGLL, previously known as CLD-NK, is defined as a persistent increase in circulating NK cells ($>2 \times 10^9$/L) without an established cause. NK-LGLL involvement is usually limited to peripheral blood and bone marrow; only rare cases of splenomegaly, hepatomegaly, lymphadenopathy, and skin involvement have been reported. The majority of patients are adults with a median age of 60, and there is no known gender or ethnic predilection. The disease is usually associated with an indolent clinical course.

The etiology of NK-LGLL is not completely understood. A retroviral antigen or a cellular protein with homology to a viral antigen has been postulated, as sera from patients with chronic NK lymphocytosis were found to react to an epitope of the human T cell lymphotropic virus (HTLV) I/II transmembrane envelope protein (*Blood.* 1997;90(5):1977). However, other studies have shown no correlation with retroviral or EBV infection (*Br J Haematol.* 2022; 196:507-522). Activating mutations of STAT3, all occurring in exons 20 and 21, which encode the SRC homology 2 (SH2) domain, have been reported in 30% to 50% of cases and TET2 mutation has been reported in approximately 25% to 30%; concurrent presence of STAT3 and TET2 mutation is not uncommon (*Br J Haematol.* 2022;196:507-522). An association with autoimmune disease, other solid tumors, hematopoietic neoplasms, and neuropathy has been reported.

The diagnostic criteria are summarized in Table 21.1-3.

Clinical Features

Clinically, the majority of the patients are asymptomatic; however, symptoms may occur due to cytopenia or other comorbidities (although not as frequently as in T-LGLL).

TABLE 21.1-3 WHO-HAEM5 Diagnostic Criteria for NK-LGLL

Essential	Desirable
• Increased circulating NK cells, typically greater than 2×10^9/L and persisting greater than 6 mo • Flow cytometric immunophenotyping showing an aberrant NK-cell population, negative for surface CD3 and CD8 positive, CD16 positive • "Restricted KIR expression" = Uniform expression or complete absence of KIRs (CD158a, CD158b, CD158e) • Intrasinusoidal bone marrow or splenic infiltration by cytotoxic CD8-positive lymphocytes with NK-cell lineage confirmed by flow cytometry and/or the presence of STAT3 and/or TET2 mutations	• NK lymphocytosis with indolent clinical presentation • Lack of nuclear EBV positivity • *CCL22* mutations may define a distinct subtype of NK-LGLL.

Diagnosis of NK-LGLL can be made in the absence of peripheral blood NK-cell count of $>2 \times 10^9$/L if there is immunophenotypic evidence of abnormal NK-cell population with documented evidence of aberrant KIR expression pattern.
EBV, Epstein-Barr virus; KIR, killer cell immunoglobulin-like receptor; NK, natural killer; NK-LGLL, NK-cell large granular lymphocytic leukemia.
Based on the WHO Classification of Tumours Editorial Board. Haematolymphoid tumours [Internet]. Lyon (France): International Agency for Research on Cancer; 2024 (WHO classification of tumours series, 5th ed.; vol. 11). Available from: https://tumourclassification.iarc.who.int/chapters/63.

Morphology

- **Peripheral blood:** Cellular morphology is indistinguishable from T-LGLL (e-Figure 21.1-6A).
- **Bone marrow:** Microscopic examination usually demonstrates an intrasinusoidal, and less commonly an interstitial, lymphocytic infiltrate morphologically similar to T-LGLL.
- **Spleen:** Although rare, intrasinusoidal red pulp involvement by NK-LGLL has been reported.

Immunophenotype

The neoplastic cells in NK-LGLL are of NK-cell origin and therefore positive for cytoplasmic CD3, CD16, and CD56, and show variable CD8 expression with loss of CD2; complete loss of CD56 has been reported. Cytotoxic granule proteins (TIA-1, granzyme B, and granzyme M) are helpful markers that can be detected by both IHC and flow cytometry. Uniform bright expression of the CD94/NKG2A heterodimer can be seen.

Also helpful is an abnormal pattern of expression of killer cell immunoglobulin-like receptors (ie, KIRs, specifically CD158a, CD158b, and CD158e). Almost all cases of NK-LGLL show KIR aberrancies manifested as complete lack of expression or restricted KIR isoform expression. Restricted KIR isoform expression is reportedly associated with negative CD56 expression (*Blood Rev.* 2023;20:101058) (e-Figure 21.1-6B).

Epstein-Barr encoding region (EBER) in situ hybridization (ISH) is negative.

Genetic Features

There is little evidence for recurrent cytogenetic abnormalities in NK-LGLL. However, activating mutations of *STAT3*, all occurring in exons 20 and 21 which encode the SH2 domain, have been reported in 30% to 50% of cases; *TET2* mutation has been reported in approximately 25% to 30% of cases, and concurrent presence of *STAT3* and *TET2* mutations is not uncommon. Other mutated genes include *CCL22* encoding chemokine (C-C motif) ligand 22 (approximately 22% of cases) and *TNFAIP3* and PI3K pathway mutations. *CCL22* mutation is mutually exclusive of *STAT3 and STAT5B* mutations and has not been reported in T-LGLL cases.

Differential Diagnosis

The differential diagnosis for NK-LGLL is similar to that for T-LGLL, and flow cytometry immunophenotyping is required to distinguish T-LGLL from NK-LGLL. If flow cytometry is not performed, but other criteria for diagnosis are present, it is recommended that a diagnosis of LGL disorder, not further classifiable, should be considered. It should also be noted that uniform CD16 expression and absence of CD5 expression can be present in normal γ/δ T cells; however, these should not be greater than 50% of the total T-cell pool.

Prognosis and Treatment

In more than 50% of cases, NK-LGLL is an indolent disease, and spontaneous regression occurs in some cases. Patients presenting with symptomatic cytopenias and/or recurrent infection may require therapy.

> **Key Points**
>
> - NK-LGLL is defined as a persistent increase in circulating NK cells ($>2 \times 10^9$/L) without an established cause.
> - The disease has an indolent clinical course.
> - Activating mutations of *STAT3*, *TET2*, or both; *CCL22* mutation; and *TNFAIP3* and PI3K pathway genes are linked to the pathogenesis of NK-LGLL.
> - Neoplastic cells express abnormal NK-cell receptors with bright CD94/NKG2A expression, weak to absent CD161 expression, variable CD56 and CD8 expression, and complete loss of detectable KIR or restricted KIR isoform expression.
> - Positive expression of CD16 and cytoplasmic CD3 with negative surface CD3, CD2, and CD7 expression is often seen.
>
> **Diagnostic Caveat**
>
> - NK-LGLL is clinically and histopathologically indistinguishable from T-LGLL; distinction can only be made by immunophenotypic analysis, preferably by flow cytometry. Complications from cytopenias and/or infection portend a poor prognosis.

IV. AGGRESSIVE NK-CELL LEUKEMIA

Aggressive NK-cell leukemia (ANKL) is a rare systemic malignant neoplasm, mainly affecting young patients (mean age 39 years) presenting with a fulminant clinical course. It can involve any organ system or multiple sites such as peripheral blood, bone marrow, liver, and spleen. In contrast to the usual leukemias, ANKL may show sparse atypical cells in the peripheral blood or in bone marrow. There is a strong association with Asian descent and with EBV infection, the latter of which is reported in approximately 90% of the cases, implying a possible etiologic role (*Virchows Arch.* 2023;482:227-244). EBV (LMP-1)-positive ANKL shows an EBV (LMP-1)-related increase in IL-10, which activates the JAK/STAT pathway and stimulates STAT3 phosphorylation and downstream activation of C-MYC.

The diagnostic criteria are summarized in Table 21.1-4.

Intravascular NK-/T-cell lymphoma (IVNKTCL), currently tentatively categorized under ANKL, is a highly aggressive disease that involves the CNS and skin without mass lesions. It is also associated with EBV (LMP-1) infection, and somatic mutation in echogenic regulators has been reported.

Clinical Features

ANKL is more prevalent among young to middle-aged adults of Asian and native American descent. It generally manifests as an acute symptomatic disease with coagulopathy, disseminated intravascular coagulation, lymphadenopathy, hepatosplenomegaly, and symptoms of liver failure. Mucocutaneous involvement is rare.

Morphology

- **Peripheral blood:** Circulating cells mimic LGLs with a moderate amount of pale basophilic cytoplasm containing azurophilic granules (e-Figure 21.1-7A). Typically, the nuclei are large with folds and irregular contours, open chromatin, and variably prominent nucleoli.
- **Bone marrow:** Bone marrow aspirates show variable number of leukemic cells, as well as reactive histiocytes with increased hemophagocytosis. Core biopsies show both interstitial and sinusoidal infiltration by the neoplastic cells.

TABLE 21.1-4 WHO-HAEM5 Diagnostic Criteria for ANKL

Essential

- Acute fulminant presentation, with fever, hepatosplenomegaly, lymphadenopathy, and a leukemic blood picture
- Systemic involvement with multiorgan infiltration of clonal NK cells
- Atypical lymphocytosis has NK-cell immunophenotype.
- Germline TCR genes or lack of TCR protein expression by immunohistochemistry

Desirable

- EBER positivity (exclude other EBV-associated T-/NK-cell malignancies[a])
- Hemophagocytic lymphohistiocytosis

ANKL, aggressive NK-cell leukemia; EBER, Epstein-Barr encoding region; EBV, Epstein-Barr virus; NK, natural killer; TCR, T-cell receptor.
[a]EBV-associated hemophagocytosis, chronic active EBV infection of T cells or NK cells, systemic EBV-positive T-cell lymphoma, NK/T-cell lymphoma, nasal and extranodal types.
Based on the WHO Classification of Tumours Editorial Board. Haematolymphoid tumours [Internet]. Lyon (France): International Agency for Research on Cancer; 2024 (WHO classification of tumours series, 5th ed.; vol. 11). Available from: https://tumourclassification.iarc.who.int/chapters/63.

- **Spleen:** Red pulp involvement is present with an angiocentric growth pattern and variable necrosis.
- **Liver:** Involvement of portal areas and sinuses is typically seen.

Immunophenotype

The immunophenotype is identical to that of extranodal NK-/T-cell lymphoma (EN-KTL; CD2 positive, surface CD3 negative, cytoplasmic CD3ε positive, CD56 positive, cytotoxic markers positive). CD16 expression is seen in 50% of cases. The TCR genes are typically in the germline configuration. CD8 and CD11b can be expressed, and CD57 is usually negative. Loss of NK-cell receptors, specifically KIRs (CD158a, CD158b, CD158e) or a restrictive expression pattern of KIRs can be detected by performing flow cytometry (*PLoS One.* 2016;11:e0158827) (e-Figure 21.1-7B). From 80% to 100% of cases will be EBV (LMP-1) positive by ISH, but the EBV-negative subset shows clinicopathologic features that are similar to the EBV-positive cases.

Genetic Features

Whole-genome and exon sequencing have shown aberrations in *JAK/STAT* (*STAT3, STAT5B, STAT5A, JAK2, JAK3, STAT6, SOCS1, SOCS3,* and *PTPN11*) and the *RAS/MAPK* pathways, as well as mutations in histone modifiers (*TET2, CREBBP, KMT2D, BCOR, SET2D,* and *GFI1*), cell cycle regulators (*TP53, ASXL1, ASXL2,* and *BRINP3*), DNA damage repair proteins, RNA helicase (*DDX3X*), messenger RNA splicing (*PRPF40B*), and immune checkpoint molecules (*CD274* [*PD-L1*]/*PDCD1LG2* [*PD-L2*]). Array-based comparative genomic hybridization (aCGH) has shown gains of 1q23.1-q23.2 and 1q31.3-q44, and loss of 7p15.1-q22.3 and 17p13.1.

Differential Diagnosis

- **CLD-NK:** Clinically, CLD-NK is an indolent disease, and the cells show aberrant loss of CD3 and CD5, with strong positivity for NK-cell markers.
- **Mature T-cell neoplasms with leukemic presentation**
  - **NK-LGLL:** NK-LGLL has an indolent clinical course and may harbor *STAT3* and/or *TET2* mutations. By morphonology the neoplastic cells are indistinguishable from ANKL. EBER is negative.
  - **T-LGLL:** Clinically T-LGLL is an indolent disease with reported spontaneous remission. Immunophenotypically, TLGL shows strong CD3 positivity and is almost always CD8+/CD4− with coexpression of CD57, and EBER is negative.
  - **Sézary syndrome:** This T-cell malignancy has loss of CD7 and CD26 expression in CD4-positive T cells. Cytotoxic markers and EBER are negative.
  - **ATLL:** Endemic distribution of HTLV-1. As a T-cell malignancy, it has positive pan-T-cell markers and aberrant loss of CD7 expression. EBER is negative.
  - **HSTL:** The neoplastic cells are TCRγδ-rearranged T cells that are typically small to medium in size, mostly KIR+, CD2+, CD3+, CD7+, CD38+, and have variable expression of CD16, CD56, and CD94. EBER is negative. Circulating neoplastic cells are uncommon.
  - **ENKTL:** As with ANKL, ENKTL has a strong association with EBV infection and the morphologic findings can overlap, making the diagnosis challenging. Clinically, ENKTL has a less aggressive presentation with upper aerodigestive tract (most commonly the nasal cavity) involvement. Bone marrow disease in ENKTL frequently exhibits geographic necrosis.

Prognosis and Treatment

ANKL has poor outcomes complicated by coagulopathy and multiorgan failure, and the response to conventional chemotherapy is minimal. Some studies have shown benefits of L-asparaginase-containing treatment. Allogeneic hematopoietic stem cell transplant may be curative.

Key Points

- ANKL is a rare and aggressive neoplasm with involvement of peripheral blood and bone marrow, and a fulminant clinical course with multiorgan failure and disseminated intravascular coagulation.
- Acute systemic presentation, as well as NK-cell immunophenotype and lack of TCR clonal rearrangement, is required for diagnosis.
- Approximately 90% of cases are EBV positive.

Diagnostic Caveats

- By morphology, the neoplastic cells in ANKL are indistinguishable from a normal LGL and a variety of T-/NK-cell malignancies (ENKTL, NK-LGLL, T-LGLL, and HSTL) but differ in clinical, immunophenotypic, and genotypic features.
- Intravascular NK-/T-cell lymphoma (IVNKTCL) is tentatively categorized under ANKL; however, it commonly involves the CNS and skin, and does not form a mass.

V. ADULT T-CELL LEUKEMIA/LYMPHOMA

ATLL is a mature T-cell malignancy closely linked to the prevalence of HTLV-1, which is endemic in southwestern Japan, the Caribbean basin, parts of Central Africa, and Iran. ATLL is the very first retrovirus with proven human disease association and, usually, a long latency period between viral infection and malignant transformation. The closest normal counterpart of the neoplastic cells is FOXP3+ T-regulatory cells.

ATLL can involve multiple nodal and extranodal sites, including the skin, lungs, liver, gastrointestinal tract, and the CNS. The skin is the most frequently involved extranodal site. The diagnostic criteria are summarized in Table 21.1-5.

Clinical Features

Clinically, ATLL is subdivided into four subtypes: acute, lymphomatous, smoldering, and chronic. Patients with the acute and lymphomatous subtypes usually have an aggressive clinical course. In contrast, the smoldering and chronic subtypes generally present as cutaneous or pulmonary lesions without visceral or bone marrow involvement and/or leukocytosis, organomegaly without an elevated lactate dehydrogenase (LDH), and visceral involvement.

Many patients have associated immunodeficiency and frequent opportunistic infections such as *Pneumocystis jiroveci* and *Strongyloides stercoralis*. A positive HTLV-1 serology test can be used as a surrogate marker for viral integration, mainly in areas of low viral prevalence; however, certain cytologic features are highly characteristic and may suggest a diagnosis even if the studies for HTLV-1 are not performed (*Mod Pathol.* 2021;34:51-58).

Morphology

- **Peripheral blood:** Circulating atypical lymphocytes have multilobulated nuclei, condensed chromatin, and multiple nuclear convolutions, known as "flower cells." Basophilic cytoplasm and hyperchromasia are used in distinguishing the cells from SS.

TABLE 21.1-5 WHO-HAEM5 Diagnostic Criteria for ATLL

Essential	Desirable
1. Atypical lymphocytosis with mature T-cell immunophenotype	1. Presence of flower cells—atypical lymphoid cells with prominent nuclear lobulation and convolutions
2. Lymphoma develops in a HTLV-1 carrier—diagnosis performed by detection of HTLV-1 antibody followed by confirmatory tests to diagnose HTLV-1	2. Demonstration of monoclonal integration of proviral HTLV-1 DNA

ATLL, adult T-cell leukemia/lymphoma; HTLV-1, human T-cell lymphotropic virus type 1.
Based on the WHO Classification of Tumours Editorial Board. Haematolymphoid tumours [Internet]. Lyon (France): International Agency for Research on Cancer; 2024 (WHO classification of tumours series, 5th ed.; vol. 11). Available from: https://tumourclassification.iarc.who.int/chapters/63.

- **Bone marrow:** Involvement is typically not prominent; however, when present, it can be interstitial, sinusoidal, or diffuse.
- **Lymph nodes:** Lymph nodes typically show diffuse architectural effacement and a variety of different morphologies, with pleomorphic to round and uniform cells, to giant cells with convoluted and cerebriform nuclear contours. Reed-Sternberg (RS)-like cells can also be seen (e-Figure 21.1-8).
- **Skin:** The lymphoid infiltrates can mimic mycosis fungoides with epidermotropism and Pautrier microabscesses, and may cause diagnostic challenges with many other inflammatory disorders. The smoldering and chronic forms of ATLL may resemble chronic dermatitis.

Immunophenotype

The neoplastic cells in ATLL are typically TCR-$\alpha\beta$-rearranged T cells with expression of CD2, CD3, CD4 (approximately 90%), CD5, CD25, CCR4 (approximately 80%), FOXP3 (in a subset of cases), and aberrant loss of CD7. CD8 positivity is rarely reported. Enlarged EBV-positive Hodgkin-like B cells may be seen interspersed among the neoplastic T cells (e-Figure 21.1-9).

Genetic Features

The viral protein TAX plays a role in early malignant transformation. After viral integration into the host genome, TAX interacts with several proteins, leading to activation of oncogenic signaling pathways such as NF-κB and PI3K pathways. In addition, TAX inactivates p53. Another viral protein HBZ has vital functions in the maintenance of the T-cell lymphoma clone.

Mutations in the JAK/STAT and TCR/NF-κB pathways, epigenetic and histone-modifying genes (including *EP300* and *SPEN*), and multiple tumor suppressor genes (including *TP53* and *APC*) have been reported. *TP53* mutations are generally associated with poor prognosis.

Prognosis and Treatment

The acute and lymphomatous subtypes of ATLL are usually treated with intensive combination chemotherapy regimens, often with limited benefit. Other treatment options are dependent on a number of factors including patient age and comorbidities; first-line agents may include an anthracycline-based regimen, and/or monoclonal antibody-based therapies, and drugs active against other retroviruses. The chronic and smoldering subtypes are usually monitored without chemotherapy. Other molecular targeted therapies, such as CCR4 and allogeneic transplantation, have also shown promise.

Differential Diagnosis

- **T-LGLL:** The atypical lymphocytes in T-LGLL have abundant granular cytoplasm, usually with a CD8+/CD16+/CD57+ immunophenotype.
- **T-PLL:** The atypical lymphocytes in T-PLL exhibit cytoplasmic projections, clumped chromatin, and variably prominent central nucleolus. By IHC, these cells are positive for CD52 and TCL1.
- **Peripheral T-cell lymphoma not otherwise specified:** This disorder is usually not associated with hypocalcemia and systemic disease, and HTLV-1 serology is negative.

- **Angioimmunoblastic T-cell lymphoma:** The neoplastic cells usually have a TFH phenotype (positive for pan-T-cell markers, CD10, CXCL13, BCL6, and PD-1) with expanded follicular dendritic cell meshworks.
- **Anaplastic large cell lymphoma (ALCL):** The neoplastic cells are CD30+ and are negative for HTLV-1. ALK IHC can help in diagnosis of ALK+ ALCL.
- **Cutaneous T-cell lymphoma/mycosis fungoides:** The neoplastic cells show variable CD25 expression and are negative for FOXP3 and HTLV-1 expression.
- **T-cell lymphoblastic leukemia/lymphoma:** Usually distinguishable by morphologic and immunophenotypic findings. Blasts are positive for CD34, TdT, CD1a, cytoplasmic CD3, but are negative for FOXP3 and HTLV-1.

Key Points

- ATLL is a mature T-cell lymphoma most likely derived from FOXP3+ T-regulatory cells.
- The characteristic phenotype is CD4+, CD8−, and CD25+ monoclonal $\alpha\beta$ T cells.
- The morphology of ATLL is variable and is best seen in peripheral blood smears.
- The lymphoma cells show monoclonal integration of HTLV-1 virus.

Diagnostic Caveats

- RS-like cells can be seen in some cases.
- CD25 expression is not highly specific for ATLL.
- A small subset of ATLL cases are CD4−, CD8−, or double positive.
- HTLV-1 positivity does not prove the diagnosis of ATLL.

ACKNOWLEDGMENT

We would like to thank David Woolston for review and editing.

SUGGESTED READINGS

T-Cell Prolymphocytic Leukemia

Rose A, Zhang L, Jain AG, et al. Delineation of clinical course, outcomes, and prognostic factors in patients with T-cell prolymphocytic leukemia. *Am J Hematol.* 2023;98(6):913-921.

Staber PB, Herling M, Bellido M, et al. Consensus criteria for diagnosis, staging, and treatment response assessment of T-cell prolymphocytic leukemia. *Blood.* 2019;134(14):1132-1143.

T-Cell Large Granular Lymphocytic Leukemia

Pflug N. T-LGLL: variety is the spice of this leukemia. *Blood.* 2023;141(9):967-969.

Rahul E, Ningombam A, Acharya S, Tanwar P, Ranjan A, Chopra A. Large granular lymphocytic leukemia: a brief review. *Am J Blood Res.* 2022;12(1):17-32.

NK-Cell Large Granular Lymphocytic Leukemia

Magnano L, Rivero A, Matutes E. Large granular lymphocytic leukemia: current state of diagnosis, pathogenesis and treatment. *Curr Oncol Rep.* 2022;24(5):633-644.

Semenzato G, Calabretto G, Barilà G, Gasparini VR, Teramo A, Zambello R. Not all LGL leukemias are created equal. *Blood Rev.* 2023;60:101058

Aggressive NK-Cell Leukemia

Fujikura K, Yamashita D, Yoshida M, Ishikawa T, Itoh T, Imai Y. Cytogenetic complexity and heterogeneity in intravascular lymphoma. *J Clin Pathol*. 2021;74(4):244-250.

Zanelli M, Parente P, Sanguedolce F, et al. Intravascular NK/T-cell lymphoma: what we know about this diagnostically challenging, aggressive disease. *Cancers (Basel)*. 2022;14(21):5458.

Adult T-Cell Leukemia/Lymphoma

Nishi Y, Miyagi T, Yamaguchi S, et al. A comprehensive study of the immunophenotype and its clinicopathologic significance in adult T-cell leukemia/lymphoma. *Mod Pathol*. 2023;36(8):100169.

Yasunaga JI. Viral, genetic, and immune factors in the oncogenesis of adult T-cell leukemia/lymphoma. *Int J Hematol*. 2023;117(4):504-511.

21.2 Intestinal T/NK-Cell Lymphoproliferative Disorders and Lymphomas

Saja Asakrah and Zaid Mahdi

I. INDOLENT T-CELL LYMPHOMA OF THE GASTROINTESTINAL TRACT

Indolent T-cell lymphoma of the gastrointestinal tract (ITCL-GI) was previously referred to as indolent T-cell lymphoproliferative disorder of the GI tract. The name has been updated by the WHO-HAEM5, replacing the term "lymphoproliferative disorder" with "lymphoma" to reflect disease-associated morbidity and the ability to disseminate (*Leukemia*. 2022;36:1720-1748; *Leukemia*. 2023;37:1944-1951). ITCL-GI is an indolent lymphoma with a chronic relapsing clinical course. It is characterized by clonal T-cell proliferation composed of small mature lymphocytes infiltrating the lamina propria without significant epitheliotropism. It is more common in men and usually presents in adulthood (*Cancers (Basel)*. 2021;13:2790). The diagnostic criteria are summarized in Table 21.2-1.

TABLE 21.2-1 WHO-HAEM5 Diagnostic Criteria for Indolent T-Cell Lymphoma of the Gastrointestinal Tract

Essential	Desirable
• Nondestructive infiltrate composed of small mature lymphocytes, usually limited to the GI mucosa without significant epitheliotropism • Phenotype: T cells with expression of TCR$\alpha\beta$ • Low Ki67 (usually <10%)	• Clonal TCR rearrangements (useful in distinguishing from inflammatory infiltrate)

GI, gastrointestinal; TCR, T-cell receptor.
Based on the WHO Classification of Tumours Editorial Board. Haematolymphoid tumours [Internet]. Lyon (France): International Agency for Research on Cancer; 2024 (WHO classification of tumours series, 5th ed.; vol. 11). Available from: https://tumourclassification.iarc.who.int/chapters/63.

Clinical Features

- **Clinical Presentation:** Patients typically present with GI symptoms similar to inflammatory bowel disease.
- **Sites of Involvement:** Any GI location can be involved; the small intestine and colon are the most common sites. Mesenteric lymphadenopathy can occur; however, peripheral lymphadenopathy is not seen. Dissemination to other sites can occur with progressive/transformed disease.

Morphology

The infiltrate is typically nondestructive, expands the lamina propria, and is composed of small mature monotonous lymphocytes. Focal involvement of muscularis mucosa and submucosa can also occur. Although significant epitheliotropism is not present, focal infiltration of crypt epithelium can be seen. Villous architecture is usually preserved in small intestinal diseases. Epithelioid granulomas can be present (*Blood.* 2013;122:3599-3606).

Immunophenotype

Most cases are positive for CD3 (cluster of differentiation 3), TCR$\alpha\beta$ (T-cell receptor), and either CD4 or CD8, with CD4 expression being more common (*Hematol Oncol.* 2017;35:3-16). Expression of CD5 and CD7 can be reduced or lost. A CD4 (+)/CD8 (+) and CD4 (−)/CD8 (−) immunophenotype is seen in a small subset (*Haematologica.* 2020;105:1895-1906). T-cell intracellular antigen (TIA) is expressed in CD8-positive cases. Ki-67 is low (usually <10%), and Epstein-Barr virus (EBV) is negative. CD30 expression is seen in transformed cases (*PLoS One.* 2013;8:e68343).

Genetic Features

ITCL-GI cases demonstrate clonal *TRB/TRG* rearrangements (*Haematologica.* 2020;105:1895-1906). Frequent alterations of *JAK-STAT* pathway genes and mutations in epigenetic modifier genes (*TET2, DNMT3A, KMT2D*) have been reported (*Blood.* 2018;131:2262). Distinct genetic alterations of the *JAK-STAT* pathway are associated with certain immunophenotypic subtypes; CD4$^+$ cases are associated with recurrent *STAT3::JAK2* fusions and a subset of CD8$^+$ cases show structural alterations involving the 3' untranslated region of the *IL2* gene (*Haematologica.* 2020;105:1895-1906).

Prognosis and Treatment

ITCL-GI is a chronic disease with poor response to chemotherapy; however, despite the chronic relapsing clinical course, survival is prolonged with conservative management. Rarely, progressive disease with dissemination and transformation to aggressive lymphoma can occur (*Int J Surg Pathol.* 2019;27:102-107).

Differential Diagnosis

- **Inflammatory conditions:** Benign inflammatory conditions are composed of a polymorphic infiltrate with a variable proportion of CD4 and CD8 + T cells; ITCL-GI shows a monotonous infiltrate usually with predominant expression of either CD4 or CD8 + T cells and clonal TCR rearrangements are detected.
- Other intestinal T-cell lymphomas (see Table 21.2-6)

Key Points

- ITCL-GI is characterized by a clonal T-cell proliferation composed of small mature lymphocytes, most commonly involving the small intestine and colon, and usually confined to the mucosa without significant epitheliotropism.
- The tumor cells have low proliferation (10% Ki-67), express CD3 and TCR, and are usually positive for either CD4 or CD8.

Diagnostic Caveats

- Inflammatory GI disorders can mimic ITCL-GI. Detection of clonal TCR gene rearrangements can be helpful to distinguish ITCL-GI from inflammatory conditions.

II. INDOLENT NATURAL KILLER CELL LYMPHOPROLIFERATIVE DISORDER OF THE GASTROINTESTINAL TRACT

Natural killer cell lymphoproliferative disorder (NKLPD) is an indolent natural killer (NK) cell proliferation involving the intestinal tract mucosa and it is of unknown etiology. Typically, there is no preceding history of celiac disease (CD) or other inflammatory gastrointestinal (GI) disorders. It is commonly diagnosed in fifth and sixth decades; however, it has infrequently been reported in pediatric and young patients (*Blood*. 2019;134:986-991; *Am J Clin Pathol*. 2019;151:75-85). Previously, it was not recognized as an entity in the WHO, was known as lymphomatoid gastropathy or NK-cell enteropathy, and was thought to be a reactive disorder partly due to the lack of evidence of clonality. However, given the recent molecular findings supporting its neoplastic process, it is included as an entity in the WHO-HAEM5. Dissemination and progression to an aggressive disease have not been reported; thus, it is designated as a "lymphoproliferative disorder" rather than a lymphoma. The diagnostic criteria are summarized in Table 21.2-2.

TABLE 21.2-2 WHO-HAEM5 Diagnostic Criteria for Indolent NK-Cell Lymphoproliferative Disorder of the Gastrointestinal Tract

Essential	Desirable
• Nondestructive infiltrate composed of medium to large mature lymphocytes, usually limited to the GI mucosa without significant epitheliotropism • Phenotype: NK cells with expression of CD56 and lacing the expression of surface CD3, CD5, and TCR including TCRγδ and TCRαβ • No angioinvasion • EBV is negative in the atypical cells	• Lack of clonal TCR rearrangements (useful in distinguishing it from T-cell lymphomas)

EBV, Epstein-Barr virus; GI, gastrointestinal; NK, natural killer; TCR, T-cell receptor.
Based on the WHO Classification of Tumours Editorial Board. Haematolymphoid tumours [Internet]. Lyon (France): International Agency for Research on Cancer; 2024 (WHO classification of tumours series, 5th ed.; vol. 11). Available from: https://tumourclassification.iarc.who.int/chapters/63.

Clinical Features
- **Clinical Presentation:** Patients are either asymptomatic with a lesion identified during screening colonoscopy, or complain of vague symptoms such as reflux, abdominal pain/discomfort, and diarrhea. Subsequent diagnostic tests may show blood in the stool and features of diverticulosis. Endoscopic findings may include superficial ulcers, erosions, and less frequently polyps. These lesions either spontaneously regress or follow a chronic, relapsing clinical course.
- **Sites of Involvement:** NKLPD can affect any site along the GI tract including stomach, duodenum, terminal ileum, and colon.

Morphology
Microscopically, NKLPD manifests as an expansion of the lamina propria with confluent medium to large lymphocytes with irregular nuclei, inconspicuous nucleoli, finely clumped chromatin, and a moderate amount of pale cytoplasm (histiocyte-like appearance) (e-Figure 21.2-1). The lesion should lack glandular destruction, angiocentricity, angioinvasion, necrosis, brisk mitosis, overt epitheliotropism, or destruction of the muscularis propria. A subset of the atypical cells may show coarse eosinophilic cytoplasmic granules. Inflammatory cells including plasma cells and eosinophils may be present, particularly at the periphery (*Am J Clin Pathol.* 2019;151:75-85).

Immunophenotype
The atypical NK cells express cytoplasmic CD3, CD56 (e-Figure 21.2-1), cytotoxic markers (TIA1 and granzyme B) and are negative for surface CD3, CD5, CD4, TCRαβ, and TCRγδ. CD2, CD7, and CD8 staining is variable. EBV by Epstein-Bar virus encoded small RNA in situ hybridization (ISH) is negative. The Ki-67 proliferation index may vary from one case to another and ranges between 25% and 95%.

Genetic Features
NKLPD typically does not show a clonal pattern by TCR γ or β gene rearrangement PCR (polymerase chain reaction) testing.

Targeted next-generation sequencing (NGS) panels covering genes known to be mutated in hematologic malignancies demonstrate recurrent *JAK3* gene mutations in 30% of cases with increased downstream STAT5 (signal transducer and activator of transcription 5) phosphorylation (*Blood.* 2019;134:986-991). In a limited case study, other mutations were identified in a number of genes including *PTPRS, AURKB, AXL, ERBB4, IGF1R, PIK3CB, CUL3, CHEK2, RUNX1T1, CIC, SMARCB1,* and *SETD5.*

Prognosis and Treatment
NK-cell enteropathy has an indolent clinical course that sometimes does not require treatment and spontaneously regresses. However, it is difficult to eradicate in persistent and symptomatic cases as it poorly responds to conventional chemotherapy. The newly identified *JAK3* mutations and activation of STAT5 pathway may represent a potential therapeutic target.

Differential Diagnosis
Other CD56-positive T cell or NK/T-cell CD56 lymphomas involving the GI tract including Monomorphic epitheliotropic intestinal T-cell lymphoma (MEATL) and extranodal NK/T-cell lymphoma (ENKTCL) (see Table 21.2-6)

> **Key Points**
>
> - It is an indolent NK-cell proliferation that is confined to the lamina propria and does not extend beyond the muscularis mucosa.
> - The atypical cells show NK-cell phenotype and lack clonality by T-cell gene rearrangement studies.
>
> **Diagnostic Caveats**
>
> - It is essential to differentiate NKLPD from NK/T-cell lymphoma arising in the gastrointestinal tract given the significant difference in clinical course and management. Sometimes NKLPD shows a high and misleading Ki-67 proliferation index and necrosis mimicking NK/T-cell lymphoma. However, other diagnostic features of NK/T-cell lymphoma are absent including angiodestruction, and diffuse EBV positivity by EBER ISH.

III. ENTEROPATHY-ASSOCIATED T-CELL LYMPHOMA

Enteropathy-associated T-cell lymphoma (EATL) is a rare and aggressive primary intestinal T-cell lymphoma that originates from intraepithelial (IEL) T cells. EATL diagnosis is either proceeded by, or established simultaneously with, the diagnosis of CD. It is more frequent in people of northern European descent and it is mostly associated with CD-related HLA (human leukocyte antigen) genotype (HLA-DQ2). It is a recognized entity in the previous and current WHO. The diagnostic criteria are summarized in Table 21.2-3.

> **Key Points**
>
> - EATL is an aggressive primary T-cell lymphoma and a recognized complication of celiac disease that may or may not be proceeded by RCD II.
> - The tumor cells are pleomorphic and express cCD3, CD103, and cytotoxic markers.
>
> **Diagnostic Caveats**
>
> - A history of celiac disease is not always available at the time of diagnosis.
> - Inflammatory cells can be so prominent that they obscure the neoplastic cells.
> - Granulomas are sometimes present causing confusion with Crohn's disease.
> - The neoplastic cells may show prominent anaplastic/large cell morphologic features and CD30 expression mimicking anaplastic large cell lymphoma (ALCL). A negative ALK will exclude ALK-positive ALCL. However, it is exceedingly difficult to distinguish such cases from ALK-negative ALCL.
> - EATL is an EBV-negative lymphoma, but sometimes few EBV-positive reactive lymphocytes are seen in the background and should not be confused with EBV-positive NK/T-cell lymphoma or angioimmunoblastic T-cell lymphoma (AITL).

Clinical Features

- **Clinical Presentation:** Clinical symptoms include abdominal pain (most commonly), intestinal obstruction, intestinal perforation, weight loss, and diarrhea with insensitivity to gluten-free diets.
- **Sites of Involvement:** Most common sites of involvement are the small intestine (90% of cases, particularly the jejunum), followed by the large intestine and

TABLE 21.2-3   WHO-HAEM5 Diagnostic Criteria for Enteropathy-Associated T-Cell Lymphoma

Essential

- Associated with CD and CD-related HLA genotype
- Destructive infiltrate composes of atypical pleomorphic medium to large lymphocytes and background inflammatory cells
- Uninvolved intestinal mucosa shows features of CD (villous atrophy, crypt hyperplasia, intraepithelial lymphocytosis).
- Phenotype: T cells with cytotoxic markers
- EBV is negative in the atypical cells.

Desirable

- Clonal TCR rearrangements (useful in distinguishing it from inflammatory infiltrate)
- CD103 staining supports its origin from IELs.
- CD30 is positive in large cells.

CD, celiac disease; EBV, Epstein-Barr virus; HLA, human leukocyte antigen; TCR, T-cell receptor.
Based on the WHO Classification of Tumours Editorial Board. Haematolymphoid tumours [Internet]. Lyon (France): International Agency for Research on Cancer; 2024 (WHO classification of tumours series, 5th ed.; vol. 11). Available from: https://tumourclassification.iarc.who.int/chapters/63.

stomach. Multiple lesions occur in 32% to 54% of cases. Reported extraintestinal sites involved by EATL include lymph nodes, bone marrow, liver, spleen, skin, lung, and central nervous system (CNS). EATL may be processed by refractory celiac disease (RCD), which is defined by irresponsiveness to gluten-free diet over 12 months, or it may arise de novo. RCD can be classified as type 1 (normal IEL lymphocyte phenotype) or type 2 (abnormal "clonal" IEL lymphocyte phenotype) (see Table 21.2-4 and e-Figure 21.2-2) (*Front Oncol.* 2023;13:1273305).

Morphology

Grossly, EATL may present as ulcerating nodules, stricture, or rarely as a mass lesion. Microscopically, it typically manifests as a polymorphic infiltration with intermediate to large malignant lymphoid cells mixed with reactive inflammatory cells including eosinophils, plasma cells, and histiocytes with variable intensity (e-Figure 21.2-3) (*Blood.* 2011;118:148-155). Granulomas are sometimes present, which can cause confusion with Crohn's disease. Other histologic features that also can be seen include angio-vascular proliferation, angio-vascular invasion, necrosis, and intraepithelial spread of tumor cells. Histopathologic changes typical of CD (villous atrophy, crypt hyperplasia, and IELs) may be seen in adjacent uninvolved intestinal segments. Infrequently, EATL presents as a monomorphic proliferation with a uniform immunoblastic/anaplastic appearance with prominent central nucleoli (e-Figure 21.2-4) (*Blood.* 2011;118:148-155).

Immunophenotype

The malignant cells are typically positive for cytoplasmic CD3, intraepithelial homing integrin CD103, and cytotoxic markers (TIA-1, granzyme B, and perforin). They are typically negative for surface CD3, CD5, CD4, CD8, CD56, TCRαβ, and TCRγδ. However, in a small subset of cases, CD8, intracellular TCR β (BF1), and TCR γ chain

TABLE 21.2-4 Comparison Between RCD I, RCD II, and EATL

	RCD I	RCD II	EATL
Disease behavior	Persistent auto-inflammatory immune response, gluten independent	Low-grade lymphoma (EATL in situ), gluten independent	High-grade lymphoma
Morphology	Mucosal pathologic changes are the same as in uncomplicated CD.	Villous atrophy is usually severe. The abnormal IELs lack significant cytologic atypia, and they can disseminate along the entire GI tract (or to extra-GI sites), with frequent infiltration of the lamina propria.	Atypical pleomorphic medium-sized cells with immunoblastic/anaplastic morphology that spread in the lamina propria and/or submucosa to transmural. The tumor may have a pronounced inflammatory background.
Immunophenotype[a]	sCD3+, cCD3+, CD5−/+, CD8+, CD103+	sCD3−, cCD3+, CD5−, CD8−, CD103+, CD30−	CD3+, CD5−, CD7+, CD4−, CD8−, CD56−, and CD103+, CD30+ in large cells[b]
T-cell receptor	Polyclonal	Monoclonal	Monoclonal
Progression to EATL	Low risk of EATL development (3%-14% within ~5 y)	High risk of EATL development (30%-52% within ~5 y)	

CD, ceCD, celiac disease; EATL, enteropathy-associated T-cell lymphoma; GI, gastrointestinal; IEL, intraepithelial; RCD, refractory celiac disease.
[a]A threshold of more than 20% of abnormal cells by flow cytometry is recommended in discriminating between RCD II from RCD I, and more than 50% of CD8−/CD4− T cells by immunohistochemical stains is recommended in discriminating RCD II IELs from reactive TCR g/d IELs.
[b]CD30 expression is considered an indicator of transformation to EATL.[b]CD30 expression is considered an indicator of transformation to EATL.

expression have been reported. CD30 is positive in cases with large cell morphology. Neoplastic cells are negative for anaplastic lymphoma kinase (ALK) and EBV.

Genetic Features

Studies using array-based approaches have identified recurrent chromosomal structural changes. For example, segmental gain of chromosome 9q or alternatively losses of chromosome 16q are noted in more than 80% of EATL cases. Other structural aberrations that have been reported include +1q (73%), +5q (80%), +8q (*MYC* gene) (27%), −9p (18%), −17p (*TP53* gene) (23%), and loss of heterozygosity (LOH) at 9p21 targeting the *CDKN2A/B* gene (56%). Targeted NGS studies have reported frequent mutations in the JAK (Janus kinase)/STAT pathway including activating mutations in *STAT5B* (26.5%-29%), *JAK1* (14.7%-23%), *JAK3* (23%-27.3%), and *STAT3* (12.1%-16%). *SETD2* was the most frequently silenced gene in EATL (32%) (*J Exp Med.* 2017;214:1371-1386).

Prognosis and Treatment

EATL has a poor prognosis and a poor response to conventional chemotherapeutic regimens such as the widely used CHOP (cyclophosphamide, hydroxydaunorubicin, oncovin, and prednisolone). Five-year survival rates range between 11% and 20% (*Blood.* 2011;118:148-155). Cases treated with autologous stem cell transplant (ASCT) following intensive chemotherapy, or CD30-targeted therapies (eg, brentuximab, vedotin) in CD30-positive cases have shown better survival outcomes.

Differential Diagnosis

- Inflammatory conditions: Both EATL and chronic inflammatory intestinal conditions may present with intestinal perforation, mucosal ulceration, and very prominent transmural mixed inflammatory cells. However, the T-lymphocytes in inflammatory conditions do not show overt cytologic atypia or phenotypic aberrancies and typically show a non-clonal pattern by TCR γ gene rearrangement PCR studies.
- Other intestinal T-cell lymphomas (see Table 21.2-6)

MONOMORPHIC EPITHELIOTROPIC INTESTINAL T-CELL LYMPHOMA

Monomorphic epitheliotropic intestinal T-cell lymphoma (MEITL) is a rare aggressive primary T-cell lymphoma derived from IELs and has no reported association with CD or celiac-related HLA genotype. It is more frequent in Asian and Hispanic populations than in Western and European populations. It is more common in the older adults with a median age 58 to 62 (age range: 23-89) with a male:female ratio of approximately 2:1. It is a recognized entity in the WHO and previously was known as enteropathy associated with T-cell lymphoma type II. The diagnostic criteria are summarized in Table 21.2-5.

Clinical Features

- **Clinical Presentation:** MEITL has an acute clinical presentation in more than 50% of cases with signs and symptoms that may include abdominal pain, perforation, diarrhea, weight loss, and features of obstruction (abdominal distention and vomiting) (*Cancers (Basel).* 2021;13:5774; *Ann Hematol.* 2019;98:2541-2550).
- **Sites of Involvement:** The small intestine, including the jejunum and ileum, is most frequently involved. The large intestine and stomach are less frequently involved. Cases with small intestine involvement, with or without large intestine involvement, tend to have a more advanced clinical course as opposed to those with an isolated large intestine involvement. Multifocal intestinal involvement at initial presentation is noted in 20% to 58% of cases. The disease may extend to abdominal/inguinal lymph nodes, omentum, lung, bone marrow, pelvic and abdominal organs, and the CNS (*Cancers (Basel).* 2021;13:5774; *Ann Hematol.* 2019;98:2541-2550).

TABLE 21.2-5 WHO-HAEM5 Diagnostic Criteria for Monomorphic Epitheliotropic Intestinal T-Cell Lymphoma

Essential

- No association with celiac disease or celiac disease-related HLA genotype, or histologic evidence of celiac disease in uninvolved mucosa
- Destructive infiltrate composes of atypical medium to large lymphocytes (typically monomorphic).
- Phenotype: T cells with cytotoxic markers
- EBV is negative in the atypical cells.

Desirable

- Clonal TCR rearrangements (useful in distinguishing it from inflammatory infiltrate)
- CD103 staining supports its origin from IELs.
- CD56 expression
- High MATK nuclear staining

EBV, Epstein-Barr virus; HLA, human leukocyte antigen; IEL, intraepithelial; MATK, megakaryocyte-associated tyrosine; TCR, T-cell receptor.
Modified from the WHO-HAEM5.

Morphology

Grossly, MEITL presents as single or multiple tumors with ulceration and occasional mesenteric lymph node involvement. Strictures are uncommon. Microscopically, MEITL is characterized by a dense monomorphic atypical lymphoid proliferation that is typically transmural. The lymphocytes are small to intermediate in size with round to slightly irregular nuclear contours, inconspicuous nucleoli, and a moderate amount of pale cytoplasm (monocytoid appearance) (e-Figure 21.2-5). Background inflammatory cells (plasma cells, eosinophils, small lymphocytes) may be present, but they are not prominent. The mucosal surface at the periphery of the lymphoma typically shows prominent IEL dissemination of the tumor cells and a variable degree of villous atrophy and crypt hyperplasia. An increase in IELs, with no overt cytologic atypia of the lymphocytes or changes in villous architecture, is frequently seen in noncontingent mucosa (*Cancers (Basel)*. 2021;13:5774).

Immunophenotype

Neoplastic cells typically express CD3, TIA-1 (e-Figure 21.2-5), CD8, and CD56 and lack CD5 and CD4 expression. Other cytotoxic markers including granzyme B and perforin are variably expressed. CD20 expression has been reported in approximately 20% of cases; however, other pan B-cell markers are negative. CD30 is usually negative. TCRγδ expression is noted in 78% of MEITL cases (*Cancers (Basel)*. 2021;13:5774). Cases with silent TCR expression (ie, negative for both TCRγδ and TCRαβ) are noted in 6% to 33% of cases. EBER ISH is typically negative. CD103 may or may not be positive. Prominent nuclear staining of megakaryocyte-associated tyrosine (MATK) (>80% of neoplastic cells) is observed in MEITL when compared to other T-cell lymphomas including EATL (*Leukemia*. 2011;25:555-557).

Genetic Features

MEITL is characterized by a clonal T-cell expansion by TCR γ gene rearrangement PCR testing. The disease also shares similar structural chromosomal abnormalities with EATL but with different frequencies. Gains at 9q and 8q24 (*MYC* gene amplification) are observed in 70% to 80% and 29% to 73% of cases, respectively. Gains at 1q and 5q are less common in MEITL than in EATL. Alterations leading to loss of function in *SETD2* (a tumor suppressor that encodes a lysine *N*-methyltransferase required for histone H3 lysine 36 trimethylation [H3K36me3]) are frequent. Also, like EATL, activating mutations in components of the JAK-STAT pathway is recurrent, with higher frequencies of mutations in *JAK3* and *STAT5B* genes (*Cancers (Basel)*. 2021;13:5774).

Prognosis and Treatment

There is no standardized treatment for MEITL. Similar to EATL, response to CHOP therapy is poor. Overall, 1- and 5-year survival are reported to be 36% to 57% and 32%, respectively (*Cancers (Basel)*. 2021;13:5774; *Ann Hematol*. 2019;98:2541-2550).

Differential Diagnosis

- Other intestinal T-cell lymphomas (Table 21.2-6)

Key Points

- MEITL is a high aggressive intestinal T-cell lymphoma not associated with celiac disease.
- It is characterized by a monomorphic deeply invasive lymphoid proliferation that typically expresses CD3, CD8, TIA-1, and CD56.

Diagnostic Caveats

- Abnormal expression of CD20 may lead to a misdiagnosis of B-cell lymphoma. Therefore, more than one B and T cell marker should be evaluated to avoid this pitfall.
- CD56 negativity may lead to difficulty in differentiating MEITL from EATL. A history of celiac disease and a polymorphic morphology would support EATL. Moreover, high levels of MATK nuclear staining would support MEITL over EATL.
- Cases with negative or partial CD8 expression may have immunophenotypic features indistinguishable from i-NKLPD. A positive clonal TCR gene rearrangement PCR test and a deep neoplastic lymphoid invasion beyond the muscularis mucosa would support MEITL.

IV. INTESTINAL T-CELL LYMPHOMA, NOS

Intestinal T-cell lymphoma, NOS (ITCL-NOS) is an aggressive T-cell lymphoma primarily involving the GI tract. The diagnosis is made after the exclusion of defined types of T- and NK-cell lymphoma involving the GI tract (see Table 21.2-6). The neoplastic cells are typically medium to large and involve the mucosa with frequent transmural infiltration. The prognosis is typically poor.

TABLE 21.2-6 Differential Diagnosis of Gastrointestinal T-Cell Lymphoma and NK- Lymphoma/Lymphoproliferative Disorder

Entity	EATL	MEITL	ALCL	ENKTC	ATLL	ITCL-GI	i-NKLPD
Clinical course	Aggressive	Aggressive	Aggressive	Aggressive	Aggressive	Indolent, low risk of progression	Indolent, no transformation
Morphology	• An infiltrate of pleomorphic medium-sized to large lymphoid cells • Variable inflammatory background • Uninvolved intestinal mucosa shows features of CD	• Dense infiltration by relatively monotonous medium-sized or occasionally large lymphoma cells • Typically lacking necrosis • Epitheliotropism is common. • No histologic evidence of CD in uninvolved mucosa	Diffuse and cohesive infiltrates of tumor cells, which are large including the presence of "hallmark cells."	• Infiltration of tissues by lymphoma cells with variable morphology and sizes • Angiocentric growth and necrosis	Infiltration of tissues by lymphoma cells with variable morphology and sizes, generally, medium to large in size, with nuclear pleomorphism and prominent convolutions and lobulation.	Nondestructive, predominantly non-epitheliotropic infiltrate of small mature lymphocytes confined to the GI mucosa	Nondestructive, predominantly non-epitheliotropic infiltrate of medium mature lymphocytes with occasional eosinophilic cytoplasmic granules, confined to the GI mucosa • No angiocentricity

	T-lineage, often with a CD4−, CD8− phenotype, with expression of cytotoxic markers	T-lineage, commonly CD3+, CD5−, CD4−, CD8+, with cytotoxic markers	Most express at least one T-cell marker. Cytotoxic markers are positive in a large subset of cases. EMA is positive in <50% of cases.	NK-cell phenotype or cytotoxic T-cell phenotype	T-lineage commonly CD4+ and CD25+	NK-cell phenotype	T-lineage (CD4+, CD8+; CD4+, CD8−; or CD4−/CD8−), with TCRαβ expression
CD56	Negative	Commonly positive	Positive in a small subset of cases	Commonly positive	Commonly negative	Commonly negative	Positive
CD103	Typically, positive	Typically, positive	Typically, negative	Typically, negative	Positive in a subset of cases (48%)	Typically, negative	Typically, negative
CD30	Positive (usually in cases of large cell or anaplastic morphology)	Negative	Positive (strong and uniform)	Variable	Variable	Negative	Negative

(*continued*)

TABLE 21.2-6　Differential Diagnosis of Gastrointestinal T-Cell Lymphoma and NK- Lymphoma/Lymphoproliferative Disorder *(continued)*

Entity	EATL	MEITL	ALCL	ENKTC	ATLL	ITCL-GI	i-NKLPD
MATK	No nuclear staining	Extensive nuclear expression (>80% of cells)	No nuclear staining	Variable amount of nuclear staining (20%-80%)	Unknown	Unknown	Unknown
ALK	Negative	Negative	Positive in 24% of GI-ALCL (ref)	Negative	Negative	Negative	Negative
Ki-67 index	Typically, high	Typically, high	Typically, high	Typically, high	Typically, high	Typically, low (<10%)	Variable, range 10%-90%
EBV (EBER) ISH	Negative	Negative	Negative	Diffusely positive in malignant cells	Negative	Negative	Negative
HTLV-1 antibody	Negative	Negative	Negative	Negative	Positive	Negative	Negative

ALCL, anaplastic large cell lymphoma; ALK, anaplastic lymphoma kinase; ATLL, adult T-cell leukemia/lymphoma; CD, celiac disease; EATL, enteropathy-associated T-cell lymphoma; EBV, Epstein-Barr virus; EMA, epithelial membrane antigen; ENKTCL, extranodal NK/T-cell lymphoma; GI, gastrointestinal; HTLV, human T-cell lymphotropic virus; i-NKLPD, indolent NK-cell lymphoproliferative disorder of the gastrointestinal tract; ISH, in situ hybridization; ITCL-GI, indolent T-cell lymphoma of the gastrointestinal tract; MATK, megakaryocyte-associated tyrosine; MEITL, monomorphic epitheliotropic intestinal T-cell lymphoma; NK, natural killer.

21.3 Hepatosplenic T-Cell Lymphoma

Omar M. Al-Rusan, Tanya Sajan Ponnatt, and Brooj Abro

Hepatosplenic T-cell lymphoma (HSTCL) is a rare aggressive extranodal lymphoma of cytotoxic T-cell lineage characterized by involvement of the liver, spleen, and bone marrow. It most commonly affects young adults (median age ~35 years). A recent study reported an increased incidence in older patients (>60 years) (*Am J Hematol.* 2020;95:151). The etiology is still largely unknown. Some cases are associated with immunodeficiency states and autoimmune disorders (*Hum Pathol.* 2018;74:5-16). The diagnostic criteria for HSTCL are summarized in Table 21.3-1.

Clinical Features

- **Clinical presentation:** Patients often present with hepatosplenomegaly and B symptoms. Common laboratory findings include cytopenias (most commonly thrombocytopenia), elevated lactate dehydrogenase (LDH), β_2-microglobulin, and elevated liver enzymes. Lymphadenopathy is typically absent.
- **Sites of involvement:** As the name implies, the liver and spleen are primarily involved. Bone marrow infiltration is nearly always present. Peripheral blood involvement can be present; however, lymphocytosis is uncommon. Other sites, such as lymph nodes and skin, are occasionally involved (*Virchows Arch.* 2016;469:591; *Hum Pathol.* 2018;74:5-16).

Morphology

HSTCL typically consists of small- to medium-sized lymphoid cells with irregular nuclear contours, inconspicuous nucleoli, and clear agranular cytoplasm. Blastoid morphology and marked pleomorphism may be present in some cases (*Blood.* 2003;102:4261). The diagnosis is usually made on bone marrow examination, which shows increased cellularity and a sinusoidal pattern of infiltrate (e-Figure 21.3-1). The

TABLE 21.3-1 Diagnostic Criteria for HSTCL

Essential

- Extranodal cytotoxic T-cell lymphoma with sinusoidal involvement of bone marrow, liver, or spleen
- Lymphoma cells are small to intermediate in size without intracytoplasmic granules.

Desirable

- Characteristic immunophenotype: $CD4^-$, $CD5^{-/+}$, $CD8^{-/+}$, $CD56^{+/-}$
- Detection of isochromosome (7q) and trisomy 8

HSTCL, hepatosplenic T-cell lymphoma.
Based on the WHO Classification of Tumours Editorial Board. Haematolymphoid tumours [Internet]. Lyon (France): International Agency for Research on Cancer; 2024 (WHO classification of tumours series, 5th ed.; vol. 11). Available from: https://tumourclassification.iarc.who.int/chapters/63.

findings may be subtle on hematoxylin and eosin (H&E) sections. Additionally, the background bone marrow may show dysplastic changes (*Hum Pathol*. 2016;50:109). Sinusoidal involvement is also prominent in the liver. In the spleen, the lymphoma cells primarily infiltrate the red pulp sinuses and cords, and the white pulp is atrophic. Hemophagocytosis may be present.

Immunophenotype

HSTCL is characterized by a cytotoxic T-cell phenotype. The tumor cells most commonly express CD3, CD2, TIA, granzyme M, and are typically negative for CD4. CD8 and CD5 are positive in a minority of cases. Natural killer (NK) cell markers such as CD56 and CD16 are often positive, and CD57 is negative. Granzyme B expression is present in a subset of cases. The majority of cases express T-cell receptor gamma/delta (TCR$\gamma\delta$), while some express T-cell receptor alpha/beta (TCR$\alpha\beta$). A small subset may lack T-cell receptor expression and are classified as TCR "null" or "silent" (*Am J Surg Pathol*. 2016;40:676). Epstein-Barr virus (EBV) in situ hybridization (EBER) is negative.

Genetic Features

Clonal TCR gene rearrangements are usually detected. Frequent cytogenetic abnormalities include isochromosome 7q (~70%) and/or trisomy 8 (~50%) (*Am J Surg Pathol*. 2017;41:82). Notably, approximately 40% of HSTCL cases have somatic mutations affecting the *STAT5B* gene, leading to constitutive activation of the *JAK-STAT* signaling pathway. Other mutations that have been reported include *SETD2*, *STAT3*, *INO80*, and *PIK3CD* (*Cancer Discov*. 2017;7:369).

Prognosis and Treatment

The prognosis for HSTCL is dismal, with a median survival of less than 1 to 2 years (*Clin Lymphoma Myeloma Leuk*. 2021;21:106). Most treatment regimens include aggressive combination chemotherapy, typically involving purine analogs and anthracyclines (*Blood*. 2020;136:2018). Hematopoietic stem cell transplant can be considered in some patients (*Leukemia*. 2015;29:686). HSTCL with the TCR$\alpha\beta$ phenotype is reported to have worse outcomes (*Am J Surg Pathol*. 2001;25:285).

Differential Diagnosis

- **T-cell large granular lymphocytic leukemia (T-LGLL):** Characterized by an indolent clinical course (most patients are asymptomatic). Lymphoma cells have abundant cytoplasmic azurophilic granules and are usually positive for CD8, CD57, and TCR$\alpha\beta$.
- Other mature T-cell lymphomas involving the bone marrow, liver, and/or spleen should be excluded using flow cytometry, immunohistochemical studies, and EBV in situ hybridization (EBER).

SUGGESTED READINGS

Vega F, Amador C, Chadburn A, et al. American registry of pathology expert opinions: recommendations for the diagnostic workup of mature T cell neoplasms. *Ann Diagn Pathol*. 2020;49:151623.

Yabe M, Miranda RN, Medeiros LJ. Hepatosplenic T-cell lymphoma: a review of clinicopathologic features, pathogenesis, and prognostic factors. *Hum Pathol*. 2018;74:5-16.

> **Key Points**
>
> - HSTCL is a mature extranodal T-cell lymphoma with a cytotoxic phenotype characterized by involvement of the liver, spleen, and bone marrow.
> - The diagnosis is commonly made on bone marrow examination, which shows a sinusoidal pattern of involvement.
> - Characteristic immunophenotype: CD3$^+$, CD2$^+$, TIA$^+$, granzyme M$^+$, TCRγδ$^+$, CD4$^-$, CD8$^{-/+}$, CD5$^{-/+}$, CD56$^{+/-}$, CD16$^{+/-}$, CD57$^{-/+}$
>
> **Diagnostic Caveats**
>
> - The findings on bone marrow biopsy may be subtle on H&E sections.
> - Clinical suspicion for HSTCL may not be high initially, as it lacks the typical presentation of a lymphoma (eg, lymphadenopathy).
> - Other T-cell lymphomas should be excluded, especially T-LGL, which also shows a sinusoidal pattern of infiltrate and is an indolent lymphoma whereas, HSTCL has an aggressive clinical course with poor outcomes.

21.4 Epstein Bar Virus-Positive NK-/T-Cell Lymphomas

Tiffany Javadi and Brooj Abro

I. EXTRANODAL NK-/T-CELL LYMPHOMA

According to the WHO-HAEM5, extranodal natural killer (NK-)/T-cell lymphoma (ENKTL) can be further categorized into two clinical subtypes, nasal-type and nonnasal, based on the site of primary tumor. The nasal subtype is more common, accounting for 80% of ENKTL cases, while the nonnasal subtype makes up the remaining 20%. The tumor cells are positive for Epstein-Barr virus (EBV), exhibit a cytotoxic NK-/T-cell phenotype, and are frequently associated with angiodestruction and prominent necrosis. ENKTL is more common in men (male-to-female ratio of ~3:1) and typically affects adults from Southeast Asia and indigenous populations of Central and South America. The diagnostic criteria for extranodal NK-/T-cell lymphoma are summarized in Table 21.4-1.

Clinical Features

- **Clinical presentation:** Patients with nasal ENKTL present with nasal obstruction, discharge, bleeding, facial swelling, proptosis, sinus infection, and vision problems, which may vary depending on the extent of invasion. In advanced stages, patients display clinical symptoms specific to the organ(s) involved. Hemophagocytic syndrome and pancytopenia can be seen with bone marrow involvement (*Front Oncol.* 2021;11:704962). Patients with nonnasal ENKTL usually present with clinical symptoms similar to those with advanced-stage nasal ENKTL (*Ann Hematol.* 2009;2:185-187).
- **Sites of involvement:** Nasal-type ENKTL primarily affects the nasal cavity, nasopharynx, and paranasal sinuses, with less frequent involvement of the upper

TABLE 21.4-1 WHO-HAEM5 Diagnostic Criteria for Extranodal NK-/T-Cell Lymphoma

Essential
- Tumor cells with variable morphology and cytotoxic NK-/T-cell phenotype
- The majority of tumor cells are EBER+.
- Involvement of extranodal sites

Desirable
- Angiocentric/angioinvasive tumor with necrosis

EBER, EBV-encoded small RNA; NK, natural killer.
Based on the WHO Classification of Tumours Editorial Board. Haematolymphoid tumours [Internet]. Lyon (France): International Agency for Research on Cancer; 2024 (WHO classification of tumours series, 5th ed.; vol. 11). Available from: https://tumourclassification.iarc.who.int/chapters/63.

aerodigestive tract. Lesions in the nasal cavity can extend into the face and orbit, causing destruction of the hard palate and visual symptoms. Regional lymph-node involvement and systemic spread can occur, most commonly to the skin, gastrointestinal tract, testis, soft tissue, liver, spleen, or bone marrow. Nonnasal ENKTL is multifocal, with primary sites similar to those involved in advanced stages of nasal ENKTL. If nasal involvement is discovered, these cases should be reclassified as advanced-stage nasal-type ENKTL.

Morphology

ENKTL usually consists of a diffuse polymorphic infiltrate. The range of tumor cell size varies, spanning from small to medium, large, and even anaplastic cells. Most commonly, the tumor shows medium-sized cells or a combination of small and large cells (e-Figure 21.4-1). The tumor cells display irregularly folded nuclei with inconspicuous nucleoli, granular chromatin, and moderate pale-to-clear cytoplasm. Admixed inflammatory cells composed of small lymphocytes, plasma cells, histiocytes, and eosinophils are often seen. Mitoses and apoptotic bodies are frequent. Angiocentric and angiodestructive growth and extensive coagulative necrosis are often observed but not always present (e-Figure 21.4-2). When mucosal and cutaneous sites are involved, ulceration, inflammation, and pseudoepitheliomatous hyperplasia may be present, mimicking squamous cell carcinoma.

Immunophenotype

ENKTL is characterized by tumor cells of cytotoxic NK- or T-cell lineage, with most of the tumor cells testing positive for EBV-encoded small RNA (EBER) by in situ hybridization. Determining NK- versus T-cell lineage is not always possible and does not have therapeutic or prognostic significance (*Mod Pathol*. 2016;29:430-443). The tumor cells are typically positive for CD43, CD45, cytoplasmic CD3, CD2, cytotoxic markers (granzyme-B, TIA-1, perforin), and CD56. Approximately 50% of cases show variable expression of CD30 (*Am J Surg Pathol*. 2013;37:14-23). Surface CD3 and other NK- and T-cell markers (CD5, CD4, CD8, CD16, CD57, TCR-αβ, and TCR-γδ) are often negative. However, T-cell lineage ENKTL may express CD5, CD8, and TCR-αβ or TCR-γδ. A small subset of cases are negative for CD56, and CD56-negative phenotype is more common in T-cell lineage ENKTL (*Am J Surg*

Pathol. 2012;36:481-499). Other reported positive markers in ENKTL include PD-1, CXCL13, MUM1, and CD25, among others (*Am J Surg Pathol.* 2012;36:481-499).

Genetic Features

Clonal TCR gene rearrangements are observed in T-cell lineage tumors. The deletion of 6q21-25 is the most common cytogenetic abnormality. Frequently mutated genes include the RNA helicase gene *DDX3X*; genes associated with the JAK-STAT signaling pathway (eg, *STAT3, STAT5B*); epigenetic modifiers such as *MLL2, ARID1A, EP300,* and *ASXL3;* and tumor suppressor genes like *TP53* and *MGA*, among others (*Nat Genet.* 2015;47:1061-1066).

Prognosis and Treatment

ENKTL is an aggressive disease. Early-stage disease has better outcomes, and treatment options include chemotherapy and radiation. Studies have shown that administering L-asparaginase–based chemotherapy regimens sequentially, followed by radiotherapy, results in long-lasting remission in up to 80% of patients with stage I/II cancer (*Ann Oncol.* 2018;29:256-263). Several factors have been incorporated into a prognostic index for ENTKTL (PINK-E), which predict poor outcomes: age over 60 years, stage III or IV disease, distant lymph-node involvement, nonnasal-type disease, and detectable plasma EBV DNA (*Lancet Oncol.* 2016;17:389-400).

Differential Diagnosis

The differential diagnosis includes other EBV-positive T- and NK-cell lymphomas, such as EBV+ nodal T-/NK-cell lymphoma and aggressive NK-cell leukemia (ANKL). Unlike ENKTL, EBV+ nodal T-/NK-cell lymphoma primarily manifests as a nodal disease, usually without angioinvasion or coagulative necrosis. The tumor cells often exhibit large size with centroblastoid morphology (resembling diffuse large B-cell lymphoma [DLBCL]), and T-cell lineage is more common (see details later). ANKL presents with prominent systemic symptoms and involvement of blood and bone marrow (see Table 21.4-2).

Key Points

- Clinically, ENKTL can be divided into nasal and nonnasal subtypes, with the former accounting for ~80% of the cases.
- ENKTL is characterized by tumor cells with a cytotoxic NK-/T-cell phenotype and consistent EBV positivity.
- The tumor cells vary in morphology and are frequently associated with necrosis and angiodestruction.

Diagnostic Caveats

- Some cases of ENKTL that appear to be nonnasal at presentation may show occult nasal involvement upon careful clinical and radiologic evaluation. Such cases should be classified as nasal-type ENKTL.

II. EBV-POSITIVE NODAL T-/NK-CELL LYMPHOMA

EBV-positive nodal T- and NK-cell lymphoma (EBV+ NTNKL) is now recognized as a distinct entity by both the WHO-HAEM5 and International Consensus Classification (ICC). Previously, in the WHO-HAEM4R, such cases were merged under

TABLE 21.4-2   WHO-HAEM5 Diagnostic Criteria for EBV+ Nodal T- and NK-Cell Lymphoma

Essential

- Cytotoxic T- or NK-cell lineage and the majority of tumor cells are EBER-positive.
- Lymph nodes are primarily involved with limited extranodal involvement and no nasal involvement.
- Exclusion of other NK-/T-cell lymphoproliferative disorders and lymphomas associated with EBV and immune deficiency

EBER, EBV-encoded small RNA; EBV, Epstein-Barr virus; NK, natural killer.

Based on the WHO Classification of Tumours Editorial Board. Haematolymphoid tumours [Internet]. Lyon (France): International Agency for Research on Cancer; 2024 (WHO classification of tumours series, 5th ed.; vol. 11). Available from: https://tumourclassification.iarc.who.int/chapters/63.

---

the peripheral T-cell lymphoma (PTCL), not otherwise specified (NOS) category. As suggested by its name, EBV-positive NTNKL predominantly manifests in the lymph nodes, with most of the tumor cells testing positive for EBV. The tumor cells often show a cytotoxic T-cell phenotype and, rarely, an NK-cell phenotype. This rare lymphoma typically affects East Asian adults, with a higher prevalence in males. The diagnostic challenge lies in excluding morphologic mimics such as extranodal NK-/T-cell lymphoma (ENKTL), immune deficiency–associated NK-/T-cell lymphoproliferative disorders, EBV-positive lymphoproliferative diseases of childhood, and NK-cell leukemia with secondary nodal involvement. The diagnostic criteria for ENKTL are summarized in Table 21.4-1.

Clinical Features

- **Clinical presentation:** Most patients present with advanced disease stage, systemic lymphadenopathy, and constitutional B symptoms. Clinical features may include splenomegaly, hepatomegaly, and elevated liver enzymes. Thrombocytopenia is the most frequently reported hematologic abnormality at presentation, followed by anemia and leukopenia (*Hum Pathol.* 2015;46(7):981-990).
- **Sites of involvement:** EBV+ NTNKL primarily involves the lymph nodes. It can also involve one or more extranodal sites, with the liver and/or bone marrow being the most common. Lack of nasal involvement is an essential criterion outlined by the WHO.

Morphology

Typically, a diffuse infiltrate of medium to large cells with centroblastoid features (resembling DLBCL) is identified on biopsy of an involved lymph node. In contrast, tumor cells in ENKTL typically show irregularly shaped nuclei. Pleomorphic or mixed-cell morphology is occasionally observed. Angiocentric growth and coagulative necrosis are usually lacking (*Am J Surg Pathol.* 2015;39:462).

Immunophenotype

EBV+ NTNKL is usually of T-cell lineage and commonly shows expression of CD3, CD2, and TCR-β and cytotoxic molecules such as TIA1, granzyme-B, and perforin. TCR-γ is expressed by a minority of cases, and a subset of cases are negative for both TCR-β and TCR-γ. CD8 is positive in most cases (>60%), whereas CD56 is positive in a small subset of cases (<30%). Most of the tumor cells are positive for EBV. Typically, CD4 and CD5 are negative; however, in a few instances, these markers may be expressed (*Hum Pathol.* 2015;46(7):981-990). NK-cell lineage cases are negative for TCR protein expression and clonal *TCR* gene rearrangements.

Genetic Features

Demonstration of clonal TCR gene rearrangements supports T-cell lineage (negative in NK-cell lineage tumors). Most cases show loss of 14q11.2 (correlates with loss of TCR loci and T-cell lineage), and other cytogenetic abnormalities have also been identified (*Haematologica.* 2018;103:278-287). A recent study showed that EBV+ NTNKL cases frequently demonstrate mutations involving *TET2*, *PIK3CD,* and *STAT3* genes. This study also showed that, in comparison to PTCL-NOS and ENKTL, EBV-positive T-/NK-cell lymphoma shows low genomic instability, upregulation of immune pathways, and downregulation of EBV miRNA (*Haematologica.* 2022;107:1864-1879).

Prognosis and Treatment

The clinical course of EBV+ NTNKL is extremely aggressive, with a poor response to conventional chemotherapy regimens and an overall median survival of less than 12 months (*Int J Hematol.* 2016;5:591-595). The overall prognosis tends to be worse than that of ENKTL and PTCL-NOS.

Differential Diagnosis

The differential diagnosis includes other EBV+ T- and NK-cell lymphomas/leukemias. A combination of histologic, immunophenotypic, and clinical features, including demographics, disease presentation, and sites of involvement, is essential to reach a definitive diagnosis (see Table 21.4-3).

Key Points and Diagnostic Caveats

- Previously merged under the PTCL-NOS category, EBV+ NTNKL is now considered a distinct entity by the WHO-HAEM5 and ICC.
- The tumor cells typically show centroblastoid morphology and are positive for EBER.
- The disease is primarily nodal.
- The diagnosis requires the exclusion of other EBV+ T-/NK-cell lymphomas.

TABLE 21.4-3 Key Features of EBV-Positive T- and NK-Cell Lymphomas/Leukemias

	Clinical Features	Phenotype
Extranodal NK-/T-cell lymphoma	• Commonly affects middle-aged adults • Extranodal disease • Majority (~80%) have nasal involvement.	• NK-cell lineage > T-cell lineage • Usually CD4$^-$ and CD8$^-$ • CD56$^+$ in majority
EBV+ nodal T-/NK-cell lymphoma	• Most patients are older adults (>60 years) • Primarily nodal disease • No nasal involvement	• T-cell lineage > NK-cell lineage • CD8$^+$ > CD4$^+$ in T-cell lineage • CD56$^+$ in minority of cases
Aggressive NK-cell leukemia	• Children and young adults • Systemic disease • Commonly involves liver, spleen, and bone marrow	• NK-cell lineage • CD4$^-$ and CD8$^-$ • CD56$^+$
Systemic chronic active EBV disease	• No nasal involvement • Commonly associated with hemophagocytic lymphohistiocytosis (HLH)	• T-cell lineage > NK-cell lineage • CD4$^+$ > CD8$^+$ in T-cell lineage • CD56$^+$ in NK-cell lineage
Systemic EBV+ T-cell lymphoma of childhood		• T-cell lineage • CD8 > CD4 • CD56$^-$

EBV, Epstein-Barr virus; NK, natural killer.

SUGGESTED READINGS

Ng SB, Chung TH, Kato S, et al. Epstein-Barr virus-associated primary nodal T/NK-cell lymphoma shows a distinct molecular signature and copy number changes. *Haematologica*. 2018;103(2):278-287.

Tse E, Kwong YL. The diagnosis and management of NK/T-cell lymphomas. *J Hematol Oncol*. 2017;10(1):85.

21.5 Anaplastic Large Cell Lymphomas

Alnoor and John L. Frater

Historically, a group of hematopoietic neoplasms with strong Ki-1 expression (CD30 antigen) was recognized as Ki-lymphoma regardless of B-cell, T-cell, or null phenotype. Later, this term was replaced by anaplastic large cell lymphoma (ALCL) and was recognized as a distinct category of T-cell lymphoma by the WHO Classification. Subsequently, it was discovered that the expression of anaplastic lymphoma kinase (ALK), a hybrid protein product of *NPM1::ALK* translocation or t(2;5)(p23;q35), is positive in a subset of ALCL cases. As a result, ALCLs were divided into two subgroups: ALK-positive ALCL and ALK-negative ALCL, a relatively heterogeneous disease with morphologic and immunophenotypic features that overlap with the former. Other distinct types of ALCL include breast implant–associated ALCL (BIA-ALCL) and primary cutaneous ALCL (discussed in Chapter 21.6).

The common feature among all these neoplasms is the uniform strong expression of CD30 by immunohistochemistry (IHC). However, it should be noted that CD30 can be expressed by other nonhematopoietic and hematopoietic neoplasms. Most notably, ALK-negative ALCL must be distinguished from peripheral T-cell lymphoma, not otherwise specified (PTCL, NOS), which may also express CD30.

I. ANAPLASTIC LYMPHOMA KINASE–POSITIVE ANAPLASTIC LARGE CELL LYMPHOMA

ALK-positive ALCL is a mature T-cell lymphoma with uniform strong CD30 and ALK expression. It is a rare lymphoma that is relatively common in pediatric and young patients. The diagnostic criteria are summarized in Table 21.5-1.

TABLE 21.5-1 WHO-HAEM5 Diagnostic Criteria for ALK-Positive Anaplastic Large Cell Lymphoma

Essential	Desirable
• ALK expression in lymphoma cells • Characteristic strong uniform expression of CD30 in lymphoma cells	• For cases that show downregulation or deletion of most T-cell-associated antigens, demonstration of clonal T-cell populations by TCR gene rearrangement may confirm the neoplastic process.

ALK, anaplastic lymphoma kinase.
Based on the WHO Classification of Tumours Editorial Board. Haemolymphoid tumours [Internet]. Lyon (France): International Agency for Research on Cancer; 2024 (WHO classification of tumours series, 5th ed.; vol. 11). Available from: https://tumourclassification.iarc.who.int/chapters/63.

Clinical Features

- **Clinical presentation:** Patients with ALK-positive ALCL usually present with advanced clinical stages (stages III and IV). The median age is 30 years, with male predominance. About 75% of patients show B symptoms. Occasionally, leukemic presentations have been reported (*J Pediatr Hematol Oncol.* 2008;30(9):696-700).
- **Sites of involvement:** Lymph nodes are commonly involved. Extranodal sites often include skin, soft tissue, lungs, and, less frequently, mediastinum. Bone marrow involvement is seen in 10% to 30% of cases. Central nervous system is rarely involved.

Morphology

- **Lymph nodes:** The morphologic spectrum of ALCL is variable. In lymph nodes, the neoplastic cells show various patterns of involvement, including paracortical, perifollicular, sinusoidal, intravascular, and diffuse. These cells are large pleomorphic, with amphophilic cytoplasm and single to multiple nuclei. The hallmark cell is called "horseshoe" cell due to its kidney-shaped nucleus, multiple prominent nucleoli, and perinuclear large eosinophilic Golgi region (e-Figure 21.5A). Necrosis can be present.
- **Bone marrow:** Bone marrow involvement can be subtle, and the neoplastic cells are observed in clusters in a sinusoidal or interstitial pattern.
- **Blood:** Neoplastic cells are medium to large atypical-appearing lymphocytes with irregular and variable numbers of nuclei.
- **Uncommon histologic variants:** Small cell variant (perivascular pattern of growth pattern), lymphohistiocytic variant (diffuse histiocytic infiltration), and Hodgkin-like

Immunophenotype

The neoplastic cells characteristically express uniform and strong CD30 (cell membrane and Golgi pattern) (e-Figure 21.5B) and ALK (e-Figure 21.5C). The ALK expression pattern can correlate with underlying genetic alterations (summarized in Table 21.5-2). CD2, CD4, and CD43 are commonly expressed T-cell-associated antigens. Lack of T-cell antigen expression is common, including loss of CD3; sometimes, leading to a "null" immunophenotype. Other positive markers include cytotoxic stains (TIA-1, granzyme B, and perforin), MUM1, CD25, clusterin, BCL6, aberrant epithelial markers including epithelial membrane antigen (EMA) and cytokeratins, myeloid-associated antigens (CD13 and CD33), and CD56. Epstein-Barr virus (EBV)-encoded small RNA (EBER) is always negative. B-cell markers and CD15 are usually absent. The neoplastic cells may lack CD45, betaF1, and TCR-δ.

Genetic Features

The *ALK* gene rearrangement (chromosome 2p23) is the primary pathogenic event with over 20 partner genes (*Semin Diagn Pathol.* 2020;37(1):57-71). The most observed fusion is t(2;5)(p23;q35) or *NPM1::ALK*, which results in the abnormal activation of numerous downstream cell signaling pathways (*Mol Cell Biol.* 1998;18(12):6951-6961). T-cell receptor gene rearrangement is often positive and can be helpful in cases with a null immunophenotype.

TABLE 21.5-2 ALK Expression Pattern in ALCL With an Underlying Genetic Abnormality

Chromosomal Abnormality	*ALK* Partner Gene	ALK Staining Pattern
t(2;5)(p23;q35)	NPM1	Nucleus and cytoplasmic
t(1;2)(q25;p23)	TPM3	Strong cytoplasmic and membrane
Inv(2)(p23q53)	ATIC	Diffuse cytoplasmic
t(2;3)(p23;q21)	TFG	Diffuse cytoplasmic
t(2;17)(p23;q23)	CLTC	Granular cytoplasmic
t(2;X)(p23;q11.12)	MSN	Membranous
t(2;19)(p23;p13.1)	TPM4	Diffuse cytoplasmic
t(2;22)(p23;q11.2)	MYH9	Diffuse cytoplasmic
t(2;9)(p23;q33-34)	TRAF1	Diffuse cytoplasmic
t(2;11)(2p23;11q12.3)	EEF1G	Diffuse cytoplasmic
t(2;17)(p23;q25)	RNF213/ALO17	Diffuse cytoplasmic

ALCL, anaplastic large cell lymphoma; ALK, anaplastic lymphoma kinase.
Based on the WHO Classification of Tumours Editorial Board. Haematolymphoid tumours [Internet]. Lyon (France): International Agency for Research on Cancer; 2024 (WHO classification of tumours series, 5th ed.; vol. 11). Available from: https://tumourclassification.iarc.who.int/chapters/63.

Prognosis and Treatment

The long-term survival is up to 80% (*Haematologica.* 2019;104(12):e562-e565). Poor prognostic factors include disease progression while receiving chemotherapy, central nervous system (CNS) involvement, and leukemic presentation.

Key Points

- Mature T-cell lymphoma is composed of cohesive pleomorphic neoplastic cells with abundant cytoplasm, multilobated nuclei, and often contains hallmark cells.
- Must express CD30 (uniform and strong) and ALK
- Loss of T-cell antigen(s) including CD3 is not an uncommon feature.
- t(2;5)(p23;q35)/*ALK::NPM1* is the frequent genetic alteration.
- Overall, ALK-positive ALCL is associated with good prognosis.

Diagnostic Caveats

- Must be differentiated from CD30-positive lymphomas including classic Hodgkin lymphoma; PTCL, NOS; and ALK-negative ALCL
- ALK expression is also seen in solid tumors including lung adenocarcinoma.

II. ANAPLASTIC LYMPHOMA KINASE–NEGATIVE ANAPLASTIC LARGE CELL LYMPHOMA

ALK-negative ALCL is a systemic mature T-cell lymphoma with uniform strong CD30 expression that lacks ALK expression or *ALK* rearrangement. The diagnostic criteria are summarized in Table 21.5-3.

TABLE 21.5-3 WHO-HAEM5 Diagnostic Criteria for ALK-Negative Anaplastic Large Cell Lymphoma

Essential

- **Morphology:** Complete or partial infiltration of lymph node or extranodal tissue by large pleomorphic cells with lobated nuclei, distinct nucleoli, including "hallmark cells"
- **Immunophenotype:**
  1. Uniform strong expression of CD30
  2. Absence of ALK protein expression or *ALK* rearrangement
  3. Negative for EBV

Desirable

- Expression of T-cell markers and cytotoxic markers, albeit with frequent losses
- Clonal rearrangement of TCR gene

ALK, anaplastic lymphoma kinase; EBV, Epstein-Barr virus.
Based on the WHO Classification of Tumours Editorial Board. Haematolymphoid tumours [Internet]. Lyon (France): International Agency for Research on Cancer; 2024 (WHO classification of tumours series, 5th ed.; vol. 11). Available from: https://tumourclassification.iarc.who.int/chapters/63.

Clinical Features

- **Clinical presentation:** Most ALK-negative ALCLs occur in adults with a median age of 54 years and with no clear male or female predominance. Patients usually present with a higher-stage disease (stage III or IV).
- **Sites of involvement:** ALK-negative ALCL is a systemic disease and usually presents with lymph node and/or extranodal involvement. Skin involvement by ALK-negative ALCL must be distinguished from primary cutaneous ALCL.

Morphology

The morphologic features are similar to ALK-positive ALCL as described previously, including the presence of hallmark cells and cohesive sinusoidal or diffuse infiltrates of large pleomorphic neoplastic cells with lobated vesicular nuclei and prominent nucleoli. A characteristic "doughnut cell" can be seen in ALK-negative ALCL with *DUSP22* rearrangement. A "starry-sky" appearance is occasionally observed with a high mitotic rate.

Immunophenotype

The neoplastic cells show a uniform strong CD30 expression with membranous and Golgi pattern. ALK expression is negative. More than half of all cases express one or more T-cell antigens. CD3, CD2, and CD4 expression is common, while CD8 expression is rare. Frequent loss of T-cell antigen(s) expression is not uncommon, and occasionally, a complete loss of all T-cell markers, null phenotype, is observed. In null-phenotype cases, the diagnosis of a classic Hodgkin lymphoma (CHL) must be ruled out. PAX5 is a useful marker in such cases; however, rare cases have aberrant B-cell marker expression, and molecular testing can be helpful in ambiguous cases. Clusterin and MUM1 are frequently expressed, with EMA expression observed in less than 50% of cases. One or more cytotoxic markers, granzyme, TIA-1, and perforin, are expressed in ALK-negative ALCL but rarely in *DUSP22*-rearranged tumors. LEF1 is specially expressed in *DUSP22*-rearranged tumors (*Am J Surg Pathol.* 2021;45(4):550-557). EBER expression is consistently negative (Hematopathology, Chapter 37, 673-691.e5).

Genetic Features

Most cases show T-cell receptor gene rearrangement. Recurrent rearrangements of the *DUSP22-IRF4* locus at 6p25.3 occur in 30% of cases, and these cases lack STAT3 activation. *TP63* rearrangements as an inv(3)(q26q28) involving *TBL1XR1* have been reported in 5% to 8% of ALK-negative ALCL (*Blood.* 2012;120(11):2280-2289; *Blood.* 2014;124(9):1473-1480).

Prognosis and Treatment

The prognosis of systemic ALK-negative ALCL is better than CD30-expressing PTCL, NOS and worse than ALK-positive ALCL using conventional chromotherapy. *DUSP22*-rearranged tumors have a survival similar to ALK-positive ALCL; however, some cases have an adverse prognosis in recent studies. Interleukin-2α (IL-2α) overexpression, *TP63* rearrangements, and *TP53* loss are associated with poor outcomes.

> **Key Points**
>
> - A mature T-cell lymphoma is composed of cohesive pleomorphic neoplastic cells with abundant cytoplasm, and multilobated nuclei that contain hallmark cells.
> - Must express CD30 (uniform and strong) and negative for ALK expression and rearrangement
> - Loss of T-cell antigen(s) including null phenotype can be seen.
> - *DUSP22* or *TP63* rearrangements are seen in a subset of cases.
> - Overall survival is poorer than ALK-positive ALCL.
>
> **Diagnostic Caveats**
>
> - Must be differentiated from other CD30-positive lymphomas including classic Hodgkin lymphoma; PTCL, NOS; primary cutaneous ALCL; and ALK-positive ALCL.
> - Cases with cohesive morphology and null phenotype can mimic carcinoma and require comprehensive IHC evaluation for a definitive diagnosis.
> - T- and B-cell clonality studies can be helpful in cases with ambiguous antigen expression (T- and B-cell markers).

III. BREAST IMPLANT–ASSOCIATED ANAPLASTIC LARGE CELL LYMPHOMA

BIA-ALCL is a CD30-positive mature T-cell lymphoma that arises in association with breast implant that lacks ALK expression or *ALK* rearrangement. The diagnostic criteria are summarized in Table 21.5-4.

Clinical Features

- **Clinical presentation:** The median time from implant placement to the diagnosis of BIA-ALCL is approximately 10 years (range: 2-32 years) (*J Clin Oncol.* 2014;32(2):114-120). Most patients present with seroma, a peri-implant

TABLE 21.5-4 WHO-HAEM5 Diagnostic Criteria Breast Implant–Associated Anaplastic Large Cell Lymphoma

Essential	Desirable
• Presence of breast implant; CD30+ lymphoma cells with anaplastic features • Proven T-cell lineage supported by expression of one or more T-lineage markers and/or clonal TCR gene rearrangement	• Identification of lymphoma cells on luminal side of capsule on properly oriented sections

Based on the WHO Classification of Tumours Editorial Board. Haematolymphoid tumours [Internet]. Lyon (France): International Agency for Research on Cancer; 2024 (WHO classification of tumours series, 5th ed.; vol. 11). Available from: https://tumourclassification.iarc.who.int/chapters/63.

fluid accumulation. A subset of patients presents with mass lesions and regional lymphadenopathy.

- **Sites of involvement:** BIA-ALCL is limited to peri-implant fibrous capsule in most cases. In some cases, the lymphoma presents as a mass infiltrating the breast and adjacent soft tissue. Regional lymph nodes may be involved; however, systemic disease is rare.

Morphology

The capsulectomy specimen shows the neoplastic cells usually line the inner surface of the capsule in a fibrinonecrotic background (e-Figure 21.5D). In higher stages of the disease, the neoplastic cells can be seen infiltrating beyond the capsule into the adjacent breast parenchyma and soft tissue. These cells are large and pleomorphic with abundant eosinophilic, amphophilic, or clear cytoplasm, oval to multilobed nuclei, and variable-sized prominent nucleoli. The hallmark cells may be seen. Reactive mixed inflammatory infiltrates of histiocytes and eosinophils are also seen. Lymph node involvement is frequently sinusoidal, and some cases mimic classic CHL.

Immunophenotype

The neoplastic cells show uniform strong CD30 expression. ALK and EBER are always negative. The T-cell-associated markers (CD3, CD5, and CD7) are frequently lost. The neoplastic cells commonly express CD4, CD43, MUM1, GATA3, cytotoxic markers (TIA1 and granzyme B), CD25, and EMA (variable). CD8-positive or CD4/CD8 double-positive cases are rare. Approximately 20% of cases express either α-β or γ-δ T-cell receptor protein.

Genetic Features

Somatic mutations of *STAT3, STAT5B, JAK1, JAK2, SOCS1*, and *SOCS3* and/or amplifications of the JAK/STAT signaling pathway are common genetic alterations in BIA-ALCL (*J Clin Oncol.* 2014;32(2):114-120). The characteristic loss of 20q13.12-13.2 is considered specific for BIA-ALCL (*Blood.* 2020;136(25):2927-2932).

Staging

- T1: Tumor in fluid or confined at the inner surface of the capsule
- T2: Superficial infiltration of the capsule
- T3: Deep infiltration of the capsule with lymphoma cells admixed with inflammatory cells
- T4: Extension beyond the limits of capsule, into the soft tissue or into breast parenchyma

Clinical stages IIB-III-IV include regional (N1) and distant lymph node involvement and disseminated disease (M1).

Prognosis and Treatment

The complete excision of the capsule and implant is curative in nearly 100% of patients with effusion only (*J Clin Oncol.* 2016;34(2):160-168). The 5-year overall survival rate is 83.7% for patients with disease beyond the capsule, and 75% for patients with lymph node involvement (*Am J Surg Pathol.* 2018;42(3):293-305). The poor outcome is in patients with advanced disease with a nonresectable mass and disseminated disease.

> ### Key Points
>
> - BIA-ALCL are mature T-cell lymphomas that arise in association with breast implants that express uniform strong CD30 and lack ALK expression or *ALK* rearrangement.
> - Morphologically similar to other ALCL types. Null immunophenotype is frequently observed.
> - Loss of 20q13.12-13.2 is the characteristic finding.
> - Careful gross and morphologic examination is required for accurate staging.
> - Excellent prognosis
>
> **Diagnostic Caveats**
>
> - Can mimic carcinoma, and diagnosis can be challenging in cases with loss of lymphoid markers
> - EBV-positive fibrin-associated large B-cell lymphomas can involve breast implants. BIA-ALCL is EBER negative.
> - Must be differentiated from systemic ALCL involving the breast

SUGGESTED READINGS

Campo E, Jaffe ES, Cook JR, et al. The International Consensus Classification of mature lymphoid neoplasms: a report from the Clinical Advisory Committee [published correction appears in *Blood.* 2023;141(4):437]. *Blood.* 2022;140(11):1229-1253. doi:10.1182/blood.2022015851

Falini B, Stain H, Lamant-Rochaix L, et al. Anaplastic large cell lymphoma, ALK-positive. In: Swerdlow SH, Campo E, Harris NL, et al. eds. *World Health Organization Classification of Tumours of Haematopoietic and Lymphoid Tissues* (pp. 413–418). Lyon: IARC Press; 2017.

WHO Classification of Tumours Editorial Board. Haematolymphoid tumours [Internet; beta version ahead of print]: In: *WHO Classification of Tumours Series.* 5th ed. Vol 11. International Agency for Research on Cancer; 2022 [cited 2023/06/19]. https://tumourclassification.iarc.who.int/chapters/63

21.6 Primary Cutaneous T-Cell Lymphoproliferative Disorders/Lymphomas

Carina A. Dehner and Leigh A. Compton

I. MYCOSIS FUNGOIDES

Mycosis fungoides (MF) is the most common form of cutaneous lymphoma. While it is more common in adults, it is also the most common primary cutaneous lymphoma in children and adolescents. It is typically a chronic, slowly progressing disease that displays characteristic clinical features of scaly patches, plaques, and tumors, each of which has histopathologic correlates. Although there are numerous variants of mycosis fungoides, only the more classic and common varieties will be discussed here. The diagnostic criteria are summarized in Table 21.6-1.

Clinical Features

- **Clinical Presentation:** Patients often present with nonspecific findings of a scaly rash that may be mistaken for a reactive dermatitis, especially eczematous dermatitis. This phase of the disease may last for years. Patch-stage disease manifests as finely scaling and erythematous patches on sun-protected skin, particularly on the trunk and buttocks. The development of plaques (ie, plaque-stage MF), defined as lesions raised above the skin surface, and tumor nodules (ie, tumor-stage MF) are associated with a worse prognosis. Typically, progression from patch- to

TABLE 21.6-1 WHO-HAEM5 Diagnostic Criteria for MF

Essential	Desirable
Early (patch) stage • Patches and plaques that persist or worsen over time, particularly in sun-protected areas • Cutaneous infiltration (preferentially involving the epidermis) by small- to medium-sized atypical T cells with cerebriform nuclei. **Tumor stage** • Concurrent or previous findings demonstrating classic histologic features of early MF	• Loss of T-cell antigens • Demonstration of clonal TCR gene rearrangements

MF, mycosis fungoides.
Based on the WHO Classification of Tumours Editorial Board. Haematolymphoid tumours [Internet]. Lyon (France): International Agency for Research on Cancer; 2024 (WHO classification of tumours series, 5th ed.; vol. 11). Available from: https://tumourclassification.iarc.who.int/chapters/63.

plaque- and tumor-stage MF takes year to decades and many patients never progress. Patients with plaque- or tumor-stage MF may continue to have or develop scaly patches.
- **Sites of Involvement:** MF is considered a primary cutaneous T-cell lymphoma, primarily presenting in the skin but extension to lymph nodes in clinically more advanced stages (*Cancer*. 1980;45:137-148) may occur. Similarly, bone marrow involvement is only noted in advanced disease, in which case it shows overlapping features with the systemic erythrodermic form of MF called Sézary syndrome (SS).

Morphology

Early lesions of MF may show nonspecific and nondiagnostic findings of parakeratotic scale and a sparse to patchy lymphocytic infiltrate, mostly situated in the upper dermis with or without epidermal involvement. Definitive diagnostic features may take years to develop, and it is not unusual for a patient to undergo several biopsies before receiving a diagnosis. Patch- and plaque-stage MF both show a lichenoid infiltrate of lymphocytes and histiocytes in the upper dermis and an intraepidermal infiltrate of variably enlarged and atypical lymphocytes, a feature known as epidermotropism (e-Figure 21.6-1A and B). Lesional lymphocytes may be present as single cells with the epidermis, aligned at the dermoepidermal junction ("lymphocyte tagging") or form clusters within epidermis known as Pautrier microabscesses. Mild acanthosis, superficial dermal fibrosis, basal vacuolar change, and increased postcapillary venules may be additional supportive features. Tumor-stage MF shows a dense dermal infiltrate of neoplastic cells. Epidermotropism is variable. Unlike patch- and plaque-stage MF, numerous eosinophils may be present in tumor-stage disease. A clinical history of MF is important when diagnosing tumor-stage disease, given significant histopathologic overlap with other forms of cutaneous lymphoma and systemic lymphoma involving the skin.

Large cell transformation, defined as greater than or equal to 25% tumor cells being 4 times larger than a regular lymphocyte (*Pathology*. 2014;46:610-616), is an important prognostic feature and should be commented on in the setting of tumor-stage MF. Folliculotropic and syringotropic variants of MF show prominent intraepithelial involvement of hair follicles and sweat gland units, respectively. The morphology of MF involving lymph nodes is unfortunately nonspecific and requires correlation with clinical and laboratory findings from flow cytometric analysis and TCR gene rearrangement studies for clonality.

Immunophenotype

Typically, neoplastic lymphocytes are positive for pan-T-cell markers such as CD2, CD3, and CD5. Most commonly, cells are CD4-positive and CD8-negative, but CD8-positive and CD4/CD8-double-negative MF may be encountered (*Yonago Acta Med* 2019; 62:153-158; *Am J Surg Pathol*. 2002;26:225-231). Loss of CD7 expression is typical. Abundant CD30 expression was once thought to be associated with a worse prognosis, but this remains unclear. Regardless, CD30 expression should be examined as it may suggest treatment response to the anti-CD30 monoclonal antibody therapy, brentuximab vedotin (*JAMA Dermatol*. 2015;151:73-77).

Genetic Features
- Presence of clonal TCR gene rearrangements: In difficult cases with nondiagnostic morphologic features, identification of the same T-cell clone across specimens can support a diagnosis.
- Inactivation of *CDKN2A* or *PTEN* in a subset

Prognosis and Treatment
The overall prognosis of MF is good, and only a minority of patients die of the disease. Extent of the disease and stage (patch, plaque, or tumor) are important prognostic features.

While patients with limited, localized disease do extremely well, those with extracutaneous involvement show a significantly worse outcome (*Blood.* 2012;119:1643-1649). As previously mentioned, the presence of plaques and tumors also portends a worse prognosis. Factors such as age older than 60 years, elevated lactate dehydrogenase (LDH) levels and large cell transformation are additional adverse prognostic factors (*Clin Lymphoma Myeloma Leuk.* 2015;15:e105-e112). Treatment of MF varies by stage and extent of disease. First-line therapies include topical corticosteroids, phototherapy, and topical chemotherapeutic agents. With disease progression, radiation, systemic chemotherapy, and/or other systemic therapies are utilized.

Differential Diagnosis
- **Inflammatory dermatoses:** Eczematous dermatitis, drug eruptions, and tinea corporis in particular may have overlapping histopathologic features. Abundant eosinophils, marked epidermal changes (spongiosis, interface change), the presence of fungal hyphae which may require a Periodic acid-Schiff (PAS) stain, and the absence of a clonal T-cell population by gene rearrangement studies can be helpful features to suggest a reactive process over MF.
- **Lymphomatoid papulosis (LyP):** Type B LyP can show identical histopathologic features but differs in its clinical presentation as one or multiple self-resolving papules or nodules.
- **Cutaneous Anaplastic Large Cell Lymphoma (ALCL):** Large cell transformation in MF may show overlapping histopathologic features with cutaneous ALCL due to the presence of large CD30-positive T cells; the presence or absence of a clinical history of MF is essential for accurate diagnosis.

Key Points

- The most common form of cutaneous lymphoma, MF presents as patches, plaques, and tumors on sun-protected skin.
- Typically, a chronic, slowly progressing disease
- Patch- and plaque-stage disease show an intraepidermal infiltrate of atypical lymphocytes with a variable immunoprofile but most commonly CD2+, CD3+, CD4+, and CD8−.
- Prognosis depends on the stage and extent of the disease.

Diagnostic Caveats
- Early-stage disease may be difficult to diagnose by histopathology, and definitive diagnosis may require multiple biopsies spanning years. Histopathologic features that

are not fully diagnostic of MF in the context of clinical suspicion are often signed out as "atypical T-lymphoid infiltrate." Identification of identical T-cell clones by gene rearrangement studies across multiple specimens may be helpful in these cases, but a clonal result in any one specimen is not diagnostic.

II. SÉZARY SYNDROME

SS is a clinical entity defined by the triad of erythroderma, circulating malignant T cells in the peripheral blood, and generalized lymphadenopathy. Neoplastic cells present in skin, blood, and lymph nodes are all clonally related. The diagnostic criteria are summarized in Table 21.6-2.

Clinical Features
- **Clinical Presentation:** Most commonly, SS presents de novo, but some patients had a prior history of MF ("SS preceded by MF") (*J Am Acad Dermatol*. 2002;46:95-106; *Blood*. 2016;127:3142-3153). Patients develop rapid-onset erythroderma, defined as diffuse redness and scaling involving all or most of the skin surface area, and lymphadenopathy.
- **Sites of Involvement:** Extracutaneous involvement may be seen, in particular nodal, pulmonary, hepatic, splenic, and brain involvement. Interestingly, the bone marrow is relatively spared.

Morphology
- **Skin:** Similar to MF, there may be an epidermotropic population of atypical lymphocytes, but the histopathologic findings are often subtle and may be nondiagnostic. The diagnostic Sézary cells display cerebriform and hyperchromatic nuclei, but these features may be difficult to discern. Lesional Sézary cells may be more prominent in the superficial dermis.

TABLE 21.6-2 WHO-HAEM5 Diagnostic Criteria for SS

Essential

- **Cutaneous involvement:** Erythroderma involving >80% body surface area
- **Blood involvement:** Clonal TCR gene rearrangements and either of the three findings below:
  1. Absolute Sézary cell count ≥1,000/μL
  2. CD4/CD8 ratio >10; CD4+/CD7− cells ≥40%
  3. CD4+/CD26− cells ≥30%

SS, Sézary syndrome.
Based on the WHO Classification of Tumours Editorial Board. Haematolymphoid tumours [Internet]. Lyon (France): International Agency for Research on Cancer; 2024 (WHO classification of tumours series, 5th ed.; vol. 11). Available from: https://tumourclassification.iarc.who.int/chapters/63.

- **Lymph nodes:** Partial to total effacement of lymph node architecture by Sézary cells; extranodal extension commonly seen; dermatopathic changes such as increased interdigitating dendritic and Langerhans cells with occasional melanophages are common.
- **Peripheral blood:** May show Sézary cells; diagnostic at $\geq 1 \times 10^9/L$
- **Bone marrow:** Typically, minimal to absent involvement by Sézary cells.

Flow Cytometry

- Sézary cells may be detected in the peripheral blood and lymph nodes by flow cytometry, which has become the standard method of detection over manual counts. Typically, there is a markedly elevated population of CD4-positive cells that show loss of CD7 or CD26 expression.

Genetic Features

- Given the sometimes subtle histopathologic features in skin biopsies, identification of a T-cell clone by gene rearrangement studies that is identical to one or more clones found in the peripheral blood and lymph nodes is supportive of a diagnosis.

Prognosis and Treatment

Compared to MF, SS is an aggressive disease with a median survival of only 32 to 36 months (*J Am Acad Dermatol.* 2012;67:1189-1199). Lymph node and visceral involvement are associated with a worse outcome (*Eur J Cancer.* 2013;49:2859-2868). Treatment varies by clinical stage, but the general approach includes extracorporeal photopheresis, methotrexate, interferons, or retinoids. These may be combined with phototherapy. If solid organ involvement is identified, systemic chemotherapy or histone deacetylase (HDAC) inhibitors may be used (*Clin J Oncol Nurs.* 2012;16:195-204).

Differential Diagnosis

Nonneoplastic erythroderma: Causes include erythrodermic psoriasis, eczema, and drug eruptions (anticonvulsants, β-blockers, etc); features such as marked epidermal changes or numerous eosinophils can support a reactive process but are not always present. Accordingly, skin biopsies in patients with erythroderma may be nondiagnostic.

Key Points

- Clinical entity defined by erythroderma, circulating Sézary cells in the peripheral blood, and lymphadenopathy
- Sézary syndrome may arise de novo or, rarely, follow a diagnosis of MF and has a poor prognosis.
- Skin biopsies may show Sézary cells, defined by cerebriform and hyperchromatic nuclei and CD4+/CD7− immunophenotype, in the epidermis and dermis.

Diagnostic Caveats
- The identification of Sézary cells in the skin by morphology may be difficult, and the findings may altogether be nondiagnostic.
- Similarly, the histopathologic features of reactive dermatoses that cause erythroderma may be subtle and/or nonspecific and nondiagnostic.

III. PRIMARY CUTANEOUS CD30-POSITIVE T-CELL LYMPHOPROLIFERATIVE DISORDERS

A. Lymphomatoid Papulosis

LyP is a chronic skin eruption characterized by papules and nodules with a predilection for the trunk and extremities. While LyP is a clonal T-cell proliferation that may share histopathologic features with lymphomas, by definition, lesions self-resolve. Therefore, clinicopathologic correlation is essential for accurate diagnosis. The diagnostic criteria are summarized in Table 21.6-3.

Clinical Features

- **Clinical Presentation:** Patients present with papular and/or nodular skin lesions in various stages that resolve in weeks to months. The number of lesions a patient may have at any instance is highly variable, ranging from one to many, as is the time between the development of new lesions. Patients may suffer from this condition for years. About 20% of patients have a preceding lymphoma or will develop lymphoma (most commonly MF, cutaneous ALCL, or Hodgkin lymphoma) (*Blood.* 2000;95:3653-3661; *J Am Acad Dermatol.* 2012;66:928-937).

TABLE 21.6-3 WHO-HAEM5 Diagnostic Criteria for LyP

Essential	Desirable
• Cutaneous infiltrate consisting of predominantly medium-sized atypical lymphocytes • Presence of CD30-positive T cells • Papulonodular skin lesions that spontaneously regress (weeks to months) • Exclusion of other lymphomas	• Demonstration of clonal TCR gene rearrangements can be helpful in some cases.

LyP, lymphomatoid papulosis.
Based on the WHO Classification of Tumours Editorial Board. Haematolymphoid tumours [Internet]. Lyon (France): International Agency for Research on Cancer; 2024 (WHO classification of tumours series, 5th ed.; vol. 11). Available from: https://tumourclassification.iarc.who.int/chapters/63.

- **Sites of Involvement:** Lesions are usually present on the trunk and extremities. Rare cases of oral mucosal involvement have been reported (*Mod Pathol.* 2012;25:983-992).

Morphology

Classically, five subtypes (outlined below) have been recognized, but several more have been recently accepted and the list continues to grow. These subtypes serve to aid the pathologist in appreciating the broad histopathologic spectrum of LyP and its overlap with cutaneous T-cell lymphomas; they are not of prognostic utility. Multiple subtypes may arise within a single patient.

> **Type A:** Most common type (>80%), characterized by clusters of large, atypical Reed-Sternberg-like lymphoid cells in a background of mixed inflammatory cells (small lymphocytes, histiocytes, and granulocytes) (e-Figure 21.6-2A)
>
> **Type B:** MF-like type, characterized by a lichenoid and epidermotropic lymphoid infiltrate
>
> **Type C:** ALCL-like type, characterized by cohesive sheets of large lymphoid cells with relatively few background inflammatory cells
>
> **Type D:** Primary cutaneous aggressive epidermotropic CD8+ cytotoxic T-cell lymphoma (PCAETL)-like, characterized by a markedly epidermotropic lymphoid infiltrate
>
> **Type E:** Angioinvasive type, characterized by a perivascular and angioinvasive lymphoid infiltrate with associated ulceration and tissue necrosis

Immunophenotype

The presence of CD30-positive T cells is the hallmark of LyP (e-Figure 21.6-2B). Lesional cells may be CD4-positive (e-Figure 21.6-2C), as is typically seen in types A, B, and C; CD8-positive as seen in type D; or CD4 and CD8-double-negative, requiring staining for additional T-cell markers (CD2, CD5). Lesional cells in type E may stain for either CD4 or CD8. Of note, many have reported the lesional cells in type B LyP may stain negative for CD30, but this is not universally accepted.

Genetic Features

- Clonality by TCR gene rearrangement studies is present. In patients with concurrent lymphoma, clones may be identical across both diseases (*J Invest Dermatol.* 1996;106:696-700).

Prognosis and Treatment

The prognosis of LyP is excellent with approximately 100% 5-year overall survival. Rarely, patients die due to their concurrent lymphoma. Therapy serves to control symptoms as needed, and steroids, ultraviolet light therapy, and methotrexate may be effective.

Differential Diagnosis

LyP may share histopathologic features with multiple T-cell lymphomas, the two lymphomas entering the differential diagnosis most commonly are detailed below.

- **Primary cutaneous or systemic ALCL with cutaneous involvement:** Morphology very similar, clinical course different as LyP presents with multiple, waxing and waning lesions, while ALCL presents as single nodules; t(2:5) (p23;q35) may be positive in ALCL, not in LyP.
- **MF with large cell transformation:** Morphology including epidermotropism may be identical; however, self-regressing lesions favor ALCL; classical clinical course of MF (patches > plaques > tumor stage) is not seen in LyP.

Key Points

- Clonal, CD30-positive T-cell proliferation that shares histopathologic features with T-cell lymphoma but is defined by its distinct, self-resolving clinical behavior
- May display multiple histopathologic patterns that serve to aid the pathologist in diagnosis but are not of prognostic or other clinical utility
- Prognosis is excellent as lesions are self-resolving.

Diagnostic Caveats

- Many forms of LyP are histologically identical to lymphomas and definitive diagnosis requires clinicopathologic correlation. If clinical history or behavior is uncertain a histopathologic differential diagnosis should be provided under a top-line diagnosis of "CD30-positive T-cell lymphoproliferative disorder."

B. Primary Cutaneous Anaplastic Large Cell Lymphoma

PC-ALCL is a T-cell lymphoma composed of large, atypical, CD30+ cells. By definition, patients should not have a history or evidence of mycosis fungoides or systemic ALCL. Like LyP, a definitive histopathologic diagnosis may be difficult when patient history or key clinical information is uncertain for the pathologist. The diagnostic criteria are summarized in Table 21.6-4.

TABLE 21.6-4 WHO-HAEM5 Diagnostic Criteria for PC-ALCL

Essential

- Lesions are limited to the skin/mucosa.
- Morphology: Anaplastic/pleomorphic/immunoblastic
- Expression of CD30 in majority of the cells (>75%)
- Exclusion of MF and LyP

LyP, lymphomatoid papulosis; MF, mycosis fungoides; PC-ALCL, primary cutaneous anaplastic large cell lymphoma.
Based on the WHO Classification of Tumours Editorial Board. Haematolymphoid tumours [Internet]. Lyon (France): International Agency for Research on Cancer; 2024 (WHO classification of tumours series, 5th ed.; vol. 11). Available from: https://tumourclassification.iarc.who.int/chapters/63.

Clinical Features

- **Clinical Presentation:** Patients present with solitary or localized tumor nodules often with superficial ulceration. Multifocality has been described in approximately 20% of cases (*Blood*. 2000;95:3653-3661). Partial spontaneous regression may occur.
- **Sites of Involvement:** Localized skin lesions may present at any part of the body with rare cases showing extracutaneous dissemination to regional lymph nodes (*Blood*. 2005;105:3768-3785).

Morphology

Nodules and sheets of atypical cells are present in the dermis and upper subcutis (e-Figure 21.6-3A). Typically, the cells are large and round with irregularly shaped nuclei, prominent nucleoli, and abundant cytoplasm (e-Figure 21.6-3B), but there is an accepted cytomorphologic spectrum with respect to cell size and atypical features. There is variability in the presence and extent of a background inflammatory infiltrate. Pseudoepitheliomatous hyperplasia, ulceration, and/or dermal necrosis may be present.

Immunophenotype

Tumor cells stain strongly positive for CD30 (e-Figure 21.6-3C). Expression of CD4 is variable, as are expression of pan T-cell markers CD2, CD3, and CD5, as well as the cytotoxic markers, TIA-1 and granzyme; accordingly, multiple stains may be needed to confirm T-cell origin. EMA, CD15, and anaplastic lymphoma kinase (ALK), markers, which may be expressed in systemic ALCL, are typically negative in PC-ALCL; however, negative staining does not confirm primary cutaneous disease.

Genetic Features

PC-ALCL does not show the typical translocation t(2;5)(p23;q35) resulting in *NPM::ALK* fusion that is found in systemic ALCL, but alterations in the *ALK* gene by fluorescence in situ hybridization (FISH) and positive nuclear and cytoplasmic ALK staining have been described in rare cases of PC-ALCL. Translocations involving the *DUSP22-IRF 5* locus on 6p25.2 have been described in PC-ALCL but may also be seen in systemic ALCL, LyP, and transformed mycosis fungoides and, therefore, is not a diagnostic finding.

Prognosis and Treatment

PC-ALCL is associated with a better outcome than most cutaneous T-cell lymphomas showing an over 90% 5-year survival rate. Age of less than 60 years, spontaneous regression, and presence of *DUSP22* are favorable prognostic factors, while *TP63* mutation is considered to be a poor prognostic factor. Local recurrence confined to skin lesions or regional lymph nodes is not associated with a worse prognosis.

Differential Diagnosis

- **LyP, type C:** Histologically identical, and distinction requires clinicopathologic correlation.
- **MF with large cell transformation:** May show overlapping histopathologic features, including epidermotropism; distinction requires clinicopathologic

correction, particularly a history of MF or cutaneous lesions (patches, plaques) compatible with MF.

> **Key Points**
>
> - Sheets of large anaplastic cells that stain positive for CD30
> - Expression of other T-cell markers is variable, often requiring utilization of multiple stains to demonstrate T-cell origin.
> - EMA, CD15, and ALK are typically negative in primary cutaneous ALCL. These markers may be positive in some cases of systemic ALCL.
> - Very good prognosis
>
> **Diagnostic Caveats**
>
> - Because PC-ALCL may be indistinguishable from type C LyP and cutaneous involvement by systemic ALCL on histopathologic grounds, a differential diagnosis should be provided under a top-line diagnosis of "CD30-positive T-cell lymphoproliferative disorder" for new diagnoses and when relevant clinical information is unavailable.

IV. SUBCUTANEOUS PANNICULITIS-LIKE T-CELL LYMPHOMA

Subcutaneous panniculitis-like T-cell lymphoma (SPTCL) is a CD8-positive cytotoxic lymphoma that involves subcutaneous fat lobules and is comprised of cells that express T-cell receptor αβ subtypes. The diagnostic criteria are summarized in Table 21.6-5.

TABLE 21.6-5 WHO-HAEM5 Diagnostic Criteria for SPTCL

Essential	Desirable
• Infiltrate of atypical lymphocytes within the subcutaneous fat lobules. • Atypical cells are positive for CD3, CD8, and βF1.	• Atypical cells are negative for γ-δ and EBV expression.

EBV, Epstein-Barr virus; SPTCL, subcutaneous panniculitis-like T-cell lymphoma.
Based on the WHO Classification of Tumours Editorial Board. Haematolymphoid tumours [Internet]. Lyon (France): International Agency for Research on Cancer; 2024 (WHO classification of tumours series, 5th ed.; vol. 11). Available from: https://tumourclassification.iarc.who.int/chapters/63.

Clinical Features

- **Clinical Presentation:** Patients present with single or multiple nonulcerated, painless subcutaneous nodules. About half may suffer from B symptoms and laboratory abnormalities, such as anemia, elevated liver enzymes, and inflammatory markers (C-reactive protein [CRP], erythrocyte sedimentation rate [ESR]). Approximately

15% to 20% will develop signs and findings diagnostic of hemophagocytic syndrome (HPS).
- **Sites of Involvement**: SPTCL most commonly involves the extremities and trunk. Hepatosplenomegaly may be present in the setting of HPS. Lymph node and bone marrow involvement are extremely uncommon.

Morphology

SPTCL is characterized by an infiltrate of atypical lymphocytes within the subcutaneous fat lobules (e-Figure 21.6-4A). Cells display mild to marked atypia with irregular nuclear contours and scant cytoplasms. Atypical cells that rim individual adipocytes are a classic but nonspecific feature of SPTCL (e-Figure 21.6-4B and C). Karyorrhexis and fat necrosis are usually prominent, and some cases show evidence of angioinvasion.

Immunophenotype

The neoplastic cells express CD3, CD8, and the cytotoxic markers granzyme B, TIA-1, and perforin, and are negative for CD4. Loss of pan-T-cell antigens such as CD2, CD5, and CD7 may be seen. CD30 is usually negative, and CD56 may be positive in rare cells. Cells stain positive for βF1, a surrogate for the T-cell receptor $\alpha\beta$ phenotype.

Genetic Features

Clonality by T-cell receptor gene rearrangement studies is usually present. Mutations involving *HAVCR2* have been shown to be associated with severe HPS in SPTCL (*Blood.* 2020;135:1058-1061).

Prognosis and Treatment

SPTCL is a relatively indolent disease with a 5-year overall survival of about 80%. Rarely, it spreads to lymph nodes many years after initial diagnosis. Presence of HPS is a poor prognostic factor lowering the medium survival to about 2 years. While treatment usually involves immunosuppressive agents or systemic corticosteroids, chemotherapy is utilized in cases that display more aggressive behavior or with evidence of HPS (*Am J Surg Pathol.* 2016;40:745-754).

Key Points

- CD8-positive, cytotoxic T-cell lymphoma involving the subcutaneous fat lobules
- Classic rimming of individual adipocytes within the subcutaneous fat lobules
- SPTCL must be distinguished from PGDTCL; SPTCL is positive for βF1, a surrogate immunohistochemical marker for $\alpha\beta$ T-cell receptors subtypes and negative for and γ-δ subtypes.
- SPTCL with associated HPS carriers has a poor prognosis.

Diagnostic Caveats

- SPTCL and γ-δ T-cell lymphoma may have overlapping histopathologic features but must be distinguished from one another due to significant differences in clinical outcomes and treatment.

V. PRIMARY CUTANEOUS γ-δ T-CELL LYMPHOMA

Primary cutaneous γ-δ T-cell lymphoma (PCGD-TCL) is a rare, aggressive cytotoxic T-cell lymphoma of T-cell receptor γ-δ phenotype that primarily involves the skin and subcutis. The diagnostic criteria are summarized in Table 21.6-6.

Clinical Features
- **Clinical Presentation:** The clinical presentation can be variable, with patients presenting with solitary to widespread patches, plaques, and nodules, often with ulceration.
- **Sites of Involvement:** PCGD-TCL most commonly occurs on the extremities, but other sites may be affected. Metastatic spread to the lungs, liver, kidneys, oral mucosa, and brain is common; however, lymph nodes, bone marrow, and spleen are usually spared.

Morphology
Different than SPTCL, PCGD-TCL has three main histologic patterns of involvement: epidermotropic, dermal, and subcutaneous. More than one histologic pattern may be present in the same patient, possibly in the same biopsy. Epidermotropism ranges from mild to marked, mimicking MF or pagetoid reticulosis. Subcutaneous infiltrates may be indistinguishable from SPTCL by morphology in that they involve the fat lobule and display identical rimming of single adipocytes.

Dermal involvement is much more commonly seen than in SPTCL.

Immunophenotype
The neoplastic cells, by definition, express T-cell γ-δ receptor subtypes and are otherwise positive for CD3, CD2, CD56, and cytotoxic markers granzyme, TIA-1, and perforin. Most tumors stain negative for CD4 and CD8, but some cases express CD8. Rare cases of co-expression of TCR γ and βF1 have been reported (*Am J Surg Pathol.* 2013;37:375-384).

TABLE 21.6-6　WHO-HAEM5 Diagnostic Criteria for PCGD-TCL

Essential	Desirable
• Atypical lymphoid infiltrate involving skin/subcutis	• Phenotype: CD4 and CD8 negative or CD4 negative and CD8 positive
• Atypical cells are positive for CD3 and γ-δ, and negative for EBV.	• Exclusion of extracutaneous disease at presentation
• Exclusion of other lymphomas (eg, MF, LyP)	

EBV, Epstein-Barr virus; LyP, lymphomatoid papulosis; MF, mycosis fungoides; PCGD-TCL, primary cutaneous γ-δ T-cell lymphoma.
Based on the WHO Classification of Tumours Editorial Board. Haematolymphoid tumours [Internet]. Lyon (France): International Agency for Research on Cancer; 2024 (WHO classification of tumours series, 5th ed.; vol. 11). Available from: https://tumourclassification.iarc.who.int/chapters/63.

Genetic Features

Clonality by T-cell receptor gene rearrangement studies (TRG [T cell receptor gamma] or TRD [T cell receptor delta]) is present. Activating mutations in *STAT5B* and *STAT3* can be seen.

Prognosis and Treatment

PCGD-TCL is an aggressive, chemotherapeutic-resistant T-cell lymphoma with a poor prognosis. The median survival time is 15 months. Subcutaneous disease is considered a poor prognostic factor, as well as the presence of HPS. Children seem to have a more indolent course.

Key Points

- An aggressive T-cell lymphoma comprised of cytotoxic cells that express γ-δ T-cell receptors and carries a poor prognosis
- There are three histopathologic patterns that are not exclusive of one another: epidermotropic, dermal, and subcutaneous.
- The immunophenotype otherwise is CD3+, CD4−, CD8+/−, CD56+, TIA-1/granzyme/perforin+.

Diagnostic Caveats

- MF and LyP rarely express γ-δ T-cell receptors and should be distinguished from PCGD-TCL due to significant differences in prognosis. Clinical history, tumor morphology, and immunohistochemical profiles may distinguish these entities.

VI. PRIMARY CUTANEOUS AGGRESSIVE EPIDERMOTROPIC CD8+ CYTOTOXIC T-CELL LYMPHOMA

PCAETL is a rare disease characterized by atypical CD8-positive cytotoxic T cells with marked epidermotropism, a T-cell receptor αβ phenotype, and a poor prognosis. The diagnostic criteria are summarized in Table 21.6-7.

TABLE 21.6-7   WHO-HAEM5 Diagnostic Criteria for PCAETL

Essential	Desirable
• Cutaneous infiltrate (epidermotropic/adnexotropic) consisting of atypical pleomorphic lymphocytes with cytotoxic phenotype and βF1+ • Persistent lesions (do not regress spontaneously)	• Demonstration of genetic alterations involving the JAK2 pathway

PCAETL, primary cutaneous aggressive epidermotropic CD8+ cytotoxic T-cell lymphoma.
Based on the WHO Classification of Tumours Editorial Board. Haematolymphoid tumours [Internet]. Lyon (France): International Agency for Research on Cancer; 2024 (WHO classification of tumours series, 5th ed.; vol. 11). Available from: https://tumourclassification.iarc.who.int/chapters/63.

Clinical Features
- **Clinical Presentation:** Patients present with numerous generalized ulcerated patches, plaques, and nodules, often ulcerated. Disease progression is rapid with peculiar involvement of the testis, lung, and central nervous system (CNS) and sparing of lymph nodes.
- **Sites of Involvement:** There is a wide cutaneous distribution, and mucosal involvement is common.

Morphology
There is a lichenoid, nodular, or diffuse infiltrate of atypical lymphocytes that may vary in size and degree of pleomorphism. There is often epidermotropism that can be marked or subtle and focal, but this feature is not required for diagnosis.

The epidermis may show additional changes such as acanthosis, dyskeratosis, and spongiosis. Adnexal involvement and angioinvasion may be present.

Immunophenotype
The neoplastic cells are usually βF1-positive, CD3+, CD8+, CD4−, granzyme B–positive, perforin-positive, TIA1+, CD45RA+, and CD45RO− phenotype. Most cases are negative for CD5, CD2, and CD30, with variable expression of CD7.

Genetic Features
Clonality by T-cell receptor gene rearrangement studies is present. Dysregulation of the JAK-STAT pathway has been demonstrated (*Haematologica.* 2022;107(3):702-714).

Prognosis and Treatment
These lymphomas are extremely aggressive with a median survival of only about 1 year. Neither the presence of localized versus diffuse lesions nor cytologic atypia correlates with outcomes. Systemic chemotherapy is the standard treatment.

Key Points
- Aggressive cytotoxic lymphoma with a poor prognosis
- Often shows an epidermotropism, but not required for diagnosis
- Cell are βF1-positive, CD3+, CD8+, CD4−, granzyme B/perforin+, TIA1+, CD45RA+, CD45RO− phenotype.
- Metastatic spread to the brain, kidney, and lungs is common.

Diagnostic Caveats
- Primary cutaneous aggressive epidermotropic CD8+ cytotoxic T-cell lymphoma may be indistinguishable from type D LyP and CD8-positive MF on histopathologic grounds alone, and diagnosis requires clinical correlation.

VII. PRIMARY CUTANEOUS ACRAL CD8-POSITIVE T-CELL LYMPHOPROLIFERATIVE DISORDER

Previously recognized as a rare lymphoma, this entity with a curious predilection for acral sites was recently reclassified as a lymphoproliferative disorder, given its benign clinical behavior. The diagnostic criteria are summarized in Table 21.6-8.

Clinical Features
- **Clinical Presentation:** Adult patients present with a slowly growing single red papule or nodule (*J Cutan Pathol.* 2016;43:125-136).
- **Sites of Involvement:** The most common site of involvement is the ear (~60%), followed by nose and foot. Cases of bilateral involvement (both ears) have been seen. Rarely, recurrence can occur at other cutaneous sites (*Br J Dermatol.* 2015;172:1573-1580).

Morphology
Lesions present as a dermal proliferation of atypical medium-sized lymphocytes with irregular, frequently folded nuclei with small nucleoli. Mitoses and striking severe atypia are absent. A grenz zone is common with the sparing of the epidermis and adnexal structures. Angiodestruction and necrosis are virtually absent.

Immunophenotype
Tumor cells express CD3, CD8, TIA1, CD68 (Golgi dot–like staining pattern), and βF1, while CD4, granzyme B, and perforin are negative. CD2, CD5, and CD7 are usually positive. CD56, CD57, CD30, and TdT are always negative. A Ki-67 proliferation index should show a low proliferation index; otherwise, other CD8+ cutaneous lymphomas should be considered.

Genetic Features
Clonality by T-cell receptor gene rearrangement studies is present.

TABLE 21.6-8 WHO-HAEM5 Diagnostic Criteria for PCA-LPD

Essential	Desirable
- Atypical medium-sized lymphoid infiltrate typically involving the dermis without epidermotropism - Atypical cells are CD8+ cytotoxic T cells. - Papule or nodule at an acral site - Exclusion of extracutaneous involvement at presentation	- Tumor cells express CD68 (Golgi pattern). - Clonal TCR gene rearrangement - Immunocompetent - EBV is negative.

EBV, Epstein-Barr virus; PCA-LPD, primary cutaneous acral CD8-positive T-cell lymphoproliferative disorder.
Based on the WHO Classification of Tumours Editorial Board. Haematolymphoid tumours [Internet]. Lyon (France): International Agency for Research on Cancer; 2024 (WHO classification of tumours series, 5th ed.; vol. 11). Available from: https://tumourclassification.iarc.who.int/chapters/63.

Prognosis and Treatment

This lymphoproliferative disease has a very good prognosis with complete remission after excision or radiotherapy.

> **Key Points**
>
> - CD8-positive T-cell lymphoproliferative disorder involving the dermis of acral sites with an excellent prognosis
>
> **Diagnostic Caveats**
>
> - Primary cutaneous acral CD8-positive T-cell lymphoproliferative disorder may be difficult to differentiate from peripheral T-cell lymphoma, not otherwise specified (NOS), which has a significantly worse prognosis.

VIII. PRIMARY CUTANEOUS CD4+ SMALL/MEDIUM T-CELL LYMPHOPROLIFERATIVE DISORDER

Primary cutaneous CD4+ small/medium T-cell lymphoproliferative disorder (PCSM-LPD) is an indolent, clonal T-cell proliferation presenting as a solitary skin nodule or plaque in the head and neck area. This entity was downgraded from lymphoma to a lymphoproliferative disorder related to its benign clinical course and excellent prognosis. The diagnostic criteria are summarized in Table 21.6-9.

TABLE 21.6-9 WHO-HAEM5 Diagnostic Criteria for PCSM-LPD

Essential	Desirable
- Single cutaneous lesion - Location: Neck > trunk > extremities - Patterns of infiltration: Nodular/diffuse or band-like - Infiltrate predominantly consists of CD4+ small- to medium-sized pleomorphic T cells and admixed B cells. - Atypical T cells have follicular helper T cells (TFH) cell phenotype: PD1+ (strong), ICOS+/−, BCL6+/−, CXCL13+/−, and CD10−.	- Adnexotropism - Lack of lymphoid follicles - Background reactive cells

PCSM-LPD, primary cutaneous CD4+ small/medium T-cell lymphoproliferative disorder.
Based on the WHO Classification of Tumours Editorial Board. Haematolymphoid tumours [Internet]. Lyon (France): International Agency for Research on Cancer; 2024 (WHO classification of tumours series, 5th ed.; vol. 11). Available from: https://tumourclassification.iarc.who.int/chapters/63.

Clinical Features
- **Clinical Presentation:** Patients present with a single plaque or tumor and are usually asymptomatic.
- **Sites of Involvement:** Lesions are typically located in the head and neck region or the upper trunk.

Morphology
There is a dense, predominantly dermal infiltrate of small to medium-sized lymphocytes (e-Figure 21.6-5A and B) in a background of mixed inflammatory cells that may include histiocytes and eosinophils. Large cells can sometimes be present but should comprise a small minority of the neoplastic infiltrate.

Immunophenotype
Tumor cells express CD3 and CD4 and are negative for CD8 and CD30, but there may be a background of CD8-positive small lymphocytes and CD20-positive B cells. Tumor cells express PD-1 and other T-helper markers such as ICOS, CXCL13, and BCL6, but CD10 is negative (*Am J Surg Pathol*. 2020;44(7):862-872).

Genetic Features
Clonality by T-cell receptor gene rearrangement studies is present. Other specific mutations have not been described.

Prognosis and Treatment
The prognosis is excellent with 100% 5-year survival related to the disease. Preferred treatment modalities are intralesional steroid injections, excision, and radiotherapy; however, spontaneous remission may occur. Local recurrences are very uncommon.

Key Points
- Single lesions typically arising in the head and neck region
- Dense infiltrate of small- to medium-sized lymphocytes within a mixed inflammatory cell background
- Excellent prognosis with potential for spontaneous regression, thus the recent downgrade to a lymphoproliferative disorder

Diagnostic Caveats
- Lymphomas, particularly MF and cutaneous peripheral T-cell lymphoma, not otherwise specified (NOS), may show overlapping histopathologic features, and definitive diagnosis requires clinicopathologic correlation.

IX. CUTANEOUS PERIPHERAL T-CELL LYMPHOMA, NOT OTHERWISE SPECIFIED

This is a wastebasket term for any cutaneous T-cell lymphoma that does not meet diagnostic criteria for another defined entity. Ultimately, most of these lesions likely represent cutaneous involvement by systemic lymphoma, but primary cutaneous lesions may occur and are now recognized in the WHO.

SUGGESTED READINGS

Willemze R, Cerroni L, Kempf W, et al. The 2018 update of the WHO-EORTC classification for primary cutaneous lymphomas [published correction appears in *Blood*. 2019;134(13):1112]. *Blood*. 2019;133(16):1703-1714.

21.7 Lymphomas of T Follicular Helper Cell Origin

Barina Aqil and Anjum Hassan

The germinal center microenvironment is not only an essential niche for the generation of B-cell response but also considered to be critical in the development of most human lymphoid neoplasms. T follicular helper (TFH) cells are a specialized subpopulation of T helper cells responsible for guiding B cells in immune responses. TFH cells are located in the apex of the light zone in germinal centers of secondary B-cell follicles and are considered to represent the putative cell of origin for aggressive types of T-cell neoplasms, including nodal TFH lymphoma, angioimmunoblastic type (nTFHL-AI), previously described as angioimmunoblastic T-cell lymphoma (AITL); nTFHL, follicular type (nTFHL-F); and nTFHL, not otherwise specified (nTFHL-NOS). TFH cells show a unique transcript signature characterized by the expression of CD4, CD10, CXCR5, BCL-6, CD57, CXCL13, PD-1, SAP, cMAF, and CD200 (*Haematologica*. 2017;102:e148). Further studies are likely to establish whether the current defining criteria of positivity for two TFH markers in addition to CD4 are sufficient for excluding peripheral T-cell lymphoma, NOS (PTCL-NOS). Core biopsy may be sufficient for the diagnosis of nTFHL-AI, but nTFHL-F and nTFHL-NOS require excisional biopsies for a definite diagnosis. Thus, if nTFHL-NOS or nTFHL-F is being considered on a core biopsy, it is recommended to use the generic terminology of nTFHL.

I. NODAL T FOLLICULAR HELPER CELL LYMPHOMA, ANGIOIMMUNOBLASTIC TYPE

This is a unique subtype of PTCL, accounting for 2% of all non-Hodgkin lymphomas and 15% to 20% of PTCLs (*Blood*. 2017;129:1095-1102; *Cancer Treat Res*. 2019;176:99-126). The diagnostic criteria are summarized in Table 21.7-1.

Clinical Features
- **Clinical presentation:** A distinctive type of PTCL, nTFHL-AI, commonly affects middle-aged and older patients, with a median age at diagnosis of about 65 years.

TABLE 21.7-1 WHO-HAEM5 Diagnostic Criteria for nTFHL-AI

Patterns II and III and tumor cell rich

Essential
- Nodal disease
- CD4+/CD8− atypical T cells
- Extrafollicular FDC meshwork expansion and proliferation of HEV

Desirable
- Strong PD1+ along with >2 TFH markers expression
- Clonal TCR gene rearrangement with/without mutations involving *RHOA* p.G17V or *IDH2* p.R172
- EBV+ cells

Patterns I and II (partial nodal involvement)

Essential
- Nodal disease
- Perifollicular CD4+ (occasional CD4−) and CD8− atypical T cells expressing >2 TFH markers, including strong PD1
- Clonal TCR gene rearrangement with/without mutations involving *RHOA* p.G17V or *IDH2* p.R172

FDC, follicular dendritic cell; HEV, high endothelial venule; nTFHL-AI, nodal T follicular helper lymphoma-angioimmunoblastic type; TFH, T follicular helper.
Based on the WHO Classification of Tumours Editorial Board. Haematolymphoid tumours [Internet]. Lyon (France): International Agency for Research on Cancer; 2024 (WHO classification of tumours series, 5th ed.; vol. 11). Available from: https://tumourclassification.iarc.who.int/chapters/63.

Patients usually present with advanced-stage disease and systemic symptoms related to immune dysregulation and cytokine production, including autoimmune hemolytic anemia, thrombocytopenia, polyclonal hypergammaglobulinemia, hypereosinophilia, skin rash, body cavity effusions, and arthralgias (*Blood*. 2008;111: 4463-4470; *In Vivo*. 2014;28:327-332).

- **Sites of involvement:** The most common site of involvement is lymph nodes. However, extranodal involvement is observed in many patients at the time of diagnosis, with frequently involved sites including the bone marrow (BM), spleen, liver, skin, and lungs.

Morphology

Histologic features include partial or complete effacement of the lymph node architecture by a polymorphous infiltrate that is typically associated with a proliferation of follicular dendritic cells (FDCs) and a prominent arborization of high endothelial venules (HEVs). The neoplastic cells are small to medium sized with pale to clear cytoplasm seen in a background of small lymphocytes, eosinophils, plasma cells, histiocytes, and scattered large lymphoid cells (some Reed-Sternberg like, Hodgkin Reed-Sternberg [HRS] like), which are often infected by Epstein-Barr virus (EBV) (e-Figure 21.7-1A-E). *IDH2* p.R172 mutant nTFHL-AI shows conspicuous medium to large clear cells with distinct cell membranes (*Mod Pathol.* 2019;32:1123-1134).

The histologic findings are separated into three overlapping patterns as follows:

Pattern I: There is partial preservation of lymph node architecture with hyperplastic follicles and poorly developed mantle zones merging into an expanded paracortex containing a polymorphic infiltrate of lymphocytes, immunoblasts, plasma cells, histiocytes, and eosinophils within a prominent vascular network. No expanded FDC meshworks are evident.

Pattern II: There is effacement of lymph node architecture with some attenuated/atretic follicles and expanded FDCs. A similar polymorphous infiltrate and vascular proliferation as described in pattern I is also present.

Pattern III: There is no evidence of residual follicles, but a prominent proliferation of FDCs and polymorphous infiltrate is present as in patterns I and II.

Pattern I represents a perifollicular pattern of involvement, whereas patterns II and III are considered to be "typical" histology for nTFHL-AI. The "tumor cell–rich variant" of nTFHL-AI may represent histologic progression, with numerous neoplastic T cells in a reduced/absent polymorphic background.

Immunophenotype

- The neoplastic cells are positive for CD2, CD3, and CD5, with variable loss of CD7; the cells are CD4+.
- The neoplastic cells are positive for >2 of the TFH markers PD1 (CD279), ICOS, BCL6, CXCL13, and CD10. Strong PD1 staining is more specific (e-Figure 21.7-2A-J).
- *IDH2* p.R172 mutant cases are strongly positive for CD10 and CXCL13.
- Expanded FDCs are identified with CD21, CD23, and CD35 (defined as score >2, meaning they have at least perivascular or perifollicular expansion [*Haematologica.* 2017;102:e148-e151]) (e-Figure 21.7-2K).
- Variable staining of B immunoblasts is seen with CD20.
- In situ hybridization for EBV-encoded small RNA (EBER) is described in 66% to 81% of cases.
- CD30 may be positive in a subset of the neoplastic cells and also stains the HRS-like cells, which are also variably positive for CD15 and EBV.

Genetic Features

Genomic sequencing technologies have defined the mutational profile of nTFHL-AI and have revealed recurrent somatic mutations in epigenetic regulator genes, such as 10 to 11 translocation 2 (*TET2*), DNA methyltransferase 3A (*DNMT3A*), isocitrate dehydrogenase 2 (*IDH2*), and *PLCG1*; mutations in *RHOA* (of which the p.G17V mutation has been identified in up to 70% of cases); and activating mutations of the T-cell receptor signaling, including CD28. Unlike *IDH2* p.R172 mutations that seem to be seen more often in TFHL-AI, *TET2*, *DNMT3A*, and *RHOA* mutations can be found in other TFH-derived T-cell lymphomas.

Prognosis and Treatment

nTFHL-AI has a poor prognosis when treated with anthracycline-containing chemotherapy regimens CHOP and CHOEP. Histone deacetylase inhibitors, including vorinostat, romidepsin, panobinostat, and belinostat, have been approved for cutaneous T-cell lymphomas, so they may have an additive and/or synergistic activity with other agents, including topoisomerase inhibitors, bortezomib, and others.

Adverse prognosis is associated with male sex and concurrent *TET2*, *DNMT3A*, and *IDH2* mutations. The AITL score combines four covariates (age [>60 years], performance status [Eastern Co-operative Oncology Group Performance Status or ECOG PS >1], β2 microglobulin [high], and C-reactive protein [high]) and stratifies patients into low-, intermediate-, and high-risk groups (*Blood*. 2021;138:213-220). Of note, patients with a high-risk AITL score have particularly dismal outcomes, with 5-year progression-free survival (PFS) of 13%. POD24 (early progression of disease within 24 months) has been described as a powerful prognostic factor.

Differential Diagnosis

- **Classic Hodgkin lymphoma (CHL):** HRS-like cells with rosetting by neoplastic CD4$^+$ T cells may be noted in nTFHL-AI. HRS cells in CHL show downregulation of B-cell programming, CD4$^+$ T-cell rosettes show weak-to-moderate PD1 and are CD10$^-$.
- **Nodular lymphocyte-predominant B-cell lymphoma:** Usually nodular but can have a diffuse pattern with no HEV. PD1$^+$ T cells may be numerous but are CD10$^-$. Large neoplastic cells are typically CD30$^-$ and very rarely EBV$^+$.
- **EBV$^+$ large B-cell lymphoma**: Consists of sheets of large B cells with EBV positivity, while nTFHL-AI has atypical T cells with TFH phenotype with FDC expansion.
- **Polymorphic lymphoproliferative disorder**: Requires a suspicious or confirmed setting of immunodeficiency/immune dysregulation
- **Nodal/extranodal marginal zone lymphoma/plasmacytoma**: Lacks FDC hyperplasia with HEV. Plasma cells are abnormal (CD19$^-$, CD56$^{+/-}$, and cyclin D1$^{+/-}$) in plasmacytoma.
- **PTCL-NOS**: Lacks extrafollicular FDC hyperplasia and TFH phenotype
- **nTFHL-NOS**: Has a TFH phenotype without FDC hyperplasia
- **Lymphomatous adult T-cell leukemia/lymphoma**: No FDC expansion. The neoplastic cells are CD25$^+$ (strong and diffuse), but CD10$^-$ and CXCL13$^-$. HTLV-1–positive serology is present. *RHOA* p.G17 mutations are rare, and cooccurrence with *TET2* mutations is very uncommon.
- **Mycosis fungoides/Sézary syndrome involving lymph node**: May express TFH markers but has a different clinical presentation of skin rashes. Cerebriform morphology of the neoplastic cells and *RHOA* mutations may occur, but involvement of p.G17 is rare.

II. NODAL T FOLLICULAR HELPER CELL LYMPHOMA, FOLLICULAR TYPE

PTCL with a nodular/follicular pattern was previously considered a follicular variant of PTCL-NOS until the WHO-HAEM4R and lymphoid tissues, where it was recognized as a separate lymphoma entity under nodal lymphomas with TFH phenotype. The diagnostic criteria are summarized in Table 21.7-2.

Key Points

- nTFHL-AI is the most common node-based PTCL.
- nTFHL-AI is characterized by systemic disease and a polymorphous infiltrate accompanied by significant proliferation of HEV and FDCs.
- Neoplastic cells should be positive for at least two or more of the TFH markers, PD1 (CD279), ICOS, BCL6, CXCL13, and CD10; strong PD1 staining is more specific.
- Recurrent somatic mutations in *TET2*, *DNMT3A*, and *IDH2*; mutations in *RHOA*; and activating mutations of T-cell receptor signaling including CD28 are seen.
- *IDH2* p.R172 mutant nTFHL-AI shows conspicuous medium to large clear cells with distinct cell membranes.

Diagnostic Caveats

- There are three overlapping histologic features (patterns I-III). Pattern I may be confused with reactive follicular hyperplasia and paracortical hyperplasia.
- HRS-like cells may have CD30 and CD15 expression, so can be misdiagnosed as CHL. A comprehensive evaluation is, therefore, required with respect to the size of the neoplastic cells ranging from B immunoblasts to HRS-like cells, variable CD30 staining, and haphazard distribution.
- Some cases of nTFHL-AI have epithelioid granulomas and cytotoxic T-cell expansion, which make them difficult to differentiate from PTCL-NOS, lymphoepithelioid morphologic variant (Lennert lymphoma). In these cases, it is imperative to identify neoplastic T cells with TFH phenotype, a polymorphic population, and expanded FDCs.

Clinical Features

- **Clinical presentation:** There are many similarities between nTFHL-AI and nTFHL-F beyond just their cell of origin. Most cases are seen in middle-aged and older patients, and patients usually present with advanced-stage disease and generalized lymphadenopathy. nTFHL-F has a high incidence of disseminated disease (up to 100% of cases), closer to the incidence in n TFHL-AI (99%) than PTCL-NOS (85%). Hypergammaglobulinemia and a positive Coombs test, typical of nTFHL-AI, have also been observed in several nTFHL-F cases.
- **Sites of involvement:** The most common sites of involvement are lymph nodes and extranodal sites, including skin, liver, spleen, and BM.

TABLE 21.7-2 WHO-HAEM5 Diagnostic Criteria for nTFHL-F

Essential	Desirable
• Follicular growth pattern	• Lack of polymorphous infiltrate and HEV hyperplasia
• No FDC meshwork expansion	• Clonal TCR gene rearrangement
• Predominantly CD4+/CD8− atypical T cells with strong PD1 and >2 TFH markers	

FDC, follicular dendritic cell; HEV, high endothelial venule; nTFHL-F, nodal T follicular helper, follicular type; TFH, T follicular helper.
Based on the WHO Classification of Tumours Editorial Board. Haematolymphoid tumours [Internet]. Lyon (France): International Agency for Research on Cancer; 2024 (WHO classification of tumours series, 5th ed.; vol. 11). Available from: https://tumourclassification.iarc.who.int/chapters/63.

Morphology

The lymph nodes show partial or complete effacement of the architecture by an atypical nodular/follicular infiltrate composed of medium-sized lymphoid cells with round/irregular nuclear contours and moderate/abundant clear cytoplasm. There are two distinct histologic patterns. The first pattern features neoplastic cells confined within sharply demarcated lymphoid follicles, with attenuated mantle zones mimicking follicular lymphoma (FL-like). The second pattern predominantly shows large, regular, or irregular nodules reminiscent of progressive transformation of germinal centers (PTGC-like), composed of mature IgD$^+$ B lymphocytes admixed with small aggregates of neoplastic cells displaying medium-sized nuclei with abundant clear cytoplasm. Both patterns are frequently noted in the same lymph node. The internodular/follicular areas may show few plasma cells and eosinophils but lack hyperplastic HEVs and a typical polymorphous population. Scattered B immunoblasts and HRS-like cells may also be seen.

Immunophenotype

- The expression of T cell and TFH markers is similar to nTFHL-AI.
- FDC meshworks may be expanded but are confined to the follicles, as noted with CD21, CD23, and CD35.
- In the FL-like pattern, CD10$^+$ and BCL6$^+$ neoplastic cells within the nodules/follicles may mimic FL. Careful evaluation of T-cell phenotype and the presence of at least two, if not more, of the TFH markers is required (see "Diagnostic Caveats" section).
- HRS-like cells seen in the PTGC-like pattern are often CD30+ and show variable expression of CD15, EBV, and other B-cell antigens. Neoplastic T cells are surrounded by IgD$^+$ B cells in a PTGC-like pattern.
- EBV has been observed in 68% of the nTFHL-F cases with a pattern reminiscent of B immunoblasts, a finding closer to that reported in most nTFHL-AI than in PTCL-NOS.

Genetic Features

Translocations involving chromosomes 5q33 (*ITK*) and 9q22 (*SYK*) resulting in an *ITK::SYK* fusion transcript have been reported. *ITK* belongs to a group of five related kinases comprising the Tec family and affects T-cell development and T-cell receptor signaling. *SYK* is a nonreceptor protein kinase that is a key regulator of multiple biochemical signal transduction pathways (*Leukemia*. 2006;20:313-318; *Leukemia*. 2008;22:1139-1143; *Am J Surg Pathol*. 2009;33:682-690).

RHOA mutations, including c.G50T, p.Gly17Val, c.G50A, p.Gly17Glu, c.A52G, p.Lys18Glu, c.T102C, p.Tyr34Tyr, c.G145T, and p.Asp49Tyr, have been reported (*Pathol Int*. 2020;70:653-660), and the incidence of *RHOA* p.G17V mutation is comparable to nTFHL-AI (*Haematologica*. 2017;102:e149). In addition, *TET2*, *DNMT3A*, and *IDH2* mutations are also seen.

Prognosis and Treatment

Patients are usually treated with anthracycline-containing chemotherapy regimens CHOP, CHOEP, and DHAP. Prognosis is uncertain due to limited data on this rare entity, although approximately 50% to 60% of patients die within 2 years of diagnosis.

III. NODAL T FOLLICULAR HELPER LYMPHOMA, NOT OTHERWISE SPECIFIED

This disease is a nodal peripheral T-cell neoplasm that has expression of CD4 and at least two TFH markers, but which does not fulfill the required criteria for nTFHL-AI or nTFHL-F. The diagnostic criteria are summarized in Table 21.7-3.

Key Points

- There are two growth patterns: FL-like and PTGC-like.
- The neoplastic cells are medium sized with round/irregular nuclear contours and moderate/abundant clear cytoplasm.
- There is no background polymorphous population or HEV proliferation.
- The neoplastic T cells are positive for the pan–T-cell antigens CD2, CD3, and CD5, with variable loss of CD7, and are mostly CD4+. All cases express at least two or more of the TFH markers.
- FDC meshworks may be expanded but remain confined to the follicles.
- Some cases of nTFHL-F show an *ITK::SYK* translocation.
- The incidence of *RHOA* p.G17V mutation is comparable to nTFHL-AI.

Diagnostic Caveats

- In the FL-like pattern, CD10+ and BCL6+ neoplastic cells within the nodules/follicles may be misdiagnosed as FL. It is imperative to compare CD10 and other TFH markers with CD20.
- Lack of polymorphous population, lack of HEV proliferation, and the presence of FDC meshworks confined to the follicles are important for differentiation from nTFHL-AI.

Clinical Features

- **Clinical presentation:** Cases of nTFHL-NOS present as advanced-stage disease with generalized lymphadenopathy and demonstrate similar clinical characteristics

TABLE 21.7-3 WHO-HAEM5 Diagnostic Criteria for nTFHL-NOS

Essential	Desirable
• Effaced lymph node architecture/T-zone pattern by atypical T cells • No extrafollicular FDC meshwork expansion, perifollicular distribution of neoplastic T cells, and follicular growth pattern • Predominantly CD4+/CD8− atypical T cells with strong PD1 and >2 TFH markers	• Clonal TCR gene rearrangement and/or mutation involving *RHOA* p.G17V

FDC, follicular dendritic cell; nTFHL-NOS, nodal T follicular helper, not otherwise specified; TFH, T follicular helper.
Based on the WHO Classification of Tumours Editorial Board. Haematolymphoid tumours [Internet]. Lyon (France): International Agency for Research on Cancer; 2024 (WHO classification of tumours series, 5th ed.; vol. 11). Available from: https://tumourclassification.iarc.who.int/chapters/63.

as of nTFHL-AI, including hypergammaglobulinemia and a positive Coombs test.
- **Sites of involvement:** There is involvement of lymph nodes, BM, liver, and spleen.

Morphology

nTFHL-NOS shows diffuse effacement of lymph node architecture by medium- to large-sized atypical lymphoid cells. There is no polymorphous background population, no HEV proliferation, and no FDC expansion outside the follicles. There is a "T-zone" pattern of involvement (*Am J Surg Pathol.* 2019;43:1282-1290).

Immunophenotype

- The neoplastic cells are mostly CD4+ and express at least two or more of the TFH markers PD1 (CD279), ICOS, BCL6, CXCL13, and CD10.
- ICOS is the most frequently positive marker in nTFHL-NOS (*Am J Surg Pathol.* 2019;43(9):1282-1290).
- No FDC expansion is noted with CD21, CD23, and CD35.

Genetic Features

Mutations characteristic of nTFHL-AI, such as *RHOA*, *TET2*, and *DNMT3A*, are also reported in nTFHL-NOS. *IDH2* mutations are rare in comparison to nTFHL-AI (*Haematologica.* 2017;102:e148-e151).

Prognosis and Treatment

Due to the rarity of the entity, the clinical data for response to treatment and outcome are somewhat limited, but reportedly not very different from nTFHL-AI (*Exp Hematol Oncol.* 2021;10:33).

Differential Diagnosis

- **nTFHL-AI (tumor rich):** The presence of FDC expansion is the only distinguishing finding from nTFHL-NOS, so definitive diagnosis of nTFHL-NOS is only possible on the excisional biopsy.
- **PTCL-NOS**: The variable expression of TFH markers in nTFHL-NOS with less specific strong expression of PD1 results in the inclusion of some cases in PTCL-NOS. Molecular studies showing the *RHOA* p.G17V mutation would support the diagnosis of nTFHL-NOS over PTCL-NOS.

Key Points

- nTFHL-NOS is characterized by disseminated disease similar to nTFHL-AI.
- There is diffuse effacement of lymph node architecture/T-zone pattern by medium to large lymphoid cells.
- A polymorphous population, HEV proliferation, and a follicular growth pattern are all lacking.
- The neoplastic T cells are mostly CD4+ and express at least two of the TFH markers; ICOS is most often positive.
- Lack of extrafollicular FDC hyperplasia.
- *IDH2* mutations are rare in comparison to nTFHL-AI

Diagnostic Caveats
- nTFHL-NOS is a diagnosis of exclusion, so an excisional biopsy is required for definitive diagnosis.
- Morphology evaluation to confirm the absence of a follicular growth pattern, a polymorphous infiltrate, and HEV proliferation is required to rule out nTFHL-AI and nTFHL-F.
- Detection of *RHOA* p.G17V mutation, observed in up to 60% of nTFHL-NOS, is a useful tool that supports the diagnosis of an nTFHL over PTCL-NOS.

SUGGESTED READINGS

Advani RH, Skyrpets T, Civallero M, et al. Outcomes and prognostic factors in angioimmunoblastic T-cell lymphoma: final report from the international T-cell Project. *Blood.* 2021;138(3):213-220.

Attygalle AD, Chuang SS, Diss TC, et al. Distinguishing angioimmunoblastic T-cell lymphoma from peripheral T-cell lymphoma, unspecified, using morphology, immunophenotype and molecular genetics. *Histopathology.* 2007;50:498-508.

de Leval L, Rickman DS, Thielen C, et al. The gene expression profile of nodal peripheral T-cell lymphoma demonstrates a molecular link between angioimmunoblastic T-cell lymphoma (AITL) and follicular helper T (TFH) cells. *Blood.* 2007;109:4952-4963.

de Leval L, Savilo E, Longtine J, et al. Peripheral T-cell lymphoma with follicular involvement and a CD4+/bcl-6+ phenotype. *Am J Surg Pathol.* 2001;25:395-400.

Dobay MP, Lemmonnier F, Missiaglia E, et al. Integrative clinicopathological and molecular analyses of angioimmunoblastic T-cell lymphoma and other nodal lymphomas of follicular helper T-cell origin. *Haematologica.* 2017;102:e148.

Feldman AL, Sun DX, Law ME, et al. Overexpression of Syk tyrosine kinase in peripheral T-cell lymphomas. *Leukemia.* 2008;22:1139-1143.

Huang Y, Moreau A, Dupuis J, et al. Peripheral T-cell lymphomas with a follicular growth pattern are derived from follicular helper T cells (TFH) and may show overlapping features with angioimmunoblastic T-cell lymphomas. *Am J Surg Pathol.* 2009;33(5):682-690.

Odejide O, Weigert O, Lane AA, et al. A targeted mutational landscape of angioimmunoblastic T-cell lymphoma. *Blood.* 2014;123(9):1293-1296.

21.8 Peripheral T-Cell Lymphoma, Not Otherwise Specified

Karen L. Fang, Brooj Abro, and John L. Frater

Peripheral T-cell lymphoma, not otherwise specified (PTCL-NOS), is primarily a diagnosis of exclusion and includes all mature T-cell neoplasms not defined by other features, such as specific morphology, genetic findings, clinical scenarios, and sites of involvement. It comprises approximately 30% to 50% of PTCLs and is aggressive, with generally poor response to standard chemotherapy. It is more common in males than females (ratio ~2:1) and may affect patients of all ages but is most common in older adults (*J Natl Cancer Inst.* 2000;92(15):1240-1251).

TABLE 21.8-1 Diagnostic Criteria for PTCL-NOS

Essential
- Morphologic, immunophenotypically aberrant, or monoclonal T-cell population
- No more than one T follicular helper cell marker is positive (CD10, BCL6, CXCR5, SAP, ICOS, CXCL13, MAF).
- EBER is negative in T cells.
- All other nodal or extranodal mature T- and NK-cell lymphomas have been excluded.

Desirable
- Clonal TCR gene rearrangement
- PTCL-TBX21 or PTCL-GATA3 designation is clear.

EBER, Epstein-Barr virus-encoded small RNA; NK, natural killer; PTCL-NOS, peripheral T-cell lymphoma, not otherwise specified.
Based on the WHO Classification of Tumours Editorial Board. Haematolymphoid tumours [Internet]. Lyon (France): International Agency for Research on Cancer; 2024 (WHO classification of tumours series, 5th ed.; vol. 11). Available from: https://tumourclassification.iarc.who.int/chapters/63.

The median age at diagnosis is ~60 years (*Ann Oncol.* 2002;13(1):140-149). The primary cell of origin is the activated mature T cell, with the CD4(+), CD8(−) phenotype being the most common. All neoplasms of T follicular helper cell immunophenotype, as well as Epstein-Barr virus (EBV)-positive nodal T-cell lymphoma, are now defined as specific entities and fall outside the definition PTCL-NOS. This "not otherwise specified" (NOS) category is expected to continue to shrink as additional separate entities are defined. As of now, there are several subcategories within PTCL-NOS, including lymphoepithelioid lymphoma (also known as Lennert lymphoma) and the emerging molecular subtypes of PTCL with overexpression of TBX21 (PTCL-TBX21) and PTCL with overexpression of GATA3 (PTCL-GATA3) (*Blood.* 2019;133(15):1664-1676). There has also been mention of a PTCL-NOS with cytotoxic phenotype (CD8(+)), primarily in cases reported from Asia (*Mod Pathol.* 2022;35(8):1126-1136). The diagnostic criteria are summarized in Table 21.8-1.

Clinical Features

- **Clinical presentation:** Most patients present with lymph node enlargement, frequently also with B symptoms, including fatigue, night sweats, and weight loss as well as poor performance status and elevated lactate dehydrogenase. Often, the disease is already widespread at diagnosis, with most patients presenting in stage III or stage IV (*J Clin Pathol.* 2008;61(11):1160-1167). Twenty-nine percent of patients display involvement of multiple extranodal sites. Hypercalcemia, hypogammaglobulinemia, and hemophagocytic lymphohistiocytosis (HLH) are rare but can occur (<10% of patients) (*Front Oncol.* 2023;13:1101441).
- **Sites of involvement:** Peripheral lymph nodes are most commonly involved, but involvement of the bone marrow, liver, spleen, and extranodal tissues (especially skin and gastrointestinal tract [e-Figure 21.8-1], lungs, or central nervous system)

is also frequently found. Leukemic presentation with peripheral blood involvement is less common but has been reported.

Morphology

PTCL-NOS does not have specific morphologic features as it is a diagnosis of exclusion. The neoplastic infiltrate usually consists of medium- to large-sized pleomorphic lymphocytes.

- **Lymph node:** Variable, but often diffuse effacement of lymph node architecture by an infiltrate of pleomorphic cells (e-Figure 21.8-1) with irregular, hyperchromatic, and/or vesicular nuclei, frequent mitotic figures, and prominent nucleoli. The infiltrate can occasionally be limited to paracortical or interfollicular distribution and can also display cells with Hodgkin Reed-Sternberg (HRS)-like or clear cell morphology. A mixed reactive background may be present, including eosinophils, histiocytes, B cells, and plasma cells. Occasional cases display a predominance of atypical small cells, but most cases consist of mixed populations of medium- to large-sized cells.
- **Skin:** Neoplastic cells with similar morphology to that found in lymph nodes, with highly variable patterns including diffuse, nodular (occasionally with central necrosis within nodules), bandlike, angiocentric, and, occasionally, even epidermotropic or with adnexal involvement
- **Spleen:** Atypical cells similar in morphologic variability to those described earlier, with various architectural patterns: micronodular, limited to T-cell–rich marginal zones, diffusely involving red and white pulp, or even limited to a single or several discrete lesions
- **Bone marrow:** Most commonly diffuse pattern of involvement, causing hypercellularity and loss of normal hematopoietic elements (e-Figure 21.8-2), but occasionally focal and nonparatrabecular. Often incites a mixed reactive cell response and increased fibrosis
- **Lymphoepithelioid lymphoma (Lennert lymphoma):** Diffuse or interfollicular growth of small, mildly atypical cells with numerous or even confluent associated clusters of epithelioid histiocytes. Histiocytes can have multinucleation and can obscure the neoplastic T cells. Clear cells, HRS-like cells, eosinophils, and plasma cells can be seen.

Immunophenotype

Pan–T-cell markers are frequently lost or downregulated, especially CD5 and CD7. The most common phenotype is CD4(+), CD8(−) (e-Figure 21.8-3). CD4/CD8 double positivity or double negativity is possible, and a significant subset, approximately 20% to 35%, of neoplasms are CD8(+), CD4(−) with expression of CD56 and cytotoxic markers (TIA-1, granzyme B, perforin). Most cases express T-cell receptor (TCR)-α/β, but cases have been found expressing TCR-γ/δ or are TCR silent (negative for α/β-TCR and γ/δ-TCR). Rare cases are positive for CD30 (scattered, variable positivity), CD20, cyclin D1, and CD15. A few scattered EBV-encoded small RNA (EBER)-positive B cells may be present.

Genetic Features

Monoclonal rearrangement of TCR genes is seen in most cases and can help distinguish the diagnosis from reactive conditions, such as infectious mononucleosis or allergic drug reactions.

The genetic findings of PTCL-NOS are usually complex, with multiple losses and gains observed across a wide range of chromosomes. Two molecular subgroups have emerged based on gene expression profile analyses. These two groups center around two differentiation regulator molecules, TBX21 and GATA3, which regulate T-cell differentiation into T helper 1 (Th1) and T helper 2 (Th2) cells, respectively. PTCL-TBX21 is associated with a better prognosis and less genomic complexity with fewer alterations in copy number than PTCL-GATA3 (*Blood*. 2022;140(11):1229-1253). Furthermore, PTCL-TBX21 seems to be associated more frequently with mutations in genes regulating DNA methylation. Lennert/lymphoepithelioid lymphoma also appears to generally fall into the PTCL-TBX21 class. More studies are required to more clearly elucidate the molecular mechanisms driving each of these forms of PTCL; perhaps, once the molecular mechanisms have been clarified, the designation of PTCL-NOS will no longer apply to these entities with disease-defining genetic aberrations.

Prognosis and Treatment

Regardless of morphology, prognosis in PTCL-NOS is poor. Response to established forms of chemotherapy is often limited, relapse is frequent, and the 5-year overall survival rate is low, at 32% (*Blood*. 2011;117(12):3402-3408). Adverse prognostic factors include advanced age, poor performance status, elevated lactate dehydrogenase (LDH), bone marrow involvement, bulky disease >10 cm, thrombocytopenia, lymphopenia, neutrophilia, hypoalbuminemia, and Ki-67 proliferative index >80% (*Front Oncol*. 2023;13:1101441).

Most patients receive anthracycline-based chemotherapy regimens, with cyclophosphamide, doxorubicin, vincristine, and prednisone (CHOP) being the most common. Five-year progression-free and treatment failure-free rates are generally between 20% and 30% (*Blood*. 2014;123(17):2636-2644). Relapse is often treated with salvage chemotherapy and autologous or allogeneic hematopoietic stem cell transplantation (HSCT), but no consensus on the type of HSCT has been established (*Leukemia*. 2022;36(5):1361-1370).

One exception to the dismal prognosis of this disease is seen in the lymphoepithelioid variant, which tends to involve extranodal tissues less often and is associated with a better overall prognosis.

Differential Diagnosis

- All other forms of (PTCL) must be ruled out. The most common other forms of PTCL include:
  - **Angioimmunoblastic T-cell lymphoma (AITL):** Expanded high endothelial venules, T follicular helper cell phenotype including CD4(+), CD10(+), CXCL13(+), BCL6(+), ICOS(+), CXCR5(+), SAP(+), MAP/c-MAP(+), and CD200 (frequently +)
  - **Anaplastic large cell lymphoma (ALCL):** Diffuse anaplastic morphology, CD30(+), ALK-1 (usually +), and CD4(+)
- If scattered large B cells or HRS-like cells are seen, the following should be excluded:
  - **Classic Hodgkin lymphoma:** Large cells are PAX5 (weak +), CD45(−), CD15(+), CD30(+); lack of clonal rearrangement of TCR genes.
  - **T-cell/histiocyte-rich large B-cell lymphoma:** Large cells are CD20(+), CD19(+), CD79a(+), and BCL6(+); lack of monoclonal T-cell population, retained pan–T-cell antigens (CD2, CD3, CD5, CD7).

> **Key Points**
> - The diagnosis of PTCL-NOS requires exclusion of all other T- and NK-cell malignancies.
> - EBV-positive nodal T-cell lymphoma and nodal T-cell lymphoma with T follicular helper cell phenotype were recently removed from this category and are now recognized as distinct entities.
> - Prognosis is usually poor, except in Lennert/lymphoepithelial lymphoma.
> - Two molecular classes are emerging: PTCL-TBX21 and PTCL-GATA3 correlate with mutations affecting differentiation controller molecules of the Th1 and Th2 lineages, respectively.
>
> **Diagnostic Caveats**
> - No more than one T follicular helper cell marker can be positive (CD10, BCL6, CXCR5, SAP, ICOS, CXCL13, MAF).
> - EBER can rarely be seen in scattered B cells but must be negative in the neoplastic T cells.
> - Most cases are CD4(+), CD8(−), but all combinations are possible.

- **Reactive paracortical lymph node hyperplasia:** Lack of aberrant immunophenotype and usually negative for clonal TCR gene rearrangements. The clinical history may help explain the etiology (reactive/infectious).

SUGGESTED READINGS

Agostinelli C, Piccaluga PP, Went P, et al. Peripheral T cell lymphoma, not otherwise specified: the stuff of genes, dreams and therapies. *J Clin Pathol.* 2008;61(11):1160-1167. doi:10.1136/jcp.2008.055335

Nicolae A, Bouilly J, Lara D, et al. Nodal cytotoxic peripheral T-cell lymphoma occurs frequently in the clinical setting of immunodysregulation and is associated with recurrent epigenetic alterations. *Mod Pathol.* 2022;35(8):1126-1136. doi:10.1038/s41379-022-01022-w

Weiss J, Reneau J, Wilcox RA. PTCL, NOS: an update on classification, risk-stratification, and treatment. *Front Oncol.* 2023;13:1101441. doi:10.3389/fonc.2023.1101441

21.9 Epstein Bar Virus-Positive NK-/T-Cell Lymphoproliferative Diseases of Childhood

Yeon-Whan Choe and Brooj Abro

Epstein-Barr virus (EBV)-positive T/natural killer (NK)-cell lymphoproliferative diseases of childhood are a group of rare EBV-associated diseases with increased frequency in Asian and Latin American populations suggesting genetic predisposition. These disorders are mostly reported in children but rarely can also affect adults. The WHO-HAEM5 and International Consensus Classification (ICC) recognize four disease entities in this category: severe mosquito bite allergy (SMBA), hydroa vacciniforme lymphoproliferative disorder (HV-LPD), systemic chronic active EBV (CAEBV) disease, and systemic EBV-positive T-cell lymphoma of childhood (SEBVTCL). These disorders may show significant clinicopathologic overlap; a detailed clinical history and comprehensive workup is essential to establishing an accurate diagnosis. An important differential diagnosis to consider is EBV infection–associated hemophagocytic lymphohistiocytosis (HLH), which is particularly difficult to distinguish from SEBVTCL. In all entities, a cytotoxic T/NK-cell infiltrate is present (can be subtle), and variable proportions of T/NK cells are positive for EBV-encoded small RNA (EBER) by in situ hybridization. Except for SEBVTCL, all entities can be derived from either T or NK cells. The key features of these disorders are summarized in Table 21.9-1.

I. SEVERE MOSQUITO BITE ALLERGY

According to the WHO-HAEM5, SMBA is a cutaneous form of CAEBV disease triggered by mosquito bites. Transient systemic symptoms may occur, including fever, lymphadenopathy, and hepatosplenomegaly. Bullae formation with intense erythema at the bite site is the typical initial skin manifestation followed by ulceration and scar formation. High levels of immunoglobulin E (IgE) and circulating EBV DNA are detected in patients with SMBA. Skin biopsy of lesions show perivascular and periadnexal dermal aggregates of variably sized atypical lymphocytes that may extend to the subcutis.

Angiodestruction and necrosis may be present. The infiltrate demonstrates a NK-cell or T-cell phenotype. SMBA is morphologically similar to HV-LPD; however, the clinical features differ (see discussion later). SMBA with persistent systemic symptoms greater than 3 months should be diagnosed as CAEBV disease. Genetic studies have detected somatic mutations in EBV-positive lymphocytes, suggesting that it is a clonal neoplastic process (*Nat Microbiol*. 2019;4:404-413). Patients have an increased risk of developing HLH and aggressive EBV-associated lymphomas such as extranodal NK/T-cell lymphoma (ENKTL) and aggressive NK-cell leukemia (ANKL). The diagnostic criteria are summarized in Table 21.9-2.

II. HYDROA VACCINIFORME LYMPHOPROLIFERATIVE DISORDER

HV-LPD is also considered a cutaneous form of CAEBV disease and includes two subtypes: classic and systemic (subtype-specific features discussed later). Skin lesions show similar histologic features as SMBA, demonstrating perivascular and periadnexal dermal aggregates of variably sized atypical lymphocytes that may extend to the subcutis. Angiodestruction and necrosis are common. The epidermis shows reticular degeneration, spongiosis, and vesicle formation. Cytotoxic T-cell phenotype is most common, and NK-cell phenotype may be seen occasionally. T-cell lineage cases most often show CD8 expression; however, cases with CD4 expression and double CD4 and CD8 expression have been reported (*J Am Acad Dermatol*. 2019;81:534-540). The lesions in the classic form show EBV+ $\gamma\delta$ T cells more often, while the systemic form commonly shows EBV+ $\alpha\beta$ T cells. Cases with NK-cell phenotype can show significant subcutaneous tissue involvement and histologic features may mimic subcutaneous panniculitis-like T-cell lymphoma. Since most cases are of T-cell lineage, demonstration of TCR gene rearrangements may be helpful. Circulating EBV DNA is detected and is higher in the systemic form. Poor prognostic factors include age of onset more than 9 years and the expression of an EBV-encoded immediate-early gene transcript, *BZLF1* mRNA, in the skin lesions (*Br J Dermatol*. 2015;172:56-63). The diagnostic criteria are summarized in Table 21.9-3.

TABLE 21.9-1 Key Features of EBV-Positive T/NK-Cell Lymphoproliferative Diseases of Childhood

	SMBA	HV-LPD	CAEBV	SEBVTCL
Clinical features	• Fever and skin lesions post mosquito bite • Disease localized to skin	• Classic: recurrent papulovesicular skin lesions in sun-exposed sites • Systemic: recurrent skin lesions including non–sun-exposed sites and systemic symptoms	• Systemic disease with multiorgan involvement • Systemic symptoms >3 mo • May have concurrent skin manifestations of SMBA or HV-LPD	• Aggressive disease with multiorgan involvement, rapid progression, and usually fatal within weeks • Some arise in the setting of CAEBV.
Morphology	• Dermal and subcutaneous infiltrate composed of variably sized lymphocytes • Perivascular distribution	• Dermal and subcutaneous infiltrate composed of variably sized lymphocytes • Perivascular distribution	• Subtle lymphocytic infiltrate in tissues with or without atypia • Liver and spleen: sinusoidal infiltrate • LNs: IM-like morphologic features	• Variable lymphocytic infiltrate in tissues. Most cases show minimal atypia. • Liver and spleen: sinusoidal infiltrate • LNs: IM-like morphologic features
Phenotype	• NK-cell (majority) or T-cell lineage	• T-cell (majority) or NK-cell lineage • T-cell cases: CD8 > CD4 • Classic form: γδ T cells • Systemic form: αβ T cells	• T-cell (majority) or NK-cell lineage • T-cell cases: CD4 > CD8	• Cytotoxic T phenotype • Loss of one or more T-cell markers (usually CD5 and CD7) • CD8 > CD4

(continued)

TABLE 21.9-1 Key Features of EBV-Positive T/NK-Cell Lymphoproliferative Diseases of Childhood (continued)

	SMBA	HV-LPD	CAEBV	SEBVTCL
Genetic features	• Lack of clonal TCRGR in NK-cell origin (majority) • *DDX3X* and other somatic mutations detected in EBV+ cells	• Clonal TCRGR in majority of cases	• Clonal TCRGR in majority of cases • *DDX3X* and other somatic mutations detected in EBV+ cells	• Clonal TCRGR • Chromosomal abnormalities
Prognosis	• Prolonged clinical course • Increased risk of developing HLH, CAEBV, and T/NK-cell lymphomas/leukemias • Expression of *BZLF1* indicates poor prognosis.	• Better prognosis in classic form, some show resolution by adolescence. • Systemic form has higher risk of developing complications and lymphoma.	• Progressive disease with poor prognosis • Complications include HLH and progression to T/NK-cell lymphomas/leukemias.	• Highly aggressive clinical course, fatal within weeks in most cases
Treatment	• Supportive treatment (steroids, antihistamines) • HSCT	• Supportive treatment, photoprotection • Systemic form may require chemotherapy and HSCT.	• HLH regimens • HSCT	• Chemotherapy followed by HSCT

SEBVTCL and EBV-associated HLH can be challenging to distinguish. Clonal TCRGR can be detected in both. The presence of chromosomal abnormalities helps establish the diagnosis of SEBVTCL.
CAEBV, chronic active EBV disease; EBV, Epstein-Barr virus; HLH, hemophagocytic lymphohistiocytosis; HSCT, hematopoietic stem cell transplant; HV-LPD, hydroa vacciniforme lymphoproliferative disorder; IM, infectious mononucleosis; LN, lymph node; SEBVTCL, systemic EBV-positive T-cell lymphoma of childhood; SMBA, severe mosquito bite allergy; TCRGR, T-cell receptor gene rearrangement.

TABLE 21.9-2 WHO-HAEM5 Diagnostic Criteria for Severe Mosquito Bite Allergy

Essential
- High fever and severe skin manifestations after mosquito bites
- Bite site biopsy showing lymphoid infiltrate with NK-cell, or less commonly T-cell, phenotype
- EBER positive

Desirable
- High circulating EBV DNA load
- Lack of T-cell receptor protein expression and/or clonal *TR* gene rearrangement in cases of NK-cell origin

EBER, EBV-encoded RNA; EBV, Epstein-Barr virus.
Based on the WHO Classification of Tumours Editorial Board. Haematolymphoid tumours [Internet]. Lyon (France): International Agency for Research on Cancer; 2024 (WHO classification of tumours series, 5th ed.; vol. 11). Available from: https://tumourclassification.iarc.who.int/chapters/63.

- **Classic HV-LPD** is characterized by skin lesions in sun-exposed sites commonly on the face, neck, upper and lower limbs. The disease is usually limited to sun-exposed skin. The skin lesions manifest as recurrent papulovesicular eruptions and may form vacciniform (pox-like) scars. The classic form is usually indolent and self-limited; however, disease recurrences can occur particularly in spring and summer. Some patients show complete resolution by adolescence. The classic form is more common in White populations (*Blood.* 2019;133:2735-2737).
- **Systemic HV-LPD** is more aggressive than the classic form and shows more extensive skin involvement including non–sun-exposed sites. Patients have systemic symptoms (fever, lymphadenopathy, hepatosplenomegaly), multiorgan involvemnt, and may develop HLH. Systemic HV-LPD is more frequently observed in individuals

TABLE 21.9-3 WHO-HAEM5 Diagnostic Criteria for Hydroa Vacciniforme Lymphoproliferative Disorder

Essential
- Classic HV-LPD: lack of persistent systemic symptoms[a] or NK-cell lymphocytosis
- Systemic HV-LPD: persistent symptoms (≥1 from the list below) or extracutaneous disease
- Papulovesicular skin eruption with or without photo-exacerbation and varioliform (pox-like) scarring
- Perivascular and periadnexal atypical lymphoid infiltrate of cytotoxic T or NK cells
- EBER positive

EBER, EBV-encoded RNA; EBV, Epstein-Barr virus; HLH, hemophagocytic lymphohistiocytosis; HV-LPD, hydroa vacciniforme lymphoproliferative disorder.
Based on the WHO Classification of Tumours Editorial Board. Haematolymphoid tumours [Internet]. Lyon (France): International Agency for Research on Cancer; 2024 (WHO classification of tumours series, 5th ed.; vol. 11). Available from: https://tumourclassification.iarc.who.int/chapters/63.
[a]Lymphadenopathy, hepatosplenomegaly, hepatitis, HLH.

of Asian and Latin American descent. Similar to SMBA, poor prognostic factors include age of onset more than 9 years and the expression of *BZLF1* (*Br J Dermatol*. 2015;172:56-63). It is critical to distinguish CAEBV without HV-LPD from systemic HV-LPD. The former is fatal without HSCT, and the latter may be treated more conservatively (*Blood*. 2019;133:2753-2764).

III. SYSTEMIC CHRONIC ACTIVE EPSTEIN-BARR VIRUS DISEASE

CAEBV disease is a chronic disorder characterized by more than 3 months duration of mild to severe infectious mononucleosis–like (IM-like) symptoms along with increased levels of EBV DNA in the blood and infiltration of organs by EBV-infected T/NK cells. B-cell-driven lymphoproliferation and underlying primary immunodeficiency exclude this diagnosis. The disease involves infiltration of EBV-positive T/NK cells in multiple organs, and symptoms include fever, lymphadenopathy, hepatosplenomegaly, cytopenia(s), enteritis, respiratory and neurologic dysfunction, etc. CAEBV disease can present with concurrent SMBA or HV-LPD. Histologically, CAEBV disease typically shows subtle lymphocytic infiltration in tissues with or without cytologic atypia. Lymph nodes may show IM-like features (paracortical hyperplasia, follicular hyperplasia, and polymorphous infiltrate). Bone marrow, liver, and spleen show sinusoidal infiltration, which may be subtle. Hemophagocytosis can be seen in patients with HLH. Most of the cases are of T-cell lineage and usually express CD4 and $\alpha\beta$ T-cell receptor (TCR$\alpha\beta$). Expression of CD8 and TCR$\gamma\delta$ is reported in a small subset (*Blood*. 2012;119:673-686). Cytotoxic markers (T-cell-restricted intracellular antigen [TIA] and granzyme) are positive. CD56 expression is most often seen in NK-cell lineage. TCR gene rearrangement studies may show clonal rearrangements (not detected in all cases). The disease generally has an aggressive course with poor prognosis and is usually fatal without HSCT. Complications include HLH and progression to NK/T-cell lymphoma/leukemia. The diagnostic criteria are summarized in Table 21.9-4.

IV. SYSTEMIC EPSTEIN-BARR VIRUS–POSITIVE T-CELL LYMPHOMA OF CHILDHOOD

SEBVTCL is an aggressive disease characterized by systemic infiltration of clonal EBV+ cytotoxic T cells. Patients are immunocompetent and may have a history of

TABLE 21.9-4 WHO-HAEM5 Diagnostic Criteria for Systemic Chronic Active EBV Disease

Essential

- Infectious mononucleosis–like symptoms persisting for >3 mo
- Increased EBV DNA in peripheral blood or EBER-positive T/NK cells in affected organs
- Absence of immunodeficiency, malignancy, or autoimmune disorders

EBER, EBV-encoded RNA; EBV, Epstein-Barr virus.
Based on the WHO Classification of Tumours Editorial Board. Haematolymphoid tumours [Internet]. Lyon (France): International Agency for Research on Cancer; 2024 (WHO classification of tumours series, 5th ed.; vol. 11). Available from: https://tumourclassification.iarc.who.int/chapters/63.

TABLE 21.9-5 WHO-HAEM5 Diagnostic Criteria for Systemic EBV-Positive T-Cell Lymphoma of Childhood

Essential	Desirable
• Multiorgan infiltration by EBV+ atypical T cells • Absence of immunodeficiency • Fever and systemic symptoms	• Clonal TCR gene rearrangements • Hemophagocytic lymphohistiocytosis (HLH) • Hepatosplenomegaly • Abnormal karyotype

EBV, Epstein-Barr virus; TCR, T-cell receptor.
Based on the WHO Classification of Tumours Editorial Board. Haematolymphoid tumours [Internet]. Lyon (France): International Agency for Research on Cancer; 2024 (WHO classification of tumours series, 5th ed.; vol. 11). Available from: https://tumourclassification.iarc.who.int/chapters/63.

CAEBV disease. Initial presentation is characterized by IM-like symptoms. The disease progresses rapidly with symptoms of multiorgan involvement and patients may develop HLH, disseminated intravascular coagulation, sepsis, and multiorgan failure.

Biopsy of involved tissue sites shows lymphocytic infiltrate with variable cytology (small- to large-sized lymphocytes with or without atypia); in many cases, the lymphocytes show minimal atypia. Histologic evaluation of lymph nodes may show IM-like features. The nodal architecture is distorted by a polymorphous infiltrate expanding the paracortex. Variable numbers of large, atypical lymphocytes may be present. Dense histiocytic infiltrate and hemophagocytosis may be seen in patients with HLH. The liver shows variable sinusoidal involvement and necrosis may be present. Spleen sections show sinusoidal infiltrate along with white pulp atrophy. All cases are of cytotoxic T-cell lineage and typically express CD8 and TIA. Loss of one or more T-cell antigens is common, particularly CD5 and CD7. Cases evolving from CAEBV disease are more often CD4 positive. The majority of the tumor cells are positive for EBER. The prognosis is poor, with rapid disease progression and death within weeks to months in many cases. HLH treatment protocols, anthracycline, etoposide, and dexamethasone-based chemotherapy regimens followed by HSCT have been effective in some cases (*Pediatr Hematol Oncol.* 2018;35:121-124). The differential diagnosis includes other EBV-associated T/NK-cell LPDs. EBV infection–associated HLH may be difficult to distinguish from SEBVTCL as both conditions show significant clinicopathologic overlap. Abnormal karyotype supports the diagnosis of SEBVTCL. The diagnostic criteria are summarized in Table 21.9-5.

SUGGESTED READINGS

Alaggio R, Amador C, Anagnostopoulos I, et al. The 5th edition of the World Health Organization classification of haematolymphoid tumours: lymphoid neoplasms. *Leukemia.* 2022;36(7):1720-1748.

El-Mallawany NK, Curry CV, Allen CE. Haemophagocytic lymphohistiocytosis and Epstein-Barr virus: a complex relationship with diverse origins, expression and outcomes. *Br J Haematol.* 2022;196(1):31-44.

Quintanilla-Martinez L, Swerdlow SH, Tousseyn T, Barrionuevo C, Nakamura S, Jaffe ES. New concepts in EBV-associated B, T, and NK cell lymphoproliferative disorders. *Virchows Arch.* 2023;482(1):227-244.

Syrykh C, Péricart S, Lamaison C, Escudié F, Brousset P, Laurent C. Epstein-Barr virus-associated T-and NK-cell lymphoproliferative diseases: a review of clinical and pathological features. *Cancers (Basel).* 2021;13(13):3315.

PART 3: Immunodeficiency-Associated Lymphoproliferative Disorders

22. Overview and Classification of Immunodeficiency-Associated Lymphoproliferative Disorders

Brooj Abro

I. CLASSIFICATION OF IMMUNODEFICIENCY-ASSOCIATED LYMPHOPROLIFERATIVE DISORDERS ACCORDING TO THE WHO-HAEM4R

In the WHO-HAEM4R, immunodeficiency-associated lymphoproliferative disorders (IA-LPDs) were classified based on the type of underlying immune deficiency and divided into four main categories: (1) LPDs associated with primary immune disorders, (2) post-transplant lymphoproliferative disorder (PTLD), (3) lymphomas associated with HIV infection, and (4) other iatrogenic IA-LPDs. While this classification scheme focuses on the underlying immune deficiency, it recognized that IA-LPDs share similar pathogenic and histologic features across various immune deficiency settings.

II. UPDATES TO THE CLASSIFICATION OF IMMUNODEFICIENCY-ASSOCIATED LYMPHOPROLIFERATIVE DISORDERS

WHO-HAEM5 has slightly modified the name IA-LPDs and added the term "dysregulation" to recognize "immune dysregulation" settings without an established diagnosis of immune deficiency that can also lead to LPDs. Therefore, the name has been updated to "immune deficiency/dysregulation-associated lymphoproliferative disorders" (IDD-LPDs). In an attempt to standardize the classification and terminology of IDD-LPDs across various IDD settings, the Society for Hematopathology/European Association for Hematopathology Workshop 2015 (*Blood*. 2018;132:1871) proposed a three-part unifying nomenclature (listed herein), and the WHO-HAEM5 has adopted this nomenclature.

1. The name of histologic lesion (eg, plasmacytic hyperplasia)
2. The presence or absence of oncogenic virus(es) (eg, $EBV^{+/-}$, $HHV8^{+/-}$)
3. The type of IDD (eg, HIV)

To classify IDD-LPDs using this nomenclature, the type of histologic lesion, Epstein-Barr virus/human herpesvirus-8 (EBV/HHV8) status, and the type of IDD should be noted. Histologic lesions in IDD settings can be classified as hyperplasias, polymorphic LPDs, and lymphomas. The types of immune deficiencies can be broadly categorized into primary immune deficiencies (PIDs)/inborn errors of immunity (IEI) and acquired immunodeficiency in HIV infection, status post-transplant, or secondary to various immunosuppressant drugs. For example, if a patient with a transplant history has EBV$^+$ polymorphous LPD, the diagnostic terminology per the new WHO classification would be "polymorphous LPD, EBV$^+$, post-transplant." Diagnosing lymphomas in the IDD setting requires fulfilling the same criteria as corresponding lymphomas in immunocompetent patients.

The WHO-HAEM5 has unified the nomenclature to harmonize the terminology used across various IDD settings. The ICC also recognizes similarities in histologic features of LPDs across various IDD settings; however, the consensus was to retain PTLD as a subgroup partly due to differences in clinical management (*Blood*. 2022;140:1229). The overall diagnostic criteria and workup (evaluation of histologic lesion and EBV status, etc) for PTLD are similar in the WHO-HAEM5 and ICC. The WHO classification of IDD-LPDs and updates are summarized in Table 22.1.

TABLE 22.1 WHO Classification of Immune Deficiency/Dysregulation-Associated Lymphoproliferative Disorders (IDD-LPDs)

WHO-HAEM5	WHO-HAEM4R
Hyperplasias arising in IDD	Not previously included, encompassing nondestructive PTLD, among others
Polymorphic LPDs arising in IDD	Not previously included, encompassing polymorphic PTLD, other iatrogenic IA-LPDs, among others
EBV$^+$ MCU[a]	Same
Lymphomas arising in IDD	Not previously included, encompassing monomorphic PTLD, CHL-PTLD, lymphomas associated with HIV infection, among others
IEI-LPDs	LPDs associated with primary immune disorders

CHL, classic Hodgkin lymphoma; IA-LPD, immunodeficiency-associated lymphoproliferative disorder; IDD, immune deficiency/dysregulation; IEI, inborn error of immunity; MCU, mucocutaneous ulcer; PTLD, post-transplant lymphoproliferative disorder.
[a]Discussed in Chapter 19.10. The rest of the entities are discussed in Chapters 23 and 24.
Modified from Alaggio R, Amador C, Anagnostopoulos I, et al. The 5th edition of the World Health Organization classification of haematolymphoid tumours: lymphoid neoplasms. *Leukemia*. 2022;36(7):1720-1748.

SUGGESTED READINGS

Natkunam Y, Gratzinger D, Chadburn A, et al. Immunodeficiency-associated lymphoproliferative disorders: time for reappraisal? *Blood*. 2018;132(18):1871-1878.

Quintanilla-Martinez L, Swerdlow SH, Tousseyn T, Barrionuevo C, Nakamura S, Jaffe ES. New concepts in EBV-associated B, T, and NK cell lymphoproliferative disorders. *Virchows Arch*. 2023;482(1):227-244.

23 Lymphoid Proliferations and Lymphomas Associated With Immune Deficiency/Dysregulation

Anne L. Chen and Brooj Abro

Lymphoid proliferations and lymphomas associated with immune deficiency and dysregulation (IDD) encompass a wide range of lymphoid lesions that occur in various IDD settings, most commonly described in the post-transplant setting. These lesions may arise soon after transplant (within 1-2 years) or several years later. Early lesions are more likely to be positive for Epstein-Barr virus (EBV), and late lesions tend to be EBV⁻. Other IDD settings include HIV infection, iatrogenic (eg, methotrexate therapy), immune senescence, and primary immune deficiencies. The WHO-HAEM5 recommends the use of the following nomenclature when reporting these lesions: (1) the type of histologic lesion, (2) the presence or absence of EBV/HHV8 (human herpesvirus-8), and (3) the type of immunodeficiency. The types of lymphoid lesions in IDD include hyperplasias, polymorphic lymphoproliferative disorders (P-LPDs), EBV⁺ mucocutaneous ulcer (EBVMCU), and lymphomas. EBVMCU is discussed in Chapter 19.10. The rest are discussed in this chapter.

I. HYPERPLASIAS ARISING IN SETTINGS OF IMMUNE DEFICIENCY/DYSREGULATION

Hyperplasias arising in the setting of immune deficiency/dysregulation (H-IDD) are nonclonal proliferations of lymphocytes and/or plasma cells in the setting of various IDDs. The involved tissue shows a preserved architecture. The term "nondestructive post-transplant lymphoproliferative disorder" was used by the WHO-HAEM4R to describe these disorders in the post-transplant setting. The ICC retains this terminology. EBV is positive in most H-IDDs and is usually demonstrated by performing Epstein-Barr virus encoded small RNA in situ hybridization (EBER-ISH) on the affected tissue. The presence of EBV is typically required to establish an association between hyperplasia and IDD since the morphologic features are nonspecific. The diagnostic criteria are summarized in Table 23.1.

Clinical Features

- **Clinical presentation**: Signs and symptoms are nonspecific and variable, depending on the site(s) of involvement. Patients may present with flulike symptoms and lymphadenopathy.
- **Sites of involvement:** Many sites can be involved, including tonsils, adenoids, mucosal sites, lymph nodes, spleen, and other extranodal sites. Tonsils and adenoids

TABLE 23.1 WHO-HAEM5 Diagnostic Criteria for Hyperplasias Arising in Settings of Immune Deficiency/Dysregulation (IDD)

Essential

- Confirmation of IDD or high clinical suspicion
- Preserved architecture
- Heterogeneous proliferations (lymphoid and/or plasmacytic) without significant atypia
- One of the following features:
    1. EBV/EBER+ in hyperplasias
    2. KSHV/HHV8+ in multicentric Castleman disease
    3. Other specific features related to IDD such as CD4−/CD8− T-cell proliferation in ALPS

ALPS, autoimmune lymphoproliferative syndrome; EBER, Epstein-Barr virus–encoded region; EBV, Epstein-Barr virus; HHV8, human herpesvirus-8; KSHV, Kaposi sarcoma–associated herpesvirus.
Based on the WHO Classification of Tumours Editorial Board. Haematolymphoid tumours [Internet]. Lyon (France): International Agency for Research on Cancer; 2024 (WHO classification of tumours series, 5th ed.; vol. 11). Available from: https://tumourclassification.iarc.who.int/chapters/63.

are most commonly involved in the post-transplant setting. Patients with underlying HIV infection, autoimmune disease, or therapy-related IDD may present with generalized lymphadenopathy.

Morphology and Immunophenotype

Regardless of etiology and subtype, the defining feature of H-IDDs is the lack of architectural effacement; some architectural distortion, however, may be present. Common H-IDD morphologic subtypes recognized by the WHO-HAEM5 include follicular hyperplasia (FH), plasmacytic hyperplasia (PCH), infectious mononucleosis-like hyperplasia (IMH), and Kaposi sarcoma–associated herpesvirus (KSHV)/HHV8+ multicentric Castleman disease. T-cell proliferations can also occur. A more detailed list of subtypes is described in the WHO-HAEM5 (see reference in "Suggested Readings" section).

- **FH:** Scattered EBV+ lymphocytes are present in lymphoid tissue with reactive hyperplastic follicles, usually in interfollicular areas, but can also be seen within germinal centers (GCs) (e-Figure 23.1). The GCs show nonneoplastic immunophenotype (positive for GC markers CD10 and BCL6 and negative for BCL2). Castleman-like features may be present.
- **PCH:** Lymphoid tissue shows increased plasma cells, usually in interfollicular areas and scattered EBV+ cells. The plasma cells in PCH have a normal immunophenotype and are polytypic.
- **IMH:** IMH is characterized by paracortical hyperplasia composed of a pleomorphic infiltrate consisting of B cells of varying sizes intermixed with reactive predominantly CD8+ T cells. Immunoblasts and scattered Hodgkin Reed-Sternberg-like (HRS-like) cells may be present. B cells show variable expression of CD20. Immunoblasts and HRS-like cells are usually positive for CD20 (variable), CD45,

CD30, and MUM1. EBV is positive in scattered B cells (both small and large cells may be positive).
- **KSHV/HHV8+ multicentric Castleman disease**: This entity is discussed in Chapter 19.9 (B-cell Lymphoproliferative Disorders Associated with HHV-8).

Genetic Features

B-cell hyperplasias usually do not show clonal *IGH/IGK* gene rearrangements. Rarely, small clonal peaks may be detected. TCR gene rearrangement testing may show clonal peaks secondary to reactive T-cell proliferation (a polyclonal background is generally present). Clonal and nonclonal karyotype abnormalities have been reported (*Hematol Oncol.* 2011;29:81-90). A recent study identified recurrent mutations involving *NOTCH1* in patients with FH associated with IDD (*Front Oncol.* 2022;11:790481).

Prognosis and Treatment

Although many cases are self-limiting and regress without intervention, some cases may require cessation of the offending therapy or immune reconstitution may be necessary.

Differential Diagnosis

The differential diagnosis is broad depending on the type of lesion and includes many reactive conditions. An established history of an underlying IDD and exclusion of other reactive conditions is essential in diagnosing H-IDD.

II. POLYMORPHIC LYMPHOPROLIFERATIVE DISORDERS ARISING IN IMMUNE DEFICIENCY/DYSREGULATION

P-LPDs arising in IDD are mass-forming lesions composed of heterogeneous B-cell proliferations typically driven by EBV, either monoclonal or oligoclonal, that efface the background tissue architecture and do not meet criteria for the diagnosis of lymphoma. B cells typically show a wide spectrum of differentiation, and scattered HRS-like cells may be present. P-LPDs are most commonly diagnosed in patients who have undergone stem cell or solid organ transplantation. The incidence in other IDD settings is lower and not as well documented. The diagnostic criteria are summarized in Table 23.2.

Clinical Features

- **Clinical presentation:** Patients may present with lymphadenopathy and other signs/symptoms depending on the site(s) of involvement.
- **Sites of involvement:** Lymph nodes are most commonly involved. Other sites include bone marrow, lungs, gastrointestinal tract, liver, and central nervous system.

Morphology

The typical appearance is an architecture-effacing, heterogeneous mixture of cells consisting of lymphocytes of variable sizes, plasmacytoid lymphocytes, plasma cells, immunoblasts, and histiocytes (e-Figure 23.2). There may be a variable number of atypical large cells and HRS-like cells; however, sheets of large cells should not be present. Mitosis is frequent, and necrosis may be present. It should be noted that certain lymphomas can exhibit polymorphic morphology, such as EBV$^+$ diffuse large B-cell lymphoma (DLBCL) or T-cell histiocyte-rich large B-cell lymphoma. Therefore, the diagnosis of P-LPD should not be made if the overall characteristics meet the diagnostic criteria for a lymphoma.

TABLE 23.2 WHO-HAEM5 Diagnostic Criteria for Polymorphic Lymphoproliferative Disorders Arising in Immune Deficiency/Dysregulation (IDD)

Essential	Desirable
- Confirmation of IDD or high clinical suspicion - Architectural effacement - Polymorphous B-cell infiltrate with atypical large cells variably positive for CD20 and CD30 and positive for PAX5 - EBV⁺ cells in tissue	- *IGH/IGK* gene rearrangement studies

EBV, Epstein-Barr virus.
Based on the WHO Classification of Tumours Editorial Board. Haematolymphoid tumours [Internet]. Lyon (France): International Agency for Research on Cancer; 2024 (WHO classification of tumours series, 5th ed.; vol. 11). Available from: https://tumourclassification.iarc.who.int/chapters/63.

Immunophenotype

B-lineage cells show variable expression for pan–B-cell markers depending on the degree of plasmacytic differentiation. Plasma cells and some plasmacytoid lymphocytes are negative for CD20 and express CD138 and MUM1. CD30 highlights immunoblasts and some larger cells, including HRS-like cells. Unlike HRS cells in classic Hodgkin lymphoma (CHL), HRS-like cells in P-LPD are usually positive for CD20 and CD45 and negative for CD15. EBER-ISH is usually positive in numerous lymphocytes of varying sizes (e-Figure 23.2). Kappa and lambda IHC or ISH studies may demonstrate light-chain restriction.

Genetic Features

IGH/IGK gene rearrangement studies show monoclonal or oligoclonal patterns (P-LPD in the post-transplant setting usually shows monoclonality). Synchronous lesions at different sites may have different clones. A subset of cases demonstrate cytogenetic abnormalities.

Prognosis and Treatment

Treatment options vary depending on the type of IDD and include reducing immunosuppression, immunotherapy, antiretroviral therapy in patients infected with HIV, and rituximab with or without cytotoxic therapy. The prognosis and clinical course vary; some patients show regression with a reduction in immunosuppression, while others may require chemotherapy for disease progression.

Differential Diagnosis

The differential diagnosis is broad and includes other disorders that exhibit polymorphic infiltrates:

- **IMH:** These lesions lack architectural effacement, which can aid in distinguishing them from P-LPD.
- **Small B-cell lymphomas:** Marginal zone lymphoma (MZL) and lymphoplasmacytic lymphoma (LPL) can be challenging to distinguish from P-LPD. Mutations in *MYD88* support the diagnosis of LPL. The presence of lymphoepithelial lesions in extranodal sites is indicative of MZL.

- **EBV⁺ DLBCL:** Sheets of large B cells are a feature of DLBCL; however, some cases have a polymorphous appearance (e-Figures 23.3 and 23.4). Unlike P-LPD, EBV⁺ DLBCL usually does not show a wide spectrum of B-cell differentiation, and EBV is mostly positive in large cells.
- **EBVMCU:** Ulcerated lesion limited to mucosal and cutaneous sites. Clinical findings are important to distinguish these from P-LPD.
- **CHL:** The diagnosis of CHL in an IDD setting should be made with caution, and diagnostic criteria should be applied more strictly. HRS cells in CHL are usually $CD30^+$ and $CD15^{+/-}$ and negative for CD20 and CD45; however, variable expression of these markers may be present. EBV is positive in mostly large cells. HRS-like cells in P-LPD are typically positive for CD20 and CD45 and negative for CD15. P-LPD shows EBV positivity in cells of varying sizes.
- **Nodal T follicular helper cell lymphoma, angioimmunoblastic type (nTFHL-AI):** Increased T follicular helper (TFH)-type cells and vascular and follicular dendritic cell proliferation are features of nTFHL-AI. Demonstration of TCR gene rearrangements and somatic mutations, particularly involving *RHOA*, may be helpful in difficult cases.

III. LYMPHOMAS ARISING IN IMMUNE DEFICIENCY/DYSREGULATION

Lymphomas arising in the setting of IDD are defined by the same criteria as in the non-IDD settings, and many of these cases are associated with EBV or HHV8. B-cell lymphomas are the most common. Lymphoma types in IDD settings are summarized in Table 23.3.

TABLE 23.3 Summary of Lymphoma Types and Features in Immunodeficiency/Dysregulation (IDD)

Lymphoma Types	Features[a]
Small B-cell lymphomas	
• Marginal zone lymphomas (nodal and extranodal) • Lymphoplasmacytic lymphoma (LPL)	• EBV+/− • There is significant overlap with polymorphic LPD, and the distinction can be challenging.
Large B-cell lymphomas	
• Diffuse large B-cell lymphoma (DLBCL)	• Overall, most common type • Most cases are non-GCB type • Subtypes include DLBCL-NOS, EBV⁺ DLBCL, HHV8⁺ DLBCL
• Burkitt lymphoma (BL)	• EBV−/+ • BL cases in IDD settings may show atypical morphologic features, such as pleomorphism and plasmacytic differentiation.

TABLE 23.3 Summary of Lymphoma Types and Features in Immunodeficiency/Dysregulation (IDD) (*continued*)

Lymphoma Types	Features[a]
• Plasmablastic lymphoma	• Majority of the cases are EBV+.
• Primary effusion lymphoma	• HHV8+, EBV+
Classic Hodgkin lymphoma (CHL)	• The mixed cellularity subtype is the most common. • HRS cells are usually EBV+, and the expression of B-cell markers is seen more often than in non-IDD settings. • Note: HRS-like cells can be seen in P-LPD. The distinction can be challenging in some cases.
Plasma cell neoplasms	
• Plasmacytoma	• Mostly extranodal lesions composed of clonal mature plasma cells. Lytic lesions are uncommon, and bone marrow is not involved. • EBV is positive in a subset.
• Plasma cell myeloma	• EBV is usually negative.
T-/NK-cell neoplasms	• Rare in IDD setting, and the association is unclear. • Reported types include PTCL-NOS, ALCL, nTFHL-AI, HSTCL, ENKTCL. • Usually, EBV−, except for the subtypes where EBV positivity is a diagnostic criterion (eg, ENKTCL).

ALCL, anaplastic larger cell lymphoma; EBV, Epstein-Barr virus; ENKTCL, extranodal NK-/T-cell lymphoma; GCB, germinal center B cell; HHV8, human herpesvirus-8; HRS, Hodgkin Reed-Sternberg; HSTCL, hepatosplenic T-cell lymphoma; nTFHL-AI, nodal T follicular helper cell lymphoma, angioimmunoblastic type; PTCL-NOS, peripheral T-cell lymphoma, not otherwise specified.

[a]The diagnostic criteria of these lymphomas are similar to their counterparts in immunocompetent patients (discussed in other chapters).

Key Points

- Lymphoid proliferations and lymphomas associated with IDD include hyperplasias (H-IDD), P-LPD, and lymphomas.
- These lesions are usually associated with EBV or HHV8.
- The diagnosis requires the establishment of or high suspicion of IDD background
- H-IDDs are lymphoid proliferations that usually show preserved lymphoid architecture. P-LPD causes effacement of architecture and may contain scattered large cells; however, diffuse large cells should not be present (a feature of lymphoma).
- Lymphomas in IDD require meeting the same diagnostic criteria as their counterparts in non-IDD settings.

Diagnostic Caveats
- H-IDD shows nonspecific morphology; without EBV positivity in the tissue, the association with IDD cannot be established. Other reactive causes should be ruled out.
- P-LPDs show overlapping morphologic features with other disorders, including some lymphomas (see "Differential Diagnosis" section in "Polymorphic Lymphoproliferative Disorders Arising in Immune Deficiency/Dysregulation").

SUGGESTED READINGS

Natkunam Y, Gratzinger D, Chadburn A, et al. Immunodeficiency-associated lymphoproliferative disorders: time for reappraisal? *Blood*. 2018;132(18):1871-1878.

Quintanilla-Martinez L, Swerdlow SH, Tousseyn T, Barrionuevo C, Nakamura S, Jaffe ES. New concepts in EBV-associated B, T, and NK cell lymphoproliferative disorders. *Virchows Arch*. 2023;482(1):227-244.

WHO Classification of Tumours Editorial Board. Haematolymphoid tumours [Internet; beta version ahead of print]. In: *WHO Classification of Tumours Series*. 5th ed. Vol.11. International Agency for Research on Cancer; 2022 [cited 2023 Dec 16]. https://tumourclassification.iarc.who.int/chapters/63. Refer to section: *Lymphoid proliferations and lymphomas associated with immune deficiency and dysregulation*.

24 Inborn Error of Immunity–Associated Lymphoid Proliferations and Lymphomas

Brooj Abro

As the name implies, inborn error of immunity–associated lymphoproliferative disorders (IEI-LPDs) and lymphomas arise in the setting of an underlying IEI. Patients with IEI have increased susceptibility to Epstein-Barr virus (EBV) infection; therefore, EBV-associated LPDs and lymphomas are more common in these patients compared to the general population. According to the WHO-HAEM5, the IEI-LPD subtypes are similar to those described across various immune deficiency/dysregulation settings, including hyperplasias, EBV^+ mucocutaneous ulcer (EBVMUC), polymorphous LPDs, and lymphomas.

There are several types of IEI or primary immune deficiencies (PIDs) and associated LPDs. IEI/PIDs primarily associated with antibody deficiencies such as common variable immune deficiency (CVID) are the most common, followed by combined immune deficiencies (CIDs) that are associated with defects in both humoral and cellular cell–mediated immunity. The clinical features and diagnosis of various IEIs are out of the scope of this book. Table 24.1 summarizes common IEIs/PIDs and associated LPDs and lymphomas. The diagnostic criteria for IEI-LPDs are summarized in Table 24.2.

Clinical Features

The clinical presentation varies based on the lymphoma subtype and site(s) of involvement. Lymph nodes and many extranodal sites can be involved by IEI-LPDs.

Morphology and Immunophenotype

The morphologic features of IEI-LPDs align with LPDs and lymphomas across various settings of immune dysregulation/dysfunction. Most IEI-LPDs are B-cell proliferations associated with EBV, including hyperplasias, EBVMCUs, and polymorphic LPDs (see Chapter 23). Common lymphomas reported in the IEI setting include diffuse large B-cell lymphoma (DLBCL), Burkitt lymphoma, classic Hodgkin lymphoma, and marginal zone lymphoma including nodal and extranodal (*Front Immunol.* 2019;10:777). The immunophenotype of lymphomas arising in the setting of IEI is similar to the corresponding lymphomas in immunocompetent patients.

Genetic Features

Genetic testing can be helpful in the diagnosis of the underlying IEI and associated LPD/lymphoma. While *IGH/IGK* and TCR gene rearrangement studies are useful in the diagnosis of B- and T-cell LPDs and lymphomas, the results need to be interpreted

TABLE 24.1 Common Primary Immune Deficiencies and Associated Lymphoproliferative Disorders and Lymphomas

IEI/PIDs	Associated LPDs and Lymphomas
CVID and other PIDs predominantly associated with antibody deficiencies	DLBCL and CHL (often associated with EBV), EMZL, T-LGLL, CD8$^+$ T-cell–rich proliferations
Combined immune deficiencies	DLBCL, BL, CHL, mature and immature T-cell lymphomas
Autoimmune lymphoproliferative syndrome	CHL, NLPHL, DLBCL
Familial hemophagocytic lymphohistiocytosis (HLH) and T-cell defects	Associated with HLH, lymphomas are rare.

BL, Burkitt lymphoma; CHL, classic Hodgkin lymphoma; CVID, common variable immune deficiency; DLBCL, diffuse large B-cell lymphoma; EMZL, extranodal marginal zone lymphoma; IEI, inborn error of immunity; LPDs, lymphoproliferative disorders; NLPHL, nodular lymphocyte predominant Hodgkin lymphoma; PID, primary immune deficiency; T-LGLL, T-large granular lymphocytic leukaemia (T-LGLL).
Front Immunol. 2019;10:777; WHO-HAEM5.

with caution in the setting of immune deficiency as these patients may have expanded clonal populations (*Sci Transl Med.* 2015;7:302ra135). Molecular tests recommended for the diagnosis of lymphomas in immunocompetent patients can be performed to evaluate corresponding lymphomas in the IEI setting. Germline testing is recommended for the diagnosis of underlying IEI.

TABLE 24.2 Diagnostic Criteria for Inborn Error of Immunity–Associated Lymphoproliferative Disorders (IEI-LPDs)

Essential	Desirable
• Criteria for lymphomas and EBV$^+$ LPDs are the same as described in relevant chapters for specific entities. • EBV status should be assessed. • Underlying IEI should be mentioned. • Exclusion of infectious etiology and other lymphomas is required for the diagnosis of granulomatous/CD8$^+$ T-cell lesions.	• Molecular classification including germline testing to evaluate the underlying IEI.

EBV, Epstein-Barr virus.
Based on the WHO Classification of Tumours Editorial Board. Haematolymphoid tumours [Internet]. Lyon (France): International Agency for Research on Cancer; 2024 (WHO classification of tumours series, 5th ed.; vol. 11). Available from: https://tumourclassification.iarc.who.int/chapters/63.

Prognosis and Treatment

Since IEI-LPDs include a broad spectrum of both underlying immune disorders and types of LPDs/lymphomas, the prognosis greatly varies and depends on these factors. Apart from the morbidity associated with LPDs/lymphomas, patients also suffer complications because of increased susceptibility to infections. Treatment options include chemotherapy and hematopoietic stem cell transplant, the latter potentially curative for both underlying IEI and associated LPD (*Hematol Educ Program.* 2020;2020:649).

> **Key Points**
>
> - Patients with IEI have increased susceptibility to EBV infection and increased incidence of EBV-associated LPDs and lymphomas.
> - The IEI-LPD subtypes are similar to those described across various immune deficiency/dysregulation settings, including hyperplasias, EBVMUC, polymorphous LPDs, and lymphomas.
> - The workup of IEI-LPDs should include evaluation of underlying IEI (germline testing recommended) and EBV status.
> - The diagnostic criteria of various lymphomas in the IEI setting (eg, DLBCL, BL, CHL) are similar to the corresponding lymphomas described in immunocompetent patients.

SUGGESTED READINGS

Gratzinger D, et al. Haematolymphoid tumours. In: WHO Classification of Tumours Editorial Board. *WHO Classification of Tumours Series*, 5th ed. Vol 11. Lyon (France): International Agency for Research on Cancer; 2024. Available from: https://tumourclassification.iarc.who.int/chapters/63.

Riaz IB, Faridi W, Patnaik MM, Abraham RS. A systematic review on predisposition to lymphoid (B and T cell) neoplasias in patients with primary immunodeficiencies and immune dysregulatory disorders (inborn errors of immunity). *Front Immunol.* 2019;10:777.

PART 4: Histiocytic and Dendritic Cell Neoplasms

25 Introduction to Histiocytic and Dendritic Cell Neoplasms

Carina A. Dehner, John D. Pfeifer, and Louis P. Dehner

Histiocytoses are a heterogeneous group of disorders of a previously ambiguous nature composed of macrophages, dendritic cells, or monocyte-derived cells; these various differentiated cell types are the progeny of a myeloid precursor. A consensus has emerged that several of the more thoroughly characterized clinicopathologic entities are neoplastic in nature with the demonstration of somatic mutations in the MAPK-ERK signaling pathway. A reformulated classification of histiocytic disorders is based in part on shared mutations as well as classic histopathologic and immunophenotypic features (Table 25.1). A more truncated classification has been proposed in WHO-HAEM5 (Table 25.2).

In the classification scheme proposed by the Histiocyte Society (Table 25.1), five groups or categories have been proposed on the basis of histology, phenotype, molecular alterations, and clinical and imaging characteristics. Studies continue to emerge that fill in the gaps.

I. "L" (LANGERHANS) GROUP

Langerhans cell histiocytosis (LCH) is a clonal proliferation of CD1a$^+$ dendritic cells presenting in a single site (bone, skin) or multiple sites with or without organ dysfunction. Mutations in the MAPK pathway are present in over 80% of cases; this molecular feature (*BRAF* V600E) is shared with Erdheim-Chester disease (ECD) though LCH and ECD have distinctive clinical and pathologic features in some but not all cases (20% of cases). Therefore, LCH, ECD, and extracutaneous juvenile xanthogranuloma (JXG) with *MAPK*-activating mutations or *ALK* translocations are grouped together. Note that cutaneous JXG is found in the "C" group. CD1a and CD207 (langerin) expression are restricted to LCH in contrast to ECD and JXG with restricted positivity to CD68 and CD163.

II. "C" GROUP: CUTANEOUS AND MUCOCUTANEOUS HISTIOCYTOSES

Two categories comprise the "C" group. The first category is the cutaneous non-LCH diseases composed of entities in the xanthogranuloma (XG) family (JXG/adult XG [AXG]), solitary reticulohistiocytoma (SRH), benign cephalic histiocytosis (BCH), generalized eruptive histiocytosis (GEH), and progressive nodular histiocytosis (PNH) (all of which are defined largely by their clinical setting of solitary, multiple, or

TABLE 25.1   Histiocyte Society Proposed Classification of Histiocytoses

L group
- Langerhans cell histiocytosis (LCH)
- Indeterminate cell histiocytosis
- Erdheim-Chester disease (ECD)
- Mixed LCH/ECD

C group
- Cutaneous non-LCH
  - Xanthogranuloma (XG) family: juvenile XG, adult XG, solitary reticulohistiocytoma (SRH), benign cephalic histiocytosis (BCH), generalized eruptive histiocytosis (GEH), progressive nodular histiocytosis (PNH)
  - Non-XG family: cutaneous Rosai-Dorfman disease (RDD), necrobiotic XG, other not otherwise specified (NOS)
- Cutaneous non-LCH with a major systematic component

R group
- Familial RDD
- Sporadic RDD
  - Classical RDD
  - Extranodal RDD
  - RDD with neoplasia or immune disease
  - Unclassified

M group
- Primary malignant histiocytosis
- Secondary malignant histiocytosis (following or associated with other hematologic neoplasia)

H group
- Primary: Monogenic inherited conditions leading to hemophagocytic lymphohistiocytosis (HLH)
- Secondary HLH (non-Mendelian HLH)
- HLH of unknown/uncertain origin

The Histiocyte Society classification is based on histology, phenotype, molecular alterations, and clinical and imaging characteristics.
Modified from Emile JF, Abla O, Fraitag S, et al. Revised classification of histiocytoses and neoplasms of the macrophage-dendritic cell lineages. *Blood*. 2016;127(22):2672-2681.

---

disseminated involvement and patient age [*Ann Diagn Pathol*. 2022;58:151940]); cutaneous Rosai-Dorfman disease (RDD); and necrobiotic xanthogranuloma (NXG). The second category is represented by xanthoma disseminatum (XD) as a member of the XG family and multicentric reticulohistiocytosis (MRH). Patchy S100 protein positivity is present in RDD, whereas the others are CD68, CD163, and factor XIIIa positive.

TABLE 25.2 Summary of WHO-HAEM5 Classification of Histiocytic/Dendritic Neoplasms

Plasmacytoid dendritic cell neoplasms[a]

Mature plasmacytoid dendritic cell proliferation associated with myeloid neoplasm

Blastic plasmacytoid dendritic cell neoplasm

Langerhans cell and other dendritic cell neoplasms

Langerhans cell neoplasms
- Langerhans cell histiocytosis
- Langerhans cell sarcoma

Other dendritic cell neoplasms
- Indeterminate dendritic cell tumor
- Interdigitating dendritic cell sarcoma

Histiocytic neoplasms

Juvenile xanthogranuloma

Erdheim-Chester disease

Rosai-Dorfman disease

ALK-positive histiocytosis

Histiocytic sarcoma

WHO-HAEM5 classification is based on multiple clinicopathologic parameters, with an emphasis on therapeutically and/or prognostically actionable biomarkers, and strives to keep practical worldwide applicability in perspective.

[a]Discussed in Chapter 16. All other entities listed are discussed in subsequent chapters of this section.

Modified from Khoury JD, Solary E, Abla O, et al. The 5th edition of the World Health Organization Classification of Haematolymphoid Tumours: Myeloid and Histiocytic/Dendritic Neoplasms. *Leukemia.* 2022;36(7):1703-1719.

III. "M" GROUP: MALIGNANT HISTIOCYTOSES

This group is separated into primary malignant histiocytoses, which include histiocytic sarcoma, indeterminate cell sarcoma, and Langerhans cell sarcoma, and secondary malignant histiocytoses, which occur after or simultaneously with another hematopoietic neoplasm including follicular lymphoma, hairy cell leukemia, acute lymphocytic leukemia (ALL), or other histiocytoses.

IV. "R" GROUP: ROSAI-DORFMAN DISEASE AND MISCELLANEOUS NONCUTANEOUS, NON–LANGERHANS CELL HISTIOCYTOSES

The "R" group is largely divisible into sporadic, classical (nodal, extranodal), and familial RDD (also designated "H" syndrome with a germline variant in the *SLC29A3* gene). Sporadic RDD presents with lymphadenopathy, often cervical, or as extranodal involvement in skin, nasal cavity, bone, or soft tissue (*Pathologica.* 2021;113:388-395). RDD also occurs in association with other neoplasms or immune diseases. Mutually exclusive somatic mutations in *KRAS* and *MAP2K1* have been detected in RDD.

V. "H" GROUP: HEMOPHAGOCYTIC LYMPHOHISTIOCYTOSIS AND MACROPHAGE ACTIVATION SYNDROME

Hemophagocytic lymphohistiocytosis (HLH) is an uncommon and often fatal syndrome characterized by extreme activation of the immune system with fever, cytopenia, hepatosplenomegaly, and hyperferritinemia occurring as a primary disorder in young children with one of several germline variants (*Annu Rev Med.* 2012;63:233-246). Secondary HLH is acquired and is associated with various infections, malignancies, and autoimmune disorders (known as macrophage activation syndrome), has many of the same clinical and laboratory features of primary HLH, and is seen in a broader age range than the latter.

SUMMARY

The subsequent chapters introduce a broad overview of the various histiocytoses including their current classification based on clinical and molecular features. In brief, most cases of the "L" group are diseases driven by activating mutations in the MAPK pathway. The skin is a site of predilection as in JXG and its apparent variants. Extracutaneous JXG, like its cutaneous counterpart, has variable histologic features not always accompanied by Touton giant cells. Systemic JXG and ALK1 histiocytosis have many overlapping clinicopathologic features, and may in fact represent the same entity. Malignant histiocytoses may present as a primary histiocytic tumor or can arise secondary to other hematologic neoplasms, and expression of macrophage/dendritic cell markers is a basic diagnostic feature. RDD is characterized by groups of histiocytes with abundant clear cytoplasm with emperipolesis of lymphocytes and plasma cells. HLH is a hyperreactive disorder with activation of CD8, natural killer (NK) cells, and macrophages that may be driven by genetic disorders, infections, or cancer. At one time, HLH had been regarded as "malignant histiocytosis" with its often fatal consequences. In the following chapters, the major entities are discussed in more detail.

26 Histiocytic Sarcoma

Carina A. Dehner, John S. A. Chrisinger, and Louis P. Dehner

Histiocytic sarcoma (HS) is a rare aggressive neoplasm of presumed myeloid origin with morphologic and immunophenotypic characteristics of mature macrophages (*Am J Surg Pathol.* 2004;28:1133-1144). There are a limited number of cases in the literature as one measure of its uncommon nature (*Am J Surg Pathol.* 1998;22:1386-1392; *Blood.* 2008;111:5433-5439; *Am J Surg Pathol.* 2004;28:1133-1144; *Arch Pathol Lab Med.* 2020;144:650-654; *Mod Pathol.* 2005;18:693-704). With the availability of molecular and immunohistochemistry (IHC) techniques, some cases in the past diagnosed as HS were likely high-grade B- or T-cell lymphoma, including anaplastic large cell lymphomas (ALCLs) and myeloid sarcoma (MS). Some cases of HS coexist with other hematopoietic neoplasms, such as follicular lymphoma (*Blood.* 2008;111:5433-5439) or chronic lymphocytic leukemia (CLL)/small lymphocytic lymphoma (SLL) (*Mod Pathol.* 2011;24:1421-1432); it is thought those cases may be the result of a "transdifferentiation," possibly mediated by PU.1 (SP11), a transcription factor for myeloid/monocytic and B-lymphoid gene expression during hematopoiesis (*Arch Pathol Lab Med.* 2018;142:1322-1329). The diagnostic challenge is the consideration and then the confirmation of the histiocytic phenotype while excluding the morphologic mimics such as a variety of high-grade lymphomas, carcinomas, melanoma, or sarcomas (*Arch Pathol Lab Med.* 2020;144:650-654; *Mod Pathol.* 2005;18:693-704). The diagnostic criteria are summarized in Table 26.1.

Clinical Features

- **Clinical Presentation:** A mass lesion with or without pain and constitutional signs with fever and weight loss are the spectrum of initial manifestations. The median age at presentation ranges from 50 to 60 years with a male predilection (*Arch Pathol Lab Med.* 2020;144:650-654). HS has been reported in children with Burkitt lymphoma and other hematopoietic malignancies (*Pediatr Hematol Oncol.* 2021;38:1-7; *Indian J Pathol Microbiol.* 2018;61:278-280).

TABLE 26.1 WHO-HAEM5 Diagnostic Criteria for HS

Essential criteria

- Large non-cohesive pleomorphic tumor cells with abundant eosinophilic cytoplasm, reniform/grooved/irregular nuclei, and prominent nucleoli
- Positive: ≥2 histiocytic markers
- Negative: CD1a, langerin (CD207), CD21, CD35

HS, histiocytic sarcoma.
Based on the WHO Classification of Tumours Editorial Board. Haematolymphoid tumours [Internet]. Lyon (France): International Agency for Research on Cancer; 2024 (WHO classification of tumours series, 5th ed.; vol. 11). Available from: https://tumourclassification.iarc.who.int/chapters/63.

- **Sites of Involvement:** HS commonly presents at extranodal sites, such as the gastrointestinal tract, deep soft tissues, bone, lung, nasal cavity (*Am J Surg Pathol.* 2004;28:1133-1144), and even thyroid (*Ann Hematol.* 2008;87:681-682), but primary cases in lymph nodes (*Mod Pathol.* 2005;18:693-704), spleen, central nervous system (CNS), and other visceral sites (*Am J Surg Pathol.* 2004;28:1133-1144; *Am J Clin Pathol.* 1994;102:45-54) have been reported. Rarely patients may present with multifocal involvement, also referred to as "malignant histiocytosis," but a proportion of these cases are ALCLs.

Morphology

Diffuse, non-cohesive sheets of large round to oval cells with distinct nuclear borders, prominent nucleoli, and abundant eosinophilic cytoplasm with or without fine vacuoles, involving nodal or extranodal tissues, are the basic microscopic features, but this characterization establishes the terms of the differential diagnosis (e-Figure 26.1) (*Am J Surg Pathol.* 2004;28:1133-1144; *Arch Pathol Lab Med.* 2018;142:1322-1329). A sinusoidal pattern of involvement can be seen in lymph nodes, liver, and spleen (*J Clin Exp Hematop.* 2013;53:1-8), while focal nodal involvement is usually paracortical. These neoplasms may have a spindle cell pattern with or without a round cell component to introduce a sarcoma, sarcomatoid carcinoma, and melanoma into the differential diagnosis. Hemophagocytosis may be discernible. The nuclei are often large with irregular folds and may be eccentrically placed (e-Figure 26.2). Multinucleated forms are commonly seen. Atypia may range from mild to pronounced. Accompanying inflammation is not uncommon, and inflammatory infiltrates are usually composed of small lymphocytes, plasma cells, histiocytes, and eosinophils (*Mod Pathol.* 2005;18:693-704); neutrophils have been observed in cases with CNS involvement (*Am J Surg Pathol.* 2001;25:1372-1379).

Immunophenotype

One or more histiocytic markers, such as CD163, CD68, CD11c, CD4, and lysozyme, are consistently expressed (*Arch Pathol Lab Med.* 2018;142:1322-1329) with the absence of B- and T-cell markers, CD30, EMA, CD21, CD23, CD35, CD1a, langerin, CD13, CD33, myeloperoxidase (MPO), cytokeratins, and HMB-45. S100 protein may be positive in some cases (*Cancers (Basel).* 2014;6:2275-2295; *Cancer Control.* 2014;21:290-300). Expression of several histiocytic markers serves to support the diagnosis in the presence of consistent histologic features (*J Clin Exp Hematop.* 2013;53:1-8).

Genetic Features

It was initially thought that a diagnosis of HS could only be made in the absence of clonal immunoglobulin heavy chain (IGH) or T-cell receptor (TCR) gene arrangements, but more recently it has been shown that a subset of cases have clonal immunoglobulin (IG) rearrangements, particularly in cases of transdifferentiation from a low-grade B-cell lymphoma (*Mod Pathol.* 2021;34:336-347). It has also been reported in single sporadic cases (*Am J Surg Pathol.* 2009;33:863-873). *BRAF* V600E mutations were found in one case series (*Histopathology.* 2014;65:261-272) in five of eight cases; however, another study did not identify the mutation in their three cases (*Blood.* 2012;120:2700-2703). It is notable that *MAPK* signaling pathway mutations may have a role in the pathogenesis of HS-like Langerhans cell histiocytosis and other less aggressive histiocytoses (*Mod Pathol.* 2019;32:830-843). Mutations in *PTPN11* have also been detected in HS (*Int J Cancer.* 2020;147:1657-1665).

Prognosis and Treatment

HS is a highly aggressive neoplasm with advanced-stage disease at presentation and a poor outcome (*Histopathology.* 2002;41:1-29; *J Clin Exp Hematop.* 2013;53:1-8; *Mod Pathol.* 2005;18:693-704). Aggressive chemotherapy to date has not had a survival benefit (*Eur J Cancer.* 2015;51:2413-2422). A single case of a *BRAF* V600E-mutated primary CNS HS showed significant response to vemurafenib (*Neurology.* 2014;83:1478-1480). A subset of cases, in particular those with clinically localized disease or those with small tumor size (<3.5 cm), seemed to show a favorable long-term outcome (*Am J Surg Pathol.* 2004;28:1133-1144).

Differential Diagnosis

- **Langerhans cell histiocytosis:** Cells are cytologically bland and positive for S100 protein, CD1a, and langerin; eosinophils are common; Birbeck granules on electron microscopy (EM)
- **MS:** Usually associated with acute myeloid leukemia (AML), myeloproliferative neoplasm (MPN), or myelodysplastic syndrome (MDS); cells less pleomorphic, may be positive for MPO favoring monocytic rather than histiocytic lineage. Useful differentiating markers include CD117, CD34, CD33, CD43 (*Ann Med Surg (Lond).* 2021;72:102894; *Blood Rev.* 2021;47:100773). CD68 and CD163 are expressed in HS and MS.
- **Rosai-Dorfman disease:** Often massive lymphadenopathy, emperipolesis, cells positive for S100 protein, while negative for CD68 and CD1a
- **Anaplastic large cell lymphoma:** Sinusoidal pattern in lymph nodes; "hallmark" cells; positive for CD30; if *ALK* rearranged may be positive for ALK IHC

Key Points

- Diagnosis of HS is a diagnosis of exclusion requiring evaluation of morphology, immunophenotype, and genetic studies in close context with clinical presentation.
- HS may arise sporadically or as a result of transdifferentiation from a low-grade B-cell lymphoma like CLL/SLL or other hematopoietic neoplasms.
- Positivity of CD163 is the most helpful marker for histiocytic differentiation.
- Tumor size (<3.5 cm) and localized disease are thought to be associated with favorable outcome.

Diagnostic Caveats

- Many other tumors may express CD68, which is by no means a specific marker for HS (eg, ALCL may be positive for CD68).
- Histiocytes often express CD31, which could lead to confusion with angiosarcoma; features such as vasoformation and positivity for additional vascular markers (ERG, CD34) are helpful to differentiate.
- HS may be positive for CD4 and CD43, which may lead to confusion with ALCL.

SUGGESTED READINGS

Hung YP, Qian X. Histiocytic sarcoma. *Arch Pathol Lab Med.* 2020;144(5):650-654.
Skala SL, Lucas DR, Dewar R. Histiocytic sarcoma: review, discussion of transformation from B-cell lymphoma, and differential diagnosis. *Arch Pathol Lab Med.* 2018;142(11):1322-1329.

27 Langerhans Cell Tumors

Carina A. Dehner, John S. A. Chrisinger, and Louis P. Dehner

Langerhans cell histiocytosis (LCH) is one of two Langerhans cell (LC) neoplasms; the other is Langerhans cell sarcoma (LCS). The LC is a member of a heterogeneous set of innate immune cells including monocyte-derived dendritic cell (DC) and plasmacytoid DC, which are antigen-presenting cells. In addition to their bone marrow derivation, they also arise in the fetal yolk sac and liver (*Immunity.* 2021;54:2305-2320). The diagnostic criteria for LCH and LCS are summarized in Table 27.1.

Clinical Features

LCH has three principal clinical manifestations: those cases with single (usually bone and skin), multifocal (local risk), and multifocal (high-risk) site involvement with liver, spleen, and bone marrow involvement (*Arch Pathol Lab Med.* 2015;139:1211-1214; *N Engl J Med.* 2018;379:856-868). It remains clinically relevant to consider LCH in terms of its solitary, multifocal, and disseminated manifestations in terms of management and outcome. As more has been learned about the mitogen-activated protein

TABLE 27.1 WHO-HAEM5 Diagnostic Criteria for LCH and LCS

Essential	Desirable
LCH	
• Large round to oval histiocytes with grooved to convoluted nuclei • Langerhans cell phenotype: positive for $CD1a^+$, $CD207^+$ (in the appropriate clinical and histologic context)	• Mutation analysis in the MAPK pathway
LCS	
• Pleomorphic histiocytes with high-grade cytology • Increased mitoses • Immunoreactivity for the following (can be focal): CD1a, S100, and CD207	• Rapid tumor progression • Molecular alteration (preferably in the MAPK pathway)

LCH, Langerhans cell histiocytosis; LCS, Langerhans cell sarcoma; MAPK, mitogen-activated protein kinase.
Based on the WHO Classification of Tumours Editorial Board. Haematolymphoid tumours [Internet]. Lyon (France): International Agency for Research on Cancer; 2024 (WHO classification of tumours series, 5th ed.; vol. 11). Available from: https://tumourclassification.iarc.who.int/chapters/63.

kinase (MAPK) pathway mutations, there is a correlation between the differentiated state of the myeloid precursor and the stage of the disease at presentation; the more primitive cells are associated with disseminated, high-risk organ involvement in the infant and young child with LCH (*Nat Immunol.* 2020;21:1-7; *Hematol Oncol.* 2021;39 Suppl 1:15-23).

Approximately 50% or more of cases present before 10 years of age with one of the three clinical patterns, but a minority of cases are known to occur in adults (*Ann Hematol.* 2022;101:265-272). Adults with LCH are more likely than children to have another hematologic malignancy (*Eur J Cancer.* 2022;172:138-145). Single-site LCH includes the skin, bone, and lung where infantile cutaneous LCH is known to undergo spontaneous regression; bone lesion(s) are usually solitary, and reticulonodular lesions are often associated with spontaneous pneumothorax. Multifocal lesions in a single organ system (multiple bone lesions) or multiple low-risk organs have a favorable outcome. LCH of the central nervous system (CNS) with a low fraction of LCs is associated with neurodegenerative manifestations (*Neuro Oncol.* 2021;23:1433-1446).

Morphology

Dense sheets or aggregates of loosely arrayed, relatively uniform, ovoid cells (e-Figure 27.1) with abundant pale, eosinophilic cytoplasm and nuclei with nuclear grooves with a "coffee bean" or reniform shape are characteristic of LCHs (e-Figure 27.2). Accompanying eosinophils are variably prominent from case to case; small lymphocytes, plasma cells, and even neutrophils, especially in sites with accompanying ulceration, are inconsistently present (e-Figure 27.3). Mitotic figures are frequently noted but atypical forms are not present, but otherwise LCS should be considered in the presence of appreciable atypia (e-Figure 27.4). Necrosis and fibrosis can be encountered in long-standing lesions (*Arch Pathol Lab Med.* 1983;107:59-63). Clusters or singly dispersed osteoclast-like multinucleated giant cells may be found, especially in bone lesions.

LCS has histologic similarities to histiocytic sarcoma, myeloid sarcoma, and other malignant-appearing neoplasms with epithelioid features (e-Figure 27.5). Nuclear grooves may or may not be present. It is with the demonstration of CD1a and/or CD207 that LCS emerges as the diagnosis.

Immunophenotype

As with any suspected histiocytic lesion, CD68 and CD163 immunoreactivity confirms the "histiocytic" nature of the cells in question (e-Figure 27.6). CD1a (e-Figure 27.7) and CD207 (langerin) (e-Figure 27.8) are the specific markers of LCs, but do not differentiate neoplastic cells from reactive LCs as in the case of dermatopathic lymphadenopathy (DL). *BRAF V600E* mutation–specific antibody is positive in at least 50% of cases of LCH. As noted, LCS has an identical immunophenotype to that of LCH, but the staining pattern is often more focal and variable. S100 protein has been largely superseded since its expression is also patchy in Rosai-Dorfman disease (RDD) and juvenile xanthogranuloma (JXG).

Genetic Features

Approximately 60% to 65% of cases have a *BRAF V600E* mutation, particularly in younger individuals (*Blood.* 2020;135:1319-1331); however, other MAPK pathway mutations have been detected in the remaining cases of LCH. Next-generation sequencing studies have found *MAP2K1* mutations in 12% to 15% of cases with wild-type *BRAF*, supporting the mutually exclusive nature of *MAP2K1* and *BRAF*, both of which are important in LCH pathogenesis and represent drug-targetable options (*N Engl J Med.* 2018;379:856-868; *Hematol Oncol.* 2021;39 Suppl 1:15-23; *Nat Rev Dis Primers.* 2021;7:73).

Prognosis and Treatment

The clinical course is highly dependent on the extent of disease, in particular if there is involvement of bone marrow, liver, or spleen (*J Am Acad Dermatol.* 2018;78:1035-1044). In the case of unifocal LCH, the survival is >99% in young children, but is 65% to 70% in multifocal disease with organ dysfunction. Children tend to do better than adults (*Pediatr Blood Cancer.* 2015;62:982-987). Multisystem disease and disease reactivation after initial treatment have been linked to increased morbidity (*J Pediatr Hematol Oncol.* 2014;36:125-133). Disease reactivation occurs in about 30% of cases (*Br J Haematol.* 2016;174:887-898). *BRAF* mutation status does not appear to correlate with prognosis (*Am J Surg Pathol.* 2014;38:1644-1648).

LCS is associated with a poor outcome with a disease-specific survival of 27.2 months (18.3 disease-free months) in a study of 66 cases (*Cancer Treat Rev.* 2015;41:320-331).

Differential Diagnosis

Langerhans Cell Histiocytosis

- **Rosai-Dorfman disease:** Capsular and pericapsular inflammation with fibrosis, emperipolesis, cells positive for S100 protein, while nonreactive for CD68, CD1a, and langerin
- **Erdheim-Chester disease:** Presents as sclerotic bone lesions; large foamy, lipid-filled histiocytes with centrally placed nuclei, lymphocytic aggregates, and fibrosis; histiocytes are CD68 positive, while negative for CD1a, S100 protein, and langerin
- Non-LCH including *JXG*, *multicentric reticulohistiocytosis*, and *xanthoma disseminatum*
- **Langerhans cell hyperplasia:** Has an interfollicular-paracortical growth pattern of LC and is seen in DL (*Mod Pathol.* 2020;33:1104-1121); MUM1/IRF4 expression in the absence of CD207 is helpful in differentiating LCH and LC hyperplasia in DL (*Am J Surg Pathol.* 2022;46:1514-1523).

Langerhans Cell Sarcoma

- **Follicular DC sarcoma:** Neoplastic cells are spindled or epithelioid with whorled and fascicular growth pattern; clinical course can be very indolent; positive for CD21, CD23, fascin, and clusterin
- **Histiocytic sarcoma:** Will be positive for CD68, CD163, and lysozyme; lacks Birbeck granules on electron microscopy (EM), negative for CD1a and langerin

---

Key Points

- LCH is clinically heterogeneous and its outcome depends highly on the extent of disease.
- LCs have very distinct nuclear features, including nuclear grooves, leading to a "coffee bean" appearance with an eosinophil-rich infiltrate.

- Immunohistochemical studies can be extremely useful, with langerin and CD1a being reasonably specific for this diagnosis.
- *BRAF V600E* mutations are found in about 50% of cases, while others may show mutations in *MAP2K1*.

Diagnostic Caveats

- JXG may express S100 protein; however, CD1a is reliably negative in those.
- Some cases of LCH may show extensive epidermotropism resembling mycosis fungoides; however, cytomorphology and immunophenotype are distinctly different.
- Certain inflammatory processes including scabies or contact dermatitis are associated with LC hyperplasia; however, knowing the clinical context is usually helpful to avoid misclassification.

SUGGESTED READINGS

Allen CE, Beverley PCL, Collin M, et al. The coming of age of Langerhans cell histiocytosis. *Nat Immunol.* 2020;21(1):1-7.

Allen CE, Merad M, McClain KL. Langerhans-cell histiocytosis. *N Engl J Med.* 2018;379(9):856-868.

Howard JE, Dwivedi RC, Masterson L, Jani P. Langerhans cell sarcoma: a systematic review. *Cancer Treat Rev.* 2015;41(4):320-331.

28 Juvenile Xanthogranuloma

Carina A. Dehner, John S. A. Chrisinger, and Louis P. Dehner

Juvenile xanthogranuloma (JXG), the most common of the "C" group histiocytic disorders, is classified as a "histiocytic neoplasm" in the WHO Classification (*Leukemia*. 2022;36:1703-1719) (the diagnostic criteria is listed in Table 28.1). Though distinct from Langerhans cell histiocytosis (LCH) in terms of morphology and immunophenotype, there are similarities in terms of its predilection for early childhood and the spectrum of clinical manifestations from solitary, multifocal, and disseminated disease. Like LCH, it may present infrequently in adults.

Clinical Features

A solitary erythematous to yellowish cutaneous nodule with a preference for the head and neck region is known to occur in a child, usually less than 5 years. Multiple cutaneous lesions noted at birth or within several months of age with or without extracutaneous manifestations such as hepatomegaly with or without splenomegaly and accompanying hepatic failure and pancytopenia are among the other manifestations of multifocal or disseminated JXG (DSJXG) (*Am J Surg Pathol*. 2003;27:579-593; *Rofo*. 1985;143:604-605; *Front Pediatr*. 2021;9:672547). Fetal hydrops is also reported (*BMC Pediatr*. 2021;21:161). In some cases, the skin nodules, less often plaques, are the only clinically apparent lesions, whereas there is rarely only visceral involvement. Yet another clinical presentation is one or more intracranial lesions without other apparent sites of JXG. Soft tissue, bone, pancreas, lung, and testis as solitary or multifocal lesions characterize the distribution of DSJXG. In the absence of skin lesions available for biopsy, infection, myeloid leukemia, neuroblastoma, and other histiocytic disorders in a young child are the other clinical considerations.

TABLE 28.1 WHO-HAEM5 Diagnostic Criteria for JXG

Essential	Desirable
• Circumscribed lesion	• Presence of Touton giant cells
• Histiocytic infiltrate without significant nuclear atypia	• Exclude Erdheim-Chester disease.
• Positive: CD68/CD163/factor XIII	
• Negative: CD1a, CD207 (langerin), and ALK	

JXG, juvenile xanthogranuloma.
Based on the WHO Classification of Tumours Editorial Board. Haematolymphoid tumours [Internet]. Lyon (France): International Agency for Research on Cancer; 2024 (WHO classification of tumours series, 5th ed.; vol. 11). Available from: https://tumourclassification.iarc.who.int/chapters/63.

Benign cephalic histiocytosis, another clinical type of JXG, is restricted to the skin and affects children under 1 year of age. Though the eruption of maculopapules begins in the head (cephalic) with involvement of the neck, the lesions become generalized on the trunk and extremities (*Pediatr Dermatol.* 2017;34:392-397). There is eventual spontaneous resolution over a period of months to a few years. A possibly related entity is generalized eruptive histiocytosis, also confined to the skin, which presents on the trunk and extremities, mainly in adults but is also reported in children (*J Am Acad Dermatol.* 2004;50:116-120). Symmetric erythematous papules on the trunk and extremities eventually resolve. NTRK1 fusion has been detected in one case (*Dermatol Online J.* 2016;22). Progressive nodular histiocytosis, also confined to the skin, presents in a somewhat similar fashion as the previous two entities except for the nodules in addition to cutaneous papules and involvement of mucous membranes mainly in adults (*Case Rep Pathol.* 2021;2021:5531820). Xanthoma dissemination is the only one of the previous variants that has systemic manifestations, including the central nervous system and respiratory and intestinal tracts (*Lancet.* 2018;391:251).

Regardless of the particular clinical presentation, the pathologic findings are similar to those of JXG including a transitional spindle cell pattern and the presence of xanthomatized mononuclear and multinucleated cells.

Morphology

The histologic spectrum of JXG has been thoroughly documented in the skin as the most common site of involvement (*Ann Diagn Pathol.* 2022;58:151940). A predominantly mononuclear infiltrate with a diffuse or mixed diffuse and nodular pattern and a varying number of multinucleated cells with and without Touton-type features and xanthomatized mononuclear and multinucleated cells are the characteristic findings in the skin (e-Figure 28.1). Touton-type giant cells are variable in number from case to case and infrequent in extracutaneous sites. A mononuclear dominant infiltrate with or without intermixed spindle cells is also encountered in extracutaneous sites so as not to immediately suggest JXG but rather a fibrohistiocytic tumor (e-Figure 28.2).

Immunophenotype

Like all of the histiocytic disorders, the mononuclear and spindle cells of JXG are immunoreactive for CD68 and CD163, with a more intense staining reaction for the latter. Factor XIIIa and fascin, dendritic cell markers, are reliable but display inconsistent staining intensity from case to case. CD4 and CD11c are more reliable and uniform in immunoreactivity (*Am J Dermatopathol.* 2022;44(7):493-498). The absence of CD1a and CD207 positivity excludes LCH. A JXG-specific marker awaits identification.

Molecular Genetics

Unlike LCH and Erdheim-Chester disease (ECD) with their shared *BRAF* and other *MAPK* pathway mutations, JXG has been a molecular genetic enigma with the exception of central nervous system-JXG and less common sites with a *BRAF* V600E mutation (*Head Neck Pathol.* 2022;16:407-415. *Acta Neuropathol Commun.* 2019;7:168). However, mutations in *CSF1R, MAP2K1, NRAS,* and *NTRK1* have been detected in individual cases (*Nat Rev Dis Primers.* 2021;7:73). It is possible that some cases of DSJXG are examples of ALK+ histiocytosis since the latter is reported in infants and children with the clinicopathologic and immunophenotypic features that had been interpreted as JXG (*Blood.* 2022;139:256-280). Any case of putative DSJXG should have appropriate molecular testing.

Prognosis and Treatment

The prognosis is usually good, with favorable outcomes in localized lesions. Liver and bone marrow involvement has been associated with serious, if not fatal, consequences, which is similar to the experience in LCH (*Blood.* 2020;135:1319-1331). Risk assignment categories with treatment and prognostic implications are not available.

Differential Diagnosis

- **LCH:** Cells have nuclear grooves and are positive for CD1a and CD207; LCH lacks Touton-type giant cells and xanthomatized cells.
- **Rosai-Dorfman disease:** Larger histiocytes with pale cytoplasm; emperipolesis often plasma cells and patchy positivity for S100 protein.

Key Points

- LCH is clinically heterogeneous, and its outcome depends highly on the extent of disease.
- Langerhans cells have very distinct nuclear features, including nuclear grooves leading to a "coffee bean" appearance with an eosinophil-rich infiltrate.
- Immunohistochemical studies can be extremely useful, with langerin and CD1a being reasonably specific for this diagnosis.
- *BRAF*V600E mutations are found in about 50% of cases, while others may show mutations in *MAP2K1*.

Diagnostic Caveats

- JXG may express S100 protein; however, CD1a and CD207 are reliably negative in those.
- Some cases of LCH may show extensive epidermotropism resembling mycosis fungoides; however, cytomorphology and immunophenotype are distinctly different.
- Certain inflammatory processes including scabies or contact dermatitis are associated with Langerhans cell hyperplasia; however, knowing the clinical context is usually helpful to avoid misclassification.

SUGGESTED READINGS

Dehner LP. Juvenile xanthogranulomas in the first two decades of life: a clinicopathologic study of 174 cases with cutaneous and extracutaneous manifestations. *Am J Surg Pathol.* 2003;27(5):579-593.

McClain KL, Bigenwald C, Collin M, et al. Histiocytic disorders. *Nat Rev Dis Primers.* 2021;7(1):73.

So N, Liu R, Hogeling M. Juvenile xanthogranulomas: examining single, multiple, and extracutaneous presentations. *Pediatr Dermatol.* 2020;37(4):637-644.

29 Rosai-Dorfman Disease

Krithika Shenoy, Carina A. Dehner, and Louis P. Dehner

Rosai-Dorfman disease (RDD), also known as sinus histiocytosis with massive lymphadenopathy, is a rare non–Langerhans cell histiocytosis (LCH) characterized by a histiocytic proliferation in groups "R" and "L" (skin only) with variably prominent emperipolesis (engulfment of one cell type by another). Its etiology has largely remained uncertain with a suspected infectious cause until some recent studies. The estimated incidence is 100 cases per year in the United States, with a prevalence of 1:200,000. It is more common in children and adults within the first three decades of life with a slight male predilection (*Blood.* 2018;131(26):2877-2890; *Pediatr Radiol.* 1990;20(6):425-432). RDD is now regarded as a likely neoplastic histiocytic disorder on the basis of its mutational status that has altered the pathogenetic concept of this and other histiocytoses. The diagnostic criteria are summarized in Table 29.1.

Clinical Features

Classic RDD has a nodal-based presentation with enlarged, painless, bilateral cervical lymphadenopathy and less often mediastinal, axillary, and inguinal lymph node enlargement. Retroperitoneal lymph node involvement is uncommon. Constitutional symptoms include intermittent fevers, night sweats, and weight loss, which occur in a minority of cases to mimic infection or lymphoma. Extranodal disease is seen in 30% to 40% of cases, with manifestation in the skin (10%-52%), bone (5%-25%), central nervous system, head and neck (11%), and nervous system (5%-8%) (*J Clin Pathol.* 2020;73(11):697-705; *Haematologica.* 2020;105(2):348-357). RDD can occur either in isolation or with various immune dysregulation disorders (immunoglobulin G4 [IgG4] disease, autoimmune lymphoproliferative syndrome), autoimmune conditions, hereditary basis (germline variant in SLC2gA3 in H syndrome), and malignant disorders, including myelodysplastic syndrome and Hodgkin lymphoma (*Pathologica.* 2021;113(5):388-395).

TABLE 29.1 WHO-HAEM5 Diagnostic Criteria for RDD

Essential	Desirable
• Large histiocytes with abundant pale cytoplasm, often with emperipolesis • Abundant plasma cells • Positive patchy staining for S100	• Positive expression of OCT-2 and cyclin D1 (can be helpful in challenging cases)

RDD, Rosai-Dorfman disease.
Based on the WHO Classification of Tumours Editorial Board. Haematolymphoid tumours [Internet]. Lyon (France): International Agency for Research on Cancer; 2024 (WHO classification of tumours series, 5th ed.; vol. 11). Available from: https://tumourclassification.iarc.who.int/chapters/63.

Morphology

- **Nodal RDD:** Cortical follicles are retained with expansion of the medullary sinuses by large, pale staining histiocytes with finely vacuolated cytoplasm and a variable number of cytoplasmic lymphocytes (emperipolesis). Plasma cells as individual cells or clustered groups are a common feature whose presence is a useful feature in the diagnosis. Sclerosis or fibrosis is present in varying degrees in 75% of cases and, in some instances, may substantially alter the basic microscopic features. These features can be especially problematic in extranodal sites. Well-formed granulomas are uncommon. In regard to plasma cells, RDD and IgG4-related disease are potential clinical and pathologic mimics (*Lancet.* 2021;398:1213-1214; *Australas J Dermatol.* 2022;63(3):372-375).
- **Extranodal RDD:** Groups of vacuolated histiocytes are uncommon, whereas the histiocytes are more dispersed among a mixed population of plasma cells, lymphocytes, and a fibrous background. In bone as an example, chronic osteomyelitis may be the initial impression. Histiocytes may be sparse, and emperipolesis may be absent. Fibrosis may be a prominent component.

Immunophenotype

The histiocytes demonstrate a patchy pattern of S100 positivity, whereas CD68 and CD163 are diffusely positive but not especially helpful. CD1a and CD207 are nonreactive, but transcription factor PU.1 and OCT-2 have been reported as coexpressed in RDD (*Am J Clin Pathol.* 2022;158(6):672-677). Plasma cells are polytypic. A subset of RDD cases have an elevated IgG4/IgG ratio, which creates some ambiguity with IgG4-related disease (*Am J Clin Pathol.* 2013;139:622-632).

Molecular Features

KRAS and *MAP2K1* are mutually exclusive mutations as well as *ARAF*, CSF1R, and NRFS mutations in RDD (*Mod Pathol.* 2017;30(10):1367-1377; *Blood.* 2018;131(26):2877-2890).

Prognosis and Treatment

Spontaneous regression is a common outcome, but in some cases, systemic therapy may be indicated (*Hematologica.* 2020;105(2):348-357).

Differential Diagnosis

The differential diagnosis includes other histiocytic neoplasms such as LCH and Erdheim-Chester disease (ECD). In LCH, the tumor cells are positive for S100, CD1a, and langerin/CD207. ECD is characterized by foamy histiocytes, and Touton giant cells are frequently present. There are rare cases of concurrent RDD, LCH, and ECD.

SUGGESTED READINGS

Emile JF, Abla O, Fraitag S, et al. Revised classification of histiocytoses and neoplasms of the macrophage-dendritic cell lineages. *Blood.* 2016;127(22):2672-2681.

30 Other Histiocytic/Dendritic Cell Neoplasms

30.1 Dendritic Cell and Dendritic Cell–Like Neoplasms

Carina A Dehner, Cody Weimholt, and Louis P. Dehner

Owing to the fact that histiocytes are derived from a common myeloid precursor, this has resulted in the reclassification of these neoplasms with characteristic immunophenotypes and molecular genetic attributes into one of two nosologic categories. Two neoplasms previously assigned to the general group of dendritic cell (DC) tumors, the follicular dendritic cell sarcoma (FDCS), and fibroblastic reticular cell tumor (FRCT), have been reclassified into a separate category termed "stromal-derived neoplasms of lymphoid tissues." The fact remains that there is considerable morphologic and immunohistochemical (IHC) overlap among these tumors, which were formerly unified under the rubric of DC tumors.

I. INDETERMINATE DENDRITIC CELL TUMOR

Indeterminate dendritic cell tumor (IDCT), also known as indeterminate cell histiocytosis (ICS), represents a neoplastic proliferation of indeterminate DCs (postulated to be precursors of Langerhans cells [LCs]); it is included among the "L" group disorders and is a rare entity, with approximately 100 extant cases (*Surg Pathol Clin.* 2019;12:805-829). The diagnostic criteria for IDCT are summarized in Table 30.1-1.

TABLE 30.1-1 Diagnostic Criteria for IDCT

Essential	Desirable
• Infiltrate consisting of cells resembling Langerhans cells • Positive: S100 and CD1a • Negative: CD207/langerin • Clinical features of multisystem LCH absent	• Ki-67 assessment

IDCT, indeterminate dendritic cell tumor; LCH, Langerhans cell histiocytosis.
Based on the WHO Classification of Tumours Editorial Board. Haematolymphoid tumours [Internet]. Lyon (France): International Agency for Research on Cancer; 2024 (WHO classification of tumours series, 5th ed.; vol. 11). Available from: https://tumourclassification.iarc.who.int/chapters/63.

Clinical Features

IDCT typically presents in adults (median age 49.5 years; range 0-88), showing a slight male predominance. In 90% of cases, the lesions are localized to the skin as multiple rather than solitary papulonodular lesions, while less than 10% of cases involve nodal disease; one case presented in spleen and another case was disseminated at presentation (*J Cutan Pathol.* 2017;44:958-963). Primary bone and pancreatic tumors have also been described (*Hemasphere.* 2020;5:e511; *J Surg Case Rep.* 2020;rjaa208).

Morphology

IDCT has many of the same features as Langerhans cell histiocytosis (LCH), with somewhat irregular nuclei with prominent nuclear grooves, however, with greater nuclear variability and pleomorphism. Eosinophils are usually not encountered. Small lymphocytes are more common in contrast to LCH. There is also a greater tendency for spindle cell formation, and multinucleated giant cells can be present. Cutaneous lesions are generally dermal-based and may extend into the subcutis.

Immunophenotype

S100 protein and CD1a are both expressed, but CD207 (langerin) is nonreactive. The cells are also negative for specific B-cell and T-cell markers, as well as CD30, CD163, CD21, CD23, and CD35, but they may rarely stain for CD45, CD68, and lysozyme.

Genetic Features

Several cases have reportedly harbored *ETV3-NCOA2* fusions (*Blood.* 2015;126:2344-2345). *BRAF* V600E mutations have been detected in a few cases (*Ann Diagn Pathol.* 2015;19:113-116; *J Cutan Pathol.* 2017;44:958-963).

Prognosis and Treatment

The clinical course of IDCT is highly variable; however, cases limited to the skin generally have a favorable outcome. Approximately 15% of cases have been associated with hematologic malignancies, such as follicular lymphoma, acute myeloid leukemia (*J Dermatol Surg Oncol.* 1985;11:1111-1119), chronic lymphocytic leukemia (CLL)/small lymphocytic lymphoma (SLL), angioimmunoblastic T-cell lymphoma, acute lymphoblastic leukemia, and acute mast cell leukemia (*Am J Dermatopathol.* 2018;40:736-748). One case with widespread disease harbored a *BRAF* V600E mutation, and the patient had a favorable response to BRAF/MEK inhibitor therapy (*J Cutan Pathol.* 2017;44:958-963). Another case was successfully managed with systemic steroid therapy (*J Dermatol.* 2018;45:1444-1447).

Differential Diagnosis

LCH/sarcoma has Birbeck granules and is CD207-reactive. Juvenile xanthogranuloma (JXG) is negative for CD1a, langerin, and S100 protein.

II. INTERDIGITATING DENDRITIC CELL SARCOMA

Interdigitating dendritic cell sarcoma (IDCS), a neoplasm derived from interdigitating DCs which normally reside in the paracortical region of lymph nodes or other secondary lymphoid tissues as presenting antigens to T cells, is included in the "L" group. The diagnostic criteria for IDCS are summarized in Table 30.1-2.

| TABLE 30.1-2 | Diagnostic Criteria for IDCS |

Essential

- Spindle/epithelioid cell proliferation
- Cells with abundant cytoplasm, indistinct cell borders, and vesicular nuclei, with or without nuclear grooves
- Positive: S100 and one or more hematolymphoid markers
- Negative: LC, FDC, and melanocytic markers

FDC, follicular dendritic cell; IDCS, interdigitating dendritic cell sarcoma; LC, Langerhans cell.
Based on the WHO Classification of Tumours Editorial Board. Haematolymphoid tumours [Internet]. Lyon (France): International Agency for Research on Cancer; 2024 (WHO classification of tumours series, 5th ed.; vol. 11). Available from: https://tumourclassification.iarc.who.int/chapters/63.

Clinical Features

An analysis of 127 cases revealed a wide age range (median of 58 years), a slight male predominance, and presentation as a painless mass (*Ann Hematol.* 2019;98:2641-2651). Most cases (65%-70%) present with localized disease, often affecting cervical and axillary lymph nodes. Primary extranodal sites have included the skin, soft tissue, and viscera, with disseminated disease occurring in 30% of cases. Similar to IDCT, there is an association with other hematologic malignancies (12.6%), typically CLL/SLL. Some studies have suggested a common clonal origin, indicating a "transdifferentiation" of a lymphoma to IDCS (*Blood.* 2008;111:5433-5439; *Am J Clin Pathol.* 2009;132:928-939).

Morphology

A fascicular growth pattern with occasional whorls of spindled to ovoid cells with abundant, eosinophilic cytoplasm, indistinct cell borders, and small nucleoli is the principal microscopic finding. Most tumors display uniform, nuclear atypia, but a small subset of cases has prominent pleomorphism. Small T-lymphocytes are intermixed with the more spindled to ovoid cells.

Immunophenotype

The neoplastic cells are diffusely positive for S100 protein and vimentin. Focal expression of CD45, CD68, and lysozyme can be seen. CD1a, CD21, CD23, CD35, and langerin are nonreactive.

Genetic Features

Some tumors have clonal immunoglobulin (IG) rearrangements, particularly in cases with concurrent low-grade B-cell lymphoma (*Am J Surg Pathol.* 2009;33:863-873).

Prognosis and Treatment

The clinical course is variable; some tumors behave very aggressive, spreading to the lung, liver, and lymph nodes, while other cases are indolent when the presentation is localized to the lymph nodes (*Am J Clin Pathol.* 2001;115:589-597). Adverse prognostic factors are larger tumors, increased mitotic activity, and histiocytic sarcoma-like areas with marked pleomorphism and anaplasia (*Case Rep Otolaryngol.* 2013;2013:913157). Currently, there is no known specific therapy. Surgical resection appears to be the most effective treatment, with radiotherapy and chemotherapy showing little survival benefit (*Ann Hematol.* 2019;98:2641-2651).

Differential Diagnosis

Given the rarity of this neoplasm and its somewhat generic spindle cell and even epithelioid features, a broad IHC panel is often necessary. A fibrohistiocytic tumor is a likely initial consideration in the soft tissues, but metastatic melanoma in a lymph node is also a reasonable consideration, especially with S100 protein positivity, although SOX10 is nonreactive. Histiocytic sarcoma is usually characterized by large, more epithelioid-appearing cells and has strong and diffuse CD163 positivity with limited S100 protein staining. FDCS is morphologically similar but is positive for CD21, CD23, CD35, and podoplanin and lacks strong S100 protein staining.

III. DENDRITIC CELL–LIKE TUMORS (STROMAL-DERIVED NEOPLASMS OF LYMPHOID TISSUES)

The following three neoplasms are currently classified as "stromal-derived neoplasms of lymphoid tissues," as mesenchymal DC neoplasms: FDCS, Epstein-Barr virus (EBV)-positive inflammatory dendritic cell sarcoma (EBV+IFDCS), and FRCT (*Leukemia.* 2022;36:1720-1748). These neoplasms are regarded as nonhematopoietic-derived tumors, unlike the histiocytic DC neoplasms of hematopoietic stem cell origin (*Blood.* 2018;132:1106-1113).

IV. FOLLICULAR DENDRITIC CELL SARCOMA

FDCS is the neoplastic transformation of follicular dendritic cells (FDCs), normally residing in the germinal center follicles where they present antigens to B cells. The diagnostic criteria for FDCS are summarized in Table 30.1-3.

Clinical Features

A slow-growing, painless mass has a broad anatomic distribution and age range (9-90 years) (median age of 50 years) (*Crit Rev Oncol Hematol.* 2013;88:253-271). Most tumors arise in extranodal sites, with only 15% in lymph nodes, and another

TABLE 30.1-3 Diagnostic Criteria for FDCS

Essential

- Spindled/ovoid cells with syncytial appearance
- Storiform/fascicular/whorled growth pattern
- Small background lymphocytes
- Positive: Two or more FDC markers
- Negative: S100 and lymphocyte-specific markers

FDC, follicular dendritic cell; FDCS, follicular dendritic cell sarcoma.
Based on the WHO Classification of Tumours Editorial Board. Haematolymphoid tumours [Internet]. Lyon (France): International Agency for Research on Cancer; 2024 (WHO classification of tumours series, 5th ed.; vol. 11). Available from: https://tumourclassification.iarc.who.int/chapters/63.

5.5% in both nodal and extranodal sites (*Pathologica*. 2021;113:316-329). Single-site involvement characterizes over 80% of cases (*Crit Rev Oncol Hematol*. 2013;88:253-271). About 10% to 15% arise in a background of hyaline-vascular Castleman disease (*Histopathology*. 2001;38:510-518; *An Bras Dermatol*. 2019;94:578-581).

Morphology

Compact ovoid to spindled cells with vesicular chromatin and small nucleoli, pale eosinophilic cytoplasm, and long, slender fibrillary processes are commonly arranged either in whorls or fascicles, with scattered multinucleated cells (e-Figures 30.1-1 and 30.1-2) (*Am J Clin Pathol*. 2020;154:S93-S94). An infiltrate of small lymphocytes and plasma cells is present in the background of the tumor cells in most cases, similar in that respect to IDCS (e-Figure 30.1-3). Most cases have relatively bland features without overt atypia, with some exceptions of high-grade transformation (e-Figures 30.1-4 to 30.1-6) (*Ear Nose Throat J*. 2010;89:E14-E17).

Immunophenotype

Like normal FDC markers, most tumors express CD21, CD23 (e-Figure 30.1-7), and CD35, as well as clusterin (e-Figure 30.1-8), podoplanin (D2-40), and CXCL13 (*Am J Surg Pathol*. 2004;28:988-998; *J Pathol*. 2008;216:356-364; *Am J Clin Pathol*. 2007;128:776-782). Epithelial membrane antigen (EMA) may be expressed focally in about 50% of cases, and S100 protein in 10% of cases (*Cancer*. 1997;79:294-313; *Semin Diagn Pathol*. 2016;33:262-276). Intermixed nonneoplastic lymphocytes are usually a mix of B and T cells. In cases associated with myasthenia gravis, terminal deoxynucleotidyl transferase (TdT)–positive T cells are present (*Am J Surg Pathol*. 2010;34:742-745).

Genetic Features

Mutations in nuclear factor kappa B (NF-κB) regulatory genes, *BRAF* V600E, *CDKN2A,* and *RB1* have been reported in some cases (*Mod Pathol*. 2016;29:67-74).

Prognosis and Treatment

Local recurrence and distant metastasis are reported in 28% and 27%, respectively, with adverse outcomes associated with age over 40, absence of a lymphoplasmacytic infiltrate, tumor size exceeding 6 cm, and mitotic rates of 5 or more per 10 high-power fields (*Crit Rev Oncol Hematol*. 2013;88:253-271). Surgery, with or without adjuvant therapy, is the treatment of choice.

Differential Diagnosis

IDCS is very similar microscopically to FDCS but is negative for CD21, CD23, CD35, and clusterin. It shows diffuse positivity for S100 and lacks well-formed desmosomes under electron microscopy. Metastatic sarcomatoid carcinoma is positive for keratins and negative for CD21, CD23, and CD35.

V. EBV-POSITIVE INFLAMMATORY FOLLICULAR DENDRITIC CELL SARCOMA

EBV+IFDCS, also known as inflammatory pseudotumor-like follicular/fibroblastic DC sarcoma or inflammatory pseudotumor-like FDCS, is a variant of FDCS consistently associated with EBV. EBV+IFDCS is a more indolent tumor compared to conventional FDCS (*Am J Surg Pathol*. 2001;25:721-731; *Am J Surg Pathol*. 1996;20:747-753). The diagnostic criteria for EBV+IFDCS are summarized in Table 30.1-4.

TABLE 30.1-4	Diagnostic Criteria for EBV+IFDCS

Essential

- Spindle/ovoid cells with indistinct cells borders, vesicular nuclei, and distinct nucleoli
- Background lymphoplasmacytic infiltrate
- Positive: FDC markers and EBER (rarely fibroblastic/myoid markers)

EBER, EBV-encoded RNA; EBV+IFDCS, EBV-positive inflammatory dendritic cell sarcoma; FDC, follicular dendritic cell.
Based on the WHO Classification of Tumours Editorial Board. Haematolymphoid tumours [Internet]. Lyon (France): International Agency for Research on Cancer; 2024 (WHO classification of tumours series, 5th ed.; vol. 11). Available from: https://tumourclassification.iarc.who.int/chapters/63.

Clinical Features

Young to middle-aged adults are mainly affected, with a possible predilection for Asian females. Initially thought to only involve the liver or spleen, it may also present as a polypoid lesion in the colon or as a mesenteric or tonsillar mass (*Histopathology.* 2020;77:832-840; *Am J Surg Pathol.* 2021;45:765-772). Unlike FDCS, systemic manifestations such as weight loss, fever, abdominal pain, hematochezia, and tonsillar obstructive symptoms are documented. Other neoplasms with similar constitutional systemic manifestations are angiomatoid fibrous histiocytoma and anaplastic lymphoma kinase (ALK)-1–positive inflammatory myofibroblastic tumor.

Morphology

A well-circumscribed tumor with a dense lymphoplasmacytic infiltrate (e-Figure 30.1-9) and spindled to oval-shaped tumor cells, with poorly defined cell borders, scant cytoplasm, and small nucleoli, are the histologic features (e-Figure 30.1-10). In some cases, focal nuclear atypia can be seen, with some tumor cells resembling Reed-Sternberg and Hodgkin cells. Some cases may show hemorrhage and necrosis (*Am J Surg Pathol.* 2001;25:721-731; *Am J Surg Pathol.* 2021;45:765-772).

Immunophenotype

The neoplastic cells are positive for the FDC markers, including CD21, CD23, CD35, and clusterin, with occasional cases showing focal S100 protein and/or EMA expression. Smooth muscle actin (SMA) is positive in the majority of cases (e-Figure 30.1-11). In contrast to conventional FDCS, EBV-encoded RNA (EBER) is positive (e-Figure 30.1-12).

Genetic Features

The presence of clonal EBV genomic material has been reported.

Prognosis and Treatment

Complete surgical excision is the treatment of choice for EBV+IFDCS. EBV+IFDCS is more indolent than conventional FDCS. When disease is limited to spleen, splenectomy is seemingly curative, unlike the experience with liver involvement, which may lead to local recurrence and dissemination in 20% of cases (*Int J Clin Exp Pathol.* 2014;7:2421-2429).

Differential Diagnosis

FDCS is histologically identical but negative for EBER. Inflammatory myofibroblastic tumor (IMT) and EBV-FDCS are very similar and both may be SMA positive, but IMT is positive for ALK and nonreactive for EBER. FDC markers should be performed.

VI. FIBROBLASTIC RETICULAR CELL TUMOR

FRCT, also known as cytokeratin-positive interstitial reticulum cell tumor, is the least common of the "dendritic cell" tumors, with only a small number of reported cases (*Am J Surg Pathol.* 1998;22:1048-1058; *Histopathology.* 2003;43:491-494). These tumors are derived from fibroblastic reticular cells (RCs), a subset of which are cytokeratin-positive. The diagnostic criteria for FRCT are summarized in Table 30.1-5.

Clinical Features

These tumors most commonly present in lymph nodes of the upper body; however, other sites such as the spleen or liver may also be involved.

Morphology

A multinodular pattern of tumor cells replaces the normal lymph node follicles; the tumor cells are uniformly large, ovoid in shape, with smooth nuclear membranes, a central nucleolus, and abundant eosinophilic cytoplasm. Lymphocytes and plasma cells are scattered throughout the background. Nuclear atypia has been reported in some cases (*Hum Pathol.* 2003;34:954-957).

Immunophenotype

The tumor cells are variably positive for desmin, keratin, and SMA, while negative for S100 protein and EBER by in situ hybridization. FDC markers are rarely positive (*Am J Surg Pathol.* 2015;39:573-580; *Hum Pathol.* 2016;49:15-21). Desmin and keratin highlight the cytoplasmic processes, which can provide useful clues for diagnosis.

Genetic Features

Cytogenetic analysis has failed to demonstrate karyotypic abnormalities, but targeted next-generation sequencing (NGS) has detected a mutation in the *JAK3* gene (*Am J Surg Pathol.* 2015;39:573-580; *Hum Pathol.* 2016;49:15-21).

TABLE 30.1-5 Diagnostic Criteria for FRCT

Essential

- Spindle/ovoid cells with whorled/fascicular/sheet-like pattern
- Background small lymphocytes
- Positive: One or more of the following: cytokeratin, actin, desmin (delicate cell processes highlighted)
- Negative: FDC markers and S100

FDC, follicular dendritic cell; FRCT, fibroblastic reticular cell tumor.
Based on the WHO Classification of Tumours Editorial Board. Haematolymphoid tumours [Internet]. Lyon (France): International Agency for Research on Cancer; 2024 (WHO classification of tumours series, 5th ed.; vol. 11). Available from: https://tumourclassification.iarc.who.int/chapters/63.

Prognosis and Treatment

FRCT has an unpredictable clinical course, ranging from indolent to aggressive behavior, with metastatic spread observed in some cases (*Am J Surg Pathol*. 1998; 22:1048-1058; *Histopathology*. 2003;43:491-494).

Differential Diagnosis

Both metastatic sarcomatoid carcinoma and FRCT are keratin-positive, but carcinoma is negative for SMA and desmin. Clinical information is crucial. FDCS is negative for keratins and positive for CD21, CD23, and CD35.

SUGGESTED READINGS

Ge R, Liu C, Yin X, et al. Clinicopathologic characteristics of inflammatory pseudotumor-like follicular dendritic cell sarcoma. *Int J Clin Exp Pathol*. 2014;7(5):2421-2429.

Muhammed A, Ahmed ARH, Maysa H, Mohamed AES, Abd-ElLateef AA, Elnakib E. New insights inside the interdigitating dendritic cell sarcoma-pooled analysis and review of literature. *Ann Hematol*. 2019;98(12):2641-2651.

Ratzinger G, Burgdorf WH, Metze D, Zelger BG, Zelger B. Indeterminate cell histiocytosis: fact or fiction? *J Cutan Pathol*. 2005;32(8):552-560.

Saygin C, Uzunaslan D, Ozguroglu M, Senocak M, Tuzuner N. Dendritic cell sarcoma: a pooled analysis including 462 cases with presentation of our case series. *Crit Rev Oncol Hematol*. 2013;88(2):253-271.

30.2 Erdheim-Chester Disease

Carina A. Dehner, John S. A. Chrisinger, and Louis P. Dehner

Erdheim-Chester disease (ECD) is a multisystemic histiocytic disorder whose characteristic lesions are found in the distal femora and tibiae with osteosclerotic changes. Despite the lesional cells are non–Langerhans cell histiocytes (LCHs), this disorder is categorized in the "L" group due to the shared *BRAF* mutation, which has superseded the phenotype in this case. The diagnostic criteria are summarized in Table 30.2-1.

Clinical Features

ECD is predominantly an adult disorder, diagnosed around the age of 55 years, with a higher incidence in males (3:1), although it is rarely seen in children. There may be

TABLE 30.2-1 Diagnostic Criteria for ECD

Essential	Desirable
• Infiltrate consisting of foamy histiocytes in the appropriate clinical setting	• MAPK pathway mutations

ECD, Erdheim-Chester disease; MAPK, mitogen-activated protein kinase.
Based on the WHO Classification of Tumours Editorial Board. Haematolymphoid tumours [Internet]. Lyon (France): International Agency for Research on Cancer; 2024 (WHO classification of tumours series, 5th ed.; vol. 11). Available from: https://tumourclassification.iarc.who.int/chapters/63.

overlapping features with LCH. Its multisystemic manifestations serve as a clinical challenge with site-related symptoms such as bone pain, exophthalmos, xanthelasmas, and diabetes insipidus. Central nervous system (CNS) involvement can lead to neurodegenerative changes like LCH. Cardiac and pulmonary manifestations can divert attention to causes other than ECD. A retroperitoneal mass with compression of the aorta and urinary tract, with so-called "hairy kidneys" and obstructive uropathy, presents differential diagnoses of retroperitoneal fibrosis (IgG4-related disease or idiopathic), lymphoma, and metastatic disease (*Mayo Clin Proc.* 2019;94:2054-2071).

Imaging Findings

Imaging studies are central to the diagnosis of ECD because of the characteristic bilateral and symmetrical sclerosis of the diaphysis and metaphysis of femora and tibiae with sparing of the epiphyses; these findings are enhanced with 99Tc bone scintigraphy, which shows usually high uptake. Infiltration of the right atrium, "coated" aorta, and "hairy" kidneys reflect retroperitoneal involvement and pachymeningitis by positron emission tomography/computed tomography/magnetic resonance imaging (PET/CT/MRI).

Morphology

In a broad morphologic context, the histologic features have "fibrohistiocytic" features, reflecting in part the histologic spectrum (*Mod Pathol.* 2018;31:581-597). The histiocytes present as xanthomatized mononuclear cells and Touton-type multinucleated xanthomatized cells. Plasma cells, neutrophils, and lymphocytes in variable numbers, with or without a fibrous stroma, are also seen (e-Figure 30.2-1). The character of histiocytic infiltrate accounts for the earlier consideration of ECD as "adult" juvenile xanthogranuloma (JXG), which is a reasonable interpretation. Bone marrow fibrosis with trabecular remodeling and a more fibrous pattern in soft tissues may lead to an interpretation of a reactive fibro-inflammatory process, but the deposits of cholesterol cleft can indicate ECD as the diagnosis. The relationship to other histiocytic disorders is illustrated in cases of ECD with composite features of LCH or Rosai-Dorfman disease (RDD) (*Nat Rev Dis Primers.* 2021;7:73; *J Pediatr Hematol Oncol.* 2021;43:e375-e379).

Immunophenotype

The histiocytes are positive for CD163, CD68, factor XIIIa, and BRAF in those cases with a *BRAFV600E* mutation. They are negative for CD1a and CD207, except in those cases of mixed ECD/LCH. Expression of phosphorylated extracellular signal-regulated kinase (ERK) is frequently observed due to mutations in the mitogen-activated protein kinase (MAPK) pathway.

Genetic Features

BRAF p.V600E mutations are present in 50% to 60% of ECD cases (*Blood.* 2020;135:1311-1318; *Blood.* 2012;120:2700-2703). Additionally, activating mutations in the RAS-RAF-MEK-ERK signaling pathway, including *NRAS, KRAS, PIK3CA,* or *MAP2K1,* have also been identified. Many of these mutations have also been identified in JXG. The argument can be made that several of the histiocytic disorders are not so much differentiated on the basis of their mutations but rather on their pathologic and immunophenotypic features.

Prognosis and Treatment

In the past, the clinical outcome for ECD was poor, with a 3-year survival of less than 50%. However, targeted therapy has resulted in a 5-year survival approaching 80% (*Blood.* 2020;135:1929-1945; *Haematologica.* 2020;105:e5-e8).

Differential Diagnosis

- **LCH:** Histiocytes lack xanthomatized features, have nuclear grooves, are accompanied by eosinophils in variable numbers, and are positive for CD1a and CD207.
- **RDD:** Histiocytes are larger with pale, nonxanthomatized cytoplasm; emperipolesis is observed and accompanied by plasma cells (like ECD). Groups of S-100 protein positive histiocytes are present (ECD histiocytes are S100 negative).
- **IgG4-related disease:** Storiform fibrosis is present (not in ECD), and there is higher IgG:IgG4 ratio. IgG4-related disease lacks the *BRAFV600E* mutation seen in ECD.

Key Points

- ECD is a chronic disease that may affect several organ systems, in which case it has a poor outcome.
- *BRAFV600E* mutations occur in approximately 50% of cases.

Diagnostic Caveats

- ECD and JXG may be histologically identical, and clinical context and molecular testing may be very helpful. Some cases of systemic JXG in children may be ECD in the presence of *BRAFV600E* mutation.
- ECD may occur in patient with LCH or RDD, which may make the diagnosis more difficult.

SUGGESTED READINGS

Emile JF, Abla O, Fraitag S, et al. Revised classification of histiocytoses and neoplasms of the macrophage-dendritic cell lineages. *Blood.* 2016;127(22):2672-2681.

Goyal G, Heaney ML, Collin M, et al. Erdheim-Chester disease: consensus recommendations for evaluation, diagnosis, and treatment in the molecular era. *Blood.* 2020;135(22):1929-1945.

30.3 ALK-Positive Histiocytosis

John D. Pfeifer

ALK-positive histiocytosis, first described in 2008 (*Blood.* 2008;112:2965-2968), is quite a rare condition. Initially described as a multisystem disease with hematopoietic and liver involvement, it is now recognized to show a broader clinicopathologic spectrum (*Blood.* 2022;139:256-279). Based on mitogen-activated protein kinase (MAPK) pathway activation, through a translocation involving the *ALK* gene, the

TABLE 30.3-1 WHO-HAEM5 Diagnostic Criteria for ALK-Positive Histiocytosis

Essential

- Tissue infiltration by aggregates and sheets of histiocytes lacking high-grade dysplasia
- Positive immunostaining for two or more histiocytic markers, including CD163, CD68, CD14, CD4, and lysozyme
- Positive immunostaining for ALK, which can be focal and weak sometimes

Desirable

- Histiocytosis showing irregular nuclear foldings
- *ALK* gene translocation

Based on the WHO Classification of Tumours Editorial Board. Haematolymphoid tumours [Internet]. Lyon (France): International Agency for Research on Cancer; 2024 (WHO classification of tumours series, 5th ed.; vol. 11). Available from: https://tumourclassification.iarc.who.int/chapters/63.

disease is included in the "L" group. Current diagnostic criteria for ALK-positive histiocytosis are summarized in Table 30.3-1.

Clinical Features

ALK-positive histiocytosis is categorized based on disease localization, specifically multisystem disease with systemic hematopoietic involvement, multisystem (other) with involvement of two or more organ systems, and single system. Infants with multisystem disease with liver, spleen, and/or hematopoietic involvement account for 15% of cases, with a median age of 1.5 months; older patients with multisystemic disease account for 26% of cases, with a median age of 14.5 years; and patients with single-system disease account for 59% of cases, with a median age of 7 years (*Blood*. 2022;139:256-279). There is a female predilection in all three clinical phenotypic groups. Overall, about 21% of cases occur in adults, and almost half of all patients have neurologic involvement.

Morphology

ALK-positive histiocytosis has variable morphologic features. Most cases are densely cellular without lipidized histiocytes; some of these cases feature histiocytes with more spindled or epithelioid morphology. Only about a third of cases have classic xanthogranulomatous features with plump foamy histiocytes and variable number of Touton giant cells. The histiocytes themselves often have ovoid nuclei with slight folding or indentation, minimal atypia, and minimal mitotic activity. Because the morphology is not entirely diagnostic (and shows significant overlap with Erdheim-Chester disease (ECD), juvenile xanthogranuloma [JXG], and Rosai-Dorfman disease), ALK immunostaining is important for diagnosis, as discussed later.

Bone marrow involvement usually takes the form of plump histiocytes with a xanthogranulomatous pattern in a normo- to hypercellular background with relatively preserved hematopoiesis, and is usually not a diffuse infiltrative process. Liver involvement is characterized by histiocytic infiltration of the sinusoids and portal tracts, and involved skin shows a noncircumscribed, nonepidermotropic infiltrate composed of sheets of histiocytes.

Immunophenotype

The neoplastic histiocytes in ALK-positive histiocytosis are positive for macrophage markers such as CD163, CD68, CD14, CD4, and lysozyme, and the diagnostic criteria for the disease include expression of at least two of these macrophage/histiocyte markers by the lesional cells.

By definition, the neoplastic histiocytes also show ALK immunoreactivity (generally as a reflection of an underlying *ALK* translocation), although the pattern of ALK staining within the histiocytes does not seem to correlate with the partner gene involved in the rearrangement (*Blood*. 2022;139:256-279). The pattern of ALK staining is usually cytoplasmic, less commonly membranous, or a Golgi dot pattern. Consequently, ALK immunostaining can be a useful screen for cases of histiocytic proliferations that do not conform to defined entities (*Leukemia*. 2022;36:1703-1719). Some groups have proposed that, with the exception of classic infantile systemic disease, a positive ALK immunostain is not diagnostic in the absence of molecular confirmation of an *ALK* rearrangement, and that cases of noninfantile histiocytosis that show ALK immunoreactivity but do not harbor *ALK* rearrangements, or that harbor *ALK* rearrangements with ALK immunopositivity in cells that are not immunoreactive for macrophage/histiocyte markers, should not be grouped within ALK-positive histiocytosis (*Blood*. 2022;139:256-279).

Genetic Features

ALK-positive histiocytosis is characterized by the presence of *ALK* gene translocation. The most common fusion is *KIF5B-ALK* (present in approximately 85% of cases). Other less common fusions include *CLTC-ALK*, *TPM3-ALK*, *TFG-ALK*, *EML4-ALK*, and *DCTN1-ALK*. These translocations result in ligand-independent constitutive activation of the MAPK and phosphoinositide 3-kinase (PIK3) intracellular signaling pathways (*Nature*. 2019;567:521-524).

Prognosis and Treatment

The multisystem disease that occurs in infants typically has a protracted course, although about a third of patients in this clinical group eventually have spontaneous regression of the disease with only supportive care. Patients in other clinical groups are generally reported to have favorable outcomes with conventional chemotherapy and/or surgical therapy.

However, the prognosis and treatment of ALK-positive histiocytosis have been fundamentally changed by the recognition that the genetic alterations of the *ALK* gene lead to activation of the MAPK signaling pathway, and the availability of highly effective therapies targeting the pathway including both BRAF and MEK inhibitors. In a recent study, robust and durable responses were seen in 100% of patients treated with ALK inhibition (*Blood*. 2022;139:256-279).

Differential Diagnosis

Clinically, the differential diagnosis of ALK-positive histiocytosis includes ECD, JXG, and Rosai-Dorfman disease. Despite some differences in the clinical features between these diseases, there is significant overlap (reviewed in *Leukemia*. 2022;36:1703-1719), and in particular, it remains unsettled whether ALK-positive histiocytosis is distinct from systemic JXG (*Haematologica*. 2019;104:e534-e536). Similarly, the morphology of ALK-positive histiocytosis is not entirely diagnostic and shows significant overlap with ECD, JXG, and Rosai-Dorfman disease.

> **Key Points**
> - ALK-positive histiocytosis is an entity associated with *ALK* fusions.
> - The clinical features and morphology of ALK-positive histiocytosis overlap significantly with JXG, ECD, and Rosai-Dorfman disease.
> - ALK inhibition induces durable responses in patients with ALK-positive histiocytosis.
>
> **Diagnostic Caveats**
> - ALK immunostaining can be a useful screening tool for cases of histiocytic proliferations that do not conform to other defined entities.
> - The most common fusion is *KIF5B-ALK*, but approximately 15% of cases harbor other translocations. Therefore, genetic testing for *ALK* rearrangements is most informative when it is comprehensive.

SUGGESTED READINGS

Chakraborty R, Abdel-Wahab O, Durham BH. MAP-kinase-driven hematopoietic neoplasms: a decade of progress in the molecular age. *Cold Spring Harb Perspect Med* 2021;11:a034892.

Chan JKC, Lamant L, Algar E, et al. ALK+ histiocytosis: a novel type of systemic histiocytic proliferative disorder of early infancy. *Blood*. 2008;112:2965-2968.

Kemps PG, Picarsic J, Durham BH, et al. ALK-positive histiocytosis: a new clinicopathologic spectrum highlighting neurologic involvement and responses to ALK inhibition. *Blood*. 2022;139:256-280.

Khoury JD, Solary E, Abla O, et al. The 5th edition of the World Health Organization Classification of haematolymphoid tumours: myeloid and histiocytic/dendritic neoplasms. *Leukemia*. 2022;36:1703-1719.

SECTION IV

Ancillary Techniques

31 Immunohistochemistry and Histochemistry

John D. Pfeifer and Brooj Abro

I. IMMUNOHISTOCHEMISTRY

Immunohistochemistry (IHC) is an essential tool in the workup and diagnosis of hematologic neoplasms, and it is often used in conjunction with flow cytometry (FC) (discussed in Chapter 32) for immunophenotyping. IHC studies are typically performed on tissue sections to highlight the pattern, location, and intensity of antigen expression in various cell populations, and in recent years, mutation-specific antibodies have been introduced as a supplement to or replacement for molecular analysis. Two major advantages of IHC over FC are the ability to perform IHC studies on formalin-fixed paraffin-embedded (FFPE) tissue and the ability to assess cells in an architectural context.

Immunostains can be performed on standard histologic tissue sections as well as cytology specimens. While some antigens require the use of fresh tissue or tissue preserved with ethanol-based fixatives, in routine practice virtually all immunostains are performed on FFPE tissue. Immediate fixation in neutral pH formalin for 12 to 48 hours at room temperature is optimal; extended formalin fixation can induce cross-links that may mask some epitopes, resulting in loss of immunoreactivity. Acid decalcification of bone samples can also cause loss of immunoreactivity. Antigen retrieval techniques can be used to "unmask" some epitopes from FFPE (and acid-decalcified tissue); heat treatment (so-called heat-induced antigen retrieval) is the most commonly used approach.

Unstained tissue sections cut onto charged slides or poly-L-lysine-coated slides are typically used for IHC, which helps ensure that the tissue does not fall off the slide during the multiple processing steps. Immunostains should be performed on freshly cut sections from the paraffin block because it is well established that unstained sections exposed to air may lose antigen immunoreactivity over the course of days to weeks.

a. The **primary antibody** is the immunoglobulin molecule that binds to the target antigen in the tissue sections and is usually a monoclonal antibody. In most clinical settings, prediluted reagents and kits are used, which simplifies the validation, standardization, and reproducibility of IHC studies. Automated immunostaining platforms are in routine use in most in most laboratories to improve throughput and to improve standardization and reproducibility of IHC procedures.
b. **Binding Approaches**
   1. **Direct conjugate-labeled antibody method:** In this method, the label is directly chemically linked to the primary antibody. Common labels include enzymes such as peroxidase and alkaline phosphatase (which is used when the target antigen is in tissues rich in myeloid cells that contain high levels of endogenous peroxidases, such as bone marrow) and fluorophores such as fluorescein. A disadvantage of this approach is that it requires large amounts of primary antibody for labeling due to a lack of signal amplification.
   2. **Indirect or sandwich methods:** The primary antibody is unlabeled, and a secondary antibody reactive against the primary antibody carries the label.
   3. **Avidin-biotin or streptavidin-biotin conjugate method:** The primary antibody is conjugated to biotin, and avidin or streptavidin (which both have an extremely high affinity for biotin) is conjugated to the label. By this approach, several peroxidase molecules are delivered to the primary antibody binding site, which increases sensitivity (Figure 31.1).
   4. **Background staining** results from nonspecific binding of antibodies to tissue components and from endogenous enzymes that nonspecifically interact with the chromogenic substrates. Endogenous enzymes that cause background staining are found in normal cells, including erythrocytes, neutrophils, eosinophils, plasma cells, and neoplastic cells, and their activity can often be blocked (eg, endogenous peroxidase can be blocked by incubation with hydrogen peroxide).
c. **Chromogens** are color-producing reactants of the detection system. There are many different chromogens in routine use, but diaminobenzidine (DAB, produces a brown color) and 3-amino-9-ethylcarbazole (AEC, produces a red color) are the most common.
d. **Counterstaining** is performed to highlight the tissue architecture, which makes it possible to interpret the results of the immunostain in the context of the histopathologic findings. The nuclear stain hematoxylin is most often used (and care must be taken not to overstain the tissue sections when the target antigen is located in the nucleus).
e. So-called **antibody cocktails** can be used to detect two or more antigens at the same time. Single-color (*Am J Surg Pathol.* 2005;29:579) or two-color (*Am J Clin Pathol.* 2005;123:231) approaches are in wide use.
f. **Quantitative IHC.** IHC stains are usually manually, semi-quantitatively, scored by pathologists with respect to staining intensity and percentage of cells stained. Formalized semi-quantitative scoring is particularly important for a few markers, for example, of HER2/*neu* immunoreactivity in the setting of breast carcinoma to determine the eligibility for trastuzumab therapy (*J Clin Oncol.* 2007;25:118). Image analysis improves the consistency of quantitative IHC scoring, and it is likely that digital microscopy with image analysis will be increasingly used in this context (*Appl Immunohistochem Mol Morphol.* 2021;29:479; *Mod Pathol.* 2022;35:23).

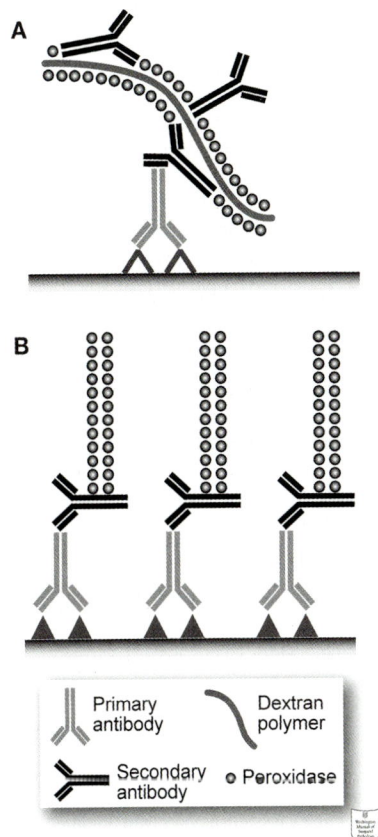

Figure 31.1. Immunohistochemical detection using the polymer method. This technique allows the linkage of numerous molecules of enzyme (either peroxidase or alkaline phosphatase) to one (**B**) or more (**A**) molecules of secondary antibody. Delivery of a large number of enzyme molecules to the antigen-primary antibody reaction site yields high sensitivity. Modified from Taylor CR, Cote RJ, eds. *Immunomicroscopy: A Diagnostic Tool for the Surgical Pathologist*. 3rd ed. Elsevier; 2006.

II. INTERPRETATION

The results of IHC must be integrated with the clinical, radiographic, gross, and histopathologic findings of the case, as well as the results of any additional ancillary tests (such as molecular genetic tests). After evaluation of positive and negative controls, the immunostained slide should be assessed for the presence of staining in the cells of interest (or the regions of intercellular matrix of interest); localization of staining in the cells (eg, cytoplasmic, nuclear, and/or membranous staining of the cells); intensity of staining; and proportion of cells that stain. Specific attention should be directed toward possible artifacts including background staining, localization of signal along tissue edges (known as edge artifact), or nonspecific staining in areas of the tissue that are necrotic or crushed.

A list of common hematopoietic cell populations that can be detected by IHC studies is provided in Table 31.1. Knowledge of the expected staining patterns for normal and neoplastic hematolymphoid cells is essential for correct interpretation of the staining results (see Tables 31.2 and 31.3).

TABLE 31.1 Hematologic Cell Populations and IHC Markers

Cell Populations	IHC Markers
Pan-hematopoietic	CD45 (LCA)[a]
Lymphoblasts	Common: CD34, TdT
	T cell: CD1a, CD3
	B cell: CD19, PAX5, CD79a, CD79a
Myeloblasts	CD34, CD117, myeloperoxidase
B cells	Pan B cell: CD19, CD20, PAX5, CD79a
	Germinal center B cells: CD10, BCL6 (BCL2 negative)
	Mantle zone B cells: CD23 and BCL2 positive
T cells	Pan T cell: CD43, CD3, CD2, CD5, CD7, CD4, and CD8; most T cells express either CD4 or CD8.
	TFH cells: CD10, BCL6, CD4, CD57, PD1, CXCL13, ICOS
Plasma cells	CD138, MUM1, kappa, lambda
Histiocytic/monocytic cells	CD163, CD68, CD4, lysozyme, CD33
Follicular dendritic cells	CD21, CD23, CD35
Myeloid cells	Myeloperoxidase, CD43, CD33
	CD34 and/or CD117 (in myeloblasts)
Erythroid cells	Glycophorin, transferrin/CD71, E-cadherin
Megakaryocytes	Factor VIII, CD61, CD41, CD42b

[a]Commonly used for screening tumors of unknown origin. Most hematopoietic tumors are positive for CD45 with some exceptions including Classic Hodgkin lymphoma, plasma cell neoplasms, and some B- and T-cell lymphomas.
IHC, immunohistochemistry; TFH, T follicular helper.

TABLE 31.2 The Staining Pattern of Commonly Used IHC Studies in Benign Lymphoid Tissue

IHC Stain	Location	Cell Populations and Pattern
CD3	Membranous and cytoplasmic	Positive in T cells: predominantly interfollicular
CD5	Membranous and cytoplasmic	Positive in T cells: predominantly interfollicular. Also positive in naïve B cells (mantle zone)
CD20	Membranous	Positive in B cells: predominantly follicular
PAX5	Nuclear	Positive in B cells: predominantly follicular
CD10	Membranous	Positive in germinal center B cells and follicular helper T cells: highlights secondary germinal centers

TABLE 31.2	The Staining Pattern of Commonly Used IHC Studies in Benign Lymphoid Tissue (*continued*)	
BCL6	Nuclear	Positive in germinal center B cells and follicular helper T cells: highlights secondary germinal centers
BCL2	Membranous	Positive in T cells and naïve B cells (primary follicles, mantle zones). Negative in germinal centers
Cyclin D1	Nuclear	Negative in lymphocytes. Epithelial cells can be positive.
CD21	Membranous	Follicular dendritic cells: meshworks within follicles
CD23	Membranous	Subset of B cells, follicular dendritic cells: meshworks within follicles
CD30	Membranous and Golgi (perinuclear dotlike staining)	Activated B cells (immunoblasts), T cells, and plasma cells
CD138	Membranous	Plasma cells
Kappa and lambda	Cytoplasmic	Plasma cells
MUM1	Nuclear	Plasma cells, activated B and T cells
CD43	Membranous	T cells, plasma cells
Ki67	Nuclear	High in normal germinal centers

IHC, immunohistochemistry.

TABLE 31.3	The Staining Pattern of Commonly Used IHC Studies in Normal Bone Marrow Core Biopsy Tissue	
IHC Stain	**Location**	**Cell Populations**
CD34	Membranous	Precursors (usually <5% of cells); vessels are also positive.
CD117	Membranous and cytoplasmic	Precursors and mast cells
Myeloperoxidase	Cytoplasmic (granular pattern)	Granulocytes
TdT	Nuclear	Hematogones
E-cadherin	Membranous	Erythroid precursors
Glycophorin-A	Membranous	Erythroid lineage cells including RBCs
CD33	Membranous	Myeloid and monocytic cells
CD41, CD42b, CD61	Membranous	Megakaryocytes

IHC, immunohistochemistry; RBC, red blood cell.

Immunohistochemical Panels for the Diagnosis of Hematologic Malignancies

IHC studies are commonly performed on FFPE sections from needle core and excisional biopsies, excisions, and cytology cell blocks. A list of recommended panels for the initial workup of commonly encountered hematologic malignancies is included in Table 31.4.

III. IN SITU HYBRIDIZATION TECHNIQUES

In situ hybridization (ISH) studies performed on FFPE tissue are analogous to IHC. For IHC, antibodies are used for the detection of specific antigens; ISH studies utilize DNA, RNA, or synthetic oligonucleotide probes that target specific genetic loci. The

TABLE 31.4 IHC Panels for the Workup of Common Hematologic Malignancies

Differential Diagnoses/ Diagnostic Consideration	IHC Panels
Reactive lymphoid hyperplasia vs low-grade B-cell lymphoma	CD3, CD5, cyclin D1, CD20, CD10, BCL6, BCL2, CD21, CD23, KI67, CD138, kappa, lambda
Small B-cell lymphoma	CD3, CD20, PAX5, CD5, Cyclin D1, CD10, BCL6, BCL2, CD21, CD23, Ki67
Large B-cell lymphoma	DLBCL/HGBCL morphology: CD3, CD20, PAX5, CD5, Cyclin D1, CD10, BCL6, BCL2, CD21, CD23, Ki67, CD30, MYC, MUM1, EBER.
	Plasmablastic morphology: add CD138, kappa, lambda, ALK, and HHV8
	Blastoid morphology: add CD34 and TdT if adequate FC analysis is not available.
Nodular lymphocyte-predominant Hodgkin lymphoma	CD20, PAX5, OCT2, BOB1, CD30, CD21, CD23, CD3, PD-1, CD57
Classic Hodgkin lymphoma	CD30, CD15, PAX5, CD20, CD45, MUM1, EBER
PTCL subtypes: nodal TFH lymphomas, EBV+ nodal T-/NK-cell lymphoma, PTCL NOS	CD20, PAX5, CD3, CD2, CD5, CD7, CD4, CD8, CD30, Ki67, TFH markers (PD-1, CD10, BCL6, ICOS, CXCL13), cytotoxic markers (TIA, granzyme B, perforin), EBER, TCRβ, TCRγδ
Anaplastic large cell lymphoma	CD3, CD2, CD5, CD7, CD4, CD8, CD20, PAX5, CD30, CD15, CD25, ALK-1, TIA, EBER

DLBCL, diffuse large B-cell lymphoma; EBV, Epstein-Barr virus; FC, flow cytometry; HGBCL, high-grade B-cell lymphoma; IHC, immunohistochemistry; NK, natural killer; PTCL NOS, peripheral T-cell lymphoma not otherwise specified; TFH, T follicular helper.

two common methods that utilize ISH are fluorescence in situ hybridization (FISH) and chromogenic in situ hybridization (CISH).

FISH techniques are discussed in detail in Chapter 34.1. In hematopathology, the most common use of FISH with FFPE tissue is the assessment of *MYC*, *BCL2*, *BCL6*, and *CCND1* rearrangements in the workup of B-cell lymphomas.

CISH techniques are also discussed in detail in Chapter 34.1. In hematopathology, the most common use of CISH with FFPE is for the detection of cytoplasmic kappa and lambda light chains in plasma cells for the assessment of clonality, and for identification of Epstein-Barr virus (EBV)-encoded small RNA (EBER) in the evaluation of EBV infection in various lymphomas and reactive conditions.

IV. HISTOCHEMICAL STAINS

Histochemical stains, as opposed to IHC stains, do not employ antibodies but instead rely on direct chemical reactions to detect specific cellular characteristics or tissue components. Histochemical stains are thus based on the chemistry of various dyes and metals, and operationally range from very simple to quite complex. Automated platforms are in routine use in in most laboratories to improve throughput and to improve standardization and reproducibility of the procedures.

In general, a histochemical stain consists of a chemical reaction that demonstrates the tissue element of interest, followed by chemical reactions that provide staining of the background uninvolved tissue elements. Histochemical stains are grouped by the tissue component they stain and include stains for carbohydrates, connective tissue, microorganisms, nerve fibers/myelin sheath, pigments and minerals, and enzymes. Of the vast array of histochemical stains, only the handful routinely encountered in hematopathology will be discussed (Table 31.5).

a. **Carbohydrates**
Although simple sugars cannot be detected by standard histochemical procedures because they are water soluble and therefore removed during tissue processing, polymers such as glycogen can be detected, as can carbohydrates linked to proteins and lipids. Naturally occurring polysaccharides can be classified into four groups based on their histochemical staining differences (Group 1, neutral polysaccharides; Group II, acid mucopolysaccharides; Group III, glycoproteins; and Group IV, glycolipids). Amyloid is usually also included because, even though it is not itself a carbohydrate, its histochemical staining properties are similar to those of polysaccharides. Histochemical stains that are encountered in hematopathology to detect and differentiate carbohydrates are Congo red and Thioflavin T.
1. **Congo red** reacts with cellulose and amyloid. The dye is a linear molecule that interacts with amyloid in a sheet-like fashion, resulting in so-called "apple-green" birefringence when subjected to polarized light, which is considered specific for amyloid in Congo red–stained tissue sections (e-Figure 31.1).
2. **Thioflavin T** is a fluorescent tissue dye that has an affinity for amyloid. Thioflavin T fluoresces yellow to yellow-green when the tissue section is viewed by fluorescent microscopy, but the dye is not as specific for amyloid as Congo red.

b. **Connective Tissue**
A wide variety of stains can be used to detect the various components of connective tissue, of which those most commonly encountered in hematopathology are the reticulin stain and the trichrome stain.

TABLE 31.5 Common Histochemical Stains

Stain	Tissue Element Demonstrated	Result
Congo red	Amyloid	Apple-green birefringence when viewed under polarized light
Thioflavin T	Amyloid	Yellow when viewed via fluorescence microscopy
Reticulin	Reticulin fibers	Black
Trichrome	Nuclei, collagen, and muscle	Black, blue, and red, respectively
Gram	Differentiating gram-positive from gram-negative bacteria	Gram-positive bacteria are blue; gram-negative bacteria are red
AFB	Acid-fast bacilli	Red
Fite AFB	*Mycobacterium leprae*	Red
Grocott methenamine silver	Fungi	Taupe to black
Warthin-Starry	Spirochetes	Black
Iron (Prussian blue)	Iron	Blue
MPO	Cellular myeloperoxidase	Intracellular blue-brown granules
Nonspecific esterase	Cellular esterases	Intracellular brown precipitate

1. **Reticulin.** For this stain, glycols are first reduced to dialdehydes by the use of an acid. The tissue is next sensitized to accept metallic silver ions with an ammoniacal silver solution, the silver ions that are attached on and around the dialdehyde groups are then reduced to metallic silver, and the tissue sections are then toned from brown to black by replacing the metallic silver with metallic gold. Sodium thiosulfate is used to remove any remaining unreacted silver in the tissue to prevent darkening of the slide over time. The end result is that reticulin fibers are stained black against a clear background (e-Figure 31.2).
2. **Trichrome.** The trichrome stain has a number of variations, all of which generally use three dyes with affinities for different connective tissue elements. The first step involves mordanting the tissue with a heavy metal fixative such as Bouin's fixative; the tissue is then dyed with a nuclear stain, most often an iron hematoxylin; an acidic dye such as acid fuchsin or biebrich scarlet is next used to stain the cytoplasm of cells, collagen, and muscle; either phosphotungstic acid or phosphomolybdic acid is used to remove the acid dye from the collagen (since the cytoplasm of cells is less permeable than collagen, with proper timing the dye can be removed from collagen without complete removal from other tissue elements); and finally, collagen is stained using aniline blue. The stain produces

tissue sections that are stained in three colors: black cell nuclei, red cell cytoplasm and muscle, and blue collagen and mucus (e-Figure 31.3).

c. **Microorganisms**

Many different stains can be performed to demonstrate microorganisms in tissue sections, including bacteria and fungi. Commonly used stains are the acid-fast bacilli (AFB) (including the Fite modification), Gram, Grocott methenamine silver (GMS), and Warthin-Starry.

1. **Gram stain.** The tissue Gram stain is similar to the standard Gram stain performed in the microbiology lab, except that after the use of crystal violet to demonstrate gram-positive bacteria by a blue color, basic fuchsin (a red dye) is used to demonstrate gram-negative organisms as well as cell nuclei. The final step involves treating the tissue with a picric acid solution to render a yellow background (the so-called Brown-Hopps method). In addition to the identification of bacteria, the tissue Gram stain can be used to demonstrate some cases of actinomycosis, *Nocardia*, coccidioidomycosis, blastomycosis, cryptococcosis, aspergillosis, rhinosporidiosis, and amebiasis (e-Figure 31.4).

2. **AFB stain.** The tissue AFB stain is a modification of the standard Ziehl-Neelsen and Kinyoun stains and takes advantage of the fact that carbol-fuchsin, a solution created by reacting basic fuchsin with phenol in alcohol, is soluble in lipids. Tissue sections are first treated with the carbol-fuchsin solution and then differentiated using acid alcohol; bacteria that have waxy, lipid-containing cell walls resist decolorization with acid alcohol and are said to be "acid fast." A methylene blue counterstain is often used to highlight other tissue elements and provide a background to highlight the red microorganisms (e-Figure 31.5). The Fite AFB stain is a modification of the standard AFB stain used when *Mycobacterium leprae* is suspected (e-Figure 31.6).

3. **GMS stain.** This stain utilizes methenamine to form a complex with silver, which is then reacted with dialdehyde groups formed by the reduction of glycol units in a process similar to that of the reticulin stain. However, the GMS stain uses a stronger oxidizer, specifically chromic acid, because the cell walls of fungi are thick and contain more carbohydrates than the basement membranes and reticulin fibers in the surrounding tissue, the stronger oxidizer creates dialdehyde groups from the carbohydrates of the fungi cell walls but leads to overoxidation and destruction of basement membranes and other tissue carbohydrates. The GMS stain utilizes a light green counterstain, resulting in fungal cell walls that are various shades of black to taupe on a light green background (e-Figure 31.7).

4. **Warthin-Starry stain.** This stain is used primarily for the demonstration of spirochetes (although other bacteria are also stained) and is based on the principle that bacteria, in general, and spirochetes, in particular, have the ability to bind silver ions. The staining procedure involves impregnation of the tissue with silver ions, with subsequent reduction of the ions to metallic silver using a developer containing hydroquinone. The stain demonstrates black spirochetes against a yellow to pale brown background and highlights their spiral morphology (e-Figures 31.8 and 31.9).

    IHC techniques for the detection of spirochetes in tissue sections are also available and, in some settings, have replaced the Warthin-Starry stain in routine clinical use. Some studies have suggested that IHC stains for *Treponema pallidum* have higher sensitivity in some settings than the Warthin-Starry stain (*J Cutan Pathol.* 2004;31:595).

d. **Pigments and Minerals**
   While a number of histochemical stains can be used to detect pigments and minerals deposited in tissues, or as inclusions or granules within cells, the stain for iron is generally the only one encountered in hematopathology.
   1. **Iron.** The Prussian blue reaction is the most common tissue stain for iron because it stains only weakly bound iron; strongly bound iron, such as iron in hemoglobin, will not stain. The principle of the stain is simple: when treated with potassium ferrocyanide in an acidic solution, ferrous ions in the tissue react to form an insoluble blue pigment. A nuclear fast red counterstain is often used to demonstrate the background tissue morphology (e-Figure 31.10).
e. **Enzymes**
   Most cytochemical stains for enzymes require the use of fresh aspirates, tissue touch preparations, peripheral blood, or frozen sections because most enzymes do not retain activity after the rigors of routine formalin fixation and paraffin processing.
   1. **Myeloperoxidase (MPO) stain.** This stain has traditionally been used to differentiate blasts in acute myeloid leukemia (AML) from those of acute lymphoblastic leukemia (ALL). Air-dried bone marrow or peripheral blood smears are fixed in formal ethanol or buffered formal acetone and then incubated with hydrogen peroxide. Under these conditions, MPO present in leukocyte granules oxidizes colorless substrates (such as benzidine or 3,3'-DAB) to insoluble blue-brown precipitates. A hematoxylin or Giemsa counterstain is used to visualize cell morphology.

      IHC stains for the detection of MPO have recently been developed, which provide many advantages since they can be performed on routinely processed FFPE tissue and cytology cell blocks. Some studies have suggested that IHC has increased the sensitivity of the detection of MPO versus cytochemical methods (*Indian J Hematol Blood Transfus*. 2018;34:233).
   2. **Nonspecific esterase stain.** This stain is employed on a cytospin preparation of cells (usually from a bone marrow aspirate), peripheral blood smear, or tissue touch preparation in which the cells are fixed by a buffered formaldehyde-based solution. When used with the substrate α-naphthyl butyrate esterase (NBE), the esterases present in monocytes/macrophages cleave the substrate to yield an intermediate that can then be coupled with hexazotized pararosaniline to produce a brown precipitate. A hematoxylin or methyl green counterstain is typically used to visualize cell morphology.

SUGGESTED READINGS

Cartun RW, Taylor CR, Dabbs DJ. Techniques of Immunohistochemistry: Principles, Pitfalls, and Standardization. In: Dabbs DJ, ed. *Diagnostic Immunohistochemistry: Theranostic and Genomic Applications*. 6th ed. Elsevier; 2021:1-46.

Suvarna KS, Layton C, Bancroft JD. *Bancroft's Theory and Practice of Histological Techniques*. 8th ed. Elsevier; 2018.

Flow Cytometry
Cara Lunn Shirai

I. BASIC PRINCIPLES

Flow cytometry (FC) is a highly versatile multi-parameter analysis technique that allows for characterization of individual cells within a heterogeneous population. FC is commonly used in a variety of clinical and research settings.

FC is accomplished using: (1) patient specimens prepared as a cell suspension and stained with fluorescence molecules, (2) instruments called flow cytometers that excite the fluorescence stains and detect emitted light signals, and (3) a downstream analysis software that is the platform for interpretation. Each of these components is described further.

The patient specimens are prepared as filtered single-cell suspensions. Peripheral blood, bone marrow, and cerebrospinal or other body fluids are already cell suspensions, but tissues require additional preparation work. Single-cell suspensions can be generated by mechanical separation processes or enzymes. Cells are stained with fluorescent dyes and fluorescently labeled antibodies that recognize cell antigens of interest. Additional steps in sample preparation may include red blood cell (RBC) lysis (unless the RBC is your target for FC analysis), fixation (which we perform after the staining step), and cell permeabilization (used for FC of intracellular antigens). There are additional specimen requirements and recommendations that depend on specimen type. FC analysis of peripheral blood and bone marrow requires specimen collection with an anticoagulant (sodium heparin, potassium-EDTA tubes, and/or acid citrate dextrose). FC of cerebrospinal fluid should be performed as soon as possible due to the short half-life of cells in this fluid. Lymph nodes and tissue masses should be placed in RPMI medium for improved viability during transport to the FC laboratory.

II. INSTRUMENTATION

The standard clinical flow cytometer is a laser-based microfluidic system that performs high-throughput analysis of cells in suspension using different wavelengths of light. Specimens are analyzed using the emissions from fluorescent dyes bound to cells and the light scattering properties inherent to the cells themselves. The working parts of a flow cytometer can be classified into three general categories: fluidics, optics, and electronics.

Fluidics

The fluidics component of the flow cytometer has one purpose: to deliver cells accurately and precisely in a single file line (think conga dance line) to the interrogation point of the flow cytometer, where cells are exposed to the excitation laser and fluorescence is detected. This delivery of single cells to the interrogation point is through hydrodynamic focusing, which allows for the confinement of the slow-flowing specimen-containing fluid by a faster flowing sheath fluid. This allows for accuracy and precision of event collection and reduces the possibility of coincident events (where two cells pass through at the same time and create artifact populations).

Optics

The optical part of the flow cytometer includes: the lasers and focusers for fluorescent molecule (fluorophore) excitation at certain wavelengths of light, the detectors to capture emitted fluorescent light, and a series of dichroic mirrors and filters for directing light to appropriate detectors for data collection.

Electronics

The electronics part of the flow cytometer converts the produced light into usable data. The detectors have photodiodes or photomultiplier tubes that collect incoming photons of light and convert them to electrons. This electronic signal is amplified, digitalized, and converted to a voltage pulse with specific magnitude (numeric values), which can be displayed in a visual format for interpretive analysis. FC analysis is performed using specialized software. There are many software programs available for this purpose, and laboratories will oftentimes opt to use the analysis software from the manufacturer of their flow cytometers. These software programs will have an Instructions for Use (IFU) guide document (often available online), and we recommend to obtain the IFU for your analysis software if you want additional assistance in using the software.

III. TYPES OF ASSAYS

There are several general approaches used in clinical FC, and the chosen approach for an assay is dependent on the information desired. These different types of assays are termed qualitative and quasi- or semi-quantitative (true quantitative measurements are rare in clinical FC since these require a standard curve). The sample preparation, performance, and interpretation of these assays are different; however, the primary type of analysis performed for hematologic malignancy is qualitative FC. Our FC panels and specimen preparation protocols are designed for this purpose. FC of hematopoietic cells can provide lineage information, indicate clonality, identify immunotherapy targets for patient treatment, and provide the immunophenotype of malignant cells to be followed over the course of a patient's treatment (particularly helpful when minimal/measurable residual disease [MRD] FC monitoring will be employed).

Quasi- or semi-quantitative FC assays include paroxysmal nocturnal hemoglobinuria (PNH) and MRD testing. Semi-quantitative assessment for immune monitoring (competency and deficiency) and CD34-expressing stem cell enumeration for hematopoietic stem cell transplants also fall under this category.

IV. GATING AND INTERPRETATION

FC gating is performed to distinguish cells of interest for further analysis by measured parameters. Gating can get quite complex, but there are important quality gates that should be used up front in most FC analyses. The following gates are commonly employed: (1) a "time" gate to allow for inclusion/exclusion of events within a sample run that may have problems (like a clog or the sample out of volume), (2) a singlet gate (to exclude coincident cell events), (3) a "live cells" gate, in which hematopoietic cells

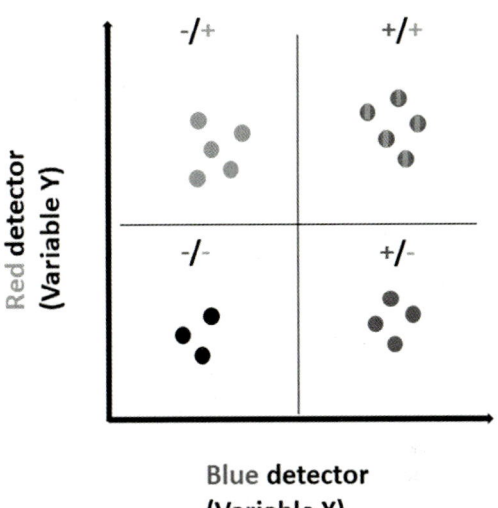

Figure 32.1. How to interpret a bivariate dot plot. Each cell is represented by a dot on the graph. The location of the cell dot on the x- and y-axes corresponds to the measured value of fluorescence signal for the independent variables displayed on these respective axes (eg, red and blue colors).

form a boot or sock shape, (4) a CD45 × side scatter (SSC) gate, where we identify basic hematopoietic populations of interest (more on this later).

Bivariate graphs are the current workhorse of general clinical FC analysis, although cluster analysis, principal component analysis, and other multidimensional approaches have been coming online to accommodate the increased amount of data we are able to collect with new and expanding technologies. Bivariate plots display independent signals on the x- and y-axes, and they should be interpreted as such. See Figure 32.1.

V. BACKGROUND SIGNALS AND ARTIFACTS

There are several sources of aberrant fluorescent signals in FC, and these should be considered during analysis and interpretation, as well as during development of new assays: autofluorescence, undesired antibody/dye binding, and spectral overlap or "spillover."

Autofluorescence

Mammalian cells have endogenous molecules that emit light upon excitation by lasers; this phenomenon is called autofluorescence. Autofluorescence is the result of excitation by lasers in the 405 to 488 spectra (violet and blue lasers). Different cells have different types and amounts of autofluorescence (neutrophils = blue FL1 and FL2 detectors, eosinophils = violet FL9 detector on the Beckman-Coulter Navios cytometer), and malignant cells may occasionally display increased and unexpected autofluorescence (eg, acute promyelocytic leukemia [APL] cells can have distinct autofluorescence due to increased primary granules and Auer rods). Autofluorescence can be expected in certain cell types and should be accounted for in the interpretation of fluorescence signals, particularly with the choice of internal negative controls for determining positivity of antigen expression.

Undesired Antibody/Dye Binding

Antibodies used in clinical FC testing should be well-vetted (eg, monoclonal antibodies from clones described by the Human Leukocyte Differentiation Antigen [HLDA] workshops), and appropriate buffers and preparation protocols should be used to avoid nonspecific and cross-reactive binding. The Fc-receptors on monocytes may bind the Fc portion of FC antibodies indiscriminately as well; however, this can be prevented by using an Fc blocking approach.

Spectral Overlap or "Spillover"

Many commonly used fluorophores have overlapping wavelength emission spectra that are broad, which can result in detection of their signal by more than one detector of a flow cytometer. This is a function of the biochemical and biophysical properties of the chosen fluorophore; therefore, common mitigation strategies are used to avoid spillover signals. Antibody choices and overall panel design can help prevent large spillovers of light from bright antigens into dim antigen detectors. However, even with carefully designed panels, spillover does occur and is dealt with via the standard process of compensation. Compensation "subtracts" the fluorescence spillover signal from the total detected fluorescence to provide a compensated "real" fluorescence signal. The need for compensation can be expected in most standard multi-parameter FC assays.

Specimen Quality Can Produce Artifacts

Specimen quality can impact the signals. Microscopic review of a cytospin made from the FC specimen should be used for quality control purposes.

VI. REPORTING OF LEUKEMIA/LYMPHOMA FLOW CYTOMETRY INTERPRETATIONS

Developing Templates

Most leukemia/lymphoma FC panels are laboratory-developed tests unique to specific institutions. This serves to standardize reporting and help ensure all pertinent information is included.

Describing Populations of Interest

Fluorescence distribution: This should be described relative to an appropriate internal negative control population identified within the sample. This requires knowledge of antigen expression (eg, a good negative control for CD19+ would be CD3+ T cells). Terms to use for fluorescence distribution are: (1) Negative = not expressed, (2) Positive = expressed, (3) Partially expressed (partial) = expressed in a subset. See e-Figure 32.1.

Fluorescence intensity: This should be described as intensity relative to the closest normal hematolymphoid population identified internal to the specimen. This parameter is presumed to correlate with the level of antigen expression. Terms to use for fluorescence intensity outside of the normal (moderate) range are: (1) Bright = more intense than closest normal population, (2) Dim = less intense than closest normal population, (3) Heterogeneous = antigen shows a spectrum of intensity (variable expression), (4) Homogeneous = antigen shows uniform intensity, important when a spectrum of expression is normal/expected. See e-Figure 32.2.

VII. IMMUNOPHENOTYPING FOR LEUKEMIA/LYMPHOMA CHARACTERIZATION

To properly interpret and describe FC results for a given tissue or fluid, you must know the expected normal expression patterns for the cell antigens in that tissue or fluid (see Table 32.1 for antigens and associated expression patterns in normal and neoplastic cells). Identifying what is different from normal (DfN) is the best way to recognize malignant cell populations, since malignancies do not display uniform immunophenotypic changes (although there are trends).

TABLE 32.1 Common Cellular Antigen Expression Patterns in Normal and Malignant Hematolymphoid Cells Useful for Flow Cytometry Analysis

Cell Antigen	Normal Distribution	Expression in Malignancy (Common or Abnormal)
CD1a	Thymocytes/immature T cells	Thymomas, some T-ALL
CD2	Pan-T-lineage cells, NK cells	T-ALL and T/NK-lymphomas (but may have reduced/loss of expression), AML, MDS, systemic mastocytosis
CD3	T-lineage cells, cytoplasmic in early T-lineage precursors/blasts	Surface expression in mature T neoplasms (can be bright, dim, or lost), cytoplasmic expression in T-ALL, or mature T/NK-cell neoplasm (surface negative)
CD4	Subset of mature T cells, monocytes	Some mature T-cell neoplasms, T-ALL, AML, BPDCN
CD5	Pan-T-lineage cells, small subset of mature B cells	T-ALL and T lymphomas (but may have reduced/loss of expression), CLL/SLL and MCL, AML
CD7	Pan-T-lineage cells, NK cells	T-ALL and T/NK-lymphomas (but may have reduced/loss of expression), AML, MDS, MPN
CD8	Subset of mature T cells, some NK cells	Some mature T-cell neoplasms, T-ALL
CD9	B-cell precursors (hematogones), activated T cells	B-ALL
CD10	B-cell precursors (hematogones), follicular B cells, immature T cells, subset of mature T cells, and mature neutrophils	B-ALL, mature B-lymphomas of germinal center origin (FL, DLBCL, BL), occasionally mature T-lymphoma, AITL, T-ALL
CD11b	Maturing myeloid and monocytic cells, NK cells	AML, MPN, MDS
CD11c	Subset of mature B cells, subset of mature T cells	HCL, often in other mature B-lineage neoplasms (dimmer)
CD13	Maturing myeloid and monocytic cells	AML, MDS, MPN, some B-ALL

(continued)

TABLE 32.1 Common Cellular Antigen Expression Patterns in Normal and Malignant Hematolymphoid Cells Useful for Flow Cytometry Analysis (*continued*)

Cell Antigen	Normal Distribution	Expression in Malignancy (Common or Abnormal)
CD14	Monocytes and myeloid cells	AML, MDS, MPN
CD15	Mature neutrophils, monocytes	AML, MDS, MPN, occasionally expressed in B-ALL, B-cell lymphomas, Reed-Sternberg cells in HL (not often detected by flow cytometry)
CD16	NK cells, NK-like T cells, mature neutrophils, subset of monocytes	AML, MDS, MPN, LGL leukemia
CD19	All B cells, including early B-precursors (hematogones), mature B cells and normal plasma cells	Retained on most malignant B-lineage cells (can be brighter or dimmer), typically absent on PCN, rarely AML
CD20	Found on mature B cells (dimmer and heterogeneous on B-cell precursors)	Retained on most mature B-lineage neoplasms (can be brighter or dimmer), occasionally B-ALL, T-cell neoplasms, and PCN
CD22	B-lineage cells (surface expression is bright on mature B cells, dimmer on B-cell precursors)	Often retained on B-lineage malignancies, can be cytoplasmic in B-ALL
CD23	Subset of B cells	Can help classify CD5+ B-cell lymphomas (CLL/SLL is CD23+, MCL is usually CD23−)
CD25	Activated B cells and T cells, NK cells	HCL, B-ALL, mature B-lymphoma, mature T-lymphoma (ATLL), systemic mastocytosis
CD26	T cells and NK cells	Sézary syndrome/CTCL
CD30	Subset of B cells, subset of T cells, virally infected lymphocytes	ALCL, some T-cell and NK-cell lymphomas, B-cell lymphomas, Reed-Sternberg cells in HL (not often detected by flow cytometry)
CD33	Maturing myeloid and monocytic cells	AML, MDS, MPN, some B-ALL
CD34	Hematopoietic stem cells, myeloblasts, B- and T-lymphoblasts	AML, MDS (increased blasts), B-ALL, T-ALL
CD36	Monocytes, maturing erythroid and megakaryocytic cells, platelets, subset of T cells	AML, MDS

TABLE 32.1 Common Cellular Antigen Expression Patterns in Normal and Malignant Hematolymphoid Cells Useful for Flow Cytometry Analysis (*continued*)

Cell Antigen	Normal Distribution	Expression in Malignancy (Common or Abnormal)
CD38	Plasma cells (bright), B-cell precursors (hematogones), subsets of B-, T-, and NK-lymphocytes, monocytes, basophils, mature neutrophils (dim), erythroid precursors	PCN (bright), B-ALL, AML, some B-cell lymphomas.
CD41	Platelets, megakaryocytes, megakaryocytic precursors	AML (may indicate megakaryocytic differentiation)
CD45	Present and variable on all hematopoietic cells (generally bright on mature cells, weaker on precursor cells and blasts), absent on late erythroids, mature RBCs, platelets, and some plasma cells	Expression can be lost or reduced in many malignant cell types, usually in immature neoplasms (but can be dim or lost in some mature neoplasms).
CD52	Mature B- and T-lymphocytes, monocytes	B- and T-cell lymphomas, B-ALL, some T-ALL
CD56	NK cells, NK-like T cells, activated monocytes, occasionally some myeloid lineage cells	T/NK-lymphomas, AML, MDS, MPN, BPDCN, some PCN
CD57	NK cells, NK-like T cells	NK-lymphomas
CD58	Expressed on most hematopoietic cells (brighter on precursor cells)	Frequently overexpressed in B-ALL
CD61	Platelets, megakaryocytes, megakaryocytic precursors	AML (may indicate megakaryocytic differentiation)
CD64	Monocytes and maturing myeloid cells	AML, MDS, MPN
CD71	Maturing erythroids and erythroid precursors (bright), some myeloid cells and activated lymphocytes	AML (may indicate erythroid lineage), MDS
CD79a	Found on most B cells and plasma cells, cytoplasmic staining in early B-precursors	B-lineage neoplasms, cytoplasmic in B-ALL
CD81	Subset of B cells, subset of T cells, most plasma cells	B-lymphomas (especially of germinal center origin), often lost in PCN and B-ALL
CD103	Subset of B cells, subset of T cells	HCL, occasionally in splenic MZL, rarely in other B- and T-lymphomas
CD117	Hematopoietic stem cells, myeloid lineage precursor cells, mast cells (bright)	AML, APL, some PCN

(*continued*)

TABLE 32.1 Common Cellular Antigen Expression Patterns in Normal and Malignant Hematolymphoid Cells Useful for Flow Cytometry Analysis (*continued*)

Cell Antigen	Normal Distribution	Expression in Malignancy (Common or Abnormal)
CD123	Basophils, plasmacytoid dendritic cells, occasionally on monocytes, dimly on myeloid precursors	BPDCN, HCL, B-ALL, AML
CD138	Plasma cells	PCN
CD200	B cells, occasional T-cell subsets	CLL/SLL, PCN, B-ALL, AML
CD235a	Maturing erythroid lineage cells and RBCs	AML (may indicate erythroid differentiation)
FMC7	Some mature B cells	Can help classify CD5+ B-cell lymphomas (typically CLL/SLL is FMC7−, MCL is FMC7+)
HLA-DR	All B cells (including B-cell precursors/hematogones), myeloid blasts, monocytes, subset of T cells	B-cell neoplasms (including B-ALL), AML, MDS, MPN
Kappa	Light chain of antibody, expressed on the surface of mature B cells, cytoplasmic on plasma cells	Restricted expression can indicate a monoclonal process (surface = mature B cell, cytoplasmic = plasma cell).
Lambda	Light chain of antibody, expressed on the surface of mature B cells, cytoplasmic on plasma cells	Restricted expression can indicate a monoclonal process (surface = mature B cell, cytoplasmic = plasma cell).
MPO	Myeloid lineage cells	Cytoplasmic in AML (antigen detection)
TCR$\alpha\beta$	Mature T cells (usually coexpress CD4 or CD8)	Mature T-cell neoplasms
TCR$\gamma\delta$	Mature T cells (usually CD4 and CD8 negative)	Mature T-cell neoplasms
TdT	B- and T-lineage precursor cells/lymphoblasts	Cytoplasmic staining in B-ALL and T-ALL, occasionally AML
TRBC1/ TRBC2	Subset of mature $\alpha\beta$ T cells	Restricted or absent surface expression can indicate a monoclonal T-cell population.

AITL, angioimmunoblastic T-cell lymphoma; ALCL, anaplastic large cell lymphoma; AML, acute myeloid leukemia; APL, acute promyelocytic leukemia; ATLL, adult T-cell leukemia/lymphoma; B-ALL, B-lymphoblastic leukemia/lymphoma; BL, Burkitt lymphoma; BPDCN, blastic plasmacytoid dendritic cell neoplasm; CLL/SLL, chronic lymphocytic leukemia/small lymphocytic lymphoma; CTCL, cutaneous T-cell lymphoma; DLBCL, diffuse large B-cell lymphoma; FL, follicular lymphoma; HCL, hairy cell leukemia; HL, Hodgkin lymphoma; LGL, large granular lymphocyte; MCL, mantle cell lymphoma; MDS, myelodysplastic syndromes; MPN, myeloproliferative neoplasm; MZL, marginal zone lymphoma; NK, natural killer; PCN, plasma cell neoplasm; RBC, red blood cell; T-ALL, T-lymphoblastic leukemia/lymphoma.

When hematopoietic cell populations are displayed on a CD45 × SSC bivariate graph, they can be grouped into four general areas that correspond to certain cell types (see e-Figure 32.3):

1. CD45 bright, low SSC = lymphocytes
2. CD45 bright, moderate SSC = monocytes
3. CD45 moderate, high SSC = granulocytes
4. CD45 dim, low SSC = heterogeneous normal (hematogones, myeloid precursors and stem cells, plasma cells, basophils, plasmacytoid dendritic cells, nucleated erythroid lineage cells) and/or malignant cells (neoplastic blasts, lymphoma cells like diffuse large B-cell lymphoma [DLBCL] or chronic lymphocytic leukemia/small lymphocytic lymphoma [CLL/SLL] cells, neoplastic plasma cells)

These four hematopoietic cell populations should add up to approximately 100% of your FC events. Calculating percentages is important in FC analysis, as it can often highlight abnormal populations that fall outside the normal ranges and gates. For example, it is recommended to add up the percentage of B cells (CD19+), T cells (CD3+), and natural killer (NK) cells (CD56+) in the lymphocyte gate, which should be approximately 100%. In a patient with a surface CD3-negative T-cell lymphoma, adding the percentages of B cells + T cells + NK cells in the lymphocyte gate equals 48%, which will highlight the other 52% of lymphocytes as abnormal lymphoma cells.

Acute Leukemia

In general, acute leukemia is a fast progressing malignancy arising from precursor cells that are immature/less differentiated, but typically display an early lineage commitment. Therefore, the FC assessment of acute leukemia utilizes antigens associated with immaturity (eg, CD34, TdT) and approaches to detect early lineage commitment (eg, cytoplasmic detection of CD3, CD79a, and CD22).

CD45 dim/low SSC gate: The CD45 dim/low SSC gate of FC was historically referred to as the "blast" gate. Acute leukemias tend to present in this area of FC scattergrams, with rare exceptions (high side scattering APL, CD45 bright expressing ALL). The percentage of blasts is typically provided in FC reports; however, the gold standard for blast enumeration is a differential count performed on the bone marrow aspirate smear (200-500 counted cells is preferred). This is especially important to remember when diagnosing acute myeloid leukemia (AML), since many guidelines require 20% or more blasts. *NOTE*: There are many types of cells that appear in the CD45 dim/low SSC gate that are not blasts, so interpret with caution (see earlier #4 for the normal contents of the CD45 dim/low SSC gate). In general, most normal hematopoietic tissues will have less than 5% of cell events in the CD45 dim/low SSC gate. If this population is greater than 5% of total cells, careful consideration of the gate's contents is needed.

Determining lineage of an acute leukemia by flow cytometry: While it is recommended that you consult the most recent guidelines from the World Health Organization (WHO) and the International Consensus Classification (ICC) for definitive diagnostic criteria, a list of antigen expression *trends* by leukemia lineage (mixed/ambiguous lineage leukemias are discussed in a separate section) is provided. In general, the more antigens of a given lineage expressed on leukemic blasts, the more reliable that lineage assignment will be. However, there are a few antigens that are very strongly associated with a given lineage (indicated by *). The (cy) symbol indicates cytoplasmic expression; TdT is also cytoplasmic, but this is understood and notation is not needed. All other expressions can be assumed surface (s).

- **B-lymphoblastic leukemia/lymphoma (B-LL):** CD19*, cyCD79a, cyCD22, CD10, HLA-DR, CD34, TdT, CD38, CD45 (dim), sCD22, CD20, CD200; may express myeloid antigens CD13, CD33, CD15, and CD123
- **T-lymphoblastic leukemia/lymphoma (T-LL):** cyCD3* (surface is less common), pan T-cell antigens (CD2, CD5, CD7), CD34, TdT, CD1, CD10, CD4, and CD8 copositive, CD4 and CD8 double-negative
  - **Early T-cell precursor (ETP)-ALL:** A unique and aggressive variant of T-LL characterized by cyCD3, CD7+, CD1a−, CD8−, CD5 dim or −, and positive for one or more stem or myeloid antigen (includes CD34, CD13, CD33, HLA-DR, CD117, CD11b)
- **Acute myeloid leukemia:** Myeloperoxidase (MPO/MPX)*, CD34, CD117, HLA-DR, CD38, CD13, CD33, may express T-/NK-cell antigens (CD7 is most common, but also CD2, CD5, and CD56), CD4, CD200
  - If blasts are MPO/MPX+, CD117+, CD34−, HLA-DR−, consider APL.
  - AML can occasionally express CD19, usually associated with t(8;21).
  - Acute erythroid leukemia (AEL) and acute megakaryocytic leukemia (AMKL) are rare acute leukemias that will share features of AML but display differentiation along the erythroid and megakaryocytic lineages, respectively. Useful antigenic markers to distinguish these entities are included in Table 32.1.
- **Acute myeloid leukemia with monocytic differentiation:** HLA-DR, CD38, CD64, CD14 (often lost/reduced in immature monocytes), CD4, CD13, CD33, CD56, CD123, α-naphthyl butyrate esterase (NBE)*
- **Acute leukemia of ambiguous lineage (ALAL):** Occasionally the leukemia cells do not show evidence of differentiation along a specific lineage.
- **Mixed phenotype acute leukemia (MPAL):** If blasts meet the lineage assignment criteria for more than one lineage, they are considered mixed. Classification description should include use of both lineages (eg, B/myeloid, T/myeloid, etc).
- Mixed lineage can be:
  - Biphenotypic—The blasts have features of both lineages, displaying strong coexpression of lineage-specific antigens.
  - Bilineal—The blast population is composed of two different cell types of a given lineage, and independently meet classification criteria for each lineage respectively.
- **Acute undifferentiated leukemia (AUL):** Blasts do not express any antigens specific for lymphoid or myeloid classification. This is a diagnosis of exclusion, thus it requires a comprehensive workup to include all antigens that can provide lineage specificity. See recent classification systems from WHO and ICC for further details.
- **Lineage switch:** Some acute leukemias can change their lineage during treatment (clonal evolution/selection of a subclone within the leukemia population), and new therapy-related leukemias can emerge (often with longer latency). While this shift is a rare occurrence (and may be associated with particular cytogenetic abnormalities, like KMT2A rearrangement), you should be aware of it and provide a comprehensive workup if evidence for this phenomenon is noted.

Non-Hodgkin Lymphoma

FC is useful in the diagnosis of non-Hodgkin lymphoma, because it can: (1) identify abnormal antigen expression patterns on tumor cells, (2) detect monoclonality of tumor cells, (3) highlight antigens expressed on tumor cells that are targetable by immunotherapy, and (4) provide prognostic information. When a surgical specimen is obtained from a patient with concern for lymphoma in the differential diagnosis, a lymphoma workup should be performed (discussed in Chapter 2).

If not enough tissue is available for surgical pathology and FC, morphology and histology studies take precedence over FC; the majority of immunophenotyping can be performed on the fixed tissue.

B-Cell Lineage

CD19 is a B-lineage antigen that is expressed on all B-committed cells (from early precursors to plasma cells). CD19 is also largely retained on malignant B cells, so it is used as an initial gate to identify B-lineage cells for leukemia/lymphoma FC analysis.

For characterization of a mature B-lineage neoplasm, several important cell surface markers are assessed: CD5, CD10, CD200 (and/or CD23 and FMC7, depending on your institution). Kappa and lambda surface light chains are also helpful for the identification of a light chain restriction in the abnormal population (a surrogate for monoclonality). CD20 is utilized to identify mature B cells. The light scattering properties (forward scatter [FSC] and SSC) of neoplastic cells may be altered/increased in larger B-lymphoma cells (DLBCL), reflecting the increased cell volume and intracellular complexity.

NOTE: The below-mentioned characterization is useful for immunophenotypic trends of B-cell lymphomas (BCLs); you *will* find rule-breakers.

- **CD5+ CD10–:** mantle cell lymphoma (MCL) and CLL/SLL, occasional DLBCL
  - **CD200:** MCL is typically CD200–, CLL/SLL is typically CD200+ (Keep in mind that cyclin D1 antigen detection by immunohistochemistry is more reliable for this differentiation.)
  - **CD23/FMC7:** MCL is typically CD23– FMC7+, CLL/SLL is typically CD23+ FMC7–
- **CD5– CD10+:** Follicular lymphoma (FL), DLBCL, Burkitt lymphoma (BL); germinal center-derived
- **CD5– CD10–:** marginal zone lymphoma (MZL), lymphoplasmacytic lymphoma (LPL), hairy cell leukemia (HCL), occasional DLBCL, other BCLs not otherwise specified (BCL-NOS)

Kappa and Lambda Surface Light Chain Expression

Monoclonal B-cell populations are identified by FC using kappa and lambda light chain–specific antibodies. CD19+ and/or CD20+ gated cell events are displayed on a bivariate plot of kappa versus lambda. In general, normal mature B cells will display a ratio of 1:1 (kappa:lambda) up to 3:1. If the kappa:lambda ratio is significantly increased or inverted, consider a possible malignancy. Keep in mind that monoclonal populations can be hiding within a polytypic light chain background and additional gating approaches may be necessary. Finally, some mature B-cell malignancies may dimly express or totally lack expression of surface light chain (eg, CLL/SLL, DLBCL, FL).

T/NK-Cell Lineage

Identification of mature T-/NK-cell leukemias and lymphomas can be more challenging than their B-lineage counterparts, as the abnormal features of malignant T/NK cells may not be as apparent by FC assessment. Additional test modalities are often needed for definitive diagnosis and classification. Assessment for T-cell lymphomas includes an initial review of pan-T-cell antigen expression (CD2, CD5, and/or CD7 should all be retained, although up to 15% of normal T cells may display loss of CD7 expression), as well as evaluation of the CD4:CD8 ratio in CD3+ T cells. The normal CD4:CD8 ratio of CD3+ T cells is 1:1, ranging up to 4:1. This ratio can be inverted without evidence of malignancy (often due to viral infections). However, a markedly skewed CD4:CD8 ratio is often seen in cases of T-cell malignancy and warrants further investigation. Malignancy can be present within the background of normal findings, so additional gating strategies may be necessary. Normal NK cells express CD16, CD56, CD57, CD11b, CD2, CD7, but are predominantly negative for CD5. Partial or complete loss of some of these NK-cell antigens can be seen in NK-lineage malignancies, as can changes in light scattering properties (often increased FSC and/or SSC) and expression of cyCD3 and myeloid antigens CD13, CD33, and CD15.

NOTE: NK-like T cells will express CD56. NK cells can express some CD8. γδT cells are negative for CD4 and CD8, may lack CD5, and can overexpress CD3, but they are normal.

T-Cell Clonality

Clonal T-cell populations have been traditionally identified through DNA sequencing of the T-cell receptor (TCR), which can be costly and have a long turnaround time for a new diagnosis. Recent identification of anti-TRBC1 and anti-TRBC2 antibodies (which specifically recognize constant regions of the *TRB* gene product when selectively incorporated into the unique TCR of a T-cell clone) make it possible to identify clonal T-cell populations by FC. This approach should be used in the context of other antigens that indicate the T cells in question are abnormal to avoid overcalling TCUS (clonal T-cell populations of undetermined significance).

Sézary Syndrome

Sézary syndrome is the leukemic form of cutaneous T-cell lymphoma (CTCL) and is characterized by more than 1×10^9 Sézary cells per liter of blood. Sézary cells are typically CD3+ CD4+ T cells that display loss of CD7 (>30%) and/or CD26 expression (>40%). FC panels for the assessment of Sézary syndrome commonly include CD3, CD4, CD8, CD7, CD26, and CD52 (which is a target of the immunotherapy alemtuzumab).

Plasma Cell Neoplasm

Plasma cells are often identified by CD38 and CD138 antigen expression in the initial FC, since normal and abnormal plasma cells generally express both. However, CD138 expression can be downregulated by refrigeration of the specimen, and detection of CD38 expression can be blocked by daratumumab immunotherapy. Since plasma cells are fully differentiated (antibody secreting) B cells, kappa and lambda light chain distribution on plasma cell populations can be utilized in FC as a surrogate for monoclonality, although the detection in plasma cells is typically cytoplasmic (cy). Normal and neoplastic plasma cell antigen expression patterns commonly identified in FC assessment are shown:

- **Normal plasma cell immunophenotype:** CD19+, CD38++, CD138+, CD20−, polytypic (cy) kappa and (cy) lambda light chains (kappa:lambda ratio <3 and >0.3), CD81+, CD45 is variable (+ to −)
- **Neoplastic plasma cell immunophenotype:** CD19−, CD38++, CD138+, monoclonal (cy) kappa or (cy) lambda, and oftentimes CD20+, CD56+, CD117+, CD200+, CD81−, CD45 is variable (+ to −)

Chronic Myeloid Neoplasms

Myelodysplastic Syndromes (MDS): In general, MDS is a diagnosis that relies on bone marrow morphology, cytogenetics, and molecular testing, in conjunction with peripheral blood cytopenias. FC can also contribute to diagnosis and prognosis, although some cases may present only nuanced changes in immunophenotype, while other cases may have cell populations of unclear classification.ABnormal developmental patterns (dysplasia) of bone marrow cells in MDS patient samples can be identified with diverse presentations: asynchronous antigen expression during maturation, non-myeloid lineage antigen expression, increased/decreased expression of normal myeloid antigens, increased/decreased levels of differentiating cell populations, increased blasts, hypogranular neutrophils, and others. Several groups have proposed scoring systems for grading the dysplasia of MDS detected by FC, although a consensus approach is still pending. In-depth knowledge of myeloid and monocytic maturation patterns in your FC panels is needed to reliably identify MDS. Monitoring for increased blasts (indicating transformation to acute leukemia) is an important function of FC in these cases.

Myeloproliferative Neoplasms (MPN): FC findings in cases of MPN often do not contribute significantly to diagnosis except in blast enumeration. Molecular and cytogenetic tests are essential and should be prioritized over FC when specimen triage is needed.

Mastocytosis

The use of FC for the identification of aberrant mast cells is an important tool in the diagnosis of systemic mastocytosis. Normal mast cells are negative for expression of CD2, CD25, and CD30, but abnormal mast cells often express one or more of these. This finding is so specific for systemic mastocytosis that it is a WHO minor criterion. Identification of mast cells can be performed by isolation of bright CD117-expressing (CD117++) cells. Flow panels should include cell surface antigens like CD34 to avoid including myeloid precursor cells in the CD117++ gate.

Paroxysmal Nocturnal Hemoglobinuria

PNH is a rare clonal hematopoietic disorder characterized by complement-mediated lysis of blood cells and is associated with mutations in the *PIGA* gene. The PIGA protein is necessary for the biosynthesis of glycosylphosphatidylinositol (GPI) anchors, which ensure cell surface expression of critical complement-inhibiting proteins. PNH-associated *PIGA* gene mutations result in a lack of GPI anchors, which lead to lysis of PNH blood cells by activation of the complement cascade.

FC is the preferred method for the assessment of PNH. CD55 and CD59 are two GPI-anchored cell surface proteins lost on PNH cells that are commonly assessed by FC, as is the direct binding of the fusion protein fluorescein-labeled proaerolysin (FLAER; a fluorophore-conjugated bacterial protein aerolysin) to the GPI anchor. PNH is reported as partial or complete loss of CD55 and/or CD59 on the surface of RBCs and white blood cells (WBCs), as is the partial or complete loss of binding of FLAER protein on the surface of WBCs. Loss of GPI-anchored cell surface proteins should be detected in at least two lineages for PNH diagnosis. RBCs, neutrophils, and monocytes are the most commonly assessed cell types. Additional GPI-anchored proteins can be assessed as well; these are a minimum starting point:

- RBC
  - Normal= CD235a+, CD59+
  - PNH= CD235a+, CD59−

- Granulocyte
  - Normal = CD45+, SSC^{hi}, CD15+, CD59+, FLAER+
  - PNH = CD45+, SSC^{hi}, CD15+, CD59−, FLAER−

VIII. MINIMAL/MEASURABLE RESIDUAL DISEASE FLOW CYTOMETRY

Evaluation of low-level disease involvement (MRD) has become standard of care for many hematologic malignancies. MRD status has been shown to correlate with patient prognosis and outcome, and MRD results are currently used in clinical decisions. FC is an effective approach to MRD detection because an abnormal cell immunophenotype can be readily identified in the context of a normal cell background (even at very low levels).

Guidelines for MRD analysis include recognizing a discrete abnormal population of at least 20 to 50 cell events. Aberrant populations in MRD are best identified using a combination of the DfN approach, as described earlier, and the leukemia-associated immunophenotype (LAIP) that was identified in the patient at diagnosis or relapse. Identification of MRD solely based on LAIP is not recommended, as antigen expression can alter due to therapy effects or clonal evolution and MRD can be missed. MRD FC interpretation requires significant expertise, including knowledge of the range of antigen expression on normal hematolymphoid populations examined in the assay across all clinical time points being assessed. The high sensitivity of an MRD assay requires collection of more cellular events than the standard qualitative leukemia/lymphoma analysis (more events = more sensitivity). For an MRD population identified at 0.01% involvement, 50 MRD events are recognized within 500,000 total cell events. The sensitivity of an MRD analysis should be provided in the pathology report.

IX. COMMON CELL ANTIGENS USED IN CLINICAL FLOW CYTOMETRY

See Table 32.1.

SUGGESTED READINGS

Craig FE, Foon KA. Flow cytometric immunophenotyping for hematologic neoplasms. *Blood*. 2008;111:3941-3967.

Davis BH, Holden JT, Bene MC, et al. 2006 Bethesda International Consensus recommendations on the flow cytometric immunophenotypic analysis of hematolymphoid neoplasia: medical indications. *Cytometry B Clin Cytom*. 2007;72B:S5-S13.

Khoury JD, Solary E, Abla O, et al. The 5th edition of the World Health Organization Classification of Haematolymphoid Tumours: myeloid and histiocytic/dendritic neoplasms. *Leukemia*. 2022;36:1703-1719.

Wood BL, Arroz M, Barnett D, et al. 2006 Bethesda International Consensus recommendations on the immunophenotypic analysis of hematolymphoid neoplasia by flow cytometry: optimal reagents and reporting for the flow cytometric diagnosis of hematopoietic neoplasia. *Cytometry B Clin Cytom*. 2007;72B:S14-S22.

33 Cytogenomics

Bahareh A. Mojarad and Julie Ann Neidich

The science of clinical cytogenomics began in 1882 with the first descriptive illustrations of human chromosomes, published by Flemming (F. C. W. Vogel, Leipzig). The three significant achievements that allow for current methodology were published in the ensuing 90 years: the preparation of chromosome spreads from peripheral blood cultures (*Exp Cell Res*. 1960;20:613), the development of hypotonic methods to obtain enhanced chromosome spreads (*Cancer Res*. 1960;20:462), and the discovery that fluorescent quinacrine compounds demonstrate a unique banding pattern for each human chromosome pair (*Hereditas*. 1971;67:89). The advancement of the field of human cytogenetics is made more remarkable by the fact that it has been just over 65 years since the correct number of human chromosomes was established. The various banding methods in current use not only permit the identification of each chromosome but also make it possible to detect specific subchromosomal alterations associated with constitutional and acquired syndromes and neoplasms.

I. TRADITIONAL CYTOGENETIC ANALYSIS

The primary application of karyotype analysis in hematopathology lies in the evaluation of neoplastic disorders affecting the bone marrow and lymph nodes. The utility of this technique in hematopathology rests on the fact that specific cytogenetic abnormalities have been recognized that are closely, and sometimes uniquely, associated with morphologically and clinically distinct subsets of leukemia and lymphoma. Cancer cytogenetic studies have greatly aided targeted therapy, prognosis, and risk-based stratification of intensity of therapy, as later discussed in Section 3.

Advantages

The power of conventional cytogenetics (ie, chromosome analysis or karyotyping) lies in its ability to simultaneously analyze the entire genome without any foreknowledge of the chromosomal regions involved in the disease process. In most cases, the type and location of an identified chromosomal abnormality are either directly diagnostic or can be used to direct additional testing. Contrary to some predictions, the advent of technologies, such as chromosomal microarray analysis or genome/exome sequencing, has not diminished the importance of traditional cytogenetics; in fact, these newer cytogenomic techniques achieve some of their greatest utility when they are utilized in conjunction with traditional clinical cytogenetics.

Limitations

The clinical utility of traditional chromosome analysis is restricted by two general features of the method. From a technical standpoint, analysis can only be performed on viable tissue specimens that contain proliferating cells (discussed in more detail later).

From a sensitivity standpoint, the analysis has a resolution of approximately 3 to 4 Mb at an 850-band level and approximately 7 to 8 Mb at a 400-band level. Traditional cytogenetic analysis is therefore only suited for detection of numerical abnormalities and gross structural rearrangements. Furthermore, this method does not have the sensitivity to detect sequence-level variants such as small deletions, duplications, amplifications, or single base-pair substitutions.

Basic Laboratory Procedures

Chromosomes that can be individually distinguished by light microscopy can only be visualized during cell division; thus, the fundamental requirement for traditional cytogenetic analysis is a tissue specimen that contains actively proliferating cells or cells that can be induced to proliferate in vitro. The general schema for obtaining metaphase chromosomes for cytogenetic analysis is shown in Figure 33.1.

- **Culture initiation:** Different specimen types have different sample and handling requirements (Table 33.1). Inappropriate handling or delays between specimen collection and culture initiation can markedly decrease the likelihood that the sample will grow in vitro. Hence, communication and coordination with the cytogenetics laboratory are essential. In vitro culture relies on a sterile microenvironment; therefore, specimens must be collected under sterile conditions. Bone marrow neoplasms consist of cell types that spontaneously proliferate in culture, although often at a low rate.

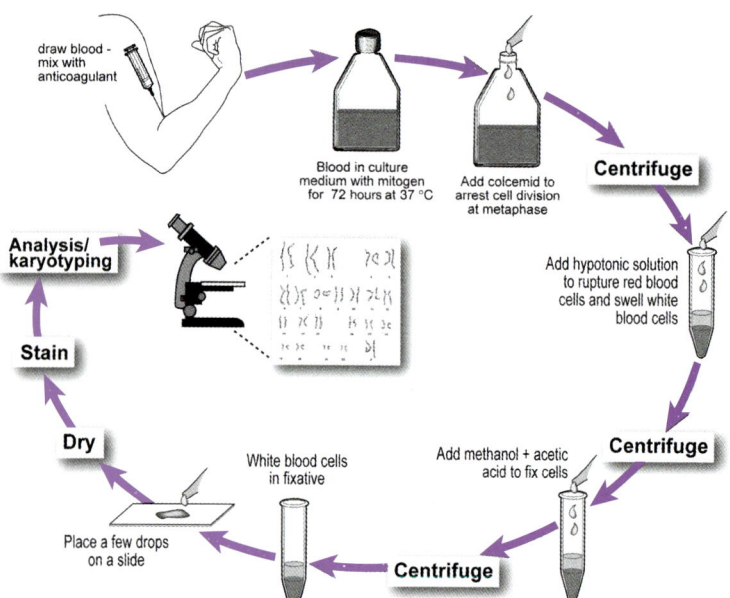

Figure 33.1. Overall scheme for the production of metaphase chromosomes for traditional cytogenetic analysis. (From Pfeifer JD, Dehner LP, Humphrey PA. *The Washington Manual of Surgical Pathology*. 3rd ed. Wolters Kluwer; 2019.)

TABLE 33.1 Specimen Requirements

Sample Type	Sample Collection
Peripheral blood	Preservative-free sodium heparin; transport refrigerated or at room temperature
Bone marrow aspirate	Preservative-free sodium heparin; the first several milliliters of the aspirate usually contain the greatest proportion of cells and is therefore the optimal sample for cytogenetic analysis; transport at room temperature

Phytohemagglutinin (PHA) stimulates the proliferation of T-lymphocytes, while lipopolysaccharide (LPS), protein A, 12-O-tetradecanoly-phorbol-13-acetate (TPA), Epstein-Barr virus (EBV), synthetic oligonucleotides, and pokeweed mitogen induce proliferation of B-lymphocytes. These stimuli are also required for the successful culture of some leukemias and lymphomas of B-cell origin.

- **Culture maintenance:** The duration of in vitro culture depends on the cell type. Since bone marrow cultures contain spontaneously proliferating cells, they can be harvested after only a 24- to 48-hour culture interval or directly after specimen collection. Peripheral blood cultures usually require a 72-hour culture interval.
- **Cell harvest:** Colcemid, a synthetic analogue of colchicine (an alkaloid from the bulb of the Mediterranean plant *Colchicum*), prevents separation of sister chromatids and is used to block proliferating cells in metaphase, thus allowing an accumulation of cells at metaphase stage. A hypotonic solution is then used to swell the cells so that, after fixation, the chromosomes are adequately spread for microscopic analysis. Since cells in culture do not proceed through the cell cycle in synchrony, chemical synchronization of cell division is often required to obtain an acceptable mitotic index. A common chemical approach involves addition of excess thymidine, which stalls cells at the S-phase of the cell cycle by decreasing the amount of deoxycytidine triphosphate (dCTP) available for DNA synthesis. When the excess thymidine is removed (or the effect of excess thymidine is eliminated by the addition of deoxycytidine), normal DNA replication resumes, and the collective release of the cells from S-phase produces a transiently high mitotic index. Alternatively, 5-fluorodeoxyuridine (which inhibits the enzyme thymidylate synthetase) can be used to stall cells at the G1/S boundary; in this method, the addition of thymidine releases the block.
- **Banding:** The different techniques that can be used to stain metaphase chromosomes can be divided into two general categories: methods that produce specific alternating light and dark regions (bands) along the length of each chromosome and methods that stain only a defined region of specific chromosomes (Table 33.2). In general, the dark bands consist of gene-poor AT-rich regions, whereas light bands comprise gene-rich GC-rich regions. The quality of staining depends on several technical factors, including sufficient separation of the chromosomes in the metaphase spread to allow clear visualization. Most modern cytogenetics laboratories use a Giemsa dye method (G-banding) as a standard for all karyotype analyses and add additional stains or fluorescent probes to reveal more detail about individual cases. Although there are no internationally accepted standards for banding resolution,

TABLE 33.2 Major Chromosome Staining and Banding Techniques

Method	Staining Pattern
Techniques that produce specific alternating band patterns along each chromosome	
Giemsa banding (G-banding)	Dark bands are AT-rich; light bands are GC-rich.
Quinacrine banding (Q-banding)	Bright regions are AT-rich.
Reverse banding (R-banding)	AT-rich regions stain lightly (have dull fluorescence), and GC-rich regions stain darkly (have bright fluorescence).
4,6-Diamidino-2-phenylindole staining (DAPI staining)	DAPI binds AT-rich regions and produced a pattern similar to Q-banding.
Techniques that stain selective chromosome regions	
Constitutive heterochromatin banding (C-banding)	Stains heterochromatin (α-satellite DNA) around the centromeres; can also be used to demonstrate some inherited polymorphisms
Telomere banding (T-banding)	A technical variation of R-banding used to stain telomeres
Silver staining for nucleolar organizer regions (NOR staining)	Stains NORs (which contain rRNA genes) on the satellite stalks of acrocentric chromosomes
Fluorescence in situ hybridization (FISH)	Staining pattern is dependent on the probe.

ideograms are used as reference points. Clinical laboratories aim for resolution at or above the 550-band level for blood chromosome analysis, while analysis of prenatal or neoplasm samples may be closer to 400 to 500 bands. Many countries, including the United States, Canada, the United Kingdom, France, Japan, and Australia, have established standards that specify the minimum requirements for the number and quality of cells that must be processed for chromosome analysis depending on sample type, although many cases require even more detailed analysis.

- **Microscopic analysis:** The method used to stain the chromosomes dictates whether bright-field microscopy or fluorescence microscopy is used to visualize the chromosomes. While conventional photography was traditionally used to produce high-resolution prints of stained chromosomes, electronic imaging systems have now become a standard.

The final step in cytogenetic analysis is the production of a karyotype, which consists of the chromosomal complement of the cell displayed in a standard sequence on the basis of size, centromere location, and banding pattern.

Assay Failure

Many of the common causes of failure to obtain a cytogenetic result (Table 33.3) can be avoided by careful selection of viable tissue with prompt specimen transport to the

TABLE 33.3 — Common Reasons for Failure of Traditional Cytogenetic Analysis

Culture Failure

No viable cells present in the sample (improper specimen handling)

Inappropriate sample (peripheral blood without blasts is submitted instead of bone marrow)

Overgrowth by nonneoplastic cells

Overgrowth by a nonrepresentative clone of tumor cells

Microbial overgrowth

Postculture Failure

Technical errors involving cell harvest, slide preparation, or staining

Misdiagnosis (an abnormality is overlooked, or an abnormality is incorrectly interpreted)

---

cytogenetics laboratory in the appropriate medium. Nonetheless, several causes of assay failure are inherent to in vitro culture and cannot be eliminated by even the most meticulous laboratory technique.

Cytogenetic analysis of hematologic neoplasms highlights a number of these intrinsic technical limitations. First, insufficient cell numbers in bone marrow aspirates, often observed in cases of acute myeloid leukemia (AML) with myelofibrosis and hypocellular AML, can make the culture susceptible to overgrowth by nonneoplastic cells or specific subclones. In such circumstances, blood cultures may be considered; however, blood cultures may not be appropriate for diagnosing all hematologic neoplasms, such as myelodysplastic syndrome (MDS). Second, in vitro culture selects for subclones within the neoplastic population that have a growth advantage, and so the karyotype may not be representative of the entire neoplasm. Third, in vitro cell death can pose a major problem to ALL samples, and multiple cultures are therefore recommended. Nevertheless, prolonged exposure to cell cycle synchronization agents can have a negative impact on metaphase yield due to cell poisoning. Fourth, bone marrow samples that have been contaminated with blood during aspiration might not have an adequate number of spontaneously dividing cells.

The overall failure rate of conventional cytogenetic analysis is difficult to quantify for many tissue types, neoplasms, and diseases. However, studies examining cytogenetic analysis of hematolymphoid neoplasms report success rates ranging from 33% to 100% in detecting characteristic chromosomal aberrations, depending on the specific diagnosis (*Am J Clin Pathol.* 2004;121:826).

II. METAPHASE FLUORESCENCE IN SITU HYBRIDIZATION

Virtually all in situ hybridization analyses are performed using probes that are directly or indirectly labeled with fluorophores. Guidelines for the use of fluorescence in situ hybridization (FISH) in clinical laboratory testing have been developed by the American College of Medical Genetics, and standardized nomenclature for reporting results has been developed (discussed in more detail later). FISH assays may be performed on nuclei obtained from a direct culture of the sample (or using formalin-fixed paraffin-embedded tissue samples, as discussed in detail in Chapter 34.1).

Metaphase FISH is essentially a modified Southern blot (as is interphase FISH), wherein the target DNA consists of chromosomes rather than membrane-bound DNA. Technically, the method involves four steps: (1) denaturation of the probes and metaphase or interphase targets by high temperature and formamide; (2) hybridization of the probe to the chromosomal target; (3) removal of unbound probe by post-hybridization washes; and (4) detection of the hybridized probe by fluorescence microscopy. A fluorochrome-based counterstain is virtually always used to help detect the chromosomes or nuclei during microscopic examination; the use of 4,6-diamidino-2-phenylindole (DAPI) as a counterstain makes it possible to localize the position of the bound probe to specific chromosomes. For more details on FISH, please refer to Chapter 34.1.

Probes

A variety of fluorophores can be directly or indirectly incorporated into FISH probes. The choice of labels is largely governed by practical issues, such as the excitation and emission filters on the microscope that will be used to view the chromosome spreads. Several probe kits have been cleared by the United States Food and Drug Administration (FDA) for in vitro diagnostic testing, although many probes for FISH are classified as analyte-specific reagents (ASRs) and are thus exempt from FDA approval. Standards and guidelines for the clinical use of ASRs have been established by the American College of Medical Genetics, including recommendations for interpreting metaphase or interphase FISH results.

1. **Repetitive sequence probes:** The most widely used repetitive sequence probes bind to α-satellite AT-rich sequences of centromeres; these probes produce strong signals since α-satellite sequences are present in hundreds of thousands of copies. Chromosome-specific centromere-specific probes have been developed for human chromosomes, based on differences in α-satellite sequences, and are particularly useful for demonstrating aneuploidy. These FISH probes can be used on both metaphase and interphase preparations, and simultaneous analysis of multiple loci is possible when a cocktail of differentially labeled probes is used in the same hybridization. Other repetitive sequence probes include probes that recognize β-satellite sequences (located on the short arms of acrocentric chromosomes) and probes that recognize the telomeric repeat sequence TTAGGG.
2. **Unique sequence probes:** Probes of this type are used to detect sequences that are present only once in the genome. They are usually derived from genomic clones but can also be produced from cDNA or by polymerase chain reaction (PCR). Different cloning vectors are used to produce unique sequence probes of different length, including plasmids for probes ranging from 1 to 10 kb long, bacteriophage λ for probes up to 25 kb long, bacterial artificial chromosomes (BACs) for probes up to about 300 kb long, and yeast artificial chromosomes (YACs) for probes ranging from 100 kb to 2 Mb long. The availability of mapped BAC libraries, originally developed as part of the Human Genome Project, has greatly simplified the production of probes for any locus (http://genome.ucsc.edu/cgi-bin/hgGateway and https://bacpacresources.org/). Unique sequence probes (also known as locus-specific identifier probes, or LSI probes) are primarily used to detect changes in the copy number of a specific locus, to confirm the presence of rearrangements involving a specific locus, or to detect so-called cryptic rearrangements that cannot be identified by examination of chromosomes stained by routine banding methods. The advantages and disadvantages

of metaphase FISH analysis using unique sequence probes directly parallel those of interphase FISH (as discussed in Chapter 34.1).

3. **Whole chromosome probes (WCPs):** WCPs, also known as chromosome painting probes or chromosome libraries, consist of thousands of overlapping probes that recognize unique and moderately repetitive sequences along the entire length of individual chromosomes. They are isolated through flow sorting of specific chromosomes, microdissection of specific chromosomes accompanied by PCR amplification, or via production of somatic cell hybrids. WCPs are used to identify rearrangements that are not evident by routine banding methods, to confirm the interpretation of aberrations identified by routine banding methods, or to establish the chromosomal origin of rearrangements that are difficult to evaluate by other approaches. These probes are designed for use with metaphase chromosome preparations because hybridization to the decondensed chromatin in interphase nuclei gives a splotchy, undefined hybridization pattern. WCPs for each human chromosome are commercially available.

III. MULTIPLEX METAPHASE FLUORESCENCE IN SITU HYBRIDIZATION

Multiplex FISH (also known as multicolor FISH) and spectral karyotyping (SKY) are related techniques where metaphase chromosome spreads are hybridized with a combination of probes labeled with different fluorophores. With N different fluorophores, $(2N - 1)$ different color combinations can be produced. Five different fluorophores provide sufficient color combinations to uniquely label WCPs so that all 24 different human chromosomes can be identified in one hybridization. In both multiplex FISH and SKY, a cocktail consisting of labeled probes for each of the 24 chromosomes is hybridized to metaphase chromosome spreads, and the fluorescent emissions are measured by computerized imaging systems. Specialized software is then used to determine the combination of fluorophores present along the length of each chromosome, which makes it possible to assemble a karyotype.

Advantages

Multiplex FISH and SKY are used to detect aneuploidy and interchromosomal rearrangements and identify marker chromosomes (chromosomal material of unknown origin). In many cases, multiplex FISH or SKY make it possible to establish the chromosomal origin of rearrangements that cannot be defined based on routine cytogenetic analysis.

Disadvantages

The lower limit for the size of individual DNA chromosomal fragments that can be visualized by either technique falls in the range of 1 to 2 Mb, although neither technique provides direct information on the involved chromosomal bands. Similarly, both multiplex FISH and SKY only reveal intrachromosomal deletions and duplications that are large enough to cause a change in the size of the affected chromosome; neither technique is designed to detect intrachromosomal rearrangements such as inversions, and neither is informative in regions with repetitive DNA. Due to the expense of the probe sets, hardware, and software, many clinical laboratories do not perform SKY or multiplex FISH assays.

Modifications of Multiplex Fluorescence In Situ Hybridization and Spectral Karyotyping

Mixtures of the so-called partial chromosome paints, each of which hybridizes to only a band or sub-band of an individual chromosome, can be used to produce a pseudo-color banded karyotype with a resolution of about 550 bands (*Cytogenet Cell Genet.* 1999;84:156). The use of partial chromosome paints makes it possible to employ multiplex FISH and SKY methodology to identify translocation breakpoints and to detect interchromosomal rearrangements. While these techniques may reveal more detail about any aberration, they are not usually available as clinical assays and are instead used as research tools.

IV. COMPARATIVE GENOMIC HYBRIDIZATION

While comparative genomic hybridization (CGH) often has a higher sensitivity than conventional cytogenetic analysis, its ability to use DNA extracted from fixed as well as fresh tumor samples is of even greater significance. This technique, therefore, makes it possible to perform a genomewide scan for copy number alterations, even in cases where conventional cytogenetic analysis is not feasible or unsuccessful. CGH essentially opens the entire formalin-fixed tissue archive to at least limited cytogenetic analysis. In a typical CGH test, genomic DNA from a tumor sample is labeled with a red fluorophore, while genomic DNA from a paired normal tissue sample is labeled with a green fluorophore. The green and red probes are then mixed and used in a single hybridization.

Metaphase Comparative Genomic Hybridization

- This technique is basically a variation of metaphase FISH used to survey the entire genome for chromosomal deletions and amplifications (*Trends Genet.* 1997;13:405). At this point, most laboratories do not perform metaphase CGH and have incorporated array CGH (see later) or other microarray methods to detect losses and gains of chromosomal material using DNA extracted from the sample. In this process, the patient's labeled probe mixture is used in a hybridization to metaphase chromosomes prepared from normal cells, and the ratio of the green to red fluorescent signals is measured along the length of each chromosome. Areas where the ratio significantly deviates from the expected one-to-one relationship indicate a change in DNA copy number in the tumor. Specifically, areas where the red to green ratio is significantly greater than 1 are areas of chromosomal gain (usually amplifications), while areas where the red to green ratio is significantly lower than 1 are areas of chromosomal loss (deletions). The smallest chromosomal alterations that can be reproducibly detected are about 2 to 3 Mb long.

Array Comparative Genomic Hybridization

- This approach utilizes a microarray consisting of an ordered arrangement of DNA molecules (features) linked to a solid matrix support. The labeled probe mixture is then hybridized to the microarray, and the ratio of the green to red fluorescent signals is measured for each feature (Figure 33.2). Because each DNA feature has been mapped to a specific region of the genome, the ratio of the green to red fluorescent signal for each feature provides information on the gain or loss of the

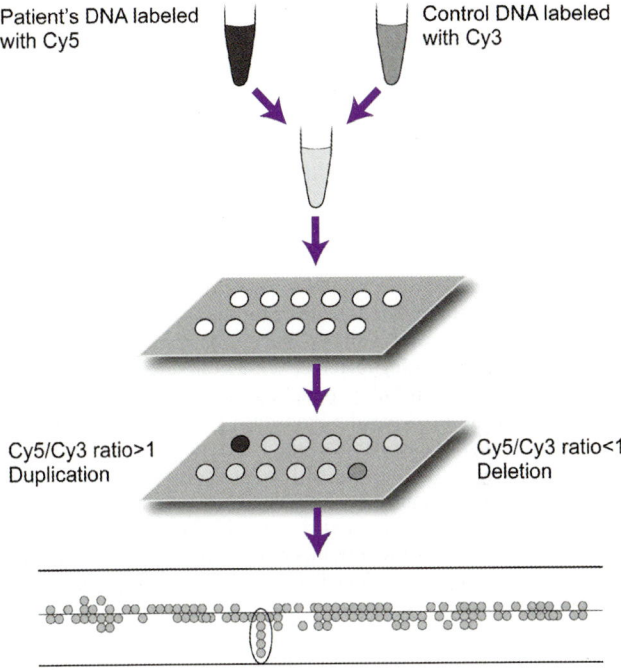

Figure 33.2. Array CGH methodology. Top. Method. A patient's DNA is labeled with a red dye, and a control genomic DNA preparation is labeled with green dye. These DNA preparations are mixed and cohybridized to an array of BACs or oligonucleotides on a glass slide. The DNA bound to each spot (known as a feature) of the array is quantified using a laser scanner. In the patient's DNA, normal regions will be indicated by a yellow balanced color; regions of duplication will be identified as red, and regions of deletion will be identified as green. **Bottom.** Data presentation. The data from each feature of the array (represented by circles) are plotted in relation to the features' positions along the chromosome and a balanced copy number (horizontal line). In this illustration, a cluster of adjacent features falling significantly below a balanced copy number result (oval) indicates the presence of a deletion. The resolution of array CGH is in theory limited only by the number of features in the array; commercially available arrays currently provide a resolution of less than 10 kb. BAC, bacterial artificial chromosome; CGH, comparative genomic hybridization. (From Pfeifer JD, Dehner LP, Humphrey PA. *The Washington Manual of Surgical Pathology*. 3rd ed. Wolters Kluwer; 2019.)

corresponding chromosomal region. The resolution of aCGH is in theory limited only by the number of features in the array, with commercially available arrays currently providing a resolution of under 10 kb. Genomic microarrays (aCGH and related microarray-based methods) are currently clinically applied to detect genomic copy number changes, as well as copy-neutral changes (uniparental disomy [UPD] and loss of heterozygosity [LOH]).

V. MICROARRAY ANALYSIS

Since the advent of the use of genomic microarrays in the clinical laboratory, the technology has rapidly become the standard of care to evaluate patients for genomic imbalance, especially in diagnostic testing for patients with congenital anomalies, developmental delay, and intellectual disabilities. However, the adaptation of genomic microarrays in cancer diagnostics is not currently widespread.

Advantages

- Microarray testing offers several advantages over traditional cytogenetic techniques. With a markedly increased resolution over conventional chromosome analysis, genomic imbalances less than 50 to 100 kb are routinely detectable using array-based copy number methodology. In addition, there is no requirement for cell viability since DNA serves as the starting material. Testing can therefore be performed on a variety of specimen types, including peripheral blood lymphocytes, bone marrow, lymph nodes, formalin-fixed paraffin-embedded tumor tissue, amniocytes, products of conception, fresh tissue samples, and buccal cells, among others.
Although BAC arrays, utilizing cloned DNA targets of approximately 160 kb, served as the first generation of aCGH diagnostics in clinical laboratories, oligonucleotide arrays (utilizing probes that are 25-75 bp long) are easier to design and manufacture and provide markedly increased probe coverage across the genome. Consequently, oligonucleotide arrays have replaced BAC arrays in clinical laboratories; their use employs two general strategies: aCGH and single-nucleotide polymorphism (SNP) analysis. Although the aim of both techniques is the detection of genomic gain or loss, the methods for doing so differ between each assay.

As discussed earlier, aCGH detects copy number imbalances through the comparison of a normal control sample against a patient sample. In contrast, SNPs are evaluated by comparing signal intensities from the assay substrate (derived from the DNA of the patient sample) to that of an in silico reference model in order to determine relative gains and losses. The ability to probe for SNPs is advantageous for several reasons. First, the approach makes it possible to perform simultaneous copy number quantification and SNP detection. Second, the use of SNP arrays allows for detection of regions with copy-neutral LOH, which may be used to identify genetic alterations in tumor samples, heterodisomy, the parental chromosome of origin for a de novo deletion or duplication, and, more generally, consanguinity and uniparental disomy. Ultimately, SNP detection helps maximize the potential for detecting disease-associated abnormalities and also offers mechanistic evidence for the molecular basis of the disease. A comparison of SNP and oligo arrays is shown in Table 33.4.

The technique of allelic discrimination by SNP analysis differs between commercially available platforms but involves hybridization of fragmented single-stranded DNA (derived from the patient sample) to arrays that contain unique nucleotide probe sequences (2 million or more). One widespread commercial approach is based on allele-specific hybridization to probes representing the possible alleles, with signal intensities corresponding to the level of binding (Figure 33.3) measured by scanning technology. The other widespread commercial approach utilizes a single-base extension technique with differentially labeled nucleotide terminators

TABLE 33.4 Comparison Between SNP and Oligo Arrays

Array Attributes	Single-Nucleotide Polymorphism (SNP) Arrays	Oligonucleotide Arrays
Number of markers	Greater than 1,000,000 markers	Less than 200,000 markers
DNA input requirement	200–500 ng	1–5 µg
Probe types	SNP and oligo probes	Oligo probes
Limits of resolution	Less than 10–20 kb	As low as 10–20 kb
Threshold for detection of mosaicism	May be as low as 5%	20%–30%
Ability to detect copy-neutral LOH	Yes	No
Ability to detect uniparental disomy	Yes	No
Ability to detect consanguinity	Yes	No
Method of assessment of copy number imbalance	Probe signal intensities (derived from the patient sample) compared to an in silico reference model	Patient sample directly hybridized against control DNA to detect relative gains and losses
Detection of balanced chromosomal rearrangements	No	No

LOH, loss of heterozygosity.

to distinguish the SNP alleles, with the signal intensity generated from this reaction used to make a base call at that SNP (Figure 33.3).

Finally, exon-level arrays have been designed to allow for the identification of very small losses and gains. These arrays concentrate probes over exons within expressed genes, usually genes of clinical interest, in order to assay for deletions and duplications as small as one exon in a gene of interest. Since deletions and duplications have been identified as pathogenic variants in numerous genes, this type of assay serves as a useful diagnostic tool, especially when used in conjunction with next-generation sequencing panels, whole-exome analysis, and whole-genome analysis.

Limitations

While copy number changes are often readily discernable, balanced chromosomal rearrangements cannot be detected with this technology, including balanced translocations, inversions, and insertions. In addition, regions containing segmental duplications, complex genomic structure, or other repetitive sequences may have limited detection. Low-level mosaicism may also not be detectable, and LOH is demonstrable only by using SNP-based platforms.

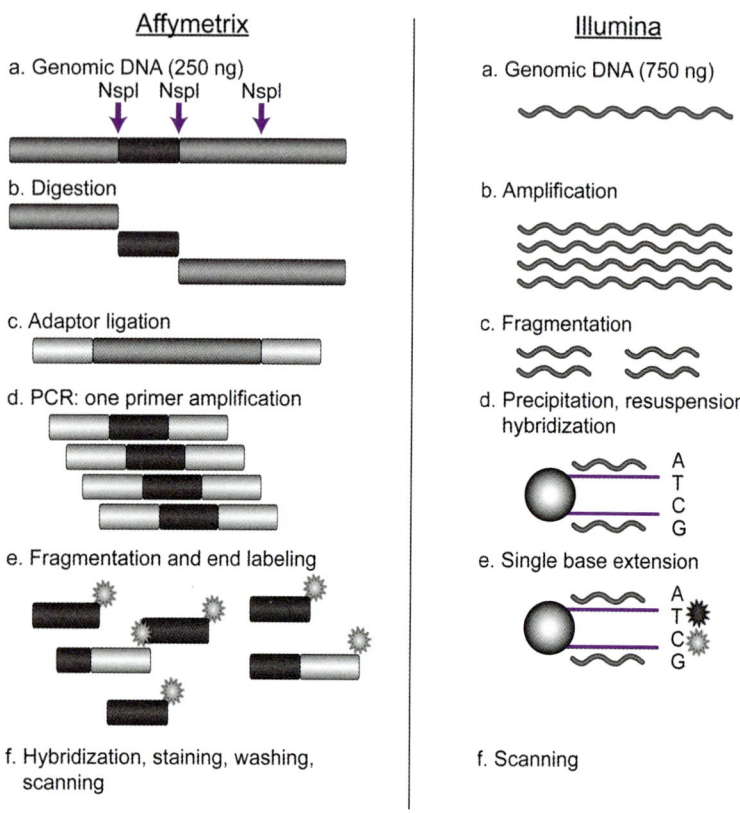

Figure 33.3. SNP array procedures. In the ThermoFisher platform (ThermoFisher; Waltham, MA), genomic DNA is digested with the *Nsp*I restriction enzyme, and the resulted DNA fragments are ligated to adaptors and subsequently amplified; the amplification products are fragmented, end-labeled, and hybridized to the array. In the Illumina platform (Illumina, Inc., San Diego, CA), the entire genome is amplified and then hybridized to a bead array; allelic discrimination is achieved by a single-base extension reaction. In both platforms, the signal intensity is measured for each probe and compared with an in silico reference to evaluate DNA copy number. (From Pfeifer JD, Dehner LP, Humphrey PA. *The Washington Manual of Surgical Pathology*. 3rd ed. Wolters Kluwer; 2019.)

VI. HUMAN CHROMOSOME NOMENCLATURE

Technical advancements, together with an ever more complete understanding of human chromosomal structure, necessitate periodic revisions of nomenclature guidelines. The current document in use is the *International System for Human Cytogenetic Nomenclature* from 2020, abbreviated as ISCN 2020, which includes ideograms for all of the chromosomes that serve as useful reference points because of their universal acceptance and availability.

TABLE 33.5 Common Symbols and Abbreviations Used in Karyotype Designations

Abbreviation or Symbol	Description
add	Additional material of unknown origin
square brackets []	Number of cells in each clone
cen	Centromere
single colon (:)	Break
double colon (::)	Break and reunion
comma (,)	Separates chromosome number, sex chromosomes, and abnormalities
del	Deletion
der	Derivative chromosome
dmin	Double minute(s)
dup	Duplication
i	Isochromosome
idem	Identical abnormalities as in prior clone
inv	Inversion
ins	Insertion
mar	Marker chromosome
minus sign (−)	Loss
multiplication sign (×)	Multiple copies, also designates copy number with ISH
plus sign (+)	Gain
question mark (?)	Uncertainty of chromosome identification or abnormality
r	Ring chromosome
rcp	Reciprocal
slash (/)	Separates cell lines or clones
semicolon (;)	Separates chromosomes and breakpoints in rearrangements involving more than one chromosome
t	Translocation

Chromosome Region and Band Designations

The centromere divides each chromosome into a short or p arm and a long or q arm. Each chromosome arm ends in a terminus, designated "pter" and "qter" for the short and long arms, respectively. A list of the most common symbols and abbreviations used to describe human karyotypes is shown in Table 33.5.

Chromosome arms are further divided into regions based on landmarks, which are consistent and distinct morphologic areas that aid in the identification of that chromosome. The regions adjacent to the centromere of the short arm and long arm are designated as p1 and q1, respectively, followed by p2 and q2, and so on. Chromosome regions are divided into bands, and the bands are divided into sub-bands, both of which are sequentially numbered. For instance, the terminal band on the long arm of chromosome 11 is denoted as 11q25, indicating chromosome 11, long arm, region 2, band 5, and is referred to as "eleven q two-five."

Description of Karyotypes

ISCN nomenclature provides rules for karyotype designations. The first item of the designation is the total number of chromosomes (including the sex chromosomes) followed by the sex chromosomes. Chromosomal abnormalities follow the sex chromosome designations using established symbols and abbreviations. The sex chromosomes are described first, followed by abnormalities in the autosomal chromosomes in numerical order. For each chromosome described, numerical changes are listed before structural aberrations. Table 33.6 provides examples of the karyotypic designation of

TABLE 33.6 Examples of Human Chromosome Nomenclature

Designation	Description
Description of karyotypes	
Constitutional sex chromosome aneuploidies	
45,X	Turner syndrome
47,XXY	Klinefelter syndrome
Autosomal chromosome aneuploidies	
47,XY,+21	Male with trisomy 21 (Down syndrome)
48,XY,+21c,+21[20]	Male with trisomy 21, with gain of an additional chromosome 21 in his tumor cells. The number in brackets designates the number of cells that were analyzed and contain the additional chromosome 21.
Abnormalities in neoplasms	
47,XX,+10,t(11;22)(q24;q12)[5/20]	Female whose tumor cells have two cytogenetic abnormalities: an additional chromosome 10, and a reciprocal translocation between the long arm (q) of chromosome 11 at region 2, band 4, and the long arm (q) of chromosome 22 at region 1, band 2. The first number in brackets designates the number of cells with the observed abnormalities and the last number designates the total number of cells that were analyzed.
Description of metaphase FISH results	
47,XY,+mar.ish der(3)(wcp3+)	In this tumor, traditional cytogenetic analysis shows a marker chromosome; metaphase FISH using a whole chromosome paint for chromosome 3 shows that the marker is derived from chromosome 3.

FISH, fluorescence in situ hybridization.

numerical and structural abnormalities detected by traditional cytogenetic analysis. The rules for designating the karyotype of constitutional abnormalities are also used for designating the abnormalities associated with neoplasms, although the biology of tumors requires additional definitions and guidelines.

Description of Fluorescence In Situ Hybridization and Microarray Results

ISCN 2020 also includes rules for designating cytogenetic findings derived from various in situ hybridization techniques (a summary of the more common symbols and abbreviations is shown in Table 33.5) as well as microarrays. For metaphase chromosome in situ hybridization, the results of conventional cytogenetic analysis (if performed) are listed first, followed by the results of in situ hybridization analysis, and finally the nomenclature for the microarray findings. Ideally, loci are designated according to the Human Genome Organization (HUGO) Gene Nomenclature Committee (http://www.genenames.org/); when HUGO designations are unavailable, probe names are used.

ACKNOWLEDGMENTS

The authors thank Patrick Mann, Shashikant Kulkarni, Hussam Al-Kateb, and Catherine Cottrell, co-authors of a related chapter in *The Washington Manual of Surgical Pathology*, 3rd edition.

SUGGESTED READINGS

Mascarello JT, Hirsch B, Kearney HM, et al. Section E9 of the American College of Medical Genetics technical standards and guidelines: fluorescence in situ hybridization. *Genet Med.* 2011;13(7):667-675. doi:10.1097/GIM.0b013e3182227295. PMID: 21738013.

McGowan-Jordan J, Simons A, Schmid M, eds. *ISCN 2020: An International System for Human Cytogenetic Nomenclature.* S Karger; 2020.

Miller DT, Adam MP, Aradhya S, et al. Consensus statement: chromosomal microarray is a first-tier clinical diagnostic test for individuals with developmental disabilities or congenital anomalies. *Am J Hum Genet.* 2010;86:749-764.

Rack KA, van den Berg E, Haferlach C, et al. European recommendations and quality assurance for cytogenomic analysis of haematological neoplasms. *Leukemia.* 2019;33:1851-1867. doi:10.1038/s41375-019-0378-z

Rooney DE, ed. *Human Cytogenetics: Constitutional Analysis: A Practical Approach.* 3rd ed. Oxford University Press; 2001.

34 Molecular Diagnostics

34.1 Interphase Fluorescence In Situ Hybridization

Jennifer K. Sehn, Yi-Shan Lee, and John D. Pfeifer

Fluorescence in situ hybridization (FISH) is a molecular technique for the evaluation of specific DNA sequences in a cellular context.[1] Fluorescently labeled probes are hybridized to DNA regions of interest based on Watson-Crick base pairing. Given the size of FISH probes (usually in the range of 100-200 kb), FISH is most commonly utilized for the evaluation of structural or numeric chromosomal abnormalities, including translocations, gene deletion/amplification, and aneusomy (e-Figures 34.1-1 through 34.1-3). FISH is not useful for the evaluation of alterations less than around 20 kb in size (such as single-nucleotide variants, small structural rearrangements, or smaller insertions/deletions).

One of the most useful features of interphase FISH is that it is performed directly on cells, allowing for the evaluation of molecular aberrations in the context of intact tissue morphology. For hematopathology, interphase FISH tests are performed on nondividing cells from formalin-fixed, alcohol-fixed, or air-dried specimens, including sections from routine surgical pathology tissue blocks, cytology smears, and blood or bone marrow smears. Importantly, while EDTA decalcification is suitable for specimens in which FISH will be performed, acid decalcification is not compatible with FISH or other DNA-based analyses.

Interphase FISH is used primarily to detect somatic cancer–associated mutations (particularly aneusomy, gene deletion/amplification, and translocations) with known diagnostic, prognostic, or therapeutic implications (Tables 34.1-1 and 34.1-2). A marked hematoxylin and eosin (H&E)-stained guide slide is usually used to specify which areas are best for interpretation, designating the regions with high tumor cellularity (mostly tumor cells, with little background inflammation, stroma, and vessels) and viability (avoiding areas of necrosis). In addition, sex chromosome (XY) FISH can be useful in evaluating engraftment in patients with sex-mismatched bone marrow transplants (e-Figure 34.1-4). FISH also can be performed on dividing (metaphase) cells from cell cultures (see Chapter 33).

---

[1]This chapter draws from Pfeifer JD, Humphrey PA, Ritter JH, Dehner LP, eds. *The Washington Manual of Surgical Pathology*. 3rd ed. Lippincott Williams & Wilkins; 2020.

TABLE 34.1-1 Examples of Diagnostic Tests Performed by Interphase FISH

Prenatal testing
- Trisomy 12, 18, 21
- XY aneusomies
- Microdeletion syndromes

Transplant pathology
- XY FISH on sex-mismatched organ transplant
- Disease relapse using known genetic alterations in primary tumor

Oncology (diagnostic, prognostic, and/or predictive markers)
- Chromosomal aneusomies
- Gene/locus deletions
- Gene amplifications
- Translocations

FISH, fluorescence in situ hybridization.

TABLE 34.1-2 Examples of Hematologic Malignancy–Associated Alterations Commonly Detected by Interphase FISH

Mutation Type	Tumor Type	Alterations/Probes	Association
Aneusomies	CLL	13q–, 11q–, 17p– (*TP53*)	Diagnostic, prognostic
Deletions/Gains	AML/MDS	–5, –7, 17p– (*TP53*)	Diagnostic, prognostic
	ALL	9p– (*CDNK2A*)	Prognostic
	Multiple myeloma	13q–, 17p– (*TP53*), 1q21 gain	Prognostic
	HGBCL	11q gain/loss	Diagnostic, prognostic
Translocations	Burkitt lymphoma	*MYC::IGH*, *MYC*	Diagnostic
	Follicular lymphoma	*IGH::BCL2*	Diagnostic
	ALCL	*ALK*, *DUSP22*	Diagnostic, prognostic, predictive
	MALT lymphoma	*BIRC3::MALT1*, *IGH::MALT1*, *MALT1*	Diagnostic
	DLBCL	*BCL2*, *MYC*, *BCL6*, *IRF4*	Diagnostic, prognostic
	HGBCL	*BCL2*, *MYC*, *BCL6*	Diagnostic, prognostic

(*continued*)

TABLE 34.1-2 Examples of Hematologic Malignancy–Associated Alterations Commonly Detected by Interphase FISH (*continued*)

Mutation Type	Tumor Type	Alterations/Probes	Association
	Mantle cell lymphoma	IGH::CCND1	Diagnostic
	Multiple myeloma	IGH::CCND1, IGH::FGFR3, IGH::MAF, IGH::MAFB	Prognostic
	CML, AML, ALL	BCR::ABL	Diagnostic, predictive
	APML	PML::RARA, RARA	Diagnostic, prognostic, predictive
	AML/MDS	RUNX1::RUNX1T1, CBFB, KMT2A, MECOM	Diagnostic, prognostic
	ALL	ETV6::RUNX1, TCF3::PBX1, KMT2A	Diagnostic, prognostic
	Myeloid and lymphoid neoplasms with eosinophilia	PDGFRA::CHIC2:: FIP1L1, PGDFRB, FGFR1	Diagnostic, prognostic, predictive

ALCL, anaplastic large cell lymphoma; ALL, acute lymphoblastic leukemia; AML, acute myeloid leukemia; APML, acute promyelocytic leukemia; BCL, B-cell lymphoma; CLL, chronic lymphocytic leukemia; CML, chronic myeloid leukemia; DLBCL, diffuse large B-cell lymphoma; FISH, fluorescence in situ hybridization; HGBCL, high-grade B-cell lymphoma; IGH, immunoglobulin heavy chain; MALT, mucosa-associated lymphoid tissue; MDS, myelodysplastic syndrome.

I. FISH APPLICATIONS AND PROBE TYPES

Aneusomy and Gene Copy Number Changes: Centromere Enumeration Probes

Centromere enumeration probes (CEPs) are highly robust probes that target repetitive DNA sequences that are specific to the centromere of each chromosome (eg, CEP7 hybridizes to the centromere of chromosome 7). They are most useful as a reference for chromosome copy number (distinguishing when there are more or fewer signals from a gene-targeted probe vs the total number of copies of that chromosome in each cell); in deletion/amplification analysis, CEP probes are used in combination with locus-specific identifier (LSI, also known as gene-specific) probes to evaluate the copy number of the locus of interest compared with the number of chromosomes present in the cell. A normal cell shows two signals for each CEP probe (representing the maternally and paternally inherited copies of each chromosome). Examples of common applications for CEP probes in hematopathology are listed in Table 34.1-2.

Chromosomal polysomy/monosomy and gene amplification/deletion are also among the common alterations detected in neoplasms by interphase FISH (Table 34.1-2). It can be difficult to distinguish specific tumor-associated polysomies and monosomies from nonspecific gains and losses that are secondary changes due to tumor genomic instability. The use of CEP reference probes helps to distinguish polysomy/monosomy (gain or loss of the entire chromosome) from true gene amplification/deletion (e-Figure 34.1-2).

Structural Variants: Break-Apart and Fusion Locus-Specific Identifier Probe Sets

Multiple types of FISH probes are available for the detection of structural variants (particularly translocations) in surgical pathology specimens, including break-apart (FISH-BA), fusion (FISH-F), and extra signal (ES-FISH). Which type of probe is employed depends on whether or not the fusion partner gene is relevant. It is important to remember that usually only one of the two cellular copies of a gene is involved in a structural aberration such as a translocation or inversion, such that tumor cells harboring a translocation also still harbor one normal copy of each gene. Examples of common applications in hematopathology for these types of probes are also listed in Table 34.1-2.

1. **Dual-color fusion probes.** Dual-color fusion probes employ two locus-specific probes with different fluorophores that target two different partners in a translocation (eg, *BCR* on 22q and *ABL* on 9q). Translocation-negative cells yield separated or "split" signals (eg, two green and two red signals; e-Figure 34.1-3A). Translocation-positive cells yield "fusion" yellow or red-green signals as the loci of interest are brought together by the translocation (eg, one fusion, one green, and one red signal; e-Figure 34.1-3B). Cells must be scored carefully to avoid overinterpretation of small populations of cells where green and red signals overlap purely by chance. Based on signal proximities in normal controls, typical conservative cutoffs for a positive FISH-F test result require the presence of fused signals in more than 30% of cells (*Mod Pathol.* 2006;19:1).
2. **Break-apart probes.** Break-apart probes are composed of two probes localizing just proximal and distal to a breakpoint of interest. In translocation-negative cells, the two probes are in proximity to one another, resulting in fusion signals. Translocation-positive cells will result in at least one pair of split signals (eg, one fusion, one green, and one red signal). Compared with dual-color fusion probes, break-apart probes offer several advantages. False-positive results are rare, as split signals should not occur purely by chance. Also, commercial break-apart probes are often more than 500 kb in size, yielding large, easily interpretable signals.

   Most importantly, the break-apart strategy identifies translocations that involve multiple partner genes, although the resulting disadvantage of break-apart probes is that they provide no information regarding the identity of the fusion partner. However, in many cases it is complicated and unnecessary to identify the partner gene in a translocation; merely identifying that the target gene is rearranged is sufficient to answer the clinical question. In normal cells, the probes are located close enough to result in one overlapping signal (which appears yellow); each normal cell will have two yellow signals (one for each copy of the chromosome) (e-Figure 34.1-3C). In cells with a rearrangement of the target gene, the probes are split (broken apart) and are seen as two signals—one red and one green; positive cells have one red, one green, and one yellow signal (split signals for the rearranged copy of the gene, and a fused signal for the other copy of the gene) (e-Figure 34.1-3D). Typical conservative cutoffs for positive FISH-BA test results require the presence of split signals in more than 15% of cells (*Mod Pathol.* 2006;19:1).

3. **Other approaches.** ES-FISH is a strategy that has been used to increase the sensitivity and decrease the false positivity rate of FISH-F. One of the probes in ES-FISH is particularly large and spans the breakpoint region. In the presence of a translocation, the large probe is split, leading to an extra signal that is smaller than the non-split, non-fused signals (eg, one fusion, one normal green, one normal red, and one ES red signal). Since it is unlikely that individual cells will contain both a fusion signal and an extra signal, the probability of scoring cells with chance overlap of red and green signals as translocation-positive is close to zero.

4. **Probe availability.** A number of companies market multicolor probe cocktails for clinical use, each with different recommendations for minimum number of nuclei counted and cutoffs for alterations. For example, a number of vendors market probes for FISH assays that have been shown to detect aneusomies and deletions that identify prognostically relevant subsets of chronic lymphocytic leukemia, acute myeloid leukemia, and myelodysplastic syndrome. Of note, many laboratories perform FISH-based testing of hematopathology specimens on a commercial basis for a wide range of diseases and chromosomal abnormalities.

II. INTERPHASE FISH NOMENCLATURE

FISH results are reported using standardized nomenclature, according to the International System for Human Cytogenomic Nomenclature (ISCN), which was most recently revised in 2020 (McGowan-Jordan J, Hastings RJ, Moore S, eds. *ISCN 2020: An International System for Human Cytogenomic Nomenclature.* Karger; 2020). A summary of the more common symbols and abbreviations is shown in Table 33.5, which emphasizes that the same nomenclature applies to metaphase and interphase FISH.

For interphase in situ hybridization, results are presented in the following order: the abbreviation nuc ish is listed first, followed by the chromosome band to which the probe maps, followed by the locus designation, a multiplication sign, and the number of signals present (Table 34.1-3). If both conventional cytogenetic analysis and metaphase in situ hybridization are performed, the results of the conventional cytogenetic analysis are listed first, followed by a period, the abbreviation ish, and then the in situ hybridization results in the same order described earlier. If conventional cytogenetic analysis is performed in conjunction with interphase in situ hybridization, the results are described on separate lines of nomenclature. Ideally, loci are designated according to Genome Database (GDB) nomenclature (http://www.gdb.org). When GDB designations are unavailable, probe names are used. If two or more probes for the same or different loci are used, they are separated by commas.

By ISCN guidelines, aneusomy or amplification/deletion is reported as the number of signals present for the probes of interest, as described earlier. A positive result for structural variants (rearrangements, translocations) is reported as con (for "connected," in cells in which fusion probes are normally present on separate chromosomes but are juxtaposed on the same chromosome in cells harboring the target

TABLE 34.1-3 Examples of Nomenclature Used for Neoplasms Evaluated by Interphase FISH

Designation	Description
nuc ish (IGH × 3, BCL2 × 3)(IGH con BCL2 × 2) [121/200]	Interphase FISH of a tumor cell using dual-color dual-fusion probes. There are three signals of IGH probes and three signals of BCL2 probes including two fusion signals in which IGH and BCL2 signals are juxtaposed (or connected), consistent with a t(14;18)(q32;q21) translocation in 121 of 200 nuclei evaluated.
nuc ish (IGH, BCL2) × 2 [200]	Interphase FISH using the same dual-color dual-fusion probes as in the above example. In this tumor, two signals of IGH probes and two signals of BCL2 probes were spatially separated and there is no fusion signals, consistent with normal hybridization pattern/negative for *IGH::BCL2* fusion.
nuc ish (MYC × 2) (5′MYC sep 3′MYC × 1) [119/200]	Interphase FISH using a *MYC* (8q24) break-apart probe set. In this tumor, a split of red and green signals was detected. This is consistent with a *MYC*-containing chromosomal rearrangement in 119 of 200 nuclei evaluated.
nun ish (MYC × 2) [200]	Interphase FISH using the same break-apart probe set as in the above example. However, in this tumor, the two probes remain juxtaposed on both copies of chromosome 8 (which provides no evidence of a rearrangement of the *MYC* locus). This is equivalent to the nomenclature described in the following example.
nuc ish (5′MYC, 3′MYC) × 2(5′MYC con 3′MYC × 2) [174/200]	Interphase FISH was performed utilizing *MYC* (8q24) break-apart probe set. In this particular case, a split of fusion signals was not detected in 174 of 200 nuclei evaluated.

BCL, B-cell lymphoma; FISH, fluorescence in situ hybridization; IGH, immunoglobulin heavy chain.

rearrangement) or sep (for "separated," in cells in which break-apart probes normally flank the gene of interest but are separated due to rearrangement).

III. LIMITATIONS

The basic steps for FISH protocols are similar to those of immunohistochemistry (IHC) and include deparaffinization, pretreatment/target retrieval, probe and target DNA denaturation, hybridization (a few hours to overnight), post-hybridization washes, detection, and microscopic interpretation/imaging. FISH is therefore typically a 2-day assay, although same-day assays are possible if the probes are particularly robust.

Several factors can complicate interpretation of FISH results.

- **Artifacts in probe hybridization** secondary to fixation and processing techniques.
- **Truncation artifact** due to the underestimation of copy number because of an incomplete DNA complement within transected nuclei, which emphasizes that it is important to assess controls cut at the same thickness.
- **Aneuploidy and polyploidy** artifacts can result in confusing signal counts. Although the simplest approach is to interpret absolute losses (<2 copies) and gains (>2 copies), relative losses and gains can also be delineated based on a reference ploidy, obtained either by flow cytometry or the assessment of multiple chromosomes by FISH.
- **Autofluorescence** is background fluorescence from the tissue itself, separate from true probe signals and frequently present at multiple wavelengths of light. This is a particularly common problem in formalin-fixed paraffin-embedded (FFPE) tissue sections.
- **Partial hybridization failure** is most problematic when combining a highly robust probe with a comparatively weak probe, such as a CEP with a small locus-specific probe.
- **Fading of fluorescent signals** over time, especially with exposure to light. In some cases, **chromogenic in situ hybridization (CISH)** can be used instead of FISH to allow for more permanent signals (*Am J Pathol.* 2000;157:1467).
  1. CISH combines the nucleic acid hybridization methods of FISH with the chromogenic substrate methods of IHC and can be designed to detect either DNA or RNA target sequences within the cells of interest. For CISH, the nucleotide probes do not incorporate a fluorescent label that is directly detected, but rather incorporate biotin or digoxigenin that is subsequently linked with the enzyme horseradish peroxidase or alkaline phosphatase for production of an insoluble product via standard IHC approaches. Use of different probes and multiple chromogenic substrates makes it possible to perform dual-color CISH.
  2. CISH performed on glass slides is much easier to score than FISH, since a standard light microscope can be used instead of a fluorescence microscope. The concordance rate between FISH and CISH demonstrates that the methods are comparable (*Breast.* 2005;15:519).

IV. USE OF INTERPHASE FISH VERSUS OTHER MOLECULAR TECHNIQUES

1. When compared with metaphase cytogenetics (see Chapter 33), interphase FISH has several advantages. One advantage is the lack of a requirement for mitotically active cells via cell culture, which removes potential artifacts due to in vitro growth selection biases such as overgrowth of nonneoplastic stromal elements. In fact, interphase FISH with CD138 enrichment is the technique of choice for cytogenetic characterization of myeloma due to low proliferative activity of neoplastic plasma cells. On the other hand, FISH is not a genomic screening tool; it provides a targeted approach for alterations that have been initially identified by more global molecular techniques, such as classic cytogenetics, loss of heterozygosity (LOH) screening, comparative genomic hybridization (CGH), array CGH (aCGH), array single-nucleotide polymorphism (SNP) analysis, and various next-generation sequencing (NGS) approaches (eg, RNA sequencing and whole-genome sequencing, as discussed in Chapter 34.3).

2. In terms of resolution, FISH is more sensitive than conventional karyotypic analysis and CGH (both of which are limited to alterations of several megabases in size) but less sensitive than polymerase chain reaction (PCR)-based assays and NGS approaches for detecting small alterations (which detect even single base pair changes). Since FISH probes are typically at least 20 kb long, and most average 100 to 200 kb long, alterations need to be fairly large for reliable detection by FISH, and consequently, FISH cannot detect small sequence changes, small deletions or insertions, or small structural changes.
3. Minimal residual disease or early recurrences are better detected by PCR or NGS of blood or fresh tissue specimens than FISH. Minimal residual disease detection usually involves the detection of as few as one abnormal cell per million normal cells, a level of sensitivity that cannot be reliably attained by FISH techniques with complicated preanalytic steps (*Arch Pathol Lab Med.* 2013;137:6; *Cytometry.* 2019;95:521). In contrast, FISH is very sensitive for identifying gene deletions or amplifications from samples of mixed cellularity, such as neoplasms with clonal heterogeneity or contaminating nonneoplastic elements. In this setting, in which morphologic analysis can be used to guide evaluation of only the cell population of interest, FISH can typically detect gains, translocations, or amplifications in as few as 5% and deletions in 15% to 30% of the cells within a sample.

34.2 Polymerase Chain Reaction and Related Techniques

Bijal A. Parikh and John D. Pfeifer

Polymerase chain reaction (PCR) is a quick, inexpensive, versatile, and highly accurate approach for analysis of a wide range of sequence variants in virtually any specimen type.[1] Because PCR-based tests are so widely used, laboratory testing guidelines and recommendations have been developed by both professional societies and regulatory agencies to assist in the design and performance of clinical PCR-based testing (Table 34.2-1).

I. SPECIMEN REQUIREMENTS, HANDLING, AND PROCESSING

Specimen requirements are dictated by the disease process, including the source of the tissue, amount of tissue, type of sample (fresh or frozen tissue, formalin-fixed paraffin-embedded [FFPE] tissue, cytology specimen, etc), and the extent of the disease in the sample. The amount of tissue required for PCR-based testing is relatively small, which contributes to the clinical utility of the technique.

---

[1] This chapter draws from Pfeifer JD, Humphrey PA, Ritter JH, Dehner LP, eds. *The Washington Manual of Surgical Pathology*. 3rd ed. Lippincott Williams & Wilkins; 2020.

TABLE 34.2-1 Selected Resources for Molecular Pathology Testing in Clinical Laboratories

Entity	Site	Tool(s)
Clinical Laboratory Improvement Amendments '88	http://www.cms.hhs.gov/clia/ Centers for Medicare and Medicaid Services	Clinical Laboratory Accreditation requirements and compliance lists 57 Federal Register 7137-7186 (1992)
College of American Pathologists (CAP)	http://www.cap.org	Laboratory Accreditation (LAP) Molecular Pathology Laboratory Inspection Checklist Proficiency Surveys • Molecular Oncology (MO) • Medical Genetics (MGL) • Pharmacogenetics (PGX) • Monitoring Engraftment (ME) • Molecular Microbiology (HIV, HCV, ID) • Microsatellite Instability (MSI) • Sarcoma Translocation (SARC) • Nucleic acid testing (viral; NAT)
Clinical and Laboratory Standards Institute (CLSI; formerly National Committee for Clinical Laboratory Standards, NCCLS)	http://www.nccls.org	Molecular Methods Guidelines • Genetic diseases • IGH & TCR Gene rearrangements • Nucleic Acid Amplification • Nucleic Acid Sequencing • Collection and Handling of Specimens • Proficiency Testing
American College of Medical Genetics (ACMG)	http://www.acmg.net	Standards and Guidelines for Clinical Genetics Laboratories Policy Statements for Molecular testing of genetic diseases
US Food and Drug Administration (FDA)	http://www.fda.gov	Medical Devices 21CFR809.30 In Vitro Diagnostic Products for Human Use • Analyte-Specific Reagents (ASRs)

TABLE 34.2-1 Selected Resources for Molecular Pathology Testing in Clinical Laboratories (*continued*)

Entity	Site	Tool(s)
Association for Molecular Pathology (AMP)	http://www.amp.org	Molecular Pathology professional organization (including genetics, hematopathology, infectious disease, solid tumors)
		CHAMP listserve for AMP members
		Test Directories
		• Solid tumors
		• Hematopathology
		• Infectious disease

Nonetheless, regardless of the PCR protocol utilized in a specific assay, two general features of the tissue sample influence the utility of the test. First, there must be a sufficient quantity of the specific target (DNA or RNA) in the sample. Second, the size or integrity of the nucleic acid molecules after isolation from the tissue can dramatically affect the sensitivity of the detection of specific alterations. Thus, nucleic acid degradation (whether due to fixation, enzymatic, heat, pH, or mechanical forces) can reduce the sensitivity of testing.

A formal review of the specimen by a pathologist is necessary to ensure the presence of abnormal cell population and to assess the quality and quantity of the specimen. Pathologic assessment is an important quality control step, since it permits evaluation of possible analytic confounders, including the percentage of nonneoplastic tissue, necrosis, and so on, and thus helps ensure that the specimen is adequate. Obtaining an approximate value of the percentage of tumor involvement in a given sample may also be useful during the interpretation of sequencing data.

It is important to recognize that **tissue heterogeneity** is different from **intratumoral heterogeneity**. Tissue heterogeneity refers to the fact that no tumor specimen is composed of 100% neoplastic cells. Instead, tumor samples contain a varying proportion of nonneoplastic cells, including stromal cells (benign parenchymal cells and fibroblasts), inflammatory cells (primarily neutrophils, lymphocytes, and macrophages), and endothelial cells (of blood vessels and lymphatics). Intratumoral heterogeneity is a term used to refer to the fact that malignant neoplasms demonstrate clonal heterogeneity. Consequently, even with a relatively pure tumor sample, the number, type, and frequency of sequence variants detected in that sample may or may not be an accurate reflection of the range and frequency of the variants elsewhere in the tumor.

1. **Tissue type:** Fresh peripheral blood, bone marrow, solid tissue biopsies, cytology specimens, enriched cell populations (eg, from flow cytometry [FC]), and FFPE tissue sections are all sources of nucleic acids for PCR. Transporting these samples

on ice and storing them refrigerated helps reduce cell lysis, minimizes nuclease activity, and reduces nucleic acid degradation.

a. **Cell suspensions:** Cell suspension–based specimens, such as bone marrow aspirates and peripheral blood, should be collected in the presence of an anticoagulant. Ethylenediaminetetraacetic acid (EDTA) is the anticoagulant of choice because it inhibits DNase activity without affecting DNA quantity. Heparin-based anticoagulants should be avoided as heparin can bind to DNA and inhibit Taq polymerases used in PCR. Following collection, the vacutainer tube should be inverted several times to ensure thorough mixing of the blood and anticoagulant (*Cell J*. 2015;17:181).

b. **Fixed tissue:** Nucleic acids extracted from fixed tissue can also be used for molecular analysis; however, both the type of fixative and length of fixation have significant effect on nucleic acid recovery. Ethanol-based fixatives provide the most consistent preservation of amplifiable nucleic acids because they prevent cross-linking of DNA, RNA, and proteins. However, most surgical pathology specimens are fixed in formaldehyde-based solutions (eg, formalin), which leads to variability in the level of nucleic acid preservation. Formaldehyde leads to several downstream effects, such as the formation of nucleic acid cross-links, the production of cyclic-based derivatives, and the promotion of oxidation and deamination reactions (*Am J Pathol*. 2002;161:1961). Consequently, nucleic acid isolation from FFPE tissue is critically dependent on fixation time. In general, nucleic acids in tissue fixed in neutral-buffered formalin for less than 12 hours can be reliably amplified.

2. **Tissue quality:**
   a. Fresh tissue and cell suspensions are the optimal specimen types for sequence analysis. The preferred method of preservation of fresh tissue, if not immediately processed for isolation of nucleic acids, is ultra-low-temperature frozen storage at -70 °C. This temperature permits indefinite preservation with virtually no effect on the quality of extracted nucleic acids and is critical for maximum recovery of intact RNA. Low-temperature frozen storage around -20 °C can adequately preserve DNA for several months.

   Cell suspensions (including hematologic specimens such as peripheral blood and bone marrow aspirates) should be collected in the presence of an anticoagulant, preferably EDTA or acid-citrate-dextrose (ACD). Heparin should be avoided because heparin carryover after nucleic acid isolation may inhibit subsequent PCR steps. Freezing of hematologic specimens presents distinct obstacles to the preparation of good-quality nucleic acid and should generally be avoided.

   b. Nucleic acids extracted from fixed tissue can also be used for sequence analysis, although the type of fixative and length of fixation both have a profound effect on their recovery. Non-cross-linking fixatives such as ethanol provide the most consistent preservation of amplifiable nucleic acids. There is more variability from tissues fixed with formalin, Zamboni and Clark fixatives, paraformaldehyde, and formalin-alcohol-acetic acid. Tissues processed with Carnoy, Zenker, Bouin, and B-5 fixatives are poor substrates for sequence analysis since little amplifiable DNA or RNA can be recovered from them.

   The effects of formalin fixation have been evaluated in some detail, not surprising given that most surgical specimens are fixed in formalin. Formaldehyde reacts with nucleic acids and proteins to form a mixture of end products that are covalently linked by methylene bridges, inducing oxidation and deamination reactions, and leads to the formation of cyclic-based derivatives. Thus, the quality of DNA and RNA isolated from formalin-fixed tissue is critically dependent on the length of fixation, with a deterioration of nucleic acids with increasing fixation time. In general, tissue fixed in neutral-buffered formalin for less than 8 hours contains DNA and RNA from which PCR products greater than 600 bp in length can be reliably amplified, but fixation extended for greater than 12 hours decreases the length of PCR products that can consistently be amplified.

3. **Tissue quantity:** Minimum sample requirements are determined by the assay methodology and the extent of target cell involvement in the tissue. A typical sequencing-based assay requires only 10 to 200 ng of DNA (about 10^3-10^4 cells).

II. GENERAL FEATURES OF POLYMERASE CHAIN REACTION–BASED NUCLEIC ACID ANALYSIS

Factors That Affect Testing on a Diagnostic Level

The intrinsic biologic variability of diseases has a significant impact on the diagnostic sensitivity and specificity of PCR-based testing, as it does with all molecular testing. Since only a subset of patients with a specific disease may harbor a characteristic mutation, more than one genetic variant may characterize a specific disease, the same mutation may be characteristic of more than one disease, a mutation characteristic of disease may be present in healthy individuals, and so on, even a molecular genetic method with perfect analytic performance will have reduced sensitivity and specificity when used for diagnostic testing of patient samples.

Another limitation of the use of PCR in routine clinical testing is a result of the fact that the technique is so sensitive that it can amplify target DNA and RNA sequences from cellular debris as well as viable cells (*Cancer*. 1997;80:1393). Consequently, the significance of PCR detection of tumor-derived nucleic acids in a patient specimen is dependent on correlation with the histopathologic findings and clinical setting.

Factors That Affect Testing on an Operational Level

Purely operational factors can introduce uncertainty into the interpretation of PCR results in routine clinical practice. If the probability that a case is subjected to additional analysis depends on the initial test result itself, clinical variables, or both, selection bias (also called verification bias, posttest referral bias, and work-up bias) is introduced into the test. Discrepant analysis (also known as discordant analysis) can also introduce uncertainty in the interpretation of test results. Finally, even mundane factors such as differences in disease prevalence can have a marked effect on the predictive value of positive and negative test results.

Polymerase Chain Reaction in Routine Testing

The technical features of PCR, biologic variability, variations in assay design, and differences in the distribution of disease in the patient populations have many implications for testing applied in routine clinical practice.

1. **Relative merit:** For clinical utility, the sequencing test should provide an improvement in patient care by providing new and independent information with the potential for clinical stratification of disease subtype, prognostic category, treatment regimen, or disease progression. The test results should complement the findings of established tests such as cytogenetics, immunohistochemistry (IHC), and FC.

And it is very important that the test results should be reported in a context that explains the data and integrates the findings with other pathology results in order to help avoid confusion caused by seemingly contradictory results from laboratory tests that possess different levels of resolution or sensitivity.

2. **Discordant cases:** Cases will arise in which there is a lack of concordance between the diagnoses suggested by PCR versus other testing methods (eg, morphologic diagnosis, IHC, cytogenetics, FC). The debate over the best approach to resolve the ambiguity presented by these types of cases reflects the fundament impact of molecular genetics on the classification of disease. The most reasonable way to handle discordant cases is to acknowledge the presence of the discrepancy and then reappraise the clinical data, pathological findings, and therapeutic implications of all the test results.

III. BASIC POLYMERASE CHAIN REACTION METHODOLOGY

Amplification

Selective amplification of the target sequence is achieved through the use of oligonucleotide primers that hybridize to the 5′ and 3′ ends of the DNA target sequence (Figure 34.2-1). In addition to the two primers and input DNA (template), the reaction mixture includes the four deoxynucleotide triphosphates, dATP, dCTP, dGTP, and dTTP, and a heat-stable (thermostable) DNA polymerase. The first step of the PCR itself involves heating the mixture to a high temperature to denature the target DNA; in the second step, the reaction is cooled to allow the primers to anneal to their complementary sequence in the target DNA; in the third step, the reaction is heated to the temperature at which the heat-stable DNA polymerase has optimal activity. As a result of this three-step denaturation, annealing, and polymerization cycle, the two primers will initiate synthesis of new DNA molecules from opposite strands of the input DNA heteroduplex. With each repetition of the three-step cycle, the newly synthesized DNA strands will also act as templates for further DNA synthesis, and so DNA duplexes in which both strands have the fixed length of the target sequence (so-called amplicons) accumulate exponentially.

PCR makes it possible to selectively amplify a specific DNA target sequence within a background of heterogeneous DNA sequences, such as total genomic DNA or cDNA derived from unfractionated cellular RNA. The sensitivity of PCR for detection of a few target molecules in a large background of unaltered DNA molecules (1 in 10^5) is one of the principle strengths of this methodology. However, each component of a PCR, including the input DNA, the oligonucleotide primers, the thermostable polymerase, the buffer, and the cycle parameters, has an effect on the sensitivity, specificity, and fidelity of the reaction.

Factors That Affect Polymerase Chain Reaction Testing on an Analytic/Technical Level

1. **Advantages of PCR**
   a. **PCR is simple, quick, and inexpensive:** A single PCR cycle, comprising melting, annealing, and extension, is usually completed within several minutes. Consequently, an entire PCR amplification of 25 to 35 cycles can be performed in just a few hours. Because of the high level of amplification achieved by PCR, the product DNA can be visualized through simple gel electrophoresis, avoiding the need for hazardous and costly radiolabeling methods.

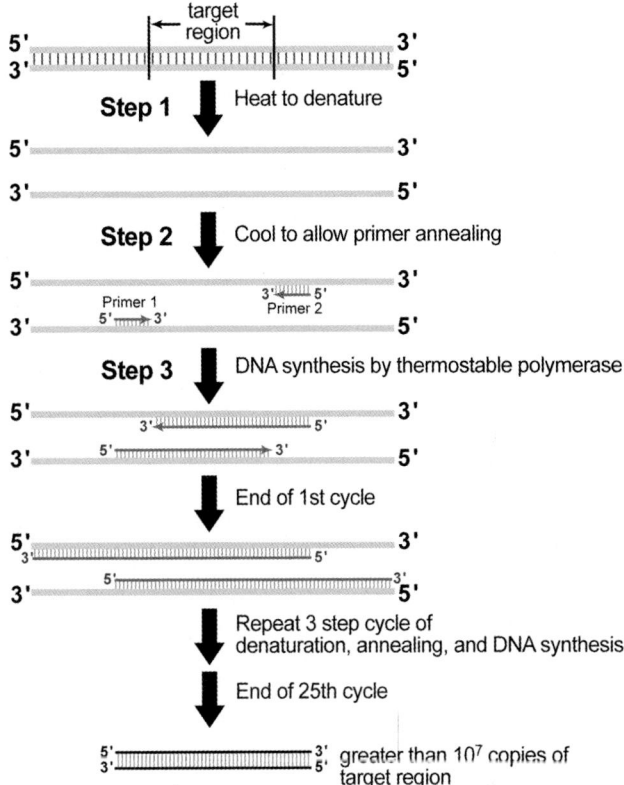

Figure 34.2-1. Schematic diagram of the polymerase chain reaction. Each cycle consists of three steps: the reaction mix is heated to denature the double-stranded DNA template; then, the reaction mix is cooled to permit annealing of oligonucleotide primers to sequences that flank the target region; finally, the reaction mix is warmed to permit the heat-stable polymerase to synthesize new DNA strands. Each newly synthesized DNA strand then acts as a template in subsequent three-step cycles of denaturation, annealing, and DNA synthesis, producing exponential amplification of the target region.

b. **PCR has high sensitivity and specificity:** When optimized, PCR can detect one abnormal cell in a background of 10^5 normal cells, and it can even be used to analyze single-copy genes from individual cells (*Methods Enzymol.* 2002;356:295; *Methods Enzymol.* 2002;356:334). PCR can also be used to detect a broad range of genetic abnormalities, ranging from gross structural alterations such as translocations to single base pair changes.

c. **PCR products are easily labeled for detection:** In primer-mediated labeling, a labeled chemical group (usually a fluorophore) is attached to the 5′ end of one or both oligonucleotide primers. Alternatively, the PCR product can be directly labeled by including one or more labeled nucleotide precursors in the PCR mix.

d. **Phenotype-genotype correlations are possible:** When performed on tissue sections, PCR provides only an indirect correlation of morphology with underlying genetic abnormalities. Microdissection techniques, in which the region of interest is carved out of the FFPE tissue blocks, scraped from tissue sections or cytology slides, or collected more precisely with a micromanipulator apparatus, provide some enrichment for morphologic-genetic correlations. More precise phenotypic-genotypic analysis is achieved by collecting individual cells by laser capture microdissection, FC, or even immunomagnetic methods. In situ PCR performed on histologic tissue sections is perhaps the ultimate method for providing morphologic localization of genotypic expression. However, the technique is so technically demanding that it has limited use in clinical laboratories.

2. **Limitations of PCR**
   a. **PCR only analyzes the target region:** Testing only provides information on the target segment amplified by the specific primer set employed.
   b. **PCR only amplifies intact target regions:** Mutations that damage a primer binding site (including insertions, deletions, and even point mutations) preclude amplification of the target region by PCR and can easily lead to errors in test interpretation. Similarly, mutations that alter the structure of the target region in ways not accounted for during primer set design (eg, large insertions, deletions, inversions, or translocations) may also preclude amplification.
   c. **Amplification bias:** PCR bias refers to the fact that some DNA templates are preferentially amplified versus other templates within the same reaction. PCR bias can be caused by differences in template length, random variations in template number (especially with very low target abundance, producing an artifact known as allele dropout), and random variations in PCR efficiency with each cycle. Amplification bias can even result from differences in the target sequence itself as small as a single base change. PCR bias can cause over 10-fold differences in amplification efficiency in some settings, a difference that can influence quantitative-PCR test results and loss of heterozygosity analysis. PCR bias can be a particularly troublesome problem in multiplex PCR.
   d. **Technical factors:** There are several technical factors that can lower the sensitivity and specificity of PCR in routine clinical practice below that obtained in optimized research settings. Nonspecific inhibitors of PCR are sometimes present in patient samples, including heparin and uncharacterized components of cerebrospinal fluid (CSF), urine, and sputum. With the extreme sensitivity of PCR, strict attention to the physical organization and methodologies of the laboratory is required to avoid cross-contamination of specimens. Nucleotide content of target sequences, especially if skewed in favor of guanine and cytosine bases (GC-rich), can affect primer binding and amplification efficiency. The lack of complexity of target regions, for example in introns, can make primer design difficult. Similarity to closely related paralogues or pseudogenes can also limit specificity, as is seen, for example, in evaluation of *SMN1/2* copy number.

However, the most important technical limitations are introduced when fixed rather than fresh tissue specimens are used for testing due to the degradation of DNA and RNA that occurs prior to and during fixation, as noted earlier. Test sensitivity and specificity are compromised by degradation since it makes it necessary to amplify shorter target sequences or employ a nested PCR approach, both of which increase the risk of amplification of nonspecific sequences and cross-contamination (*Am J Surg Pathol*. 2002;26:965).

IV. APPLICATIONS OF POLYMERASE CHAIN REACTION

Reverse Transcriptase-Polymerase Chain Reaction

Reverse transcriptase-polymerase chain reaction (RT-PCR) makes it possible to amplify RNA extracted from a tissue sample; a complementary DNA (cDNA) strand is synthesized from the RNA template using the enzyme reverse transcriptase, and the cDNA is then amplified by conventional PCR. Fresh (or fresh frozen) tissue is the preferred source of RNA for RT-PCR. RNA from fixed tissue is an acceptable substrate, even though it always suffers some degree of degradation depending on the prefixation interval, the type of fixative, the length of fixation, and the method used to isolate the RNA.

1. **Advantages of RT-PCR:** RT-PCR permits direct amplification of multiexon sequences by eliminating the intervening introns and thus greatly simplifies mutation scanning methods. Similarly, RT-PCR makes it much simpler to demonstrate the presence of translocations that create fusion genes by making it possible to directly detect the fusion transcripts encoded by the translocations (e-Figure 34.2-1). RT-PCR can also be used to detect changes in mRNA structure that result from alternative splicing, to demonstrate aberrant splicing due to mutations, and to evaluate the level of gene expression (*Ann Transl Med.* 2018;6:242).
2. **Limitations of RT-PCR:** RNA is a more technically demanding substrate with less stability than DNA. Tissue samples must be processed rapidly (ideally, within 20 minutes) to avoid mRNA degradation, especially since many mutations render transcripts more susceptible to cellular mechanisms that clear abnormal transcripts from the cell and result in unstable mRNA. The decreased stability of low-level transcripts in peripheral blood or bone marrow must be carefully considered when interpreting negative results. A nested PCR approach is often necessary when the target RNA is present at very low levels, and in this setting RT-PCR carries an increased risk of contamination and amplification of nonspecific sequences because the transfer of the first PCR product to a separate tube for the nested PCR entails transmission of a highly amplified DNA preparation.

Quantitative Polymerase Chain Reaction

An ideal PCR would generate a perfect 2-fold increase in the number of copies of amplicon in each cycle of the reaction. However, in reality, inhibitors of the reaction, accumulation of pyrophosphate molecules, decreasing polymerase activity, and reagent consumption all contribute to a plateau phase in the later stages of the reaction. During this phase, the amplicon no longer accumulates at an exponential rate (*Clin Chem Lab Med.* 2000;38:833). Reliable quantitation of PCR therefore involves more than simple measurement of the amount of product DNA present at the end of 30 to 40 cycles of the reaction. Real-time PCR, also referred to as quantitative-PCR (qPCR), employs real-time measurements of DNA accumulation (usually via fluorescence-based approaches) during the early exponential phases of PCR progress. This allows precise estimates of the initial concentration of the target sequence(s).

A wide variety of chemistries for qPCR are in routine use, including the so-called *Taq*Man (also known as 5′ exonuclease or hydrolysis real-time PCR), molecular beacon (which can be designed to distinguish targets differing by only a single nucleotide), scorpion (also known as self-probing amplicons), hybridization probe, and intercalating dye methods. Regardless of the chemistry employed, changes in fluorescence that result from target amplification are measured by a detector for each cycle of the reaction. These measurements are then used by a computer to construct an amplification plot of fluorescence versus the cycle number to quantify the concentration of the input target DNA sequence.

1. **Advantages of qPCR:** The method can be applied to both fresh tissue samples and FFPE tissue. Furthermore, phenotype-genotype correlations are possible through analysis of specific cell populations collected via microdissection, laser capture microdissection, and so on. RT-qPCR is also a robust analytic approach (e-Figure 34.2-2).
2. **Disadvantages of qPCR:** Even in optimized assays, testing can be complicated by amplification bias, which in the context of qPCR has two major sources: PCR drift, due to random fluctuations in amplification efficiency in the early cycles of the reaction when templates are present at very low concentration, and PCR selection, due to mechanisms that systematically favor amplification of some particular targets. In RT-qPCR, the reverse transcription reaction can introduce additional variables into the analysis. Additionally, when used to detect gene fusions, if specific breakpoints can vary, even a well-designed assay may fail to detect all clinically important isoforms.
3. **Use of qPCR in nonquantitative settings:** Since the probes used in qPCR (and RT-qPCR) have specificity for the target amplicon, the amplification plot not only confirms the presence of the DNA product but also confirms its identity. Intercalating dyes can also provide confirmation of both the presence and identity of the DNA product when coupled with subsequent melting curve analysis. Because qPCR eliminates the need for gel electrophoresis to demonstrate successful amplification while simultaneously confirming product identity, it is often used as a "one-step" alternative to conventional PCR or RT-PCR even when quantitation is not required.

Multiplex Polymerase Chain Reaction

Multiplex PCR is the simultaneous amplification of multiple target sequences in a single reaction through the simultaneous use of multiple primer pairs. The technique saves time and money, making it ideal for conserving templates that are in short supply. It has been successfully applied to many amplification approaches, including nested PCR and qPCR. However, even in optimized reactions, multiplex PCR may be complicated by amplification bias due to PCR drift and PCR selection. Therefore, rigorous optimization of primer design and careful titration of the relative primer concentrations among separate primer pairs are essential for achieving robust and reproducible multiplex PCR.

Methylation-Specific Polymerase Chain Reaction

Methylation of CpG sites in human DNA has been associated with transcriptional inactivation of imprinted genes, X chromosome inactivation, and developmentally regulated and tissue-specific gene regulation. Altered patterns of methylation are also characteristic of many human diseases. In some malignancies, changes in CpG methylation patterns have been associated with differences in response to specific chemotherapeutic agents and overall survival.

Some methylation-specific PCR techniques exploit the sequence differences produced when methylated CpG and unmethylated CpG sites are treated with sodium bisulfite (*Proc Natl Acad Sci USA*. 1996;93:9821). This chemical modification will not alter methyl cytosine (meC) but will depurinate cytosine to produce a transversion, which results in replacement by thymidine in subsequent DNA synthesis during PCR. Since the two strands of genomic DNA are no longer complementary after sodium bisulfite treatment, PCR with specifically designed primers for meC and T-substituted sequences makes it possible to infer the methylation status of the original untreated DNA (e-Figure 34.2-3). Methylation-specific PCR can be applied to DNA extracted from fresh tissue, FFPE tissue, and even archival cytology specimens. It is important to note that once a sequence is amplified by PCR, all methylation signals are lost.

Nested Polymerase Chain Reaction

In nested PCR, two consecutive PCRs are performed on the same DNA sample: an initial amplification of a longer target sequence followed by a second amplification of a shorter sequence contained within the first amplicon. The second PCR may involve two internal primers (fully nested) or one internal primer and one of the original primers (semi nested). Nested PCR provides a marked increase in sensitivity compared to traditional PCR and is desirable when the target sequence is present at an extremely low copy number, such as when the mutation is present in only a small subset of the cell population under study, when the nucleic acids have been degraded as a result of tissue fixation, or, in RT-PCR, when the target mRNA is expressed at an extremely low level. Since the increased sensitivity carries an increased risk of cross-contamination, reproducible nested PCR results require strict attention to laboratory techniques, rigorous use of controls, and confirmation of product identity.

Allele-Specific Polymerase Chain Reaction

Allele-specific PCR can be used to identify disease-associated mutations or genetic variations in patient samples. This approach works best when a single nucleotide variant (SNV) is the basis of the genetic difference. The reference and alternative alleles are identified through successful PCR amplification via one of the two allele-specific primers. The method also requires a common primer for both alleles to pair with the discriminatory primers. The primers can be labeled with a fluorophore for multiplexed PCR or identified via gel electrophoresis if performed in separate unlabeled reactions. This technique is highly specific and sensitive and can detect as little as a single copy of the target sequence. Depending on the assay conditions, allele-specific PCR can provide either qualitative or quantitative results.

Digital Polymerase Chain Reaction

Digital PCR partitions a traditional PCR sample into thousands of droplets or wells, each of which contains one to a few copies of the target DNA sequence. Following PCR, the number of positive reactions is quantified, thus allowing digital PCR to accurately determine the absolute quantity of target DNA in the original sample, even at low concentrations, and without reliance on a standard curve. Varieties of digital PCR include droplet digital PCR (ddPCR), chip-based digital PCR, and bead-based digital PCR. In ddPCR, the sample is partitioned into water-oil droplets, each of which contains a single DNA template and PCR mixture. Following PCR, positive and negative droplets are enumerated through fluorescence detection. Advantages of digital PCR include high precision, sensitivity, and reproducibility, as well as the ability to detect rare mutations and copy number variations (CNVs). Common uses of digital PCR include the detection and quantification of circulating tumor DNA, fetal DNA, microbial pathogens, and gene expression.

Multiplex Ligation–Dependent Probe Amplification

Multiplex ligation–dependent probe amplification (MLPA) is a technique used to detect CNVs, abnormal methylation patterns, and even single-nucleotide changes in genomic DNA samples. It is a multiplex PCR-based assay that uses pairs of target-specific oligonucleotides that are ligated (joined) and amplified only when positioned directly adjacent to each other. The resulting amplicons are discriminated by size and analyzed via capillary electrophoresis. MLPA requires careful optimization to avoid PCR bias and to ensure appropriate amplicon size differences. Data from patient samples must always be compared against reference samples. MLPA technology has successfully been leveraged to evaluate cases of Beckwith-Wiedemann syndrome, cystic fibrosis, and α-thalassemia, among other genetic disorders.

V. SEQUENCE ANALYSIS BY SANGER SEQUENCING

Cycle sequencing is similar to conventional PCR in that it employs a thermostable DNA polymerase and a temperature cycling format for DNA denaturation, annealing, and enzymatic DNA synthesis. However, only one primer (the sequencing primer) is added to the reaction mixture. The **dye terminator cycle sequencing method** for direct DNA sequencing, a derivative of so-called Sanger sequencing, is currently the most widely used cycle sequencing method for DNA sequence analyses. This technique (e-Figure 34.2-4) utilizes synthetic oligonucleotide primers complementary to a known sequence of the template strand to be analyzed and is greatly simplified by the use of fluorescently labeled, chain-terminating dideoxynucleotide triphosphates. As initially described, enzymatic extension of the primer was performed only once per sequencing reaction, but the utility of the method is greatly increased by a modification known as cycle sequencing (or linear amplification sequencing). This method can be used to effectively sequence 800 to 1,000 bases of a single stand of high-quality DNA. Tiled primers in forward and reverse orientations are often employed to cover large genes with this technique.

VI. IDENTITY DETERMINATION

Although the advantages of DNA-based identification analysis have been most widely publicized in forensics and parentage studies, this testing also has a role in the routine practice of surgical pathology, including resolution of specimen identity issues (*Am J Clin Pathol*. 2011;135:132), differentiation of synchronous and metachronous tumors from metastases, evaluation of tumors in transplant recipients, evaluation of bone marrow engraftment, diagnosis of hydatidiform moles (e-Figure 34.2-5), and demonstration of natural chimerism.

PCR-based approaches for DNA typing have greatly expanded the range of testing because they require such small amounts of DNA and can be performed on fresh, fixed, or even partially degraded specimens. Virtually all DNA typing is currently performed using short tandem repeats (STRs), which are short repetitive DNA sequences that vary in size but are stably maintained in the germline. Because these loci are highly polymorphic, and an individual may be homozygous (have only one allele) or heterozygous (have two different alleles) at each STR locus, the likelihood that two individuals chosen at random will have the same STR profile is extremely low. In practical application, STR-based typing utilizes a core set of loci chosen by the

Federal Bureau of Investigation of the United States, known as the Combined DNA Index System (CODIS). Commercial kits for either monoplex or multiplex PCR amplification of CODIS loci have greatly simplified STR typing and made the method accessible to most molecular genetic laboratories.

Short Tandem Repeat Chimerism for Bone Marrow Engraftment

The most common use of STR testing is in the analysis of chimerism following bone marrow transplant (BMT). In this setting, the recipient's hematopoietic complement of immune cells are completely replaced with donor-derived hematopoietic stem cells. While clinical indications for such transplantation vary from treating a malignant process (eg, AML, ALL) to correcting a germline disease (eg, SCID, Sickle cell disease), monitoring of donor cell engraftment is critical to guiding clinical management. If the donor and recipient have different alleles, those "informative" loci can used for chimerism analysis (e-Figure 34.2-6). At least three such informative loci are minimally required for chimerism analysis, but additional loci are helpful. In this method, PCR is performed using a mixture of labeled primers whose amplicons differ by size. The products are separated via capillary electrophoresis, and peaks corresponding to known alleles are identified. Chimerism levels are quantified by calculating the peak height (or area) of donor alleles and dividing by the sum of the height (or area) of donor and recipient alleles at that locus. The sensitivity of such a calculation approaches 2% if optimized correctly. For sex-mismatched transplants, the accuracy of STR testing closely matches with XY FISH results.

Advantages of Short Tandem Repeat Chimerism Analysis

While bone marrow specimens can be used to determine the levels of chimerism in that compartment, peripheral blood obtained through simple venipuncture can be more easily monitored and is equally sensitive for chimerism analysis. This is because the circulating leukocytes are derived directly from the bone marrow compartment and faithfully reproduce any chimerism present. In case lineage-specific chimerism is desired, peripheral blood samples can be further purified into T cell, B cell, NK cell, and myeloid components prior to STR analysis.

Challenges of Short Tandem Repeat Chimerism Analysis

The overlap of STR profiles from biologically related recipient-donor pairs can decrease the number of unique informative loci to assess chimerism. Fortunately, unless identical twins are paired, most combinations will have at least three informative loci. Calculations can become complex when one allele is shared between the pair, and the shared allele is homozygous in one of the individuals. Another limitation is noted when allele sizes are different by only one repeat, leading to the phenomenon of "stuttering" (e-Figure 34.2-6), where a minor peak one base smaller than and adjacent to the main peak appears due to polymerase slippage during amplification. Multiple transplants after incomplete graft failure can lead to emergence of complicated chimerism profiles, which can also be difficult to assess. Certain diseases, such as myelodysplastic syndrome (MDS), lead to partial chromosome loss, reinforcing the practice that all available data, including cytogenetic findings, should be incorporated into STR reports whenever possible. Finally, if the recipient's pretransplant DNA is not available for comparison, either buccal swab or skin punch fibroblasts may be requested as a surrogate. However, buccal swab DNA can be "contaminated" with host leukocytes.

VII. CLONALITY ASSAYS

Demonstration that the cells in a lesion share a common genetic alteration can be used to support classification as a neoplasm rather than as a polyclonal reactive process, although it is important to emphasize that clonal neoplasms are not necessarily malignant. Most clonality testing is migrating to assays performed via next-generating sequencing (NGS), but PCR-based testing is still used in some settings.

Assays Based on Immunoglobulin and T-Cell Receptor Genes

Most PCR clonality assays performed clinically are used to assess lymphoid infiltrates based on evaluation of immunoglobulin gene or T-cell receptor gene rearrangements. PCR primer design is an important component of these assays, because generation of immunoglobulin and T-cell receptors involves deletions, template-independent nucleotide additions, and single base pair changes. Consensus primers are designed to bind to conserved sequence regions, and multiple sets of primers are used in order to ensure that a broad range of rearrangements can be detected. Demonstration of a monoclonal or oligoclonal population of cells within an infiltrate is very often, but not always, indicative of malignancy since oligoclonal or monoclonal gene rearrangements may characterize reactive lymphoid proliferations.

Although PCR methods have traditionally been used for analysis, NGS methods have higher sensitivity and couple the identification of rearrangements with sequence-specific information. Consequently, NGS is replacing PCR in routine clinical use (see Chapter 34.3).

Clonality Assays Based on Specific Gene Mutations

This class of assays focuses on detection of specific mutations in individual genes, including single base pair changes and larger scale structural changes (such as deletions or insertions of viral genomes). Such analyses can be useful when attempting to show that two neoplasms represent independent synchronous tumors rather than one tumor with metastases.

SUGGESTED READING

Pfeifer JD. *Molecular Genetic Testing in Surgical Pathology*. Lippincott Williams & Wilkins; 2006.

34.3 Next-Generation Sequencing

Bijal A. Parikh, Robert Christopher Bell, and John D. Pfeifer

The high throughput of massively parallel sequencing methods (also known as next-generation sequencing methods or simply NGS), coupled with their low cost and high accuracy, makes them ideally suited for the analysis of patient specimens in clinical settings where diagnosis, prognosis, or choice of therapy requires the information about the presence of mutations in several different areas of the same gene, and/

or in several different genes.[1] Enthusiasm for the use of NGS is due to the fact that NGS can be used to comprehensively evaluate multiple genetic loci, the exome, and even the whole genome, when only a limited quantity of DNA is available for testing (which is of critical importance, given the increasing number of targeted chemotherapy drugs, which requires analysis of an ever-increasing number of genes, while ever smaller tissue specimens are available for testing—a result of current trends to shift from large excisional biopsies to needle or aspiration biopsies for diagnosis).

The genetic complexity of neoplasms underscores the importance of NGS's capability to evaluate the full spectrum of sequence variations in dozens to thousands of genes in a single assay. The genomes of cancer cells carry somatic (often referred to as acquired) alterations that fall into four general classes: **single nucleotide variants (SNVs), small insertions and deletions (indels,** which are generally less than a few dozen bases long), **copy number variants (CNVs),** and **structural variants (SVs,** such as translocations). Some of the mutations are so-called driver mutations because they confer selective clonal growth advantage or evasion from apoptosis and are casually involved in oncogenesis, others of which are so-called passenger mutations since they do not contribute to the development of cancer but are secondary changes with little diagnostic or therapeutic importance.

Identifying somatic driver mutations has several direct clinical applications. First, the pattern of mutations itself can be diagnostic. Second, somatic mutations can be used to predict how a patient may respond to a drug with respect to toxicity or efficacy. For example, alterations in exon 19 of *EGFR* in patients with non-small-lung cancer (NSCLC) are responsive to treatment with gefitinib, and the majority of patients with NSCLC or lung adenocarcinoma who carry inversions in *ALK* or a translocation in *ROS1* respond to treatment with crizotinib; in contrast, somatic mutations in *KRAS* predict resistance to therapy with tyrosine kinase inhibitors (TKIs) in NSCLC. Third, somatic mutations can provide prognostic information on the risk of disease progression or relapse. For example, an internal tandem duplication in the *FLT3* gene is associated with a poor prognosis in acute myeloid leukemia (AML) while mutations in nucleophosmin (*NPM1*) are associated with a favorable prognosis.

NGS tests can target a panel of genes (from several genes to several hundred genes), the exome, or the entire genome. However, as with all lab tests, the utility of the various assays is extremely dependent on the clinical setting. While clinical utility has been defined for only a few thousand different mutations in a few hundred genes, sequence analysis of the exome or entire genome is nonetheless often performed because the cost is so low, and because of the potential value of detection of unanticipated sequence variants. Laboratory testing guidelines and recommendations from both professional societies and regulatory agencies have been developed to assist in the design and performance of clinical NGS-based testing (see Table 34.2-1).

I. NGS METHODOLOGIES

Amplification-Based Methods

Similar to polymerase chain reaction (PCR), amplification-based NGS methods rely on exponential amplification of the target region using sequencing-specific primers.

---

[1] This chapter draws from Pfeifer JD, Humphrey PA, Ritter JH, Dehner LP eds. *The Washington Manual of Surgical Pathology.* 3rd ed. Lippincott Williams & Wilkins; 2020.

TABLE 34.3-1 Features of Common NGS Platforms

Platform	Read Length	Accuracy	Run Time	Bases per Run	Cost[a]	Sequencing Chemistry	Advantages	Disadvantages
Illumina (eg, MiSeq, HiSeq, NovaSeq, NextSeq)	50-600 bp	99.9%	1-11 d[b]	Up to $1,500 \times 10^9$	$5-$150	Reversible terminator	High throughput	Platforms are expensive; long TAT.
Thermo Fisher Scientific (eg, Ion GeneStudio S5, Ion Torrent Genexus)	Up to 600 bp	Up to 99.6%	4-5 h	Up to 10×10^9	$60-$750	Synthesis	Platforms are less expensive; short TAT	Homopolymer errors
PacBio	Up to >10^5	87%	1-2 h	Up to 200×10^9	$10-$40	Synthesis	Short TAT; detects methylated bases	Platform is expensive.
Nanopore	Up to >10^6	Up to 97%	2-3 d	Depends on read length	Up to $100	Membrane pore	Very long reads	Low throughput

NGS, next-generation sequencing; TAT, turnaround time.
[a]Cost per billion bases.
[b]Depends on read length.

Compared to other methods, amplification-based NGS has a relatively simpler workflow with highly reduced hands-on time and more rapid turnaround time.

1. **Workflow**
   a. **Sample collection:** This form of NGS can be performed on a variety of samples including fresh tissue, formalin fixed paraffin embedded (FFPE) tissue, fine needle aspiration samples, blood and bone marrow samples, buccal swaps, and cell pellets (*J Mol Diagn*. 2013;15:234). The highest-quality DNA is generally obtained from fresh and snap-frozen specimens (*J Mol Diagn*. 2013;15:623).
   b. **Nucleic acid preparation:** Before amplification can occur, the DNA and RNA are isolated from the sample. There are numerous methods available, automated or manual, to accomplish the step. It is important to assess the purity, integrity, and concentration of the nucleic acids before proceeding to subsequent steps. This can be accomplished through several methods, but spectrophotometry or fluorometry are the two most common.
   c. **Target enrichment:** Once the DNA or RNA is isolated, the samples need to be enriched for the regions of interest. This step is typically performed via multiplex PCR via the use of sequencing-specific primers. Regarding the primers, primer design is a very important component of assay design in order to capture desired regions while reducing sequencing errors and amplification bias.
   d. **Library preparation:** The preceding three steps are relatively similar across NGS platforms. Library preparation, however, is dependent on the platform being utilized. In this step, the post-PCR amplicons are ligated with oligonucleotide adapters that are specific to the NGS platform. Most modern applications use unique molecular identifier (UMI) adapters (often called "barcodes"), which allow for the multiplexing of specimens during a single run. This step also requires various purification steps to eliminate adapter dimers and other undesired sequences.
   e. **Library amplification:** A consequence of library preparation, mostly through purification steps, is the reduction in available DNA. To counteract this phenomenon, a limited amplification step occurs, which results in a fully double-stranded library containing only sequences with adapters complementary to the corresponding substrate adapters of the assay.
   f. **Massively parallel sequencing:** The final step in the process is massively parallel sequencing of the final amplified library. The two most commonly used platforms are Ion Torrent (Thermo Fisher Scientific) and Illumina (Illumina Inc.). Although the technologies and chemistries differ (Table 34.3-1), the end result is the generation of billions of individual base-pair data points.
2. **Advantages:** Amplification-based methods have several advantages. A major advantage is the rapid turnaround time compared to other sequencing methods. This method allows for the generation of results within a matter of hours to days instead of weeks. This method also has the advantage of multiplexing, which allows for the processing of multiple specimens within a single run. Additionally, this method is relatively simpler with less hands-on preparation time compared to more complicated and labor-intensive methods.
3. **Disadvantages:** One of the biggest disadvantages is the limit on the size of the target region due to practical issues with the number of PCR reactions that can be multiplexed in a single amplification. Second, only a subset of variant types can be detected; generally, only SNVs and small indels can be identified, while larger CNVs and SVs are more challenging. Third, as with other amplification-based tests, amplification bias, polymerase sequencing errors, contamination, and primer

binding artifacts are potential problems. This is one reason why good primer design is an important step in assay development. Fourth, amplification-based NGS requires prior knowledge of the sequence and nature of the mutations to be targeted. This method precludes the identification of novel disease-associated mutations outside the targeted regions.

Hybrid Capture–Based Methods

Hybrid capture–based NGS is a sensitive and specific method of detecting somatic alterations by utilizing DNA and RNA probes and complementary base pairing of nucleotides to capture target regions of interest. If designed appropriately, this method of NGS can detect all four classes of somatic alterations (ie, SNPs, indels, SNVs, and CNVs).

1. **Capture bait design:** The design of the capture baits (probes) is a key element in the development of a hybrid capture assay. The optimal length of the baits is largely dictated by the size of the DNA fragments within the genomic library. Generally, shorter fragments are captured at a higher frequency and specificity compared to longer ones. Overlap of the capture probes is another critical design choice as it increases the enrichment efficiency of target regions.
2. **Workflow**
   a. **Sample collection:** Specimen requirements and collection are similar to amplification-based methods.
   b. **Nucleic acid preparation:** Before library preparation can begin, the DNA needs to be fragmented. This is usually accomplished by sonication, nebulization, or endonuclease digestion.
   c. **Library preparation:** The first step of library preparation involves ligating platform-specific oligonucleotide adapters to the 3′ tail of the DNA fragments. Similar to amplification-based NGS, the adapters can be indexed to allow for multiplexing specimens. Following purification steps and prehybridization PCR, the capture probes are hybridized to the fragments and incubated for 24 to 72 hours. The final step is eluting the hybridized fragments.
   d. **Posthybridization amplification:** A limited number of PCR cycles are usually required after library preparation to optimize the number of fragments for sequencing.
   e. **Massively parallel sequencing:** The final step in the process is massively parallel sequencing of the final amplified library. The most commonly used platforms for captured-based NGS are Ion Torrent and Illumina. Although newer alternative technologies and chemistries are emerging, the end result is the generation of billions of individual base-pair data points.
3. **Advantages:** The biggest advantage of hybrid capture is the ability to capture larger target regions more easily. Additionally, this method enables the detection of all four classes of somatic alterations, including SNVs and CVs.
4. **Disadvantages:** Compared with amplification-based methods, hybrid capture requires longer and more labor-intensive library preparation. A typical library takes between 3 and 5 days (compared to 1 day for amplification-based NGS), with a large proportion allocated to probe hybridization. Ultimately, this results in a longer overall turnaround time. Hybrid capture is also sensitive to base composition (low or very high guanine–cytosine [GC] content) and areas of high homology (repetitive regions, tandem repeats, and pseudogenes), which can result in inefficient capture and coverage. This is problematic since many disease-associated

target regions are GC-rich (eg, promoter regions). Additionally, the complexity of hybrid capture can result in more computationally intensive bioinformatics pipelines that can easily overwhelm a laboratory.

II. NGS ASSAY SCOPE/TYPES OF NGS ASSAYS

Targeted Panels

1. **Design:** Panels designed to focus on specifically curated genes or genetic regions are referred to as targeted panels. These panels are typically designed to capture mutations or variants that have well-established literature or guidelines providing evidence for their diagnostics, therapeutic, and/or prognostic value. The panels can be narrowly tailored to specific cancers (only a dozen or so genes) or more broadly (hundreds of genes) across multiple diseases or malignancies. For the most part, targeted panels have been the mainstay in hematopathology NGS testing.
2. **Advantages:** The biggest advantage is in the sequencing depth of targeted panels. Amplifying specific regions allows for more parallel sequencing across the flow cell, given a constant set of flow cell primers. This has the effect of increasing the number of reads that align with the targeted gene, which increases the analytical sensitivity and the ability to detect variants with lower variant allele fractions (VAFs). Targeted panels also allow for increased multiplexing of specimens, which increases efficiency and decreases cost. Additionally, targeted panels are more likely to be reimbursed and thus more likely to be financially beneficial. Decreasing the number of targets (more focused panels) decreases the number of distracting variants of unknown significance (VUS), decreases incidental findings, simplifies the workflow, and improves turnaround time.
3. **Disadvantages:** Targeted panels can only identify alterations that are within the genes targeted and are therefore limited in their ability to identify more novel variants or variants in other genes. Additionally, targeted panels are more complicated to design and require more assay preparation when compared to whole exome (WE) or whole genome (WG) methods.

WE and WG

1. **Design:** As opposed to targeted panels, WE and WG are targeted to the whole set of exomes or the whole genome (exons plus introns). These assays are more tailored for the identification of novel/unknown variants that may or may not be associated with specific diseases or cancers. These assays also allow for the detection of CNVs and SVs.
2. **Advantages:** Up until relatively recently, the use of WE and WG in the clinical setting has been relatively limited. With the improvements in assay design, computational power, and more sophisticated informatics tools and pipelines, these assays have started to become more widely used in the clinical setting. One of the biggest advantages is the ability to detect structural changes (SV and CNVs) in addition to somatic alterations. While not having the same depth of coverage as more targeted panels, these assays are able to give a more global perspective of disease, and both WE (*Br J Haematol.* 2020;188:367) and WG (*N Engl J Med.* 2021;384:924) have the potential to supplant more traditional methods such as chromosomal analysis (karyotype) and fluorescence in situ hybridization (FISH).

WE and WG preparation is also simpler compared to targeted panels, which require probe design, more complex library preparation, and increased technologist time.
3. **Disadvantages:** First, sequencing more of the genome comes at the expense of sequencing depth, and as such, these assays are less analytically sensitive compared to targeted panels. Given this information, WE and WG have limited use in disease monitoring (such as minimal residual disease [MRD] analysis) and are best utilized at initial diagnosis. Second, there is still debate on the utility of sequencing genes without established clinical significance. This has the byproduct of increasing the number of VUS identified in addition to causing issues in reimbursement. Third, compared to targeted panels, WE and WG require substantially more bioinformatics analysis and electronic storage space, given the larger amount of sequencing that is performed. Newer technologies, such as Illumina's DRAGEN platform, have improved processing and analyzing time, but this issue should still be considered when deciding to develop a WG or WE assay.

III. BIOINFORMATICS

NGS tests are somewhat unique in that the analytic portion of the test itself consists of three individual components, specifically the sequence platform itself; the so-called wet bench procedures that are involved in the DNA library preparation; and the bioinformatics associated with the identification of sequence variants, which include reference genome alignment, variant identification, and variant annotation.

The general features of the bioinformatics analysis of neoplasms are similar to those for constitutional testing. After the sequencing reads are generated from the DNA extracted from a specimen, software tools are used to align the reads against a reference genome and identify differences between the specimen sequence and the reference. Maximum clinical utility of tumor specimen sequencing is achieved using a bioinformatic pipeline designed to detect all four classes of genomic variants (ie, SNVs, indels, CNVs, and SVs) at allele frequencies that are physiologically relevant. The four main classes of variants each require different computational approaches for sensitive and specific identification (assuming the assay is designed to permit their detection), and since various bioinformatics pipelines are known to yield different variant calls for the various classes of variants, and even for specific variants, optimization of the pipeline used for a clinical NGS test is necessary.

Alignment

A typical NGS run produces millions to billions of individual sequence reads that are largely meaningless on their own. To make the NGS assay meaningful, one of the first steps after sequencing is the process of assembling and aligning (mapping) the reads to the reference genome. Dozens of alignment algorithms have been designed (eg, Bowtie, Novoalign, Isaac), each with its own set of strengths, so deciding on the proper tool is largely at the discretion of the laboratory developing the assay. While traditionally a bottleneck in the bioinformatics process, advances in parallel and threaded computational tools (programmable gate arrays, graphic processing units, etc) have greatly sped up the alignment process. The aligner takes in an FASTQ (or sometimes FASTA) file containing the raw reads and outputs and alignment file [sequence alignment map (SAM), binary alignment map (BAM), compressed reference-oriented alignment map (CRAM)].

Variant Identification (Also Known as Variant Calling)

Following alignment, calling algorithms (eg, SAMtools, VarScan, Pindel) are used to identify specific variants or alterations based on the difference between the sequence reads and the reference genome. Most NGS pipelines utilize several callers, given that callers are generally tailored to specific variant types. For example, VarScan 2 is used for somatic SNVs whereas Pindel is largely used for indels. There are also callers designed for both structural alterations and copy number variant detection. Additionally, most pipelines utilized various filtering mechanisms that further refine the called variants depending on base quality, mapping quality, strand bias, and other metrics.

A calling algorithm's ability to identify variants is impacted by two primary factors: library complexity and depth of coverage.

1. **Library complexity:** The number of independent DNA template molecules (sometimes referred to as genome equivalents) sequenced in an NGS assay has a profound impact on the sensitivity and specificity of variant detection. Although it is possible to perform NGS analysis on picogram quantities of DNA (*Cancer Res.* 2013;73:2965; *Nat Methods.* 2014;11:18), this technical feat is accomplished by simply increasing the number of amplification cycles during library preparation. However, the information content in 1,000 sequence reads derived from one genome is quite different than the information content present in 1,000 sequence reads from 1,000 different genomes. Thus, it is essential to distinguish sequence reads that trace back to DNA molecules that were present in the original specimen (unique sequence reads) from duplicate reads, since duplicate reads can skew the bioinformatics pipeline and cause failures to detect sequence variants present in the original specimen, over- or underrepresentation of particular variants, and/or false positive variant calls resulting from PCR errors that are propagated through library preparation and sequencing.
   a. Duplicate sequence reads are easily recognized in the context of WG shotgun or hybrid capture–based NGS assays since by these methods input DNA is randomly fragmented during library preparation. Unique sequence reads are unlikely to be identical to one another and duplicate reads are easily identified based on shared mapping coordinates.
   b. In the setting of amplicon-based NGS, all reads derived from a given amplicon (those amplified from the same PCR primer set) are identical, so identifying duplicate reads is not straightforward. Of the many methods to address this issue, one of the best is to ligate UMI adapters to input DNA molecules prior to library construction because sequence reads with identical UMIs can be counted as duplicates in the bioinformatic pipeline since they were derived from the same input molecule. Unfortunately, because UMI-based methods add a layer of cost and complication to both library construction and bioinformatic analyses, they have not been uniformly adopted in the clinical setting. Many product manufacturers and laboratories tout amplicon-based assays with low DNA input in the absence of methods that facilitate the tracking of unique versus duplicate reads, which is problematic since it has been shown that library complexity is negatively affected in ways that are not consistent or predictable (*J Mol Diagn.* 2020;22:720) when DNA input is reduced.
2. **Depth of coverage:** Coverage is defined as the number of reads aligned to a given nucleotide position. Depth of coverage (DOC) or read depth is the average

number of times a given genomic position is covered by a read sequence. A sufficient DOC is a critical component of an NGS assay, especially for detecting somatic variants within a specimen sampled from a tumor. It's important to understand that tumor samples have a heterogeneous mixture of malignant cells, inflammatory cells, stromal cells, and uninvolved tissue which has the effect of diluting the pathogenic variants. The relationship between the detection of a specific variant from a sample and the DOC is relatively straightforward in that a higher number of unique sequence reads lends confidence to the base changes at a given location. In addition, higher depth makes an assay more sensitive for detecting low-level variants, which is especially important in MRD applications or stem cell transplant monitoring.

The DOC required to make accurate variant calls is also dependent on the type of variant being evaluated and whether the variant is germ line or somatically acquired (in general, a lower DOC is acceptable for constitutional testing where germ line alterations are more easily identified since they are in either a heterozygous or homozygous state). For NGS of mitochondrial DNA, an average coverage of greater than 20,000 is required to reliably detect heteroplasmic variants present at 1.5% (*Genet Med.* 2013;15:388).

There are several additional technical factors that can influence the DOC.

a. **Sequence complexity:** More complex sequences are more unique across the genome and thus are more likely to align to a specific part of the reference genomes. In contrast, target regions with high homology, a higher number of repeated sequence elements (eg, GC repeats), and pseudogenes often have coverage issues due to alignment artifacts.
b. **Target enrichment methods:** The chosen method for target enrichment can affect the DOC. Generally, amplification-based methods have higher depth compared to hybrid capture methods.
c. **Multiplexing:** The addition of multiple samples to a single flow cell has the effect of diluting the number of flow cell primers available to each sample's sequence. Additionally, in a similar fashion, larger target regions can decrease the overall DOC.

Annotation

In general terms, annotation in genomic studies is the act of adding explanatory information to the identified variants. When NGS was first used in clinical settings, this process was time-consuming and difficult, given the large number of novel variants that were being identified for the first time. Fortunately, this process has become more manageable, given the availability of public resources and databases detected for this task (Tables 34.3-2 and 34.3-3). Using these resources in combination with various classification guidelines (see later text), reporting the clinical significance of specific variants has become significantly easier.

IV. REPORTING

Variant Allele Frequency

The variant allele frequency or allelic fraction (VAF) is the relative frequency (expressed as fraction or percentage) at which a specific variant/mutation occurs at a given genomic position. For constitutional or germ line alterations, it is equivalent to the number of

TABLE 34.3-2 Selected Reference Databases and Datasets for Human Variation

Name/URL	Overview
International HapMap Project http://hapmap.ncbi.nlm.nih.gov/	International collaboration to assess common variation in multiple populations and identify haplotype blocks
1,000 Genomes Project http://www.1000genomes.org/	International collaboration to assess common variation in multiple populations using NGS approaches
NHLBI GO Exome Sequencing Project (ESP) https://esp.gs.washington.edu/drupal/	Multicenter collaboration using NGS approaches to identify variation in exomes; includes rich phenotypic data
dbSNP (Database of Short Genetic Variations) http://www.ncbi.nlm.nih.gov/snp	Archive of short (<50 bp) sequence variants; includes both common and rare variants, both germ line and somatic
dbVar http://www.ncbi.nlm.nih.gov/dbvar	Archive of longer (>50 bp) sequence variants; includes copy number changes and complex rearrangements
gnomAD (Genome Aggregation Database) https://gnomad.broadinstitute.org/	Comprehensive database of human genetic variation, containing >141,000 exomes and 15,000 genomes from diverse global populations

bp, base pair; NGS, next-generation sequencing.

TABLE 34.3-3 Selected Databases and Datasets for Variants in the Context of Phenotype

Resource	Content
OMIM http://omim.org/	Subset of variants in genes reported in human phenotypes and genes; curated from the published literature
dbGaP http://www.ncbi.nlm.nih.gov/gap	Archive of studies and datasets of genotype and phenotype; provides both unrestricted and controlled forms of access
ClinVar http://ncbi.nlm.nih.gov/clinvar/	Archive of submitted interpretations of medically related variants

(*continued*)

TABLE 34.3-3 Selected Databases and Datasets for Variants in the Context of Phenotype (*continued*)

Resource	Content
HGMD http://www.hgmd.org/	Collation of published genetic germ line variation in nuclear genes underlying or associated with human inherited disease; public and professional versions
HGVS Locus Specific Mutation Databases http://www.hgvs.org/dblist/glsdb.html	Aggregation of gene-specific databases of observed variation
COSMIC—Catalogue of somatic mutations in cancer http://cancer.sanger.ac.uk/cancergenome/projects/cosmic/	Curated catalogue of genes that undergo somatic mutation in human cancers, supported by the Wellcome Trust Sanger Institute. Contains information on neoplasms and other related samples, with somatic mutation frequencies. Data are extracted and curated from the primary literature.
The Cancer Genome Atlas (TCGA) http://cancergenome.nih.gov/abouttcga/overview	Comprehensive effort to accelerate the understanding of the molecular basis of cancer through the application of genome analysis technologies
GeneReviews http://www.ncbi.nlm.nih.gov/books/NBK1116/	Expert-authored, peer-reviewed disease descriptions presented in a standardized format, focused on clinically relevant and medically actionable information on the diagnosis, management, and genetic counseling of specific inherited conditions
PharmGKB http://www.pharmgkb.org/	Collects, curates, and disseminates information about the impact of human genetic variation on drug responses
GTEx (The Genotype-Tissue Expression [GTEx] project) browser http://www.ncbi.nlm.nih.gov/gtex/test/GTEX2/gtex.cgi/	Resource database and associated tissue bank for study of the relationship between genetic variation and gene expression in human tissues

chromosomes that carry an allele over the total population of the sample. Typically, this means approximately 0.5 (50%) or 1.0 (100%) for heterozygous or homozygous alterations, respectively. For somatic alterations, the VAF ranges from 0 (0%) to 1.0 (100%) depending on the number of malignant cells that carry the variant.

Variant Classification

Variant classification or identification is a critical component of variant interpretation as it is an indication of the clinical significance of a particular variant. Classification schemes are dependent on the type of alteration (germ line vs somatic) and on clinical or experimental evidence. Germ line variants are largely based on the pathogenicity of the particular variant and follow the American College of Medicine Genetics and Genomics (ACMG) and Association for Molecular Pathology (AMP) guidelines (*Genet Med.* 2015;17:405). Somatic alterations, on the other hand, focus on the variant's impact on clinical care including therapeutic, prognostic, diagnostic, and preventative importance. A set of guidelines created as part of a joint consensus between the American Society of Clinical Oncology (ASCO), AMP, and College of American Pathologists (CAP) is the primary tool used for somatic variant interpretation (*J Mol Diagn.* 2017;19:4).

Tier I—Variants of Strong Clinical Significance: This is the highest variant level and indicates strong evidence for the therapeutic, prognostic, and diagnostic significance of the variant. This is separated into two levels, A and B, depending on the type of evidence available.

Level A: Variants (or biomarkers) that predict response or resistance to US Food and Drug Administration (FDA)-approved therapies for a specific tumor type. Additionally, this level includes variants included as part of professional guidelines that define the variant as diagnostic or prognostic for a specific tumor type.

Level B: Variants (or biomarkers) that have been described to predict response or resistance to therapies as part of well-powered studies with consensus from experts in the field.

Tier II—Variants of Potential Clinical Significance: This tier is designed for variants that don't meet tier I guidance but appear to have the potential for being of clinical importance. This tier is further separated into levels C and D.

Level C: Variants that predict response or resistance to FDA-approved therapies for a different tumor type than the one being analyzed. These variants are also often included as part of clinical trials. This level can also be reached if several smaller studies have demonstrated the potential significance of the variant on prognosis or diagnosis.

Level D: Variants that show plausible therapeutic significance based on small studies, preclinical studies, or case reports.

Tier III—VUS: This tier is for variants that do not meet the criteria for Tier I/II or have not been demonstrated to be benign in nature. This tier usually includes novel or unique variants that have not been previously reported in population databases or the literature. Variants that fall in this category might have clinical significance, but evidence is generally lacking.

Tier IV—Benign or likely benign variants: This tier includes variants that are frequently reported in the general population and/or that have been demonstrated to be clinically insignificant.

V. RNA SEQUENCE ANALYSIS

Sequence analysis of RNA makes it possible to detect a broader range of normal variants and pathogenic changes than analysis of DNA, including the identification of changes in the coding sequences of genes (eg, SNVs and indels); alterations that occur outside of coding regions (eg, translocations within introns that cause gene fusions); changes in the level of gene expression; patterns of gene splicing; and changes in posttranscriptional modifications. RNA sequence analysis also makes it possible to evaluate populations of small noncoding RNAs that have an impact on cell growth and differentiation (eg, siRNA and miRNA).

Although other molecular methods can be used to directly or indirectly sequence RNA (including reverse transcription polymerase chain reaction [RT-PCR], quantitative RT-PCR, FISH, and microarrays), NGS approaches offer significant advantages (*J Hematol Oncol.* 2020;13:166). First, RNA sequencing via NGS (often referred to as RNAseq) can be used to address changes in a subset of RNA molecules in targeted panels or in the entire transcriptome. Second, RNAseq can be used with solid tissue, blood, or body fluids; with single cells; and for the analysis of cell-free RNA (cfRNA) (as discussed in more detail later).

Whole transcriptome analysis is frequently used for the evaluation of clinical specimens because it is comprehensive. It can be used to detect sequence variants, evaluate levels of gene expression through transcript abundance, and elucidate patterns of splicing. Whole transcriptome sequencing also has the advantage of providing information on the entire RNA landscape without a need for prior knowledge of abnormalities characteristic of a specific disease or tumor type. However, whole transcriptome analysis requires an extremely robust bioinformatic pipeline. From a technical perspective, since some transcripts are present at very low abundance, it is not well suited for all clinical assays. Consequently, targeted RNAseq assays are frequently used for the evaluation of clinical specimens. Targeted assays can be designed that evaluate from several dozen to several hundred transcripts at the same time in the same assay.

RNAseq Workflow

1. RNA is **isolated** from the specimen, followed by treatment with deoxyribonuclease (DNAase) to reduce the amount of DNA present in the sample.
2. The RNA is then **fractionated** to include the subset of RNA molecules to be evaluated (Table 34.3-4). RNA selection usually includes the depletion of rRNA, which typically represents over 90% of total cellular RNA. PolyA selection results in a population of RNA consisting predominantly of mature, processed molecules from coding regions of the DNA.
3. The RNA substrate is **reverse transcribed** to DNA using the enzyme reverse transcriptase, which makes it possible to use DNA-based NGS techniques for library generation and sequencing.

TABLE 34.3-4 Pools of RNA Commonly Used for RNAseq

Type of RNA	Isolation Method	Unprocessed RNA Content	rRNA Content (%)
Total RNA	None	High	80-90
Transcribed RNA[a]	polyA selection	Low	10-20
Transcribed RNA[b]	rRNA depletion	High	<20
Targeted RNA	Hybridization	Variable[c]	<2

[a]polyA selection for mature mRNA does not capture nascent transcripts that do not yet have polyA tails.
[b]rRNA depletion ensures the capture of mature mRNA as well as nascent transcripts (including premature mRNA that still harbors intronic sequences) as well as noncoding RNA such as small interfering RNA (siRNA) and microRNA (miRNA).
[c]Dependent on the target region.

4. **Bioinformatics analysis** of the sequence reads proceeds, in general terms, via a pipeline that parallels that for DNA-based sequencing. However, the complexities of RNA metabolism create the need for additional steps.
   a. The **RNA transcriptome** is assembled via a genome-guided approach that parallels the method used for DNA alignment to a reference genome, although the process is more complicated for RNA because many of the reads are noncontinuous due to splicing and structural changes such as translocations. Alternatively, the RNA reads can be mapped to a reference transcriptome. Several different software tools have been designed to assist assembly via either approach, most of which are optimized for one aspect of alignment, and so, as with the bioinformatics for DNA analysis, most laboratories combine multiple tools to achieve the highest-quality alignment metrics.
   b. Additional bioinformatics analysis is layered on the aligned sequences to detect sequence variants in coding regions such as SNVs and indels; structural changes such as transcripts derived from translocations that create fusion genes; splice variants; and changes in abundance.
   c. As a direct parallel with VUSs in NGS DNA sequence analysis, the significance of observed changes in RNAseq is often uncertain, but with an even further level of uncertainty in that the mechanism underlying the observed change is unknown. As an example, with respect to changes in transcript abundance, the underlying cause could be due to changes in the level of gene promoter activity, gene amplification, and/or transcript stability.

Clinical Assays

1. The clinical utility of RNAseq is well established, and it has become a routine part of the analysis of solid tumors, especially at the time of relapse. Targeted RNAseq approaches have been shown to increase the rate of detection of diagnostically relevant genetic alterations compared with RT-PCR or interphase FISH. RNAseq assays have been shown to be especially useful for detecting novel disease-associated translocations that would not be detected by RT-PCR or interphase FISH approaches (*Nat Commun.* 2019;10:1388; *J Mol Diagn.* 2021;23:1749).
2. In the setting of liquid biopsies, sufficient cfRNA can be obtained from plasma for RNAseq, although the rapid degradation of RNA offers technical challenges. Platelets have been shown to be an excellent source of RNA released due to apoptosis and necrosis of normal and tumor cells. Exosomes have been shown to be another reliable source of cfRNA.
3. Although still largely experimental, single-cell RNAseq has been shown to make it possible to reliably measure the abundance of transcripts of 1,000 to 3,000 expressed genes per cell for over 10,000 cells per assay or of more than 5,000 genes per cell of only about 1,000 cells per assay (*Blood.* 2019;133:1415). RNAseq thus has the sensitivity to not only characterize different cellular states in detail but also to detect rare populations. The approach has been particularly useful for providing novel insights into hematopoietic cell differentiation.

VI. CLONALITY ASSAYS

Demonstration that the cells in a lesion share a common genetic alteration can be used to support classification as a neoplasm rather than as a polyclonal reactive process. However, it is important to emphasize that clonal neoplasms are not necessarily malignant, and conversely, in the setting of analysis of lymphoid infiltrates, demonstration of a monoclonal or oligoclonal population of cells is not always indicative of malignancy since oligoclonal or monoclonal gene rearrangements may characterize reactive lymphoid proliferations.

Assays Based on Immunoglobulin or T-Cell Receptor Genes

Diagnosis and monitoring of B-cell and T-cell malignancies is routinely accomplished by highly sensitive molecular assays that can assess clonal rearrangements in the immunoglobulin gene (*IGH*) and/or T-cell receptor (*TCR*) loci. Demonstration of a monoclonal or oligoclonal population of cells within a lymphoid infiltrate is very often, but not always, indicative of malignancy, since oligoclonal or monoclonal gene rearrangements may also characterize reactive lymphoid proliferations. While PCR methods have historically been applied for these analyses, NGS allows for even higher sensitivity, coupling identification of rearrangements with sequence-specific information to inform diagnosis of the disease process and enable long-term MRD monitoring. In contrast to PCR, NGS takes advantage of not only amplicon size but also the amplicon's nucleotide sequence. Both Illumina and Ion Torrent sequencers can be used to evaluate *IGH* and *TCR* clonality.

Both B-cell and T-cell clonality assays require very little starting material (50 ng minimum of DNA) and can be performed on fragmented DNA, as long as the largest amplicon size of approximately 400 bases can be amplified. Control reactions are required to ensure adequate fragment lengths are present and that sequencing reactions can discriminate polyclonal (negative control) from known clonal DNA (positive control). Finally, as with most PCR-based assays, it is important to ensure that no cross-contamination has occurred (water or no template control control). With an established clinical workflow, clonality assessment by NGS can be batched and performed over 3 working days.

1. **Evaluation of B-cell clonality**

    Clinical specimens typically include FFPE tissue or bone marrow aspirates. However, any tissue source with a B-cell infiltrate can theoretically be analyzed with this approach. B-cell clonality is commonly assessed on the heavy chain (*IGH*) locus, although light chains (*IGL* or *IGK*) may also be analyzed. Similar to PCR, highly multiplexed primers target the conserved framework regions of the *IGH* locus, allowing sequence analysis across multiple V (V_H) and J (J_H) segments (e-Figure 34.3-1). There are more than 70 V_H segments, 27 diversity segments (D_H), and 6 J_H segments over 250,000 bases in the germ line configuration. Following somatic rearrangement, a stochastic but normal process in individuals with an intact immune system, specific V_H-D_H-J_H segments join with a random number of nucleotides added to the junctions. This process allows the multiplexed primers to generate amplicons only when complementary to sequences in close proximity to each other. Since this process only occurs in a subset of lymphoid cells, it is not necessary to deplete other cells to prevent nonspecific amplification. In a polyclonal process, there is no predominate V_H-D_H-J_H segment in the sample under evaluation. In a clonal process, which may or may not support malignancy, one of these rearrangements may become overrepresented.

    The calculation of the clonally rearranged sequence is expressed as a percentage of total sequenced rearrangements. Alleles are determined via homology to existing sequences in the database (IMGT, the international ImMunoGeneTics information system, http://www.imgt.org). Each laboratory must validate the threshold for reporting a finding as clonal and may range from 2% to 10%. Clonal and polyclonal results can be visualized using either vendor-supplied or in-house-developed tools (e-Figure 34.3-2).

A unique application of *IGH* sequencing is in the evaluation of hypermutation analysis in chronic lymphocytic leukemia (CLL). While the diagnosis of CLL is not dependent on NGS methods, determining if the rearrangement found is germ line or somatically mutated is of prognostic significance. During B-cell development, as the immature lymphocytes migrate through the germinal center, the normal process of somatic hypermutation allows the B-cell affinity to be appropriately tuned. CLL in which hypermutation is present carries a favorable prognosis than nonhypermutated CLL, defined as deviating greater than 2% from the germ line sequence. Before the NGS era, this analysis was much more laborious and fraught with sequencing failures. Finally, the CLL clonal rearrangement can provide detailed information on the stereotype—specific clones commonly rearranged in CLL across different individuals that are associated with prognostic importance.

2. **Evaluation of T-cell clonality**
Similar to B-cell clonality assays, FFPE, bone marrow (BM) aspirates, and even peripheral blood specimens are often assessed for T-cell clonal status. The majority of functional TCR pairs are α-β dimers. However, the process for TCR maturation requires that T-cells first rearrange both δ and γ genes prior to α and β. The δ gene is located within the α gene and is lost during α rearrangements. The β gene is rather large and only recently has it been considered for assessment of TCR clonality. Thus, the γ gene, *TCRG*, is most commonly used to assess TCR clonality and contains 14 V gene segments and 5 J gene segments over 200,000 bases. For both PCR and NGS assays, primers are designed to flank the rearrangement sites, with multiple V-γ and J-γ primer pairs employed. For NGS applications, amplification, library prep, and sequencing data are interpreted (using the IMGT database) and visualized similarly to B-cell clonality assessment (e-Figure 34.3-3).

Unlike B-cells, T-cells do not undergo a process similar to somatic hypermutation. The indications for T-cell clonality can range from investigation of large granular lymphocyte leukemia in peripheral blood specimens to cutaneous T-cell lymphoma (CTCL), including evaluation of mycosis fungoides and Sézary syndrome. For evaluation of CTCL, one or two skin biopsies are routinely submitted as FFPE tissue, along with peripheral blood for evaluation of circulating clonal cells. The diagnosis of CTCL can be challenging early in the disease when an inflammatory picture may predominate and may be indistinguishable from conditions such as eczema. Once established, treatment success can be followed through both clinical response and decreased clonal burden via NGS testing.

Clonality Assays Based on Specific Gene Mutations

This class of assays focuses on the detection of specific mutations in individual genes, including single base-pair changes and larger-scale structural changes (such as deletions or insertions of viral genomes). This type of analysis can be useful when attempting to show that two neoplasms represent independent synchronous tumors rather than one tumor with metastases.

VII. HUMAN LEUKOCYTE ANTIGEN TYPING

A growing trend in clinical evaluation of human leukocyte antigen (HLA) typing for donor-recipient histocompatibility is the use of NGS technologies. Sanger sequencing reveals only the possible nucleotides at a given position, as it is a consensus of all sequence traces. NGS, however, is able to generate allele-specific sequence data, with longer reads able to better "phase" sequence variants, avoiding *cis-trans* ambiguities that have plagued the field. NGS provides broader coverage and higher throughput, thus reducing both cost and turnaround times while providing highly accurate genotype information. Genotypes by NGS have a particular nomenclature displayed as "two-field" or "four-field" typing. The first two fields describe the allele and the version of the protein encoding it, whereas the less commonly used third and fourth fields describe synonymous differences and noncoding region differences, respectively.

Numerous commercial kits have simplified the implementation of HLA NGS in the clinical lab. The approach to sequencing genes at the HLA locus involves a "long-amplicon, short-read" strategy. Initially, DNA from the peripheral blood of a donor and a recipient is isolated and subjected to long-range PCR at the various Class I (HLA-A, B, C) and Class II (HLA-DR, DQ, DP) loci on chromosome 6 (e-Figure 34.3-4). The long amplicons, typically 5 to 6 kb, contain the necessary exons required for distinguishing different alleles. These long amplicons are next fragmented (usually by one or more restriction enzymes) to sizes small enough to sequence on commonly used Ion Torrent or Illumina sequencers, although long-read technology such as Nanopore sequencing has successfully been used in the research setting. Following fragmentation, the workflow is similar to other NGS applications, including library preparation and sequencing. The data are analyzed by comparing them against the known database of HLA alleles (IMGT) and assigning genotypes accordingly. Due to the unbiased approach to HLA typing, NGS technologies have resulted in the rapid discovery of a number of novel HLA alleles with over 25,000 Class I and 10,000 Class II alleles described to date. Using one of several commercial kits, the workflow can be performed in less than 7 hours with a typical turnaround time of 2 days from start to reporting.

VIII. LIQUID BIOPSIES

The term liquid biopsy encompasses a number of minimally invasive approaches for detecting tumor markers from blood and other body fluids and encompasses a number of analytes including formed elements (circulating tumor cells, platelets); extracellular vesicles (exosomes); and extracellular nucleic acids such as cell-free DNA (cfDNA), mRNA (cf mRNA), and miRNA (cf miRNA).

cfDNA

The extracellular nucleic acid that is most often evaluated currently is cfDNA. The majority of cfDNA originates from the nucleus and is packaged as mono- or oligonucleosomes that are present on the surface and in the lumen of vesicles; as such, most cfDNA ranges from about 40 to 200 bp in length (fragments longer than 10 kb are thought to arise from necrotic cells, and fragments shorter than 100 bp are enriched for mitochondrial DNA and bacterial DNA).

1. **Nonneoplastic settings:** cfDNA has been shown to arise from a number of processes including active secretion (eg, expulsion of nuclei by maturing erythroblasts) and release of nuclear DNA by neutrophils (in response to various stimuli). In fact, most cfDNA in healthy individuals is of hematopoietic origin (55% from white blood cells and 30% from erythrocyte progenitors), vascular endothelial cells (~10%), neurons (~2%), and hepatocytes (~1%). Physiologically, cfDNA is present in healthy individuals at 0 to 100 ng/mL but can increase in a number

of nonmalignant pathologic processes such as trauma, diabetes, trauma, sepsis, inflammatory syndromes, after exercise, and in pregnancy (*Cancer Biol Ther.* 2019;20:1057). Finally, it is important to recognize that there is a measurable level of genetic variation in cfDNA in apparently healthy individuals, including the presence of so-called driver mutations as well as passenger mutations in oncogenes. In the setting of hematopathology, this phenomenon is perhaps best illustrated by the somatic mutations that accumulate with age in normal hematopoietic cells that can drive clonal expansions in the absence of dysplasia (referred to as clonal hematopoietic mutations of indeterminate potential, or simply CHIP) (*Ann Oncol.* 2019;30:464).

2. **Neoplastic settings:** In patients with cancer, cfDNA ranges from 0 to 1,000 ng/mL (or more), and the concentration of cfDNA generally correlates with the underlying tumor burden. However, the precise mechanisms responsible for the relationship with tumor burden are complex; the correlation is a reflection of the intricacies of tumor metabolism more so than merely the number of tumor cells or the number of dying tumor cells. Of more importance, it has been shown in a variety of solid tumor cell types that detection of tumor-specific genetic (and epigenetic) changes in cfDNA can be used for disease detection, diagnosis, and prognosis; monitoring response to therapy; and monitoring of MRD. In these settings, the most sensitive and specific approach involves testing focused on specific mutations that have been previously shown to be present in the patient's tumor. It is worth mentioning that, generally, cfDNA should not be used to genotype a tumor since studies comparing paired tumor and plasma samples have shown a significant lack of concordance between the genetic profile obtained from tissue specimens versus cfDNA, with the latter showing less sensitivity, although it is unclear whether the discordance is due to technical artifacts, assay design issues, or the intrinsic biologic heterogeneity of most malignancies (*Arch Path Lab Med.* 2018;142:1242).

   While testing of patient cfDNA has been hindered by a lack of reproducibility, improvements in the methods used to purify cfDNA, timing of sample collection, and application of NGS methodologies have resulted in approaches with sufficient sensitivity and specificity for routine clinical use. In fact, in 2016, the FDA approved the first cfDNA test (for the *EGFR* mutation T790M in plasma of patients with non-small-cell lung cancer) and has more recently approved additional cfDNA tests for a broader range of mutations and indications.

   In the setting of hematopathology, analysis of cfDNA has been used clinically for the detection of tumor-specific mutations for targeted therapy and prediction of prognosis, evaluation of therapeutic efficacy, and MRD detection in acute myeloid leukemia/myelodysplastic syndromes, lymphoma, and multiple myeloma (*Cancers.* 2021;12:2078; *Leukemia.* 2022;36:2151). Further, cfDNA analysis may even have a role in screening for disease, as suggested by the detection of four cases of lymphoma and one case of myelodysplastic syndrome with excess blasts based on evaluation of CNVs via cfDNA in 1,002 individuals over age 64 years with no history of malignancy (*Ann Oncol.* 2019;30:85).

SUGGESTED READINGS

Kulkarni S, Pfeifer JD. *Clinical Genomics: A Guide to Clinical Next Generation Sequencing.* Academic Press; 2015.
Strachan T, Lucassen A. *Genetics and Genomics in Medicine.* 2nd ed. CRC Press; 2022.
Strachan T, Read AP. *Human Molecular Genetics.* 5th ed. Garland Science; 2018.

Index

Note: Page numbers followed by f and t indicate figures and tables, respectively.

A

Acute leukemia/lymphomas, 244–245
Acute leukemias of ambiguous lineage (ALAL), 267–274
   acute undifferentiated leukemia, 274
   with defining genetic abnormalities, 269
      mixed-phenotype acute leukemia with *BCR::ABL1* fusion, 269–271, 269t
      mixed-phenotype acute leukemia with *kmt2a/mll* rearrangement, 271–272
   differential diagnosis, 270–271
   European group of immunological classification of scoring system, 268
   genetic features, 270
   immunophenotypically defined, 273, 273t
   mixed-phenotype acute leukemia, rare types (MPAL-rt), 274
   with other defined genetic alterations, 272–273
   prognosis and treatment, 270
Acute myeloid leukemia (AML), 126–127, 176–196
   classification of, 180
      diagnostic differences, 180–181t
   clinical presentation, 176
   cytochemistry and immunophenotype, 177–178
      complete remission, 178
      CR with incomplete hematologic recovery, 178
      first complete remission, 178
      follow-up marrow assessment, 177
      morphologic leukemia-free state, 177–178
   defined by differentiation, 192–194, 193–194t
   with defining genetic abnormalities, 183–189, 185–186t
   genetic features, 178–179
   International Consensus classification, 180
   morphology, 176–177
   with mutated *TP53,* 192
   myelodysplasia related, 186–191, 190–191t
   not otherwise specified, 192–194
   overview, 176
   treatment, 179–180
      consolidation therapy, 179
      induction therapy, 179
      maintenance, 179
      prognosis, 180
      salvage therapy, 179–180
      types and blast requirements by diagnostic system, 182–183t
   World Health Organization classification, 180
Adipocytes, 9
Adult T-cell leukemia/lymphoma, 399–401
   clinical features, 399
   differential diagnosis, 400–401
   genetic features, 400
   immunophenotype, 400
   morphology, 399–400
   prognosis and treatment, 400
Aggressive NK-cell leukemia, 396–398
   clinical features, 396
   differential diagnosis, 398
   genetic features, 397–398
   immunophenotype, 397
   morphology, 396–397
   prognosis and treatment, 398
   WHO-HAEM5 diagnostic criteria for, 397t
ALAL. *See* Acute leukemias of ambiguous lineage (ALAL)
ALCL. *See* Anaplastic large cell lymphomas (ALCL)
Alder-Reilly anomaly, 52
ALK-positive histiocytosis, 503–505
   clinical features, 504
   differential diagnosis, 505
   genetic features, 505
   immunophenotype, 505
   morphology, 504
   prognosis and treatment, 505
α-Thalassemia, 41
AML. *See* Acute myeloid leukemia (AML)
Anaplastic large cell lymphomas (ALCL), 423–429
   anaplastic lymphoma kinase–negative anaplastic large cell lymphoma, 425–427
      clinical features, 426
      genetic features, 427
      immunophenotype, 426–427
      morphology, 426
      prognosis and treatment, 427
   anaplastic lymphoma kinase–positive anaplastic large cell lymphoma, 423–425

Anaplastic large cell lymphomas (*continued*)
  clinical features, 424
  genetic features, 424
  immunophenotype, 424
  morphology, 424
  prognosis and treatment, 425
  WHO-HAEM5 diagnostic criteria for, 423t
  breast implant–associated anaplastic large cell lymphoma, 427–429
    clinical features, 427–428
    genetic features, 428
    immunophenotype, 428
    morphology, 428
    prognosis and treatment, 429
    staging, 429
Anaplastic lymphoma kinase–negative anaplastic large cell lymphoma, 425–427
  clinical features, 426
  genetic features, 427
  immunophenotype, 426–427
  morphology, 426
  prognosis and treatment, 427
Anaplastic lymphoma kinase–positive anaplastic large cell lymphoma, 423–425
  clinical features, 424
  genetic features, 424
  immunophenotype, 424
  morphology, 424
  prognosis and treatment, 425
  WHO-HAEM5 diagnostic criteria for, 423t
Aplastic anemia, 77–78
Aspergillosis, 72
Aspirate smear, 20
Asplenia, 107
Atypical hemolytic uremic syndrome, 59
Auer rods, 52
Autoimmune disease-associated lymphadenopathy, 93–95
  autoimmune lymphoproliferative syndrome, 95
  rheumatoid arthritis-associated lymphadenopathy, 95
  sarcoidosis lymphadenopathy, 94
  SLE-associated lymphadenopathy, 94
Autoimmune disorder–associated lymphadenopathy, 344
Autoimmune lymphoproliferative syndrome, 95

B

Babesiosis, 71
Bacterial infections, 68–70
  Q fever, 68–69
  syphilis, 70
  Tick-borne illnesses, 70
  tuberculosis, 68
  Whipple disease, 69
B-ALL/LBL. *See* B-lymphoblastic leukemia/lymphoma (B-ALL/LBL)
Basophils, 2t
B-cell lymphoid proliferations and lymphomas, 244
B-cell prolymphocytic leukemia (B-PLL), 279
β-Thalassemia, 41–42
BL. *See* Burkitt lymphoma (BL)
Blastic plasmacytoid dendritic cell neoplasms (BPDCN), 236–238
  clinical features, 236
  differential diagnosis, 238
  genetic features, 238
  immunophenotype, 237
  morphology, 236–237
    bone marrow aspirate and blood smear, 236
    tissue sections, 236–237
  prognosis and treatment, 238
  WHO-HAEM5 diagnostic criteria for, 237t
Blastomycosis, 72
Blood
  cell types, 2–3t
  components, 1
  description of, 1
Blood smears, platelets and, 57
Bloom syndrome, 209
B-lymphoblastic leukemia/lymphoma (B-ALL/LBL), 249–258
  clinical features, 249, 250–251t
  cytochemical stains, 252
  differential diagnosis, 257
    Burkitt lymphoma, 257
    hematogones, 257
  immunophenotype, 252
  molecular classification of, 252–257
  morphology, 251
  overview, 249
  prognosis and treatment, 257
  subtypes, key features of, 252–257, 255–256t
  WHO-HAEM5 diagnostic criteria for, 251t
Bone marrow
  abnormalities in systemic conditions, 68–77
  amyloidosis, 76
  architecture, 3–4
  autoimmune diseases, 76–77

bacterial infections, 68–70
  Q fever, 68–69
  syphilis, 70
  Tick-borne illnesses, 70
  tuberculosis, 68
  Whipple disease, 69
biopsy. *See* Bone marrow biopsy
collagen vascular disorders, 76–77
examination of, 1
failure syndromes, 77–83
  aplastic anemia, 77–78
  Diamond-Blackfan anemia, 81–82
  dyskeratosis congenita, 80–81
  fanconi anemia, 78–80
  inherited, 79t
  Shwachman-Diamond syndrome, 82–83
fungal infections, 71–72
  aspergillosis, 72
  blastomycosis, 72
  coccidioidomycosis, 71–72
  cryptococcosis, 72
  histoplasmosis, 72
  mucormycosis, 72
  paracoccidioidomycosis, 71–72
granuloma formation, etiologies of, 69t
hemophagocytic lymphohistiocytosis, 75–76, 76t
lipid storage disorders, 74–75, 74t
  Fabry disease, 75
  Gaucher disease, 74
  Niemann-Pick disease, 74–75
parasitic and protozoal infections, 70–71
  babesiosis, 71
  filariasis, 71
  leishmaniasis, 70
  malaria, 71
  toxoplasmosis, 71
  trypanosomiasis, 70–71
viral infections, 72–74
  COVID-19, 74
  cytomegalovirus, 73
  Epstein-Barr virus, 73
  HIV/AIDS, 72–73
  parvovirus B19, 73
Bone marrow biopsy, 19f
  approaches, 19–22
    clinical history, 19–20
    complete blood count, 20
  cytogenetics, 20–21
  fluorescence in situ hybridization, 20–21
  immunophenotypic studies, 20
  microscopic examination, 20–21
    aspirate smear, 20
    clot section, 21
    core biopsy, 20–21
    iron stain, 21
    peripheral blood smear, 20
    touch preparation, 20
  molecular studies, 20–21
  procedure, 18
BPDCN. *See* Blastic plasmacytoid dendritic cell neoplasms (BPDCN)
B-PLL. *See* B-cell prolymphocytic leukemia (B-PLL)
Breast implant–associated anaplastic large cell lymphoma, 427–429
  clinical features, 427–428
  genetic features, 428
  immunophenotype, 428
  morphology, 428
  prognosis and treatment, 429
  staging, 429
Burkitt lymphoma (BL), 338–340
  clinical features, 338–339
  differential diagnosis, 340
  genetic features, 340
  immunophenotype, 339
  morphology, 339
  prognosis and treatment, 340
  WHO-HAEM5 diagnostic criteria for, 339t

C

Cancer predisposing syndromes, 204–206t
Capsule, 12
Castleman disease, 92–93, 94t
  hyaline vascular, 92
  idiopathic multicentric Castleman disease, 93
  immunophenotype, 93
  mixed/plasma cell, 93
  unicentric Castleman disease, 93
Castleman disease (CD), 92–93
Cat scratch disease (CSD), 103
CD. *See* Castleman disease (CD)
Chronic lymphocytic leukemia/small lymphocytic lymphoma (CLL/SLL), 275–279
  clinical features, 275
  differential diagnosis, 277–278
    mantle cell lymphoma, 277–278
    monoclonal B-cell lymphocytosis, 277
    small B-cell lymphomas, 278
  disease progression and transformation, 277
  genetic features, 277
  immunophenotype, 276–277
  morphology, 276

Chronic lymphocytic leukemia/small
lymphocytic lymphoma
(*continued*)
bone marrow, 276
lymph nodes and spleen, 276
peripheral blood, 276
prognosis and treatment, 277
prognostic markers in, 278t
Chronic myeloid leukemia (CML), 130
diagnosis and differential diagnosis,
131–133, 132t
genetic features, 131
morphologic and immunophenotypic
features, 130–131
Chronic myelomonocytic leukemia
(CMML), 164–165t, 164–168
clinical features, 165
differential diagnosis, 167–168
genetic features, 167
immunophenotype, 166–167
morphology, 166
prognosis and treatment, 167
Chronic neutrophilic leukemia, 146–147,
146–147t
Classic Hodgkin lymphoma (CHL),
382–385
clinical features, 382–383
differential diagnosis, 385
genetic features, 384–385
immunophenotype, 384
morphology, 384
prognosis and treatment, 385
subtypes of, 383t
WHO-HAEM5 diagnostic criteria for, 383t
CLL/SLL. *See* Chronic lymphocytic
leukemia/small lymphocytic
lymphoma (CLL/SLL)
CML. *See* Chronic myeloid leukemia (CML)
CMML. *See* Chronic myelomonocytic
leukemia (CMML)
CMV. *See* Cytomegalovirus (CMV)
Coccidioidomycosis, 71–72
Cold agglutinin disease, 358–360
clinical features, 359
differential diagnosis, 359–360
genetic features, 359
morphology and immunophenotype, 359
prognosis and treatment, 359
WHO-HAEM5 diagnostic criteria for,
359t
Cooley anemia, 42
Copper, 34
Cords of Billroth, 15
Cortex, 10–12

COVID-19, 74
bone marrow and, 74
Cryptococcosis, 72
CSD. *See* Cat scratch disease (CSD)
Cutaneous and mucocutaneous histiocytoses,
478–480
Cutaneous mastocytosis (CM), 228–230
clinical features, 228–229
genetic features, 229–230
immunophenotype, 229
morphology, 229
prognosis and treatment, 230
WHO-HAEM5 diagnostic criteria for,
229t
Cutaneous peripheral T-cell lymphoma, not
otherwise specified, 446–447
Cytogenomics, 531–545
assay failure, 534–535
comparative genomic hybridization,
538–539, 539f
array, 538–539
metaphase, 538
human chromosome nomenclature,
542–545, 544t
chromosome region and band
designations, 543–544
fluorescence in situ hybridization and
microarray results, description
of, 545
karyotypes, description of, 544–545
metaphase fluorescence in situ
hybridization, 535–537
microarray analysis, 540–542, 542f
advantages, 540–541
limitations, 541–542
multiplex metaphase fluorescence in situ
hybridization, 537–538
advantages, 537
disadvantages, 537
modifications of, 538
overview, 531
traditional cytogenetic analysis, 531–535
advantages, 531
basic laboratory procedures, 532–534,
532f, 533–534t
limitations, 531–532
Cytomegalovirus (CMV), 73
Cytomegalovirus lymphadenitis, 102–103

D

DCA. *See* Dyskeratosis congenita (DCA)
Dendritic cell and dendritic cell–like
neoplasms, 494–501

dendritic cell–like tumors, 497
EBV-positive inflammatory follicular
    dendritic cell sarcoma, 498–500
  clinical features, 499
  diagnostic criteria for, 499t
  differential diagnosis, 500
  genetic features, 499
  immunophenotype, 499
  morphology, 499
  prognosis and treatment, 499
fibroblastic reticular cell tumor, 500–501
  clinical features, 500
  genetic features, 500
  immunophenotype, 500
  morphology, 500
follicular dendritic cell sarcoma, 497–498
  clinical features, 497–498
  diagnostic criteria for, 497t
  differential diagnosis, 498
  genetic features, 498
  immunophenotype, 498
  morphology, 498
  prognosis and treatment, 498
indeterminate dendritic cell tumor,
    494–495, 495
  clinical features, 495
  diagnostic criteria for, 494t
  differential diagnosis, 495
  immunophenotype, 495
  morphology, 495
  prognosis and treatment, 495
interdigitating dendritic cell sarcoma,
    495–497
  clinical features, 496
  diagnostic criteria for, 496t
  differential diagnosis, 497
  genetic features, 496
  immunophenotype, 496
  morphology, 496
  prognosis and treatment, 496–497
Dermatopathic lymphadenopathy (DL), 87
Diamond-Blackfan anemia, 81–82
Down syndrome, 209
  myeloid proliferations associated with,
    211–214
    clinical features, 211–212
    diagnostic criteria for, 212t
    genetic features, 213
    morphology and immunophenotype,
      212–213
    overview, 211
    prognosis and treatment, 213
Drug-induced neutropenia, 45
Dyskeratosis congenita (DCA), 80–81, 208

E

Early T-precursor lymphoblastic leukemia/
    lymphoma (ETP-ALL), 263–266,
    264–265T
  clinical features, 263
  differential diagnosis, 266
  genetic features, 264–265
  immunophenotype, 263–264
  morphology, 263
  prognosis and treatment, 266
EBV. *See* Epstein-Barr virus (EBV)
EMZL. *See* Extranodal marginal zone
    lymphoma (EMZL)
Endothelial cells, 9
Enteropathy-associated T-cell lymphoma,
    406–409
  clinical presentation, 406
  comparison Between RCD I, RCD II, and
    EATL, 408t
  differential diagnosis, 409
  genetic features, 407–408
  immunophenotype, 407
  morphology, 407
  prognosis and treatment, 409
  WHO-HAEM5 diagnostic criteria for,
    407t
Eosinophilia, 215–225
Eosinophils, 2t
Epstein-Barr virus (EBV), 73, 114
Epstein-Barr virus lymphadenitis,
    101–102
Epstein-Barr virus-positive inflammatory
    follicular dendritic cell sarcoma,
    498–500
  clinical features, 499
  diagnostic criteria for, 499t
  differential diagnosis, 500
  genetic features, 499
  immunophenotype, 499
  morphology, 499
  prognosis and treatment, 499
Epstein-Barr virus–positive mucocutaneous
    ulcer, 356–358
  clinical features, 356
  diagnostic criteria for, 357t
  differential diagnosis, 357
  genetic features, 357
  immunophenotype, 357
  morphology, 357
  prognosis and treatment, 357
Epstein-Barr virus-positive nodal T-/natural
    killer- cell lymphoma, 419–422
  clinical features, 420
  differential diagnosis, 421

Epstein-Barr virus-positive nodal T-/natural killer- cell lymphoma (*continued*)
  genetic features, 421
  immunophenotype, 421
  key features of, 421–422t
  morphology, 420
Epstein Bar virus-positive natural killer-/T-cell lymphomas, 417–422
  EBV-positive nodal T-/natural killer- cell lymphoma, 419–422
    clinical features, 420
    differential diagnosis, 421
    genetic features, 421
    immunophenotype, 421
    key features of, 421–422t
    morphology, 420
    prognosis and treatment, 421
Epstein Bar virus-positive natural killer-/T-cell lymphoproliferative diseases of childhood, 459–465
  hydroa vacciniforme lymphoproliferative disorder, 460–464
    WHO-HAEM5 diagnostic criteria for, 463t
  key features of, 461–462t
  severe mosquito bite allergy, 460
    WHO-HAEM5 diagnostic criteria for, 463t
  systemic chronic active Epstein-Barr virus disease, 464
    WHO-HAEM5 diagnostic criteria for, 464t
  systemic Epstein-Barr virus–positive T-cell lymphoma of childhood, 464–465
    WHO-HAEM5 diagnostic criteria for, 465t
Erdheim-Chester disease, 487, 501–503
  clinical features, 501–502
  differential diagnosis, 503
  genetic features, 502
  imaging findings, 502
  immunophenotype, 502
  morphology, 502
  prognosis and treatment, 503
Erythrocytes (RBCs), 2t
Erythropoiesis, 4
Essential thrombocythemia (ET), 140–143, 142t
  diagnosis and differential diagnosis, 142–143
  genetic features, 142
  morphologic and immunophenotypic features, 140–142
  prognosis and treatment, 143

ETP-ALL. *See* Early T-precursor lymphoblastic leukemia/lymphoma (ETP-ALL)
Extranodal marginal zone lymphoma (EMZL), 281–283
  clinical features, 281
  common rearrangements in, 284t
  diagnostic criteria for, 283t
  etiologies implicated in, 283t
  genetic features, 284
  morphology and immunophenotype, 283
  prognosis and treatment, 284
Extranodal natural killer-/T-cell lymphoma, 417–419
  clinical features, 417–418
  differential diagnosis, 419
  genetic features, 419
  immunophenotype, 418–419
  morphology, 418
  prognosis and treatment, 419

F

Fabry disease, 75
Fanconi anemia, 78–80
FC. *See* Flow cytometry (FC)
Fibroblastic reticular cell tumor, 500–501
  clinical features, 500
  genetic features, 500
  immunophenotype, 500
  morphology, 500
Filariasis, 71
FISH. *See* Fluorescence in situ hybridization (FISH)
FL. *See* Follicular lymphoma (FL)
Flow cytometry (FC), 517–530
  background signals and artifacts, 519–520
    autofluorescence, 519–520
    specimen quality, 520
    spectral overlap or spillover, 520
    undesired antibody/dye binding, 520
  common cell antigens used in clinical flow cytometry, 521–524t, 530
  gating and interpretation, 518–519
  immunophenotyping for leukemia/lymphoma characterization, 521–524t, 521–530
    chronic myeloid neoplasms, 529
    kappa and lambda surface light chain expression, 527–528
    mastocytosis, 529
    non-hodgkin lymphoma, 526–527
    paroxysmal nocturnal hemoglobinuria, 529
    plasma cell neoplasm, 528

Sézary syndrome, 528
  T-cell clonality, 528
 instrumentation, 517–518
  electronics, 518
  fluidics, 517–518
  optics, 518
 minimal/measurable residual disease flow cytometry, 530
 reporting of leukemia/lymphoma flow cytometry interpretations, 520
 types of assays, 518
Fluorescence in situ hybridization (FISH), 20–21
Follicular dendritic cell sarcoma, 497–498
 clinical features, 497–498
 diagnostic criteria for, 497t
 differential diagnosis, 498
 genetic features, 498
 immunophenotype, 498
 morphology, 498
 prognosis and treatment, 498
Follicular lymphoma (FL), 300–309, 344–345
 classic
  bone marrow and peripheral blood, morphology in, 302–303
  cytomorphology, 302
  genetic features, 303
  grading, 302
  immunophenotype, 303
  lymph nodes and extranodal sites, morphology in, 302
 classification of, 300t
 clinical features, 301
 duodenal-type, 304–307, 307t
 follicular large B-cell lymphoma, 304
  prognosis and treatment, 304
  transformation, 304
 morphology, immunophenotype, and genetic features, 301–302
 pediatric-type, 307–308, 308t
 with predominantly diffuse growth pattern, 303–304
 in situ follicular B-cell neoplasm, 308–309, 309t
 subtypes, key features of, 305–306t
 with unusual cytological features, 303
 WHO-HAEM5 diagnostic criteria for, 300t

G

Gaucher disease, 74, 112
Germinotropic lymphoproliferative disorder (GLPD), 348–350
Germline predisposition, myeloid neoplasms and, 203–211
 clinical features, 203–210
 diagnostic criteria for, 207t
 genetic features, 210
 morphology and immunophenotype, 210
 overview, 203
 prognosis and treatment, 210
Glucose-6-phosphate dehydrogenase (G6PD), 35
Granulopoiesis, 5

H

Hairy cell leukemia, 291–293
 clinical features, 291
 differential diagnosis, 292
 genetic features, 292
 immunophenotype, 292
 key features, 298–299t
 morphology, 291–292
 prognosis and treatment, 292–293
 WHO-HAEM5 diagnostic criteria for, 292t
Hb Bart syndrome, 41
HbH disease, 41
Heavy chain diseases, 366–371
 alpha heavy chain disease, 369–371
 gamma heavy chain disease, 368–369
 Mu heavy chain disease, 366–371
Hemangioendothelioma, 114
Hemangioma, 113
Hematopoiesis, 4, 5f
 Hematopoietic lineages, 4, 5–8, 6–8f
  erythropoiesis, 4–5
  granulopoiesis, 5
  lymphopoiesis, 7
  megakaryopoiesis, 6–7
  monopoiesis, 5–6
Hemolytic uremic syndrome, 59
Hemophagocytic lymphohistiocytosis (HLH), 75–76, 76t, 481
Hemostasis
 platelet components in, 55t
Heparin-induced thrombocytopenia (HIT), 57
Hepatosplenic T-cell lymphoma, 415–417
 clinical features, 415
 differential diagnosis, 416
 genetic features, 416
 immunophenotype, 416
 morphology, 415–416
 prognosis and treatment, 416
Hereditary elliptocytosis, 37
Hereditary spherocytosis, 36

Hereditary stomatocytosis, 37
Histiocytic sarcoma (HS)
    clinical presentation, 482
    differential diagnosis, 482–484
    genetic features, 483
    immunophenotype, 483
    morphology, 483
    prognosis and treatment, 484
    sites of involvement, 483
    WHO-HAEM5 diagnostic criteria for, 482t
Histochemical stains, 513–516
    carbohydrates, 513
        Congo red, 513
        Thioflavin T, 513
    connective tissue, 513–515
        reticulin, 514
        trichrome, 514–515
    microorganisms, 515–516
        AFB stain, 515
        enzymes, 516
        GMS stain, 515
        gram stain, 515
        pigments and minerals, 516
        Warthin-Starry stain, 515
Histoplasma lymphadenitis, 105–106
Histoplasmosis, 72
HIV/AIDS, 72–73
HIV lymphadenitis, 100–101
Hodgkin lymphoma, 247
HS. *See* Histiocytic sarcoma (HS)
Human chromosome nomenclature, 542–545, 544t
    chromosome region and band designations, 543–544
    fluorescence in situ hybridization and microarray results, description of, 545
    karyotypes, description of, 544–545

I

IB-LBP. *See* Indolent B-lymphoblastic proliferations (IB-LBP)
IEI-LPDs, inborn error of immunity–associated lymphoproliferative disorders (IEI–LPDs)
IgG4-related disease, 344
IHC. *See* Immunohistochemistry (IHC)
Immune deficiency and dysregulation (IDD), lymphoid proliferations and lymphomas associated with, 468–474
    hyperplasias arising in settings of, 468–470
        clinical features, 468–469
        differential diagnosis, 470
        genetic features, 470
        morphology and immunophenotype, 469–470
        prognosis and treatment, 470
        WHO-HAEM5 diagnostic criteria for, 469t
    lymphomas arising in, 472–473
    polymorphic lymphoproliferative disorders arising in, 470–472
        clinical features, 470
        differential diagnosis, 471–472
        genetic features, 471
        immunophenotype, 471
        morphology, 470
        prognosis and treatment, 471
        WHO-HAEM5 diagnostic criteria for, 471t
    types and features, lymphoma, 473t
Immune-mediated neutropenia, 45
Immunodeficiency-associated lymphoproliferative disorders (IA-LPDs), 466–467, 467t
    classification of, 466
    updates, 466–467
Immunoglobulin G4-related disease associated lymphadenopathy (IgG4-LAD), 90
Immunohistochemistry (IHC), 507–512
    antibody cocktails, 508
    binding approaches, 508
    chromogens, 508
    counterstaining, 508
    hematologic cell populations and IHC markers, 510t
    interpretation, 509
    primary antibody, 508
    quantitative, 508
    staining patterns, 510–511t
Inborn error of immunity–associated lymphoproliferative disorders (IEI-LPDs), 475–477
    associated lymphoproliferative disorders and lymphomas, 476t
    clinical features, 475
    diagnostic criteria for, 476t
    genetic features, 475–476
    morphology and immunophenotype, 475
    primary immune deficiencies, 476t
    prognosis and treatment, 477
Indeterminate dendritic cell tumor, 494–495, 495
    clinical features, 495
    diagnostic criteria for, 494t
    differential diagnosis, 495
    immunophenotype, 495
    morphology, 495

prognosis and treatment, 495
Indolent B-lymphoblastic proliferations (IB-LBP), 88
Indolent natural killer cell lymphoproliferative disorder of the gastrointestinal tract, 404–406
  clinical presentation, 404
  differential diagnosis, 406
  genetic features, 405
  immunophenotype, 405
  morphology, 404–405
  prognosis and treatment, 405
  sites of involvement, 406
  WHO-HAEM5 diagnostic criteria for, 405t
Indolent T-cell lymphoma of the gastrointestinal tract, 402–403
  clinical features, 403
  differential diagnosis, 403
  genetic features, 403
  immunophenotype, 403
  morphology, 403
  prognosis and treatment, 403
  WHO-HAEM5 diagnostic criteria for, 402t
Indolent T-lymphoblastic proliferation (IT-LBP), 88
Infectious lymphadenopathies, 95–106
Inherited bone marrow failure syndromes (IBMFS), 207
In situ hybridization (ISH) techniques, 512–513
Interdigitating dendritic cell sarcoma, 495–497
  clinical features, 496
  diagnostic criteria for, 496t
  differential diagnosis, 497
  genetic features, 496
  immunophenotype, 496
  morphology, 496
  prognosis and treatment, 496–497
Interphase fluorescence in situ hybridization, 546–553
  applications and probe types, 548–550
  limitations, 551–552
  nomenclature, 550–551, 551t
  versus other molecular techniques, use of, 552–553
  overview, 546
Intestinal T/NK-cell lymphoproliferative disorders and lymphomas, 402–414
  enteropathy-associated T-cell lymphoma, 406–409
    clinical presentation, 406
    comparison Between RCD I, RCD II, and EATL, 408t
    differential diagnosis, 409
    genetic features, 407–408
    immunophenotype, 407
    morphology, 407
    prognosis and treatment, 409
    WHO-HAEM5 diagnostic criteria for, 407t
  indolent natural killer cell lymphoproliferative disorder of the gastrointestinal tract, 404–406
    clinical presentation, 404
    differential diagnosis, 406
    genetic features, 405
    immunophenotype, 405
    morphology, 404–405
    prognosis and treatment, 405
    sites of involvement, 404
    WHO-HAEM5 diagnostic criteria for, 405t
  indolent T-cell lymphoma of the gastrointestinal tract, 402–403
    clinical features, 403
    differential diagnosis, 403
    genetic features, 403
    immunophenotype, 403
    morphology, 403
    prognosis and treatment, 403
    WHO-HAEM5 diagnostic criteria for, 402t
  intestinal T-cell lymphoma, NOS, 411
  monomorphic epitheliotropic intestinal T-cell lymphoma, 409–411
    clinical presentation, 409
    differential diagnosis, 411, 412–414t
    genetic features, 411
    immunophenotype, 410–411
    morphology, 410
    prognosis and treatment, 411
    sites of involvement, 409–410
Iron deficiency anemia (IDA), 34
IT-LBP. *See* Indolent T-lymphoblastic proliferation (IT-LBP)

J

JML. *See* Juvenile myelomonocytic leukemia (JML)
Juvenile myelomonocytic leukemia (JML), 143–146, 144t
  diagnosis and differential diagnosis, 145–146
  genetic features, 145
  morphologic and immunophenotypic features, 144–145
  prognosis and treatment, 146

Juvenile xanthogranuloma (JXG), 489–491
  clinical features, 489–490
  differential diagnosis, 491
  immunophenotype, 490
  molecular genetics, 490
  morphology, 490
  prognosis and treatment, 491
  WHO-HAEM5 diagnostic criteria for, 489t
JXG. *See* Juvenile xanthogranuloma (JXG)

K

Kaposi Sarcoma, 113–114
Kaposi sarcoma–associated herpesvirus/human herpesvirus-8–associated multicentric Castleman disease (KSHV/HHV8-MCD), 341–347
  clinical features, 341–343
  differential diagnosis, 344–345
  genetic features, 344
  immunophenotype, 343
  morphology, 343
  pathologic grading in multicentric Castleman disease, 343t
  positive diffuse large B-cell lymphoma, 347–348
    clinical features, 347
    differential diagnosis, 349
    genetic features, 349
    immunophenotype, 347
    morphology, 347
    prognosis and treatment, 349
    WHO-HAEM5 diagnostic criteria for, 347t
  positive germinotropic lymphoproliferative disorder, 348
    clinical features, 348t
    differential diagnosis, 348
    genetic features, 348
    immunophenotype, 348
    morphology, 348
    prognosis and treatment, 348
    WHO-HAEM5 diagnostic criteria for, 348t
  prognosis and treatment, 344
  WHO-HAEM5 diagnostic criteria for, 342t
Kaposi sarcoma (KS), 341
Kikuchi-Fujimoto disease, 89–90
  necrotic phase, 90
  proliferative phase, 89–90
  xanthomatous phase, 90
Kikuchi-Fujimoto disease (KFD), 89–90
  necrotic phase, 90
  proliferative phase, 89–90
  xanthomatous phase, 90
Kimura disease, 90
Kimura disease (KD), 90

L

Langerhans cell histiocytosis (LCH), 478, 485–487, 487
  clinical features, 485–486
  differential diagnosis, 487
  genetic features, 486–487
  immunophenotype, 486
  morphology, 486
  prognosis and treatment, 487
Langerhans cell hyperplasia, 487
Langerhans cell sarcoma, 487
Large B-cell lymphomas (LBCLs), 314–337
  associated with specific anatomic sites, 327–330
  classification of, 315t
  diffuse, not otherwise specified, 316–319
    clinical features, 316
    genetic features, 319
    immunophenotype, 317–318
    morphologic subtypes of, 317t
    morphology, 316–317
    prognosis and treatment, 320
    WHO-HAEM5 diagnostic criteria for, 316t
  diffuse large B-cell lymphoma associated with chronic inflammation, 332
  fibrin-associated large B-cell lymphoma, 332
  fluid overload–associated large B-cell lymphoma, 332
  high-grade B-cell lymphomas, 320–322, 321t
  of immune-privileged sites, 327, 326t
  intravascular, 329, 330t
  with *IRF4* rearrangement, 319–320, 320t
  key features of, 333–337t
  mediastinal gray zone lymphoma, 329, 329t
  overview, 314–316
  with plasmablastic features, 330–332
    ALK-positive large B-cell lymphoma, 331, 332t
    plasmablastic lymphoma, 330–331, 331t
  with polymorphic pattern, 323–327, 323t
    Epstein-Bar virus–positive diffuse large B-cell lymphoma, 324–325, 325t
    lymphomatoid granulomatosis, 325–327, 326t
    T-cell histiocyte-rich large B-cell lymphoma, 323–324

WHO-HAEM5 diagnostic criteria for, 323t
  primary mediastinal, 328, 328t
LBCLs. *See* Large B-cell lymphomas (LBCLs)
LCH. *See* Langerhans cell histiocytosis (LCH)
Leishmaniasis, 70
Leukocytes (WBCs), 2t
Littoral cell angioma, 112–113
LPL. *See* Lymphoplasmacytic lymphoma (LPL)
Lymphangioma, 113
Lymph node, 10–14
  architecture, 10–12
    capsule, 12
    cortex, 10–12
    medullary region, 12
    paracortex, 10–12
    sinuses, 12
  autoimmune disease-associated lymphadenopathy, 93–95
    autoimmune lymphoproliferative syndrome, 95
    rheumatoid arthritis-associated lymphadenopathy, 95
    sarcoidosis lymphadenopathy, 94
    SLE-associated lymphadenopathy, 94
  biopsy. *See* Lymph node biopsy
  Castleman disease, 92–93, 94t
    hyaline vascular, 92
    idiopathic multicentric Castleman disease, 93
    immunophenotype, 93
    mixed/plasma cell, 93
    unicentric Castleman disease, 93
  clinical features, 91–92
  dermatopathic lymphadenopathy, 87
  function, 13–14t
  immunoglobulin G4-related disease associated lymphadenopathy, 90
    differential diagnosis, 92
    morphology and immunohistochemistry, 92
    rectal tonsil, 88
    tissue samples, 18
    variations in morphology, 12
  prognosis and treatment, 92
  Progressive Transformation of Germinal Centers, 89
  reactive lymphoid hyperplasia, 84–87
    florid follicular hyperplasia, 84
    marginal zone hyperplasia, 85–87
    paracortical hyperplasia, 84–85
  immunophenotype, 14–15t
  indolent B-lymphoblastic proliferations, 88
  indolent T-lymphoblastic proliferation, 88
  infectious lymphadenopathies, 95–106, 96–99t
    cat scratch disease, 103
    cytomegalovirus lymphadenitis, 102–103
    Epstein-Barr virus Lymphadenitis, 101–102
    histoplasma lymphadenitis, 105–106
    HIV lymphadenitis, 100–101
    mycobacterial lymphadenitis, 104–105
    syphilitic lymphadenitis, 103–104
    toxoplasma lymphadenitis, 105
    viral lymphadenitis, 100–103
  Kikuchi-Fujimoto disease, 89–90
    necrotic phase, 90
    proliferative phase, 89–90
    xanthomatous phase, 90
  Kimura disease, 90
  lymphoma-like lesion, 88–89
  reactive lymphoid hyperplasia
    sinus hyperplasia, 87
Lymph node biopsy
  approaches to, 22–23
  clinical history, 22
  genetic studies, 22
  immunophenotypic studies, 22
  microscopic evaluation, 22, 23t
Lymphocytes, 3t, 47–51
  iatrogenic causes, 51
  infectious causes, 50–51
  lymphocytosis, 49–50
  lymphopenia, 50
Lymphocytosis, 49–50
Lymphoid neoplasms
  eosinophilia and, 215–225
  overview and classification of, 240–248
    acute leukemia/lymphomas, 244–245
    B-cell lymphoid proliferations and lymphomas, 244
    hodgkin lymphoma, 247
    mature B-cell lymphomas, 245–247
    paraproteins, 247
    plasma cell neoplasms, 247
    T cell lymphomas, 247–248
    WHO-HAEM5 and ICC, 241–244t
Lymphoma-like lesion (LLL), 88–89
Lymphomas of T follicular helper cell origin, 447–455
  nodal T follicular helper cell lymphoma, angioimmunoblastic type, 447–450
    clinical features, 447
    differential diagnosis, 450
    genetic features, 449

Lymphomas of T follicular helper cell origin (*continued*)
  immunophenotype, 449
  morphology, 448–449
  prognosis and treatment, 450
  WHO-HAEM5 diagnostic criteria for, 448t
 nodal T follicular helper cell lymphoma, follicular type, 450–452
  clinical features, 451
  genetic features, 452
  immunophenotype, 452
  morphology, 452
  prognosis and treatment, 452
  WHO-HAEM5 diagnostic criteria for, 451t
 nodal T follicular helper lymphoma, not otherwise specified, 453–454
  clinical features, 453
  differential diagnosis, 454
  genetic features, 454
  immunophenotype, 454
  morphology, 454
  prognosis and treatment, 454
  WHO-HAEM5 diagnostic criteria for, 453t
Lymphomatoid papulosis, 435
 clinical presentation, 435
 differential diagnosis, 436
 genetic features, 436
 immunophenotype, 436
 morphology, 436
 prognosis and treatment, 436
 WHO-HAEM5 diagnostic criteria for, 435t
 features of normal/reactive and atypical mast cells, 228t
Lymphopenia, 50
Lymphoplasmacytic lymphoma (LPL), 287–290, 359
 clinical features, 288
 differential diagnosis, 290
  IgM MGUS, 290
  marginal zone lymphoma, 290
  small B-cell lymphomas, 290
 genetic features, 289
 immunophenotype, 289
 morphology, 288–289
  blood and bone marrow, 288–289
  lymph node and spleen, 289
 prognosis and treatment, 289–290
 transformation, 289
 WHO HAEM5 diagnostic criteria for, 288t
Lymphopoiesis, 7

M

Macrophage activation syndrome, 481
Malaria, 71
Malignant histiocytoses, 480
Malpighian corpuscles, 15
Mantle cell lymphoma, 310–312
 clinical features, 310
 differential diagnoses, 312
 genetic features, 311
 immunophenotype, 311
 leukemic non-nodal, 312–313, 313t
 morphology, 311
 prognosis and treatment, 313
 in situ mantle cell neoplasm, 314, 314t
 WHO-HAEM5 diagnostic criteria for, 310t
Marginal zone lymphomas (MZLs), 280–281, 360
 differential diagnosis, 281
  reactive lymphoid hyperplasia, 281
  small B-cell lymphomas, 281
 immunophenotype, 280–281
 morphology, 280
 transformation, 281
Mast cell sarcoma (MCS), 233–234
 WHO-HAEM5 diagnostic criteria for, 234t
Mastocytosis, 128–129, 227–234
 cutaneous, 228–230
  clinical features, 228–229
  genetic features, 229–230
  immunophenotype, 229
  morphology, 229
  prognosis and treatment, 230
  WHO-HAEM5 diagnostic criteria for, 229t
 features of normal/reactive and atypical mast cells, 228t
 mast cell sarcoma, 233–234
  WHO-HAEM5 diagnostic criteria for, 234t
 systemic, 230–233
  B and C findings, 232t
  clinical features, 231
  genetic features, 233
  immunophenotype, 233
  morphology, 232–233
  prognosis and treatment, 233
  WHO-HAEM5 diagnostic criteria for, 230–231t
 WHO-HAEM5 classification, 227t
Mature B-cell lymphomas, 245–247
Mature plasmacytoid dendritic cell proliferation associated (MPDCP), 239, 239t
Mature T-/NK-cell leukemias, 387–401

adult T-cell leukemia/lymphoma, 399–401
  clinical features, 399
  differential diagnosis, 400–401
  genetic features, 400
  immunophenotype, 400
  morphology, 399–400
  prognosis and treatment, 400
aggressive NK-cell leukemia, 396–398
  clinical features, 396
  differential diagnosis, 398
  genetic features, 397
  immunophenotype, 397
  morphology, 396–397
  prognosis and treatment, 398
  WHO-HAEM5 diagnostic criteria for, 397t
NK-cell large granular lymphocytic leukemia, 393–395
  clinical features, 394
  differential diagnosis, 395
  genetic features, 395
  immunophenotype, 395
  morphology, 395
  prognosis and treatment, 395
  WHO-HAEM5 diagnostic criteria for, 394t
T-cell large granular lymphocytic leukemia, 390–393
  clinical features, 390–391
  differential diagnosis, 392–393
  genetic features, 392
  immunophenotype, 392
  morphology, 392
  prognosis and treatment, 393
  WHO-HAEM5 diagnostic criteria for, 391t
T-cell prolymphocytic leukemia, 387–390
  clinical features, 387
  differential diagnosis, 389–390
  genetic features, 389
  immunophenotype, 388–389
  morphology, 387–388
  prognosis and treatment, 389
  WHO-HAEM5 diagnostic criteria for, 388t
May-Hegglin anomaly, 52
MCS. *See* Mast cell sarcoma (MCS)
MDSs. *See* Myelodysplastic neoplasms (MDSs)
Medullary region, 12
Megakaryopoiesis, 6–7
Megaloblastic anemia, 34
Metaphase fluorescence in situ hybridization, 535–537

MNs. *See* Myeloid neoplasms (MNs)
Molecular diagnostics, 546–583
  interphase fluorescence in situ hybridization, 546–553
    applications and probe types, 548–550
    limitations, 551–552
    nomenclature, 550–551, 551t
    versus other molecular techniques, use of, 552–553
    overview, 546
  next-generation sequencing, 566–583
    assay scope/types of assays, 571–572
    bioinformatics, 572–574
    clonality assays, 579–581
    human leukocyte antigen typing, 581–582
    liquid biopsies, 582–583
    methodologies, 567–571
    overview, 566–567
    reporting, 574–577
    RNA sequence analysis, 577–579
  polymerase chain reaction and related techniques, 553–566
    applications of, 561–564
    clonality assays, 565
    identity determination, 564–565
    methodology, 559–560
    nucleic acid analysis, general features, 557–559
    overview, 553
    sequence analysis by Sanger sequencing, 564
    specimen requirements, handling, and processing, 553–557
Monoclonal B-cell lymphocytosis (MBL), 279, 279t
Monocytes, 2t
Monomorphic epitheliotropic intestinal T-cell lymphoma, 409–411
  clinical presentation, 409
  differential diagnosis, 411, 412–414t
  genetic features, 411
  immunophenotype, 410–411
  morphology, 410
  prognosis and treatment, 411
  sites of involvement, 409–410
Monopoiesis, 5–6
MPNs. *See* Myeloproliferative neoplasms (MPNs)
MS. *See* Myeloid sarcoma (MS)
Mucopolysaccharidoses, 112
Mucormycosis, 72

Multiplex metaphase fluorescence in situ hybridization, 537–538
  advantages, 537
  disadvantages, 537
  modifications of, 538
Mycobacterial lymphadenitis, 104–105
Mycosis fungoides, 430
  clinical presentation, 430–431
  differential diagnosis, 432
  genetic features, 432
  immunophenotype, 431
  morphology, 431
  prognosis and treatment, 432
  sites of involvement, 431
  WHO-HAEM5 diagnostic criteria, 430t
Myelodysplastic/myeloproliferative neoplasm, not otherwise specified (MDS/MPN-NOS), 174
Myelodysplastic/myeloproliferative neoplasm with neutrophilia (MDS/MPN-N), 168–171, 169t
  clinical features, 168
  differential diagnosis, 170
  genetic features, 170
  immunophenotype, 170
  morphology, 169–170
  prognosis and treatment, 170
Myelodysplastic/myeloproliferative neoplasm with *SF3B1* mutation and thrombocytosis (MDS/MPN-*SF3B1*-T), 171–173
  clinical features, 171
  differential diagnosis, 173
  genetic features, 173
  immunophenotype, 172
  morphology, 171–172
  prognosis and treatment, 173
Myelodysplastic neoplasms (MDSs), 124–125, 124–126, 150–162, 150t
  classification, 158–159, 160–162t
  clinical and risk stratification, 162
  diagnostic criteria, 150
  genetic features, 157–158, 158t
  immunophenotypic features, 155–157
    erythroid cells, 156
    lymphoid progenitors, 156
    maturing granulocytic cells, 156
    megakaryocytes, 156–157
    monocytes, 156
    multiparameter flow cytometry, 155
    myeloid progenitors, 155–156
  laboratory hematology features, 150–151
  management, 162
  morphologic features, 152–154, 153t
    blasts, 152
    bone marrow aspirate, 153–154
    dysplasia, 152
    peripheral blood, 152–153
    trephine core biopsy, 154
Myeloid neoplasms (MNs), 116–129, 117f, 118–122t
  acute myeloid leukemia, 126–127
  cancer predisposing syndromes, 204–206t
  eosinophilia and, 215–225
  with eosinophilia and gene rearrangements, 128
  germline predisposition. *See* Germline predisposition, myeloid neoplasms and
  mastocytosis, 128–129
  myelodysplastic syndrome, 124–125
  myeloid precursor lesions overview of, 123–124
  myeloproliferative neoplasms overview of changes in, 116–123
  plasmacytoid dendritic cell neoplasm, 128
  secondary, 128
Myeloid neoplasms post-cytotoxic therapy (MN-pCT), 199–203
  clinical features, 201
  genetic features, 202
  morphology and immunophenotype, 201
  overview, 199–201
  prognosis and treatment, 202
  WHO-HAEM5 diagnostic criteria for, 200t
Myeloid precursor lesions, 149–150
  clonal cytopenia, 149–150
  clonal hematopoiesis, 149
  overview of, 123–124
Myeloid proliferations, down syndrome and, 211–214
  clinical features, 211–212
  diagnostic criteria for, 212t
  genetic features, 213
  morphology and immunophenotype, 212–213
  overview, 211
  prognosis and treatment, 213
Myeloid sarcoma (MS), 195–196, 195t
Myeloproliferative neoplasms overview of changes in, 116–123
Myeloproliferative neoplasms (MPNs), 130–148
  chronic myeloid leukemia, 130
    diagnosis and differential diagnosis, 131–133, 132t
    genetic features, 131
    morphologic and immunophenotypic features, 130–131

chronic neutrophilic leukemia, 146–147, 146–147t
essential thrombocythemia, 140–143, 142t
  diagnosis and differential diagnosis, 142–143
  genetic features, 142
  morphologic and immunophenotypic features, 140–142
  prognosis and treatment, 143
juvenile myelomonocytic leukemia, 143–146, 144t
  diagnosis and differential diagnosis, 145–146
  genetic features, 145
  morphologic and immunophenotypic features, 144–145
  prognosis and treatment, 146
overview of changes in, 116–123, 126
polycythemia vera, 133–134
  diagnosis and differential diagnosis, 134–135t
  genetic features, 134
  morphologic and immunophenotypic features, 134
  prognosis and treatment, 133, 135
primary myelofibrosis, 136–140
  diagnosis and differential diagnosis, 139
  genetic features, 139
  morphologic and immunophenotypic features, 137–138, 138t
  prognosis and treatment, 139–140
MZLs. *See* Marginal zone lymphomas (MZLs)

N

Neural cells, 9
Neutropenia, 45
  causes of, 46t
Neutrophilia, 45
Neutrophils, 2t, 44–47
  causes of neutropenia, 45–47, 46t
  drug-induced neutropenia, 45
  function, disorders of, 47, 48t
  immune-mediated neutropenia, 45
  neutropenia, 45
  neutrophilia, 45
  number, disorders of, 44–47
Next-generation sequencing (NGS), 566–583
  assay, scope/types of, 571–572
    targeted panels, 571
    WE and WG, 571–572
  bioinformatics, 572–574
    alignment, 572
    annotation, 574
    variant identification, 573–574
  clonality assays, 579–581
    based on immunoglobulin or T-cell receptor genes, 580–581
    based on specific gene mutations, 581
  human leukocyte antigen typing, 581–582
  liquid biopsies, 582–583
    cfDNA, 582–583
  methodologies, 567–571
    amplification-based methods, 567–570
    hybrid capture–based methods, 570–571
  overview, 566–567
  reporting, 574–577
    variant allele frequency, 574
    variant classification, 577
  RNA sequence analysis, 577–579
    clinical assays, 578
    workflow, 577–578
NGS. *See* Next-generation sequencing (NGS)
Niemann-Pick disease, 74–75, 112
NK-cell large granular lymphocytic leukemia, 393–395
  clinical features, 394
  differential diagnosis, 395
  genetic features, 395
  immunophenotype, 395
  morphology, 395
  prognosis and treatment, 395
  WHO-HAEM5 diagnostic criteria for, 394t
NK-lymphoblastic leukemia/lymphoma (NK-ALL/LBL), 266
NMZL. *See* Nodal marginal zone lymphoma (NMZL)
Nodal marginal zone lymphoma (NMZL), 284–285
  clinical features, 284
  diagnostic criteria for, 285t
  genetic features, 285
  morphology and immunophenotype, 285
  prognosis and treatment, 285
Nodal T follicular helper cell lymphoma, angioimmunoblastic type, 447–450
  clinical features, 447–448
  differential diagnosis, 450
  genetic features, 449
  immunophenotype, 449
  morphology, 448–449
  prognosis and treatment, 450
  WHO-HAEM5 diagnostic criteria for, 448t

Nodal T follicular helper cell lymphoma, follicular type, 450–452
  clinical features, 451
  genetic features, 452
  immunophenotype, 452
  morphology, 452
  prognosis and treatment, 452
  WHO-HAEM5 diagnostic criteria for, 451t
Nodal T follicular helper lymphoma, not otherwise specified, 453–454
  clinical features, 453
  differential diagnosis, 454
  genetic features, 454
  immunophenotype, 454
  morphology, 454
  prognosis and treatment, 454
  WHO-HAEM5 diagnostic criteria for, 453t
Nodular lymphocyte-predominant Hodgkin lymphoma (NLPHL), 378–382
  clinical features, 378
  differential diagnosis, 381
  genetic features, 381
  growth patterns in, 380t
  immunophenotype, 379t, 381
  morphology, 378–380
  prognosis and treatment, 381
  progression and transformation, 381
  WHO-HAEM5 diagnostic criteria for, 379t
Non-hematopoietic cells, 9
Non–Langerhans cell histiocytoses, 480–481

O

Osteoblasts, 9
Osteoclasts, 9
Ovalocytosis, 37

P

Paracoccidioidomycosis, 71–72
Paracortex, 10–12
Paraproteins, 247
Parvovirus B19, 73
PCNs. *See* Plasma cell neoplasms (PCNs)
PCR. *See* Polymerase chain reaction (PCR) and related techniques
Pediatric nodal marginal zone lymphoma (PNMZL), 285–287
  clinical features, 286
  diagnostic criteria for, 286t
  differential diagnosis, 286–287
    atypical marginal zone hyperplasia, 286–287
  genetic features, 286
  morphology and immunophenotype, 286
  prognosis and treatment, 286
PEL. *See* Primary effusion lymphoma (PEL)
Pelger-Huet anomaly, 52
Peliosis, 113
Periarterial lymphatic sheaths (PALS), 15
Periodic acid-Schiff (PAS) stain, 15
Peripheral blood smear, 20
Peripheral T-cell lymphoma, not otherwise specified, 455–459
  clinical features, 456–457
  diagnostic criteria for, 456t
  differential diagnosis, 458–459
  genetic features, 457–458
  immunophenotype, 457
  morphology, 457
  prognosis and treatment, 458
Perivascular cells, 9
Plasma cell neoplasms (PCNs), 247, 358–377
  with associated paraneoplastic syndrome, 375–377
  cold agglutinin disease, 358–360
    clinical features, 359
    differential diagnosis, 359–360
    genetic features, 359
    morphology and immunophenotype, 359
    prognosis and treatment, 359
    WHO-HAEM5 diagnostic criteria for, 359t
  diseases with monoclonal immunoglobulin deposition, 363–366
    immunoglobulin light chain amyloidosis, 363–365
    monoclonal immunoglobulin deposition disease, 365–366
  heavy chain diseases, 366–371
    alpha heavy chain disease, 369–371
    gamma heavy chain disease, 368–369
    Mu heavy chain disease, 367–368
  IgM monoclonal gammopathy of undetermined significance, 360–361
  monoclonal gammopathies, 358–360
    of renal significance, 362–363
  non-IgM monoclonal gammopathy of undetermined significance, 361–362
  plasma cell myeloma/multiple myeloma, 373–375
    WHO-HAEM5 diagnostic criteria for, 371t
  plasmacytoma, 371–372
Plasmacytoid dendritic cell (pDC) neoplasms, 128, 236–239

blastic, 236–238
  clinical features, 236
  differential diagnosis, 238
  genetic features, 238
  immunophenotype, 237
  morphology, 236–237
  prognosis and treatment, 238
  WHO-HAEM5 diagnostic criteria for, 237t
Platelet adhesion, 54f
Platelet aggregation, 54f
Platelet disorders, 53–66
  acquired nonneoplastic disorders, 63–64, 63t
    von Willebrand Syndrome, 64
  acquired thrombocytopenia, 57–61, 58t
    atypical hemolytic uremic syndrome, 59
    bone marrow infiltration/suppression/primary disorders, 61
    disseminated intravascular coagulation, 60
    hemolytic uremic syndrome, 59
    heparin-induced thrombocytopenia, 57
    immune thrombocytopenia purpura, 60
    posttransfusion purpura, 61
    pregnancy-associated thrombocytopenia, 60–61
    thrombotic microangiopathies, 59
    thrombotic thrombocytopenia purpura, 59
    vaccine-induced thrombocytopenia, 57–59
  acquired thrombocytosis, 62, 62t
  inherited disorders, 64–66, 65–66t
  laboratory assessment, 53–57
    blood smears, morphology on, 57
    methodology, 53–55
    preanalytical errors, 55–57
  overview, 53
Platelets, 3t
PMF. *See* Primary myelofibrosis (PMF)
PNMZL. *See* Pediatric nodal marginal zone lymphoma (PNMZL)
Polycythemia vera (PV), 133–134
  diagnosis and differential diagnosis, 134–135t
  genetic features, 134
  morphologic and immunophenotypic features, 134
  prognosis and treatment, 133, 135
Polymerase chain reaction (PCR) and related techniques, 553–566
  advantages, 558–560
  applications of, 561–564
    allele-specific polymerase chain reaction, 563
    digital polymerase chain reaction, 563
    methylation-specific polymerase chain reaction, 562–563
    multiplex ligation–dependent probe amplification, 563
    multiplex polymerase chain reaction, 562
    nested polymerase chain reaction, 563
    quantitative polymerase chain reaction, 561–562
    reverse transcriptase-polymerase chain reaction, 561
  clonality assays, 565
  identity determination, 564–565
  limitations, 560
  methodology, 559–560
    amplification, 558
    analytic/technical level, factors that affect testing on, 558–560
  nucleic acid analysis, general features, 557–559
    diagnostic level, factors that affect testing, 557
    operation level, factors that affect testing, 557
    polymerase chain reaction in routine testing, 557–558
  overview, 553
  sequence analysis by sanger sequencing, 564
  specimen requirements, handling, and processing, 553–557
    tissue quality, 556–557
    tissue quantity, 557
    tissue types, 555–556
Primary cutaneous acral CD8-positive T-cell lymphoproliferative disorder, 444–445
  clinical presentation, 444
  genetic features, 446
  immunophenotype, 444
  morphology, 444
  prognosis and treatment, 446
  sites of involvement, 444
  WHO-HAEM5 diagnostic criteria for, 444
Primary cutaneous aggressive epidermotropic CD8+ cytotoxic T-cell lymphoma, 442–443
  clinical presentation, 443
  genetic features, 443
  immunophenotype, 443
  morphology, 443
  prognosis and treatment, 443
  sites of involvement, 443

Primary cutaneous anaplastic large cell
  lymphoma, 437–439
 clinical presentation, 438
 differential diagnosis, 438–439
 genetic features, 438
 immunophenotype, 438
 morphology, 438
 prognosis and treatment, 438
 sites of involvement, 438
 WHO-HAEM5 diagnostic criteria for, 437t
Primary cutaneous B-cell lymphoproliferative
  disorders/lymphomas, 350–358
 Epstein-Barr virus–positive
   mucocutaneous ulcer, 356–357
  clinical features, 356
  diagnostic criteria for, 357t
  differential diagnosis, 357
  genetic features, 357
  immunophenotype, 357
  morphology, 357
  prognosis and treatment, 357
 primary cutaneous diffuse large B-cell
   lymphoma, leg type, 352–354
  clinical features, 353
  diagnostic criteria for, 352t
  differential diagnosis, 353
  genetic features, 353
  immunophenotype, 353
  morphology, 353
  prognosis and treatment, 353
 primary cutaneous follicle center type
   lymphoma, 354–356
  clinical features, 354
  diagnostic criteria for, 354t
  differential diagnosis, 357
  genetic features, 355
  immunophenotype, 355
  morphology, 355
  prognosis and treatment, 355–356
 primary cutaneous marginal zone
   lymphoma, 350–352
  clinical features, 351
  diagnostic criteria for, 350t
  differential diagnosis, 353
  genetic features, 351
  immunophenotype, 351
  morphology, 351
  prognosis and treatment, 351
Primary cutaneous CD30-positive T-cell
  lymphoproliferative disorders
 lymphomatoid papulosis, 435–437
  clinical presentation, 435
  differential diagnosis, 436
  genetic features, 436
  immunophenotype, 436
  morphology, 436
  prognosis and treatment, 436
  WHO-HAEM5 diagnostic criteria for,
    435t
Primary cutaneous CD4+ small/medium
  T-cell lymphoproliferative
  disorder, 445–446
 clinical presentation, 446
 genetic features, 446
 immunophenotype, 446
 morphology, 446
 prognosis and treatment, 446
 sites of involvement, 446
 WHO-HAEM5 diagnostic criteria for, 445t
Primary cutaneous diffuse large B-cell
  lymphoma, leg type, 352–354
 clinical features, 353
 diagnostic criteria for, 352t
 differential diagnosis, 353
 genetic features, 353
 immunophenotype, 353
 morphology, 353
 prognosis and treatment, 353
Primary cutaneous follicle center type
  lymphoma, 354–356
 clinical features, 354
 diagnostic criteria for, 354t
 differential diagnosis, 356
 genetic features, 355
 immunophenotype, 355
 morphology, 355
 prognosis and treatment, 355–356
Primary cutaneous g-d T-cell lymphoma,
  441–442
 clinical presentation, 441
 genetic features, 442
 immunophenotype, 441
 morphology, 441
 prognosis and treatment, 442
 sites of involvement, 441
 WHO-HAEM5 diagnostic criteria for,
   441t
Primary cutaneous marginal zone lymphoma,
  350–352
 clinical features, 351
 diagnostic criteria for, 350t
 differential diagnosis, 351–352
 genetic features, 351
 immunophenotype, 351
 morphology, 351
 prognosis and treatment, 351
Primary cutaneous T-cell lymphoproliferative
  disorders/lymphomas, 430–447
 mycosis fungoides, 430
  clinical presentation, 430–431

differential diagnosis, 432
genetic features, 432
immunophenotype, 431
morphology, 431
prognosis and treatment, 432
sites of involvement, 431
WHO-HAEM5 diagnostic criteria, 430t
Sézary syndrome
clinical presentation, 433
differential diagnosis, 434
flow cytometry, 434
genetic features, 434
morphology, 433–434
prognosis and treatment, 434
sites of involvement, 433
WHO-HAEM5 diagnostic criteria for, 433t
Primary effusion lymphoma (PEL), 345
differential diagnosis, 345
genetic features, 345
immunophenotype, 345–346
morphology, 345
prognosis and treatment, 345
WHO-HAEM5 diagnostic criteria for, 345t
Primary myelofibrosis (PMF), 136–140
diagnosis and differential diagnosis, 139
genetic features, 139
morphologic and immunophenotypic features, 137–138, 138t
prognosis and treatment, 139
Primary splenic angiosarcoma, 114
Progressive Transformation of Germinal Centers (PTGC), 89
PV. *See* Polycythemia vera (PV)
Pyruvate kinase deficiency (PKD), 35–36

Q

Q fever, 68–69

R

*RAS*opathies, 208
RDD. *See* Rosai-Dorfman disease (RDD)
Reactive lymphoid hyperplasia (RLH), 84–87
florid follicular hyperplasia, 84
marginal zone hyperplasia, 85–87
paracortical hyperplasia, 84–85
sinus hyperplasia, 87
Rectal tonsil, 88
Red blood cell disorders, 32–44
cell membrane disorders, 36–37

hereditary elliptocytosis, 37
hereditary spherocytosis, 36
hereditary stomatocytosis, 37
ovalocytosis, 37
enzyme deficiency, 35–36
glucose-6-phosphate dehydrogenase, 35
pyruvate kinase deficiency, 35–36
hemoglobin disorders, 41–43
α-Thalassemia, 41
β-Thalassemia, 41–42
sickle cell disease, 42–43, 43t
immune hemolytic anemias, 37, 38–40t
nutritional anemias, 32–35
copper, 34
folate, 32–33
iron, 34–35
vitamin B12, 33–34
rheology of, 32
Red pulp, 15
Rheumatoid arthritis-associated lymphadenopathy, 95
RLH. *See* Reactive lymphoid hyperplasia (RLH)
Rosai-Dorfman disease (RDD), 480–481, 487, 492–493
clinical features, 492
differential diagnosis, 493
immunophenotype, 493
molecular features, 493
morphology, 493
prognosis and treatment, 493
WHO-HAEM5 diagnostic criteria for, 492t

S

SAMD9 and *SAMD9L* related syndromes, 209
Sarcoidosis lymphadenopathy, 94
Sclerosing angiomatoid nodular transformation (SANT), 113
Secondary myeloid neoplasms, 198–214
classification of, 198–199
post-cytotoxic therapy, 199–203
clinical features, 201
genetic features, 202
morphology and immunophenotype, 201
overview, 199–201
prognosis and treatment, 202
WHO-HAEM5 diagnostic criteria for, 200t
Severe congenital neutropenia (SCN), 207

Sézary syndrome
  clinical presentation, 433
  differential diagnosis, 434
  flow cytometry, 434
  genetic features, 434
  morphology, 433–434
  prognosis and treatment, 434
  sites of involvement, 433
  WHO-HAEM5 diagnostic criteria for, 433t
Shwachman-Diamond syndrome (SDS), 82–83, 208
Sickle cell disease (SCD), 42–43, 43t
Sinuses, 12
SLE-associated lymphadenopathy, 94
SM. *See* Systemic mastocytosis (SM)
Spleen, 15–17, 107–115
  architecture, 16f
  congenital anomalies, 107
    accessory spleen, 107
    asplenia, 107
    splenic gonadal fusion, 107
  function, 15–17
  gross anatomy, 15
  gross examination and tissue processing, 17
    biopsy, 17
    splenectomy, 17
  hypersplenism, 108–109, 109t
  hyposplenism, 109, 110t
  metastatic tumors, 115
  microscopic anatomy, 15
    red pulp, 15
    white pulp, 15
  pseudoneoplastic lesions, 114–115
    inflammatory pseudotumor, 114
    post-chemotherapy histiocyte-rich pseudotumor, 115
    splenic cyst, 114
  reactive splenic disorders, 110–111
  splenic trauma, 107–108
    splenic rupture, 107
    splenosis, 107
  splenomegaly, 107, 108t
  storage diseases, 111–112
    Gaucher disease, 112
    mucopolysaccharidoses, 112
    Niemann-Pick disease, 112
  vascular tumors, 112–114
    Epstein-Barr virus, 114
    hemangioendothelioma, 114
    hemangioma, 113
    Kaposi Sarcoma, 113–114
    littoral cell angioma, 112–113
    lymphangioma, 113
    peliosis, 113
    primary splenic angiosarcoma, 114
    sclerosing angiomatoid nodular transformation, 113
    splenic hamartoma, 113
Splenectomy, 17
Splenic B-cell leukemias/lymphomas, 291–299, 298t
  differential diagnosis of, 297
  hairy cell leukemia, 291–293
    clinical features, 291
    differential diagnosis, 292
    genetic features, 292
    immunophenotype, 292
    key features, 298–299t
    morphology, 291–292
    prognosis and treatment, 292–293
    WHO-HAEM5 diagnostic criteria for, 292t
  with prominent nucleoli, 296, 297t
  splenic diffuse red pulp small B-cell lymphoma/ leukemia, 296, 296t, 298–299t
  splenic marginal zone lymphoma, 293–295
    clinical features, 292
    differential diagnosis, 295
    genetic features, 295
    immunophenotype, 294
    key features of, 298–299t, 298t
    morphology, 294
    prognosis and treatment, 295
    WHO-HAEM5 diagnostic criteria for, 294t
Splenic biopsies, 17
Splenic cyst, 114
Splenic diffuse red pulp small B-cell lymphoma/ leukemia, 296, 296t, 298–299t
Splenic gonadal fusion, 107
Splenic hamartoma, 113
Splenic marginal zone lymphoma, 293–295
  clinical features, 292
  differential diagnosis, 295
  genetic features, 295
  immunophenotype, 294
  key features of, 298–299t, 298t
  morphology, 294
  prognosis and treatment, 295
  WHO-HAEM5 diagnostic criteria for, 294t
Splenosis, 107
Subcutaneous panniculitis-like T-cell lymphoma, 439–440
  clinical presentation, 439–440
  genetic features, 440

immunophenotype, 440
morphology, 440
prognosis and treatment, 440
sites of involvement, 440
WHO-HAEM5 diagnostic criteria for, 439t
Syphilis, 70
Syphilitic lymphadenitis, 103–104
Systemic mastocytosis (SM), 230–233
  B and C findings, 232t
  clinical features, 231
  genetic features, 233
  immunophenotype, 233
  morphology, 232–233
  prognosis and treatment, 233
  WHO-HAEM5 diagnostic criteria for, 230–231t

T

T-cell acute lymphoblastic leukemia/lymphoma (T-ALL/LBL), 258–267
  clinical features, 258
  common genetic abnormalities in, 260t
  differential diagnosis, 261–263
    acute undifferentiated leukemia, 261
    indolent T-lymphoblastic proliferation, 263
    mature T-cell leukemia/lymphoma, 261
    thymoma, 261
  genetic features, 259
  genetic subgroups of, 260t
  immunophenotype, 259
  morphology, 259
  new provisional entities under subclassification, 262t
  prognosis and treatment, 261
  stages of T-Cell differentiation and maturation, 259t
  WHO-HAEM5 diagnostic criteria for, 258t
T-cell large granular lymphocytic leukemia, 390–393
  clinical features, 390–391
  differential diagnosis, 392–393
  genetic features, 392
  immunophenotype, 392
  morphology, 392
  prognosis and treatment, 393
  WHO-HAEM5 diagnostic criteria for, 391t
T-cell large granular lymphocytic leukemia (T-LGLL), 416
T cell lymphomas, 247–248
T-cell prolymphocytic leukemia, 387–390
  clinical features, 387
  differential diagnosis, 389–390
  genetic features, 389
  immunophenotype, 388–389
  morphology, 387–388
  prognosis and treatment, 389
  WHO-HAEM5 diagnostic criteria for, 388t
Telomere maintenance disorders, 208
Thrombocytopenia
  causes of, 58t
Thymus, 9–10
Tick-borne illnesses, 70
Toxoplasma lymphadenitis, 105
Toxoplasmosis, 71
Trypanosomiasis, 70–71
Tuberculosis, 68
Tyrosine kinase gene fusions (M/LN-eo-TK), 215–225
  clinical features of, 215–216
  differential diagnosis of, 220–222, 221–222t
  with *ETV6::ABL1* fusion
    genetic features, 225
    prognosis and treatment, 225
  with *FGFR1* rearrangement
    genetic features, 224
    prognosis and treatment, 224
  with *FLT3* rearrangement
    genetic features, 225
    prognosis and treatment, 225
  general features of, 215, 217–219
  genetic features of, 220
  with *JAK2* rearrangement
    genetic features, 224
    prognosis and treatment, 224
  morphology, 215–220
  with *PDGFRA* rearrangement, 222–223
    genetic features of, 223
    prognosis and treatment, 223
  with *PDGFRB* rearrangement
    genetic features, 223
    prognosis and treatment, 223

U

Unicentric Castleman disease (UCD), 93

V

Vaccine-induced thrombocytopenia (VITT), 57–59
Viral lymphadenitis, 100–103
Von Willebrand Syndrome, 64

W

Whipple disease, 69
White blood cell disorders, 44–52
    abnormalities, morphologic, 51–52
        Alder-Reilly anomaly, 52
        Auer rods, 52
        inflammatory changes, 51–52
        May-Hegglin anomaly, 52
        Pelger-Huet anomaly, 52
    lymphocytes, 47–51
        iatrogenic causes, 51
        infectious causes, 50–51
        lymphocytosis, 49–50
        lymphopenia, 50
    neutrophils, 44–47
        causes of neutropenia, 45–47, 46t
        drug-induced neutropenia, 45
        function, disorders of, 47, 48t
        immune-mediated neutropenia, 45
        neutropenia, 45
        neutrophilia, 45
        number, disorders of, 44–47
    overview, 44
White pulp, 15